Complications of

COLON & RECTAL SURGERY

Complications of COLON & RECTAL SURGERY

EDITED BY

Terry C. Hicks, M.D.
David E. Beck, M.D.
Frank G. Opelka, M.D.
Alan E. Timmcke, M.D.

Department of Colon and Rectal Surgery
Ochsner Clinic
New Orleans, Louisiana

with 125 illustrations

Williams & Wilkins
A WAVERLY COMPANY

BALTIMORE • PHILADELPHIA • LONDON • PARIS • BANGKOK
BUENOS AIRES • HONG KONG • MUNICH • SYDNEY • TOKYO • WROCLAW

Editor: Carroll C. Cann
Production Coordinator: Peter J. Carley
Typesetter: The Type House

ISBN 0-683-30033-4
90000>
9 780683 300338

351 West Camden Street
Baltimore, Maryland 21201-2436 USA

Rose Tree Corporate Center
1400 North Providence Road
Building II, Suite 5025
Media, Pennsylvania 19063-2043 USA

Accurate indications, adverse reactions, and dosage schedules for drugs are provided in this book, but it is possible that they may change. The reader is urged to review the package information data of the manufacturers of the medications mentioned.

Printed in Hong Kong

Library of Congress Cataloging in Publication Data

Complications of colon & rectal surgery / edited by Terry C. Hicks ...
[et al.].
p. cm.
Includes bibliographical references and index.
ISBN 0-683-30033-4
1. Colon (Anatomy)—Surgery—Complications. 2. Rectum—Surgery—Complications. I. Hicks, Terry C.
[DNLM: 1. Colonic Diseases—surgery. 2. Rectal Diseases—surgery.
3. Intraoperative Complications. 4. Postoperative Complications.
5. Surgery, Laparoscopic—adverse effects. WI 520 C737 1996]
RD544.C656 1996
617.5'547—dc20
DNLM/DLC
for Library of Congress 96-15263
CIP

The publishers have made every effort to trace the copyright holders for borrowed material. If they have inadvertently overlooked any, they will be pleased to make the necessary arrangements at the first opportunity.

To purchase additional copies of this book, call our customer service department at **(800) 638-0672** or fax orders to **(800) 447-8438.** For other book services, including chapter reprints and large quantity sales, ask for the Special Sales department.

Canadian customers should call **(800) 268-4178** or fax **(905) 470-6780.** For all other calls originating outside of the United States, please call **(410) 528-4223** or fax us at **(410) 528-8550.**

Visit Williams & Wilkins on the Internet: **http://www.wwilkins.com** or contact our customer service department at **custserv@wwilkins.com.** Williams & Wilkins customer service representatives are available from 8:30 am to 6:00 pm, EST, Monday through Friday, for telephone access.

95 96 97 98 99
1 2 3 4 5 6 7 8 9 10

To

My parents, **Nancy** and **Harold,**
for their love and support of my life goals;
my wife, **Debi,** who is truly my life partner;
my children, **Robbie** and **Kerry,** who remind me daily how
precious and fragile life is; and my nurse, **Judy,** who is my
"center of gravity" in my clinical practice

T.C.H.

My wife, **Sharon,** for her love, support, and
infinite ability to remind me of my human idiosyncrasies;
my children, **Allison, Lauren,** and **John,** for their unfailing love,
their frequent reminder of the important aspects of life, and for allowing me
to share and guide their growth and development; my residents, fellows, and colleagues,
who challenge me on a daily basis; and **J. Byron Gathright,** who has been
a mentor in the true sense of the word

D.E.B.

Duckie and **Gregg,** for every "first step"—
you provided the untiring encouragement of loving parents;
Dave, for your endless patience with the thankless job of creating
schedules and managing this group of physician-authors, a task similar to herding cats;
Terry, for including me in so many of your visions as a co-author, co-editor, my partner and
my friend (just do not close your club face); **Wilma** and **Jim,** for our trips to the bayou that
revitalized my enthusiasm and focused my thoughts (SAS-SA and F); **Mary Ann,** for her
care and concern for my patients with her ebullient spirit and continuous smile;
Susan, for her unconditional support and for giving me four of God's greatest
gifts—**Erin, Andrew, Mark,** and **Caitlin;** my deepest appreciation
to these close friends and for the efforts of all our co-authors

F.G.O.

My wife, **Terri,** and my children, **Gretchen** and **A.J.,**
for allowing me the precious time to complete this project and the use
of "their" new computer

A.E.T.

Contributors

Feran Agachan, M.D.
Research Fellow, Department of Colorectal Surgery, Cleveland Clinic Florida, Ft. Lauderdale, Florida

David E. Beck, M.D.
Chairman, Department of Colon and Rectal Surgery, Ochsner Clinic, New Orleans, Louisiana

John S. Bolton, M.D.
Clinical Assistant Professor, Louisiana State University Medical Center, Alton Ochsner Medical Foundation, New Orleans, Louisiana

Peter A. Cataldo, M.D.
Assistant Professor of Surgery, Department of Surgery, University of Vermont, Burlington, Vermont

Thomas E. Cataldo, M.D.
Clinical Fellow, Department of Colon and Rectal Surgery, Ochsner Clinic, New Orleans, Louisiana

James M. Church, M.B. Ch.B., M. Sc.
Associate Professor of Surgery, Department of Colorectal Surgery, Ohio State University; Staff Surgeon, Cleveland Clinic, Cleveland, Ohio

Kemol I. Deen, M.D.M.S, F.R.C.S.
Senior Lecturer in Surgery, University of Kelaniya, Colombo, Sri Lanka

Gregory A. DeLaurier, M.D.
Fellow in Colon and Rectal Surgery, Mayo Graduate School of Medicine, Rochester, Minnesota

D. Scott Donaldson, M.D.
Resident, Department of Urology, Ochsner Clinic, New Orleans, Louisiana

James W. Fleshman, Jr., M.D.
Associate Professor of Surgery, Washington University School of Medicine, St. Louis, Missouri

George M. Fuhrman, M.D.
Staff Surgeon and Associate Program Director, Department of General Surgery, Ochsner Clinic, New Orleans, Louisiana

J. Byron Gathright, Jr., M.D.
Chairman Emeritus, Department of Colon and Rectal Surgery, Ochsner Clinic, New Orleans, Louisiana

Charles F. Gay, Jr., J.D.
Partner, Adams and Reese Attorneys and Counselors at Law, New Orleans, Louisiana

Francis J. Harford, M.D.
Professor of Clinical Surgery, Department of Colon and Rectal Surgery, Loyola University Medical Center, Maywood, Illinois

Charles N. Headrick, M.D.
Assistant Professor of Clinical Surgery, Harbor-UCLA Medical Center, Torrance, California

Terry C. Hicks, M.D.
Assistant Chairman and Program Director, Department of Colon and Rectal Surgery, Ochsner Clinic, New Orleans, Louisiana

Lt. Col. Richard E. Karulf, M.C., USAF
Assistant Professor of Surgery, Department of Surgery, Uniformed Services University of Health Sciences, Bethesda, Maryland

Douglas A. Khoury, M.D.
Assistant Professor of Surgery, New York Medical College, Valhalla, New York

Robert R. Kuske, Jr., M.D.
Chairman, Ochsner Center for Radiation Oncology, New Orleans, Louisiana

Sergio W. Larach, M.D.
Colon and Rectal Clinic of Orlando, Orlando, Florida

Walter E. Longo, M.D.
Assistant Professor of Surgery, Head of Research, Section of Colon and Rectal Surgery, St. Louis University School of Medicine, St. Louis, Missouri

John M. MacKeigan, M.D., F.R.C.S.(C)
Associate Clinical Professor of Surgery, Michigan State University, College of Human Medicine; Staff Surgeon, Ferguson-Blodgett Digestive Disease Institute, Grand Rapids, Michigan

Peter W. Marcello, M.D.
Clinical Fellow, Department of Colon and Rectal Surgery, Lahey-Hitchcock Clinic, Burlington, Massachusetts

John J. Murray, M.D.
Staff Surgeon, Department of Colon and Rectal Surgery, Lahey-Hitchcock Clinic, Burlington, Massachusetts

Heidi Nelson, M.D.
Assistant Professor of Surgery, Mayo Medical School; Consultant, Division of Colon and Rectal Surgery, Mayo Clinic, Rochester, Minnesota

Daniel A. Ng, M.D.
Colon and Rectal Surgeon, Newport Beach, California

Frank G. Opelka, M.D.
Staff Surgeon Department of Colon and Rectal Surgery, Ochsner Clinic, New Orleans, Louisiana

Bruce A. Orkin, M.D.
Assistant Professor of Surgery; Director, Colorectal Physiology Laboratory; Program Director, Residency in Surgery Program, The George Washington University Medical Center, Washington, D.C.

Martha B. Roach, M.D.
Staff Urologist, Department of Urology, Ochsner Clinic, New Orleans, Louisiana

Patricia L. Roberts, M.D.
Staff Surgeon, Department of Colon and Rectal Surgery, Lahey-Hitchcock Clinic, Burlington, Massachusetts

David A. Rothenberger, M.D.
Clinical Professor of Surgery and Chief, Division of Colon and Rectal Surgery, University of Minnesota, Minneapolis, Minnesota

Anthony J. Senagore, M.D.
Associate Professor, Department of Surgery, Michigan State University, College of Human Medicine, East Lansing, Michigan; Director, Colon and Rectal Surgical Research, Ferguson-Blodgett Digestive Disease Institute, Grand Rapids, Michigan

Michael P. Spencer, M.D.
Assistant Professor of Surgery, Division of Colon and Rectal Surgery, University of Minnesota, Minneapolis, Minnesota

Michael J. Stamos, M.D.
Assistant Professor of Surgery, Harbor-UCLA Medical Center, Torrance, California

Charles P. Theuer, M.D.
Chief Resident, General Surgery, Harbor-UCLA Medical Center, Torrance, California

Alan G. Thorson, M.D.
Associate Professor of Surgery and Program Director, Section of Colon and Rectal Surgery, Creighton University School of Medicine, Omaha, Nebraska

Alan E. Timmcke, M.D.
Staff Surgeon, Department of Colon and Rectal Surgery, Ochsner Clinic, New Orleans, Louisiana

Carol-Ann Vasilevsky, M.D.C.M., F.R.C.S.(C)
Assistant Professor, Department of Surgery, McGill University, Montreal, Quebec, Canada

Anthony M. Vernava III, M.D.
Associate Professor of Surgery and Chief, Section of Colon and Rectal Surgery; Director, Residency Training Program in Colon and Rectal Surgery, St. Louis University School of Medicine, St. Louis, Missouri

Steven D. Wexner, M.D.
Chairman and Residency Program Director, Department of Colorectal Surgery, Cleveland Clinic Florida, Ft. Lauderdale, Florida

W. Douglas Wong, M.D., F.R.C.S.(C)
Clinical Assistant Professor and Director of Residency Program, Division of Colon and Rectal Surgery, Department of Surgery, University of Minnesota School of Medicine, St. Paul, Minnesota

Foreword

In *Complications of Colon & Rectal Surgery*, Drs. Beck, Hicks, Opelka, and Timmcke have assembled a distinguished group of contributors to cover the very broad range of topics that must be addressed to present a complete picture of these complications. These contributors are youthful, talented, and highly qualified to discuss their subjects.

The first text on complications of colon and rectal surgery is now more than 10 years old and is out of print. Advances in colon and rectal surgery dictate the need for a modern text. New techniques abound, some of them so different from earlier approaches that they might properly be called a new discipline of colon and rectal surgery.

The broad scope of this book ranges from general complications associated with surgical procedures to the specific complications unique to colon and rectal surgery. The text offers comprehensive coverage of advances in endoscopy and stapling, including instrumentation, technique, and management of associated complications. The new techniques and thus new complications of surgery for fecal incontinence are extensively discussed, as are complications related to current radiotherapy and chemotherapy methods.

The editors have not abandoned the basics, however; complications associated with surgical treatment of common diseases and frequently performed procedures, from treatment of hemorrhoids and fissures to surgery for colon cancer, are thoroughly covered. Recognizing the litigious reality of our times in health care, an excellent chapter on medicolegal issues is included.

It has been said that good surgeons can extricate themselves from intraoperative as well as postoperative complications; however, great surgeons are those who can avoid these pitfalls in the first place. This book outlines for both inexperienced and well-seasoned surgeons methods of avoiding complications and provides management guidelines for those complications which occur despite our best efforts.

Thanks are due to the editors and contributors of *Complications of Colon & Rectal Surgery*. I commend them for the clarity, timeliness, and completeness of their contributions.

J. Byron Gathright, Jr., M.D.

Chairman Emeritus, Department of Colon and Rectal Surgery, Ochsner Clinic, New Orleans, Louisiana

Preface

To provide patients with the best possible care while maintaining a successful practice, it is essential that all surgeons performing colorectal surgery be prepared to manage the inevitable problems associated with these procedures. Our goal in writing this book was to present the current knowledge and techniques for avoiding and managing the problems that do arise.

Complications of Colon & Rectal Surgery represents the collaborative efforts of many individuals. The contributing authors were selected for their knowledge of colorectal surgery and ability to present their surgical judgment and experience in written form. Although many of these contributors are relatively young, these dedicated individuals will shape the future of colorectal surgery. In addition to reviewing the available literature, they have described their personal approach to complications in colorectal surgery. Numerous technical descriptions and highlights from multiple discussions held in surgical locker rooms, morbidity and mortality conferences, and the hallways of conferences and symposiums have been included. Using this approach, we hope this text will provide initial guidance to the less experienced surgeon and stimulate additional thought and research to the more experienced surgeon.

We gratefully acknowledge the efforts of the many individuals who made this book possible. First, Drs. Bernard T. Ferrari, John E. Ray, and J. Byron Gathright, the editors of *Complications of Colon and Rectal Surgery: Prevention and Management,* whose vision and expertise initiated the first text on this important subject and trained many of the editors and contributors of this text. We especially thank our contributors, who took time from their busy schedules to produce their contributions on the prevention and management of colorectal complications. Most of the illustrations were produced by Barbara Siede, Director of Ochsner Medical Illustrations, whose exceptional ability has clarified many difficult concepts. Marion Stafford, Director of Ochsner Medical Editing, aided many of the contributors in concisely expressing their thoughts and improved the readability of the text. Our trainees and patients continue to stimulate us to find additional answers and techniques to minimize complications. Our nurses and clinic support staff assist us in patient management and help us squeeze out time for these academic projects. Finally, our thanks to Beth Campbell, Suzanne Wakefield, and staff members who supported our efforts and worked hard to make this text a reality.

Terry C. Hicks
David E. Beck
Frank G. Opelka
Alan E. Timmcke

Contents

PART I

GENERAL CONSIDERATIONS

CHAPTER 1

Preexisting Conditions

ALAN G. THORSON

Whether a physician is a general surgeon or a colorectal or other surgical specialist, the decision to operate because of a specific disease involves much more than knowledge of the disease process. Thorough examination of the patient is imperative to assess the overall potential benefit of surgery. Such examination may reveal preexisting conditions that predispose the patient to risks and complications not related directly to the primary procedure. Most such conditions may be identified with a careful history and physical examination[1]; others may require additional preoperative testing for clarification. Many may lead to modification of routine postoperative care to minimize associated risks.

The major areas in which preexisting conditions may have a significant effect on surgical outcome are reviewed, along with indications for additional workup of certain findings. For the most part, however, the details of such workups are beyond the scope of this chapter. Suggested modification of perioperative management is offered in areas in which it is believed that significant risk reduction for associated complications can be achieved.

CARDIOVASCULAR DISEASE

The overall risk for perioperative myocardial infarction is 0.15%.[2] Without a prior clinical history of heart disease, men are considered at risk beginning at age 35 years and women at age 40 years.[3] Many preoperative anesthesia protocols include an ECG for patients 40 years or older. Abnormal ST segments and ECG evidence of previous myocardial infarction are associated with increased risk for postoperative ischemic events.[4] Preoperative dysrhythmias (>5 premature ventricular contractions per minute) and P wave abnormalities are predictive of postoperative dysrhythmias.[4,5] Such findings, especially in the patient with a positive clinical history, may warrant additional preoperative cardiac tests or increased postoperative cardiac monitoring.

Patients with a positive clinical history, abnormal ECG findings, or a history of coronary artery disease should undergo preoperative exercise stress testing. Evidence of ST depression >2 mm, exercise-induced hypotension (i.e., >10 mm

Hg decrease in systolic blood pressure), more than three consecutive premature ventricular contractions, and symptomatic chest pain are considered positive indications of ischemic heart disease. Such findings at exercise stress testing are predictive of increased perioperative morbidity and mortality.[6] Not all patients, however, are candidates for exercise stress testing, because of other peripheral vascular disease, orthopedic disorders, or other limitations on exercise. In such patients, radioisotope imaging or two-dimensional echocardiography may be appropriate. Both tests have predictive value for ischemic cardiac events in the perioperative period in patients undergoing major nonvascular surgery.[7] Two-dimensional echocardiography can be performed to assess for left ventricular dysfunction and risk factors for perioperative pulmonary edema. Radioisotope imaging can be used to assess for myocardial perfusion defects and is predictive of perioperative myocardial infarction and cardiac death.[7,8]

Patients at high cardiac risk should undergo increased monitoring in the perioperative period. Standard measures used to assess peripheral organ perfusion include monitoring of urine output with a Foley catheter. An arterial catheter may be used for instantaneous blood pressure monitoring and to determine acid-base balance. Central pressures can be monitored simply with a central venous catheter. However, a pulmonary artery catheter enables evaluation of a significant amount of additional information that can be of critical value in high-risk cardiac patients, such as cardiac output, peripheral resistance, and left ventricular filling pressures, and allows tor appropriate fluid management and pharmacologic manipulation of cardiac stress factors.

The clinical history and physical examination should be focused to carefully assess for recent history of myocardial infarction or the presence of congestive heart failure (CHF).These are the two most important factors that place patients at risk for perioperative cardiac complications and death.[9-12] The risk for repeat infarction after recent infarction is significant for 6 months. Myocardial infarction occurs in 0.13% of patients undergoing surgery without prior infarction, in 27% to 38% of patients undergoing surgery within 3 months after infarction, and in 11% to 16% of patients 3 to 6 months after infarction.[9,12] This risk for repeat infarction stabilizes at about 5%, 6 months after infarction.[12] These risks can be modified with appropriate medical treatment or surgical correction of causative factors. The ECG is an important tool in the evaluation of patients who may have had a silent myocardial infarction (silent ischemia) or who are unwilling to communicate their cardiac history.

Current medication usage (e.g., digoxin, diuretics) and physical examination are important components in the evaluation of CHF. Pitting ankle edema, rales on auscultation of the chest, jugular venous distention, and an S_3 gallop rhythm all support the diagnosis of CHF. A clinical history of orthopnea, fatigability, dyspnea on exertion, and paroxysmal nocturnal dyspnea suggest CHF. The diagnosis frequently may be confirmed with a chest radiograph that shows cardiomegaly and prominent pulmonary vascularity. Surgery should be delayed until CHF is well controlled.

The finding of a heart murmur at physical examination may have particular importance in the presence of cardiac symptoms including CHF or angina. In the absence of symptoms, only the murmur of aortic stenosis (harsh systolic murmur along the right sternal border with radiation into the carotid arteries) must be carefully evaluated to avert sudden cardiac death with induction of anesthesia.[13]

Physical signs of peripheral vascular disease include slowed or absent peripheral pulses, loss of extremity hair, thinning of skin, muscle atrophy, and skin ulcerations and should raise suspicion of not only concomitant coronary artery disease but also the possibility of carotid artery disease. Careful additional history should be elicited to detect any symptoms of transient ischemic attack (TIA). The carotid bifurcations should be evaluated for the presence of bruits. The presence of either TIA or bruit should prompt further evaluation, because 30% to 40% of patients with a history of TIA will develop a serious stroke within 3 to 5 years of initial symptoms. The majority occur in the first year.[14]

PULMONARY DISEASE

Pulmonary complications are the most common cause of morbidity and mortality after abdominal surgery.[15] For this reason particular emphasis on identification of risk factors and preventive measures is appropriate to this organ system. Clearly, anorectal surgery alone does not have the same pulmonary risks as abdominal colorectal surgery.

As with cardiac evaluation, the physical examination and clinical history are important components of the preoperative pulmonary assessment. This assessment need not be complicated in most patients.[16] If there is no history of pulmonary disease and no abnormal breath sounds on auscultation of the lungs, the patient is likely at normal risk. Chronic cough, sputum production, dyspnea on exertion, wheezing, hemoptysis, or history of cigarette smoking are indications to expand the preoperative evaluation to include pulmonary function tests, chest radiography, and perhaps determination of arterial blood gas levels.

A limited pulmonary function test (spirometry) can be performed to assess tidal volume, inspiratory capacity, vital capacity (VC; both volume and flow rate), and maximum voluntary ventilation. Values 80% to 120% of predicted are considered normal. A low expiratory volume (VC) suggests loss of lung volume. A low expiratory flow rate should be rechecked after administration of a bronchodilating agent. A positive response suggests the need for bronchodilator therapy in the perioperative period. Maximum voluntary ventilation below 50% of predicted is the greatest risk factor for postoperative pulmonary complications. Consideration should be given to pulmonary consultation and more detailed tests of pulmonary function.[17]

Pulmonary endurance may be assessed by asking patients how many flights of stairs they can comfortably climb without resting. Alternatively, patients can be observed climbing stairs. Inability to climb two flights of stairs at a steady pace may indicate respiratory compromise and requires further evaluation.[18]

In the normal-risk patient, a number of steps can be taken to minimize the risk of postoperative pulmonary complications. Incisions should be made as low in the abdominal wall as possible. Deep breathing, early ambulation, and incentive spirometry all are beneficial.[19,20]

Abnormal pulmonary findings should be corrected as fully as possible before surgery. Wheezing should be treated with bronchodilator therapy (e.g., with metaproterenol, terbutaline, isoetharine, or albuterol), and bronchitis should be treated with organism-specific antibiotics, chest physiotherapy, and tracheal suctioning when necessary.

RENAL DISEASE

Common conditions that could lead to perioperative renal dysfunction can be easily evaluated before surgery. Urinalysis may identify unsuspected urinary tract infection, diabetes, or renal disease. These conditions should be evaluated and treated before surgery. Careful questioning of the patient about symptoms of dysuria, hesitancy, nocturia, and a feeling of incomplete evacuation may lead to a diagnosis of unsuspected prostatic disease with risks for postoperative renal dysfunction.

Preexisting renal disease presents a special challenge to the surgeon. Foremost is the prevention of additional injury to the patient. Adequate hydration and monitoring of urine output (0.5-1.0 ml/kg/hr) as an indication of adequate perfusion are critical. Low-dose dopamine therapy (1 to 2 μg/kg/min) may be of benefit.[21] Medications cleared by glomerular filtration must be dose adjusted in a timely manner and carefully monitored. Nephrotoxic agents (e.g., aminoglycosides) must be carefully monitored and maintained at nontoxic levels, and any effects or change in renal function must be carefully scrutinized. Particular caution must be exercised in the use of antihypertensive medications. Angiotensin-converting enzyme inhibitors should probably not be used, particularly in patients with renal vascular hypertension.[22]

Patients with uremia who are receiving dialysis add further challenge and have unique risks for complications. For example, coronary artery disease and pericarditis commonly occur in the older patient[23-25]; serosal wound healing is delayed, which leads to increased risk for anastomotic leaks[26]; and pulmonary edema and uremic pneumonitis may compromise respiratory function.[27]

Of particular interest to the colorectal surgeon are gastrointestinal manifestations of uremia: ammonia released by bacterial action on urea in the gut lumen may lead to edema, ulceration, and hemorrhage[28]; postoperative ileus may be prolonged[29]; and patients with diverticulosis are at increased risk for acute infection and perforation.[30]

Other surgical considerations include anemia, increased risk for bleeding due to use of heparin during dialysis, platelet dysfunction,[31,32] secondary hyperparathyroidism, and bone demineralization. Compromised leukocyte and immunologic function lead to increased risk for infection[33] and impaired cellular immunity.[34] Antibiotic prophylaxis may be of benefit. Finally, fluid and electrolyte abnormalities are expected. Changes occur rapidly and require intensified scrutiny to maintain balance.

Despite all of these potential problems, elective surgery can be safely performed in patients with chronic renal insufficiency or renal failure. In patients with complete renal failure, dialysis typically is performed on the day before surgery and again on postoperative day 1. Dialysis enables improvement in abnormalities of hemostasis caused by platelet dysfunction, correction of electrolyte imbalance, and removal of unsafe levels of many medications from the blood.

HEPATIC DISEASE

The liver is the body's physiologic processing center and performs many functions that have important implications for the surgical patient. It is the sole provider of albumin and a host of other plasma proteins. It is the major detoxifier of endogenous and exogenous waste products, including ammonia, steroids, and many drugs. It is of major importance in glucose metabolism and lipid synthesis. Dysfunction can lead to nutritional wasting, accumulation of toxic waste products, immunocompromise, and bleeding diatheses.

The capacity of hepatic reserve and hepatic regeneration is legendary. As a result, the early stages of liver disease may produce only subtle evidence of dysfunction, but a dysfunction that can easily be transformed into fulminant failure by seemingly minor events including the stress of anesthesia and surgery. It is the wise surgeon who can identify the subtle signs of hepatic disease in a preoperative history and at physical examination.

The history of a patient with liver disease may include anorexia, weight loss, fatigue, fever, loss of libido, and pruritus. The patient or family may note lightening of stool color coexistent with dark urine, scleral icterus, jaundice, change in sleeping pattern, apathy, agitation, restlessness, confusion, and incoordination.

The physical examination in the patient with liver disease may reveal spider telangiectasia and palmar erythema. Cirrhosis in male patients may lead to hormonal changes, with male pattern hair loss, gynecomastia, and small testes. Early cirrhosis is associated with an enlarged liver, and advanced disease with a small, shrunken liver. Asterixis (flapping tremor) is a sign of advanced disease.

The most common cause of acute hepatic failure is viral hepatitis (especially hepatitis B); the second most common cause involves the use of certain drugs (e.g., acetaminophen, halothane, isoniazid, and tetracycline) and the introduction of toxins (e.g., chlorinated hydrocarbons and aflatoxin).[35] In contrast, the most common cause of chronic liver disease (cirrhosis) in the United States is alcohol abuse. Other causes include a host of drugs (e.g., methyldopa, methotrexate, isoniazid, vitamin A, and carbon tetrachloride); infections such as hepatitis B and C, tertiary syphilis, and *Schistosoma japonicum* infection; chronic biliary obstruction; metabolic disease such as Wilson's disease and hemochromatosis; and chronic right-sided heart failure.[36]

Surgery in the patient with liver disease presents some special problems. Certain anesthetic agents, notably halothane, are more likely to cause hepatotoxicity and could contribute to postoperative exacerbation of the disease process.[37] Compromised hepatic function leads to increased risk for gastrointestinal (GI) bleeding. Because upper GI bleeding due to gastritis, peptic ulcer disease, or varices is common, upper GI tract evaluation before major surgery should be considered, especially in the patient with jaundice or cirrhosis. After surgery, gastritis is probably best controlled with antacids to maintain a pH of ≥ 5. If this can be accomplished, histamine$_2$ (H_2) blockers offer little in addition.[38] Alternatively, H_2 blockers can be used instead of antacids to elevate gastric pH.

Elevated prothrombine time (PT) is common and can usually be corrected with supplemental vitamin K. If an adequate response to vitamin K does not occur, fresh-frozen plasma can be administered. An antibiotic bowel preparation will tend to exacerbate the problem of prolonged PT, because gut bacteria are necessary for the production of prothrombin.[39] Thrombocytopenia may result from hypersplenism or as a direct result of alcohol ingestion. The latter should be treated with supplemental folate.

Lower GI bleeding may also occur and is almost always attributed to hemorrhoids; however, hemorrhoids are no more common in patients with portal hypertension or liver disease than in the population at large.[40] Abnormal clotting factors may increase the risk for bleeding from hemorrhoidal disease in these patients, or rectal varices may be present. The surgeon must be familiar with the difference in appearance between varices and hemorrhoids, because varices should be oversewn to control an acute bleeding episode, whereas hemorrhoids may need to be excised. In the long term, rectal varices are a sign of portal hypertension and can be resolved only if the underlying process is treated with a shunt procedure (e.g., a transcutaneous intrahepatic portal shunt [TIPS] procedure).

Disturbance of fluid and electrolyte balance is common in liver disease, including sodium retention, potassium loss, and the development of ascites and edema. Fluid and sodium restriction, potassium supplementation, and the judicious use of diuretics (e.g., spironolactone and furosemide) may be necessary. In a patient with marginal hepatic reserve, ascites may become a problem after

Table 1-1 Child's classification of operative risk

Criteria	Risk		
	Good (A)	**Moderate (B)**	**Poor (C)**
Serum bilirubin (mg/dl)	>2.0	2.0–3.0	>3.0
Serum albumin (mg/dl)	>3.5	3.0–3.5	<3.0
Ascites	None	Easily controlled	Not easily controlled
Encephalopathy	None	Minimal	Advanced
Nutrition	Excellent	Good	Poor

surgery even if not present before. Careful attention to detail during closure of the abdominal wound may prevent problems of leakage of ascites in the postoperative period.

Advanced liver disease is associated with poor nutritional reserve and immunocompromise.[41] Nutritional supplementation will likely be necessary, with increased caloric and protein needs.[42] Prolonged antibiotic prophylaxis and fungal prophylaxis should be considered.

Finally, as hepatic reserve decreases, the risks associated with surgery increase and should be considered before surgery is recommended. Although originally described to assess the operative risk in patients with portal hypertension undergoing shunt placement, the Child's classification may be useful in other major abdominal surgery also. It is clear that risk increases as bilirubin concentration rises, albumin level falls, malnutrition intensifies, and ascites and encephalopathy develop (Table 1-1).

METABOLIC DISEASE

The metabolic diseases are disorders in which altered chemical transformation processes result in abnormal release, storage, synthesis, or degradation of various protein, carbohydrate, lipid, or other products of metabolic activity (see box). Although a few are common, most are rare and generally will not be seen in the surgeon's general practice. Nevertheless, special considerations may be necessary if a patient with such a disease does need surgical intervention.

In glycogen storage diseases (e.g., glucose-6-phosphate deficiency, debranching enzyme deficiency), progressive glomerulosclerosis and hepatic fibrosis develop, which lead to cirrhosis. The hyperlipoproteinemias produce coronary artery disease at a young age and in some cases lead to valvular heart disease, stroke, and renal failure. The same is true of inborn errors of amino acid metabolism (e.g., homocystinuria and aminoaciduria) with cardiac, hepatic, renal, and central nervous system (CNS) complications.

METABOLIC DISEASES

Disorders of carbohydrate metabolism

Galactosemia
Glycogen storage diseases
Fructose intolerance
Primary hyperoxaluria

Disorders of lipoprotein metabolism

Hyperlipoproteinemias
Fabry's disease
Gout
Gaucher disease
Niemann-Pick disease

Inborn errors of amino acid metabolism

Hyperaminoaciduria
Hyperphenylalaninemias
Alcaptonuria
Hyperprolinemias and hydroxyprolinemias
Diseases of the urea cycle
Branched-chain aminoaciduria
Homocystinuria

Disorders of purine and pyrimidine metabolism

Gout
Disorders of purine metabolism
Disorders of pyrimidine metabolism

Inherited disorders of connective tissue

Mucopolysaccharidoses
Marfan syndrome
Ehlers-Danlos syndrome
Osteogenesis imperfecta
Pseudoxanthoma elasticum

Disorders of porphyrins or metals

Prophyrias
Wilson's disease
Hemochromatosis
Phosphorus deficiency and hypophosphatemia
Disorders of magnesium metabolism

Other hereditary disorders

Familial Mediterranean fever
Amyloid diseases
Hereditary syndromes that involve multiple organ systems

Gout is a generic term for a number of genetic and acquired conditions manifested by hyperuricemia and deposition of uric acid crystals in joints and which precipitate acute inflammatory arthritis. Acute gouty arthritis often follows a precipitating event, including surgery. Postoperative gout is manifested most commonly on the third to fifth postoperative day.[43] Treatment consists of joint rest and administration of colchicine or nonsteroidal anti-inflammatory agents. A short course of systemic steroid therapy may be administered if other treatments fail.

The connective tissue diseases are frequently complicated by valvular heart disease with associated implications for surgery and endoscopy. Vascular disease with arterial dissection and rupture are common. Type IV arterial Ehlers-Danlos syndrome is associated with intramural small bowel hemorrhage and rupture of the sigmoid colon.[44]

Disorders of porphyrins and metals include the porphyrias. The major surgical concern is proper identification of the source of associated abdominal pain so that unnecessary surgery is not performed. The symptoms include steady but poorly localized abdominal pain and may include cramping, nausea, vomiting, and constipation. The abdominal symptoms are neurologic rather than inflammatory; thus tenderness, fever, and leukocytosis are usually absent. Wilson's disease and hemochromatosis result in liver injury, dysfunction, and cirrhosis.

MALNUTRITION

Although malnutrition is a frequent preexisting condition in hospitalized surgical patients, the effect on complications is not clear. Controversy persists as to whether preoperative nutritional supplementation should be used in these patients, and specifically, in attempts to identify those patients who might benefit from both a physiologic and an economic standpoint.

It is estimated that 30% to 50% of hospitalized patients are at least moderately malnourished.[45,46] Identification of these patients is determined with the clinical history, physical examination, and laboratory findings. A history of anorexia, nausea, vomiting, diarrhea, and abdominal pain may contribute to inadequate nutritional intake before surgery. A 6% to 12% weight loss over the previous 6 months may be consistent with mild to moderate nutritional depletion, and greater than 12% weight loss with severe malnutrition. Patients who remain at or above their ideal body weight despite such weight losses can be further identified by means of serum protein levels. A serum albumin concentration <3.5 g/dl, transferrin concentration <200 g/dl, and total lymphocyte count <1200 are consistent with some level of nutritional depletion. Anthropometric measurements (e.g., triceps skinfold thickness) can be used to estimate lean muscle mass and total body fat[47] but are poor predictors of nutritional status and clinical outcome.[48,49]

If a decision is made to correct malnutrition before surgery, the enteral route is preferred if the gastrointestinal tract is functioning. Numerous types of tubes and routes of administration are available and should be selected on the basis of the particular needs of the patient. However, the data to support such a decision are at best soft.

Numerous retrospective uncontrolled studies have found benefit to postoperative morbidity and mortality from preoperative correction of nutritional deficiencies,[50] although results of prospective randomized studies have not been so promising.[51-53] In general, these studies suggest an improvement in metabolic end points of nutritional assessment but no significant improvement in postoperative morbidity or mortality. Criticisms of these studies include small patient numbers and poor study designs. Subset analysis suggests improvement in outcome may be seen in severely malnourished patients who receive prolonged, sustained nutritional support until nutritional status returns to normal[54]; the economic effects, however, are not known.

To summarize, although we know malnutrition is a common problem in surgical patients, we do not know what complications can be attributed to it. Patient selection for nutritional support has not been well defined, and the end point for that support is still speculative. It would seem that preoperative nutritional support is best limited to severely malnourished patients and, if it is utilized, that support should continue for a prolonged period before surgery.

IMMUNOCOMPROMISE

The numerous sources of immunocompromise in potential surgical patients may be primary or acquired. The defects in immunity may be primarily local, as in burns and wounds or loss of mucosal integrity, or systemic. Systemic immunocompromise may include one or any combination of cell-mediated (T cell function), humoral (B cell function), phagocytosis (neutrophils), or complement defects. Primary immunodeficiencies are relatively rare (1 in 10,000)[55] and will not be encountered in most surgical practices. Acquired immunodeficiencies are common and range from mild defects to complete loss of immune function. Age, malnutrition, obesity, malignancy, burns, sepsis, trauma, surgery, anesthesia, blood transfusion, diabetes, renal failure, liver disease, splenectomy, radiation, and foreign bodies all modify the body's response to invasion. Drugs, including chemotherapeutic agents, are probably the most frequently encountered cause of severe immunocompromise manifested by profound neutropenia.

The development of a disease that requires surgical treatment in an immunocompromised patient presents a unique challenge. For the colorectal surgeon, this may be a perianal inflammation or an intra-abdominal catastrophe. Some conditions, such as neutropenic enterocolitis,[56] are unique to the compromised state; others may simply be severe manifestations of common disease processes. For example, neutropenia has been associated with increasing severity of complications in diverticular disease of the colon.[57]

The obvious risks to immunocompromised patients are postoperative sepsis and poor wound healing. In the case of anorectal pain and inflammation, local care and antibiotic therapy should prevail, with open drainage reserved for treatment of a fluctuant mass. If bowel resection becomes necessary, diversion of the fecal stream will most frequently provide the best management, depending on the degree of contamination, preparation of the bowel, presence of peritonitis, and projected duration of the neutropenia. In general, the white blood cell count nadir occurs 10 to 20 days after initiation of chemotherapy. Administration of broad-spectrum antibiotics, use of prophylactic antifungal therapies such as oral nystatin and vaginal suppositories, and careful respiratory and hemodynamic monitoring are critical. Filgrastim, a granulocyte colony–stimulating factor, decreases the duration of neutropenia and the prevalence of infection (compared with that in control groups in patients undergoing chemotherapy for small cell carcinoma of the lung and other nonmyeloid malignancies.[58,59]

ACQUIRED IMMUNODEFICIENCY SYNDROME

In the case of acquired immunodeficiency syndrome (AIDS), one of the major potential complications of the preexisting condition is transmission of the human immunodeficiency virus (HIV) to health care workers. This risk appears low, about 0.3% to 0.5%, after exposure through needle sticks or cuts with sharp instruments while caring for patients with AIDS.[60,61] Although this risk seems low, all steps should be taken to minimize the possibility of exposure, and universal precautions should be used in the care of all patients. In brief, these precautions entail the appropriate use of barrier gowns to prevent skin and mucous membrane contact, use of gloves when handling body fluids, and washing of hands after contact with body fluids; special precautions to avoid injuries from needles, scalpels, and other sharp instruments, including disposal of needles uncapped into puncture-resistant containers; use of mouthpieces and resuscitation bags or other ventilation devices rather than mouth-to-mouth resuscitation; use of masks and protective eyewear whenever there is a possibility of aerosolization of material; and avoiding patient contact when exudative lesions or weeping dermatitis is present in a health care worker.[62] The wearing of double gloves decreases the risk of blood contact in the operating room.[63,64]

Despite the apparent low risk of transmission in the operating room, one must consider the overall exposure that does occur at this risk level. It is estimated that the average practicing surgeon in the United States has 30 parenteral exposures to blood each year.[65] Three factors determine a surgeon's lifetime risk for acquiring HIV: number of needle sticks or punctures contaminated with body fluids, prevalence of HIV-positive patients in the surgeon's practice, and number of years of practice in a surgeon's career. If risk per needle stick is 0.5% and the HIV-positive population is 10%, with 30 needle sticks per year, and a surgeon practices for 40 years, the overall lifetime risk is 60%.[66]

If a health care worker is exposed to blood products through a puncture wound or needle stick, short-term use of zidovudine (AZT) should be considered. Experimental data from animal studies suggest that administration of zidovudine in the first hours after inoculation may prevent infection.[67] The current recommended protocol is an initial dose of 1 g as soon as possible after the incident, followed by 200 mg orally every 4 to 6 hours for 4 weeks.[68]

When evaluating a patient with AIDS for surgical intervention, special attention must be paid to evidence of infectious complications that could result in a prolonged postoperative course. An absolute CD4 count <200 or a decreasing ratio of CD4 to CD8 (normal 1.8:2.2) is associated with severe immunocompromise and subsequent risk for viral, fungal, protozoal, and bacterial infections and prolonged wound healing.[69] Careful evaluation of the respiratory system should be undertaken to preclude subacute infections. A search for subtle localizing neurologic abnormalities could identify early CNS infections (especially toxoplasmosis).[70] Any identified infection should be treated before elective surgery is performed. The presence of associated infections and low CD4 counts with the need for emergency surgery has a very poor prognosis.

DIABETES

It is estimated that diabetes mellitus affects 2% to 4% of the U.S. population. Type I (insulin-dependent) diabetes comprises 7% to 10% of these cases, for an overall prevalence of 0.2% to 0.3%.[71] The prevalence increases with age: in the decade between 65 and 74 years, 16.5% of men and 14.8% of women are affected.[72] In the patient with diabetes that is recognized before surgery and well managed after surgery, mortality is equal to that in the patient without diabetes.[73] In the patient with diabetes that is not recognized before surgery and in whom hyperglycemia develops after surgery, the most serious complications can occur rapidly. For this reason, preoperative assessment of all patients should include a clinical history with questions about complaints of polyuria, polydypsia, or polyphagia. Associated weight loss with any of these could be a sign of diabetes. The presence of such symptoms should alert the physician to order a fasting blood glucose test. Repeated values >0.8 mmol/L (140 mg/dl) confirm the diagnosis of diabetes. Appropriate steps should then be taken to manage and monitor perioperative and postoperative blood glucose levels.

In patients with known diabetes, special attention should be given to evaluation of the vascular, renal, and cardiac systems. The patient with diabetes ages physiologically much faster than does the general population. It has been said that the physiologic age of the renal and cardiovascular systems in a patient with diabetes is equal to chronologic age plus the duration in years since the diagnosis of diabetes.[74] Renal disease is common in patients with diabetes, and renal failure is a frequent cause of death.

Cardiovascular disease is the major cause of death in patients with diabetes. Compared with the nondiabetic population, cardiovascular disease occurs more frequently, at a younger age, and with more severe manifestations. The reasons for this accelerated atherosclerosis are postulated to include the high prevalence of hyperlipoproteinemia in diabetic patients, abnormalities of endothelial cell function, increased platelet aggregation, and a high prevalence of hypertension.[71] A careful preoperative cardiac history and physical examination is always prudent in the diabetic patient because of these risks.

Neuropathy is the most common disabling complication of diabetes, and autonomic neuropathy is probably of most concern to the surgeon. Three major types of dysfunction are involved: gastrointestinal, cardiovascular, and genitourinary. Gastrointestinal dysfunction is manifested as gastroparesis, nocturnal diarrhea, and colonic dilatation. Impotence, retrograde ejaculation, and large amounts of postvoiding residual urine characterize genitourinary disturbances.[75] Cardiovascular symptoms include impaired vasomotor reflexes, with increased heart rate and loss of respiratory sinus arrhythmia.

In patients with cardiac autonomic neuropathy, mortality is 50% within 2.5 years of diagnosis.[76] They also are at high risk for cardiorespiratory arrest in the perioperative period. This makes preoperative recognition of this neuropathy very important to avert a serious postoperative cardiac event. Orthostatic hypotension, mild resting tachycardia, and associated symptoms of other autonomic neuropathies as described are frequently present.[77] A shortened RR interval ratio on an ECG during the Valsalva maneuver[78] or while standing[79] is diagnostic of cardiac neuropathy.

ADVANCED AGE

Age as a preexisting condition provides the perfect summary to what has been the point of the discussions so far. There is clear evidence that age has an effect on physiologic life processes: maximum heart rate slowly decreases with age[80]; arrhythmias occur with increasing frequency[81-83]; maximum oxygen uptake is decreased[84]; and exercise-induced cardiac output tends to decrease[85] except in very active patients.[86]

With age comes decreasing strength and endurance of the respiratory muscles.[87,88] Maximum oxygen consumption,[89,90] vital capacity (VC), forced expiratory flow volume in 1 minute (FEV_1), and mid-expiratory flow rate all decline.[91-94]

Renal physiology is also affected. Glomerular filtration rate declines, and the rate of decline increases with age.[95,96] The ability to concentrate urine and minimize flow in response to dehydration gradually declines.[97-99] Proteinuria and bacteriuria increase with the age of the patient.[100]

Body composition shifts, with an increase in total fat mass and decrease in lean body mass.[101,102] Even though these changes occur in the statistical sense as age advances, for any given individual it is much less clear at what chronologic age the acceleration of these changes begins.[103] For example, active athletic persons can maintain lean body mass equal to that of younger athletes well into their eighth decade.[104,105]

Operative mortality data also demonstrate this phenomenon. Although mortality does show a consistent increase with age,[106,107] there is a strong dependence on medical and physiologic status.[107-112] Operative mortality in healthy elderly patients is low and approximates that of their younger counterparts.[109-111]

Of particular interest is an evaluation of the causes of postoperative mortality. Many deaths are related to the primary procedure,[110,113,114] a large number of which are performed because of a diagnosis of cancer. But the proportion of operative deaths attributable to cancer is far fewer than the proportion of operations being performed because of cancer (25% versus 78%).[113] Careful analysis of several large studies indicates that cardiovascular and respiratory complications are responsible for the majority of postoperative deaths, deaths not directly related to the primary condition.[110,113,115,116] Other preexisting diseases such as diabetes and hepatic and renal diseases also contribute to this mortality.[11,108,117-119] Preexisting conditions, not age, contribute most to operative mortality. Therefore it is important that surgeons familiarize themselves with an appropriate evaluation for these factors so that their adverse effect on surgical outcome can be minimized.

REFERENCES

1. Hampton JR, Harrison MJG, Mitchell JRA. Relative contributions of history taking, physical examination, and laboratory investigation to diagnosis and management of medical outpatients. Br Med J 2:486, 1975.
2. Freeman WK, Gibbons RJ, Shub C. Preoperative assessment of cardiac patients undergoing noncardiac surgical procedures. Mayo Clinic Proc 64:1105, 1989.
3. Multiple Risk Factor Intervention Trial Research Group: Coronary heart disease death, nonfatal acute myocardial infarction and other clinical outcomes in the multiple risk factor intervention trial. Am J Cardiol 58:1, 1986.
4. Velanovich V. Preoperative screening electrocardiography: Predictive value for postoperative cardiac complications. South Med J 87:431, 1994.
5. Cooperman M, Pflug BP, Martin EW Jr, et al. Cardiovascular risk factors in patients with peripheral vascular disease. Surgery 84:505, 1978.
6. Older P, Smith R, Courtney P, Holn R. Preoperative evaluation of cardiac failure and ischemia in elderly patients by cardiopulmonary exercise testing. Chest 104:701, 1993.
7. Takase B, Younis LT, Byers SL, Shaw LJ, Labovitz AJ, Chaitman BR, Miller DD. Comparative prognostic value of clinical risk indexes, resting two dimensional echocardiography, and dipyridamole stress thallium-201 myocardial imaging for perioperative cardiac events in major nonvascular surgery patients. Am Heart J 126:1099, 1993.
8. Shaw L, Miller DD, Kong BA, Hilton T, Stelken A, Stock EK, Chaitman BR. Determination of perioperative cardiac risk by adenosine thallium-201 myocardial imaging. Am Heart J 124:861-869, 1992.
9. Tarhan S, Moffit EA, Taylor WF, et al. Myocardial infarction after general anesthesia. JAMA 220:1451, 1972.

10. Goldman L. Cardiac risks and complications of noncardiac surgery. Ann Intern Med 98:504, 1983.
11. Goldman L, Caldera DC, Nussbaum SR, et al. Multifactorial index of cardiac risk in noncardiac surgical procedures. N Engl J Med 297:845, 1977.
12. Steen PA, Tinker JH, Tarhan S, Myocardial re-infarction after anesthesia and surgery. JAMA 239:2566, 1978.
13. Fullerton DA, Harken AH. Cardiac insufficiency. In Willmore DW, Brennan MF, Harken AH, Holcroft JW, Meakins JL, eds. Care of the Surgical Patient. New York: Scientific American, 1988.
14. Giordano JM. Extracranial cerebrovascular disease. In Cameron JL, ed. Current Surgical Therapy, 5th ed. St. Louis: Mosby, 1995, p 639.
15. Zibrak JD, O'Donnell CR, Martin K. Indications for pulmonary function testing. Ann Intern Med 112:763, 1990.
16. Holleman DR Jr, Simel DL, Goldberg JS. Diagnosis of obstructive airways disease from the clinical examination. J Gen Intern Med 8:63, 1993.
17. Tisi GM. Preoperative evaluation of pulmonary function: Validity, indications, and benefits. Am Rev Respir Dis 119:293, 1979.
18. Bolton JWR, Weiman DS, Haynes JL, et al. Stair climbing as an indicator of pulmonary function. Chest 92:783, 1987.
19. Roukema JA, Carroll EJ, Prins GJ. The prevention of pulmonary complications after upper abdominal surgery in patients with noncompromised pulmonary status. Arch Surg 123:30, 1988.
20. Bartlett RH, Gazzaniga AB, Geraghty TR. Respiratory maneuvers to prevent postoperative pulmonary complications: A critical review. JAMA 224:1017, 1973.
21. Davis RF, Lappas DG, Kirklin JK, et al. Acute oliguria after cardiopulmonary bypass: Renal functional improvement with low-dose dopamine infusion. Crit Care Med 10:852, 1982.
22. Hricik DE, Browning PJ, Kopelman R, et al. Captopril-induced functional renal insufficiency in patients with bilateral renal artery stenoses or renal artery stenosis in a solitary kidney. N Engl J Med 308:373, 1983.
23. Lazarus JM, Lowrie EG, Hampers CL, et al. Cardiovascular disease in uremic patients on hemodialysis. Kidney Int 7:167, 1975.
24. Lindner A, Charra B, Sherrard DJ, et al. Accelerated atherosclerosis in prolonged maintenance hemodialysis. N Engl J Med 290:697, 1974.
25. Lindsay J Jr, Crawley IS, Callaway GM Jr. Chronic constrictive pericarditis following uremic hemopericardium. Am Heart J 79:390, 1970.
26. Nayman J. Effect of renal failure on wound healing in dogs: Response to hemodialysis following uremia induced by uranium nitrate. Ann Surg 164:227, 1966.
27. Bleyl U, Sander G, Schindler T. The pathology and biology of uremic pneumonitis. Intensive Care Med 7:193, 1981.
28. Mason EE. Gastrointestinal lesions occurring in uremia. Ann Intern Med 37:96, 1952.
29. Bailey GL, Griffiths H, Lock JP, et al. Gastrointestinal abnormalities in uremia [abstract]. Am Soc Nephrol 5:5, 1971.
30. Adams PL, Rutsky EA, Rostand SG, et al. Lower gastrointestinal tract dysfunction in patients receiving long-term hemodialysis. Arch Intern Med 142:303, 1982.
31. Llach F, Arieff AI, Massry SG. Renal vein thrombosis and nephrotic syndrome. Ann Intern Med 83:8, 1975.
32. Rabiner SF. The effect of dialysis on platelet function of patients with renal failure. Ann NY Acad Sci 201:234, 1972.

33. Burke JF. The use of preventive antibiotics in clinical surgery. Ann Surg 39:6, 1973.
34. Touraine JL, Touraine F, Revillard JP, et al. T-lymphocytes and serum inhibitors of cell mediated immunity in renal insufficiency. Nephron 14:195, 1975.
35. Scharschmidt BF. Acute and chronic hepatic failure. In Wyngaarden JB, Smith LH, Bennett JC, eds. Cecil Textbook of Medicine. Philadelphia: WB Saunders, 1992, pp 796.
36. Boyer TD. Cirrhosis of the liver and its major sequelae. In Wyngaarden JB, Smith LH, Bennett JC, eds. Cecil Textbook of Medicine. Philadelphia: WB Saunders, 1992, p 786.
37. Rosenberg TH, Wahlstrom T. Hepatotoxicity of halothane metabolites in vivo and inhibition of fibroblast growth in vitro. Acta Pharmacol Toxicol 29:9, 1971.
38. Priebe HJ, Skillman JJ, Bushnell LF, et al. Antacid versus cimetidine in preventing acute gastrointestinal bleeding: A randomized trial in 75 critically ill patients. N Engl J Med 302:426, 1980.
39. Frick P, Riedler G, Brogli H. Dose response and minimal daily requirement for vitamin K in man. J Appl Physiol 23:387, 1967.
40. Bernstein WC. What are hemorrhoids and what is their relationship to the portal venous system? Dis Colon Rectum 26:829, 1983.
41. Brayton RG, Stokes PE, Schwartz MS, et al. Effect of alcohol and various diseases on leukocyte mobilization, phagocytosis, and intracellular bacterial killing. N Engl J Med 282:123, 1970.
42. Rigotti P, Peters JC, Tranberg KG, et al. Effects of amino acid infusions on liver regeneration after partial hepatectomy in the rat. J Parenter Enter Nutr 10:17, 1986.
43. Wyngaarden JB. Gout. In Wyngaarden JB, Smith LH, Bennett JC, eds. Cecil Textbook of Medicine. Philadelphia: WB Saunders, 1992, pp 1107.
44. Byers PH. Ehlers-Danlos syndrome. In Wyngaarden JB, Smith LH, Bennett JC, eds. Cecil Textbook of Medicine. Philadelphia: WB Saunders, 1992, pp 1123.
45. Butterworth CE Jr, Weinsier RL. Malnutrition in hospitalized patients: Assessment and treatment. In Goodhart RS, Shils ME, eds. Modern Nutrition in Health and Disease, 6th ed. Philadelphia: Lea & Febiger, 1980.
46. Hill GL, Ticford I, Young GA, et al. Malnutrition in surgical patients: An unrecognized problem. Lancet 1:689, 1977.
47. Frisancho AR. Triceps skin fold and upper arm muscle size norms for assessment of nutritional status. Am J Clin Nutr 27:1052, 1974.
48. Bozzetti F, Migliavacca S, Gallus G, et al. "Nutritional" markers as prognostic indicators of postoperative sepsis in cancer patients. J Parenter Enter Nutr 9:464, 1985.
49. Blackburn GL, Bistrian BR, Maini BS, et al. Nutritional and metabolic assessment of the hospitalized patient. J Parenter Enter Nutr 1:11, 1977.
50. Reilly JJ, Gerhardt AL. Modern surgical nutrition. Current Probl Surg 22:1, 1985.
51. Thompson BR, Julian TB, Stremple JS. Perioperative total parenteral nutrition in patients with gastrointestinal cancer. J Surg Res 30:497, 1981.
52. Holter AR, Fischer JE. The effects of perioperative hyperalimentation on complications in patients with carcinoma and weight loss. J Surg Res 23:31, 1977.
53. Moghissi K, Hornshaw J. Teasdale PR, et al. Parenteral nutrition in carcinoma of the esophagus treated by surgery: Nitrogen balance and clinical studies. Br J Surg 64:125, 1977.
54. Vitello JM. Nutritional assessment and the role of preoperative parenteral nutrition in the colon cancer patient. Semin Surg Oncol 10:183, 1994.
55. Rosen FS, Cooper MD, Wedgewood RJP. The primary immunodeficiencies. (Parts 1 and 2). Med Prog 235:300, 1984.

56. Kemeny MM, Brennan MS. The surgical complications of chemotherapy in the cancer patient. Curr Probl Surg 24:607, 1987.
57. Tyau ES, Prystowsky JB, Joehl RJ, Nahrwold DL. Acute diverticulitis: A complicated problem in the immunocompromised patient. Arch Surg 126:855, 1991.
58. Morstyn G, Souza L, Keech J, et al. Effect of granulocyte colony-stimulating factor on neutropenia induced by cytotoxic chemotherapy. Lancet 26:667, 1988.
59. Bronchud MH, Scarffe JH, Thatcher N, et al. Phase 1/2 study of recombinant human granulocyte colony stimulating factor in patients receiving intensive chemotherapy for small cell lung cancer. Br J Cancer 56:809, 1987.
60. McCray E. Occupational risk of the acquired immunodeficiency syndrome among health care workers. N Engl J Med 314:1127, 1986.
61. Marcus R. The CDC cooperative needle stick surveillance group: Surveillance of health care workers exposed to blood from patients infected with the human immunodeficiency virus. N Engl J Med 319:1118, 1988.
62. Update: Universal precautions for prevention of transmission of human immunodeficiency virus, hepatitis B virus, and other blood borne pathogens in healthcare settings. MMWR 37:377, 1988.
63. Genberding JL, Littel C, Tarkington A. Risk of exposure of surgical personnel to patient's blood during surgery at San Francisco General Hospital. N Engl J Med 322:1788, 1990.
64. Quebbemann EJ, Telford GL, Wadsworth K, et al. Double gloving: Protecting surgeons from blood contamination in the operating room. Arch Surg 127:213, 1992.
65. Popejoy SL, Fry DE. Blood contact and exposure in the operating room. Surg Gynecol Obstet 172:480, 1991.
66. Hagen MD, Meyer KB, Kopelman RI. Human immunodeficiency virus infection in health care workers: A method for estimating individual occupational risk. Arch Intern Med 149:1541, 1989.
67. Henderson DK, Gerberding JL. Prophylactic zidovudine after occupational exposure to the human immunodeficiency virus: An interim analysis. J Infect Dis 160:321, 1989.
68. Centers for Disease Control. Public health service statement on management of occupational exposure to HIV including considerations regarding zidovudine post exposure use. MMWR 39:1, 1990.
69. Davidson TI, Allen-Mersh TG. Operating on the immunosuppressed colorectal patient. In Fielding LP, Goldberg SM, eds. Rob & Smith's Operative Surgery: Surgery of the Colon, Rectum and Anus, 5th ed. Oxford, England: Butterworth-Heinemann, 1993, p 116.
70. Price RW. Neurologic complications of HIV-I infection. In Wyngaarden JB, Smith LH, Bennett JC, eds. Cecil Textbook of Medicine. Philadelphia: WB Saunders, 1992, p 1928.
71. Olefsky JM. Diabetes mellitus. In Wyngaarden JB, Smith LH, Bennett JC, eds. Cecil Textbook of Medicine. Philadelphia: WB Saunders, 1992, p 1291.
72. Jarrett RJ. Descriptive epidemiology of diabetes types I and II. In Diabetes Mellitus. Littleton, Mass.: PSG Publishing, 1986, p 11.
73. Galloway JA, Schuman CR. Diabetes in surgery: A study of 667 cases. Am J Med 34:177, 1963.
74. Steinke J. Management of diabetes in the surgical patient. Med Clin North Am 55:939, 1971.
75. Schamburg HH. Diabetic and other endocrine neuropathies. In Wyngaarden JB, Smith LH, Bennett JC, eds. Cecil Textbook of Medicine. Philadelphia: WB Saunders, 1992, pp 2244.
76. Ewing DJ, Campbell IW, Clarke BF. Mortality in diabetic autonomic neuropathy. Lancet 1:601, 1976.

77. Fraser DM, Campbell IW, Ewing DJ, et al. Peripheral and autonomic nerve function in newly diagnosed diabetes mellitus. Diabetes 26:546, 1977.
78. Page MM, Watkins PJ. Cardiorespiratory arrest in diabetic autonomic neuropathy. Lancet 1:14, 1978.
79. Ewing DJ, Campbell IW, Murray A, et al. Immediate heart rate response to standing. Simple test for autonomic neuropathy in diabetics. Br Med J 1:145, 1978.
80. Kenney RA. Physiology of aging. Clin Geriatr Med 1:37, 1985.
81. Fisch C. Electrocardiogram in the aged: An independent marker of heart disease? Am J Med 70:4, 1981.
82. Fleg JL, Kennedy HL. Cardiac arrhythmias in a healthy elderly population: Detection by 24 hour ambulatory electrocardiography. Chest 81:302, 1982.
83. Camm AJ, Evans KE, Ward DE, et al. The rhythm of the heart in active elderly subjects. Am Heart J 99:598, 1980.
84. Julius S, Amery A, Whitlock LS, et al. Influence of age on the hemodynamic response to exercise. Circulation 36:222, 1967.
85. Conway J, Wheeler R, Sannerstedt R. Sympathetic nervous system activity during exercise in relation to age. Cardiovasc Res 5:577, 1971.
86. Rodeheffer RJ, Gerstenblith G, Becker LC, et al. Exercise cardiac output is maintained with advancing age in healthy human subjects: Cardiac dilatation and increased stroke volume compensate for a diminished heart rate. Circulation 69:203, 1984.
87. Rizzato G, Marrazini L. Thoracoabdominal mechanics in elderly men. J Appl Physiol 28:457, 1970.
88. Black LF, Hyatt RE. Maximal respiratory pressures, normal values, and relationship to age and sex. Am Rev Respir Dis 99:696, 1969.
89. Dehn MM, Bruce RA. Longitudinal variations in maximal oxygen intake with age and activity. J Appl Physiol 33:805, 1972.
90. Hodgson JL, Buskirk ER, Physical fitness and age, with emphasis on cardiovascular function in the elderly. J Am Geriatr Soc 25:385, 1977.
91. Wahba WM. Influence of aging on lung function: Clinical significance of changes from age 20. Anesth Analg 62:764, 1983.
92. Levitzky MG. Effects of aging on the respiratory system. Physiologist 27:102, 1984.
93. Knudson RJ, Lebowitz MD, Holberg CJ, et al. Changes in the normal maximal respiratory flow volume curve with growth and aging. Am Rev Respir Dis 127:725, 1983.
94. Milne JS. Longitudinal respiratory studies in older people. Thorax 33:547, 1978.
95. Rowe JW, Andres R, Tobin JD, et al. The effect of age on creatinine clearance in men: A cross sectional and longitudinal study. J Gerontol 31:155, 1976.
96. Rowe JW. Aging and renal function. Ann Rev Gerontol Geriatr 1:161, 1980.
97. Phillips PA, Rolls BJ, Ledingham JG, et al. Reduced thirst after water deprivation in healthy elderly men. N Engl J Med 311:753, 1984.
98. Rowe JW, Shock NW, DeFronzo RA. The influence of age on the renal response to water deprivation in men. Nephon 17:270, 1976.
99. Epstein M, Hollenberg NK. Age as a determinant of renal sodium conservation in normal men. J Lab Clin Med 87:411, 1976.
100. Seely JF. Renal function in the elderly. In Meakins JL, McClaran JC, eds. Surgical Care of the Elderly. Chicago: Year Book Medical Publishers, 1988, p 129.
101. Cohn SH, Vartsky D, Yasumura S, et al. Compartmental body composition based on total body nitrogen, potassium, and calcium. Am J Physiol 239:E524, 1980.

102. Forbes GB, Reina JC. Adult lean body mass declines with age: Some longitudinal observations. Metabolism 19:653, 1970.
103. Rowe JW, Kahn RL. Human aging: Usual and successful. Science 237:143, 1987.
104. Heath GW, Hagberg JM, Ehsani AA, et al. A physiological comparison of young and older endurance athletes. J Appl Physiol 51:634, 1981.
105. Wilmore JH, Miller HL, Pollock ML. Body composition and physiological characteristics of active endurance athletes in their eighth decade of life. Med Sci Sports Exerc 6:44, 1974.
106. Ziffren SE. Comparison of mortality rates for various surgical operations according to age groups, 1951-1977. J Am Geriatr Soc 27:433, 1979.
107. Farrow SC, Fowkes FG, Lunn JN, et al. Epidemiology and anesthesia. II. Factors affecting mortality in the hospital. Br J Anesth 54:811, 1982.
108. Palmberg S, Hirsjarvi E. Mortality in geriatric surgery: With special reference to the type of surgery, anesthesia, complicating diseases, and prophylaxis of thrombosis. Gerontology 25:103, 1979.
109. Marx GF, Mateo CV, Orkin LR. Computer analysis of postanesthetic deaths. Anesthesiology 39:54, 1973.
110. Djokovic JL, Hedley-Whyte J. Prediction of outcome of surgery and anesthesia in patients over 80. JAMA 242:2301, 1979.
111. Boyd JB, Bradford B Jr, Watne AL. Operative risk factors of colon resection in the elderly. Ann Surg 192:743, 1980.
112. Lewin I, Lerner AG, Green SH, et al. Physical class and physiologic status in the prediction of operative mortality in the aged sick. Ann Surg 174:217, 1971.
113. Turnbull AD, Gundy E, Howland WS, et al. Surgical mortality among the elderly: An analysis of 4,050 operations (1970-1974). Clin Bull 8:139, 1978.
114. Warner MA, Hosking MP, Lobdell CM, et al. Surgical procedures among those greater than or equal to 90 years of age: A population-based study in Olmstead County, Minnesota, 1975-1985. Ann Surg 207:380, 1988.
115. Nehme AE. Groin hernias in elderly patients: Management and prognosis. Am J Surg 146:257, 1983.
116. Puxty JA, Horan MA, Fox RA. Necropsies in the elderly. Lancet 1:1262, 1983.
117. Mohr DN. Estimation of surgical risk in the elderly: A correlated review. J Am Geriatr Soc 31:99, 1983.
118. Denney JL, Denson JF. Risk of surgery in patients over 90. Geriatrics 27:115, 1972.
119. Fowkes FG, Lunn JN, Farrow SC, et al. Epidemiology and anesthesia. III. Mortality risk in patients with coexisting physical disease. Br J Anesth 54:819, 1982.

CHAPTER 2

Bowel Preparation for Elective Colon Surgery

TERRY C. HICKS

Septic complications are an ever present danger for patients undergoing elective surgery for diseases of the large bowel and rectum. Frequently these infections are limited to the operative wound, but other potential sites include the abdominal cavity, pelvis, and bloodstream. Postoperative wound infections are reported to occur following 6.4% to 12% of elective colorectal operations.[1-5] Infections produce serious morbidity and mortality and drive up the cost of health care. Green and Wenzel[6] reported that wound infections double the duration of hospitalization. Brachman et al.[7] found that wound infections increased hospital stay by 7.4 days and increased the cost of the admission by as much as $7900.

The causes of septic complications include a myriad of factors, not all controllable, that can be categorized as preoperative, intraoperative, and postoperative. The focus of this chapter is on the preoperative period, in which appropriate mechanical bowel preparation and antibiotic use contribute to reduction of septic complications. The major consideration in the preoperative phase involves proper bowel preparation, which is heavily reliant on patient compliance. For a number of reasons, the traditional inpatient conduct of bowel preparation has been shifted to the outpatient setting. With dedicated, experienced support systems (e.g., patient education by nurses and simple preparation regimens), equivalent results can be obtained.[8,9]

MECHANICAL PREPARATION OF THE COLON

The current standard preoperative preparation of the bowel for elective colorectal surgery includes mechanical cleansing and antibiotic preparation. Appropriate bowel preparation decreases infectious complications and anastomotic disruptions, simplifies colonic surgery, and is more aesthetically pleasing to the surgeon.[10] Ideally, mechanical bowel preparation should be safe and rapid, provide good cleansing, be easily administered in both inpatient and outpatient settings, produce minimal patient discomfort, and be cost effective.[11] Although no method presently fulfills all of these criteria, reliable methods with good clinical results are available.[12,13]

The colon can be mechanically cleansed with dietary restrictions, enemas, cathartics, or lavage. Several authors have demonstrated that any cleansing method used will reduce the quantity of stool but will not significantly reduce the concentration of bacteria remaining in the colonic lumen.[14-17] Traditionally, most techniques for emptying the colon used irritant-type purgatives and enemas to remove feces, combined with dietary restrictions so as not to add to the fecal bulk. This technique was reported by Keighley[18] and DiPalma et al.[19] to produce adequate and acceptable bowel cleansing in approximately 70% of patients. The cathartic and enema cleansing methods, however, require 2 to 3 days to complete and are associated with significant physiologic side effects. In patients undergoing cathartic bowel preparation, dehydration and electrolyte imbalance often occur.[10-12]

Burbige et al.[20] reported that patients receiving the cathartic and enema preparation for colonoscopy experienced, on average, a 2-pound weight loss. Vanner et al.[21] reported laboratory evidence of dehydration (e.g., elevation in sodium and chloride levels, hematocrit, and serum osmolarity) in patients receiving oral sodium phosphate (Fleet Phospho-soda, C.B. Fleet Co., Lynchburg, Va.). Other authors who evaluated oral sodium phosphate also found subclinical depletion of intravascular volume[22] and hyperphosphatemia.[22,23] These studies confirm the overall safety of this preparation in the majority of patients if taken correctly. The physiologic alterations associated with the preparation may limit its usefulness in patients with impaired renal function. The small volume associated with a sodium phosphate preparation is appealing to many patients, and many providers use it as an alternative preparation in patients who have difficulty taking the volume of polyethylene glycol lavage preparations.

Enema preparations may contain tap water, soapsuds, saline solution, or chemicals such as mineral oil or phosphate mixtures. They work by irritating the colon or by dilution. As a single agent for bowel preparation, they are routinely unsuccessful and require concomitant cathartic administration for adequate cleansing. Enema administration is cumbersome for the nursing staff and often uncomfortable for the patient. Physiologic complications have been documented.[10-12] The use of hypertonic preparations can result in dehydration, and isotonic or hypotonic solutions may result in an increase in body fluid.[25] Use of enemas containing phosphate or water has also been associated with potassium imbalance. Patients with impaired renal function are most likely to be physiologically challenged by these preparations.

Enema use may result in mechanical complications. Perforation is uncommon in the patient with a normal GI tract but is a significant risk for those patients with inflammation or obstruction of the colon or rectum.[26] Injury may occur because of technical misadventure during insertion of the enema tube tip or from hydrostatic perforations. There is also the rare case of thermal injury if the tap water enema is not evaluated for appropriate temperature prior to instillation. Hypothermia can occur if large volumes of cool (room temperature) water are used.

The transition to oral lavage resulted in two distinct improvements: better bowel preparation and decreased time required for mechanical cleansing. Initial trials with the oral lavage technique utilized normal saline solution. After passage of a nasogastric tube, the patient received 1 L of fluid per hour. To obtain adequate cleansing, an average 7 to 10 L of normal saline solution was required.[13,27,28] Use of normal saline solution for lavage was also associated with important complications such as significant fluid and electrolyte imbalance and subsequent weight gain.[13] Because of these findings, Hares and Alexander-Williams[10] suggested that this technique not be used in patients with impaired renal or cardiovascular status. If the normal saline solution is not administered at body temperature, hypothermia may develop secondary to the large volume of solution required. The use of normal saline lavage technique was short lived because it involved insertion of a nasogastric tube, was skill and labor intensive, and was associated with the physiologic complications described.

Mannitol, a nonabsorbed osmotic agent was reported as a successful oral lavage agent by numerous authors between 1979 and 1986.[13] When used in concentrations of 10% to 15% in water, as little as 1 L cleansed the bowel adequately in approximately 50% of patients, although several authors reported significant dehydration in their patients.[10,29,30] With a 5% solution, a volume of 3 to 4 L was required, but still caused electrolyte imbalance. Mannitol is metabolized by the colonic bacterial flora, which produce potentially explosive gas. Levy[31] reported that explosive concentrations of hydrogen gas in free air ranged from 4.1% to 74%. The hydrogen concentration in the flatus of normal bowel varies from 2.9% to 21%.[32-34] La Brody et al.[35] used a 10% mannitol solution for bowel preparation before colonoscopy and found explosive concentrations of hydrogen gas in 60% of their patients. Beck et al.[30] used a 10% mannitol lavage with intravenous cefotaxamine and metronidazole and reported that 10% of their surgical patients had combustible levels of hydrogen gas in the bowel. Electrocautery-induced colonic explosions have been reported at endoscopy and surgery in patients given bowel preparations that contained mannitol. The prevalence of this complication is low compared with the total number of procedures performed in patients who have received mannitol-containing bowel preparations. In a national survey in 1987, only 4% of respondents noted that they used mannitol as an oral lavage agent because of such potential catastrophic sequelae.[12]

Mannitol has also been associated with significantly higher intracolonic counts of *Escherichia coli.* Keighley et al.[29] compared *E. coli* counts in patients receiving either a mannitol lavage preparation, a saline solution lavage preparation, or a mannitol lavage preparation along with oral antibiotics. *E. coli* overgrowth was noted in the mannitol lavage group who did not receive antibiotics. The use of oral antibiotics with mannitol lavage prevents *E. coli* overgrowth; this protection is not noted with the isolated use of parenteral antibiotics.[30]

In 1980 Davis et al.[36] described the development of a lavage solution associated with minimal water and electrolyte absorption or secretion in an effort to avoid the disadvantages of the saline solution and mannitol preparations. Their solution was composed of polyethylene glycol 3350 (PEG 3350) and electrolytes (i.e., sodium 125 mmol/L, sulfate 40 mmol/L, chloride 35 mmol/L, bicarbonate 20 mmol/L, and potassium 10 mmol/L).

DiPalma and Brady[37] reported that ingestion of 2 to 4 L (8 ounces every 10 minutes) of this solution produces excellent bowel preparation in 90% to 100% of patients, usually in less than 4 hours, without electrolyte or metabolic complications. This solution is presently produced as GoLytely (Braintree Laboratories, Braintree, Mass.) and CoLyte (Reed & Carnrick, Piscataway, N.J.) and is the lavage solution of choice for colonoscopy and elective colon surgery.[13] Some patients experience symptoms of nausea and fullness with the polyethylene glycol preparation. To alleviate these side effects, Rhodes et al.[38] proposed metoclopramide as an adjunct to the polyethylene glycol preparation. In their perspective study of 40 patients undergoing colonoscopy, they reported a decrease in patient symptoms; others, however, have found metoclopramide to be of no help in reducing nausea or abdominal cramping.[39] Some clinicians noted that polyethylene glycol preparations were associated with significant intraluminal fluid retention. Brady et al.[40] administered bisacodyl (Dulcolax; Boehrigen Ingelhem, Ridgefield, Conn.) as an adjunct to polyethylene glycol solution before colonoscopy but found no improvement in cleansing quality or residual fluid volumes. Other studies of the efficacy of bisacodyl noted significant histologic and macroscopic changes in colonic mucosa with use of this chemical.[41,42]

Special Situations

Patients with partial obstructions. The clinician frequently sees patients with a partially obstructing colonic process. In cases in which there is radiologic (excluding retrograde obstruction) and clinical confirmation that complete obstruction is not present and in patients who do not have an inflammatory bowel process, the physician can consider bowel preparation with small increments of Fleet Phospho-soda, GoLytely, or mineral oil solutions.

Intraoperative lavage. Patients who require emergency surgery or those with inadequate bowel preparation found at elective surgery are candidates for intraoperative lavage. The two major techniques are transabdominal lavage and transrectal lavage.

Stewart et al.[43] reported that a transabdominal technique in selected patients provides the opportunity for the surgeon to perform resection with a primary anastomosis. Intraoperative lavage requires insertion of a Foley-type catheter

(20 Fr) through a stab incision associated with a small purse-string suture.[44] The incision may be made in the terminal ileum or through the appendiceal orifice and the tube advanced into the cecum. The catheter balloon is then inflated and pulled back flush against the ileocecal valve or the base of the appendix. A firm, sterile, large tube (e.g., ribbed anesthesia tubing or laser plume evacuation tubing) is placed in the distal end of the mobilized colon away from the line of resection and is secured with umbilical or vascular tape. Next, the distal end of the drainage tube is directed to a bucket or closed collection system placed on the floor to avoid contamination. The Foley catheter is connected to a warm saline solution, and the colon is irrigated with 2 to 4 L of fluid (Fig. 2-1). Gentle manipulation of the bowel may be helpful to remove solid material and excess fluid. Some surgeons finish the preparation with an antimicrobial solution such as povidone-iodine. When the fluid is clear, the bowel is clamped above the taped insertion site, and a short segment of distal bowel and the tubing can be removed from the operation field. Routine resection and anastomosis can then be performed.

In the transrectal approach, a large Foley or Malecot catheter (32 Fr)[13] is positioned in the rectum, and carefully inflated if it is the Foley type. The catheter is connected to a Y system with an ingress and an egress arm. The ingress arm is connected to the warm saline solution. This technique is excellent for use in left-sided colonic resection with the proximal bowel occluded while the solution is gently instilled.[44] During instillation of fluid, the egress arm is occluded until the bowel segment is filled, then the ingress arm is occluded while the egress tube is opened to allow the fluid mixed with stool to drain into an

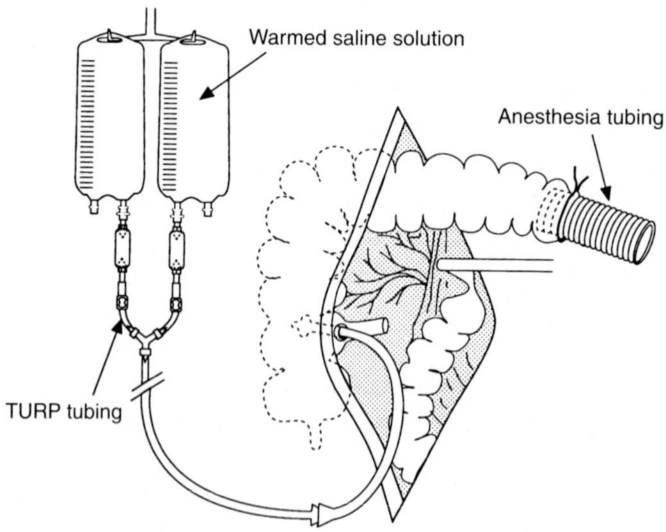

Fig. 2-1 Intraoperative lavage.

appropriate collection system. Some authors have also suggested conducting the final irrigation with an antimicrobial solution such as povidone-iodine.[45]

ANTIBIOTICS

In current practice, in the absence of obstruction there is little support for failing to use a mechanical preparation as part of the preoperative bowel preparation for colon surgery. Furthermore, it can strongly be argued that the standard of care requires that antibiotics be added to such mechanical preparation. The emptying of the colon lumen of feces, although an essential first step in an elective preparation has little effect on the bacteria. To attack the residual bacteria, antimicrobial agents have been added to the preparation regimen. In a substantive review of clinical series reported from 1965 to 1980, Baum et al.[46] showed that infection rates were significantly increased in patients given mechanical preparations alone compared with patients given mechanical preparations and prophylactic antibiotics. This evidence, combined with the work of others, led Polk and Ausobsky[47] to conclude in 1984 that "significant benefits in terms of operative mortality and infection are attendant on the use of antibiotic prophylaxis in colorectal operations, there is presently no *ethical* [emphasis added] justification for the use of placebo controls in clinical trials...or omission of appropriate antimicrobial agents in the preparation of the patient for large bowel operations."

Although today's surgeons would agree with this conclusion, the debate continues as to whether the antibiotics used should be administered enterally and selected primarily for their intraluminal activity or administered parenterally and selected for their systemic effects, or both.

Oral Antibiotics

In the selection of an appropriate oral antibiotic regimen, the surgeon must consider the normal bowel flora, the bacteriologic features of infections associated with colon operations, any synergism among bacteria found in postoperative infections, and the antibiotic sensitivity of the bacteria.

Normal colonic flora includes approximately 20 species of aerobic bacteria and more than 50 species of anaerobic bacteria. The most commonly cultured anaerobic bacterial species in postoperative infections in elective colon and rectal surgery is *Bacteroides fragilis,* followed by *Clostridia* and peptostreptococci. The most common cultured aerobic bacteria from colorectal surgical infections is *E. coli.* Other coloform bacteria found in such infections include *Klebsiella, Proteus,* and *Pseudomonas* organisms, as well as *Streptococcus faecalis* and other streptococci. Because colorectal infections are caused by endogenous bacteria that violate the colonic mucosal barrier, from either a leaking anastomosis or contamination during the original operation, the prophylactic antibiotics used should be effective against these bacteria. Nichols et al.[48,49] in 1970 began a series of studies that formed the basis for the utilization of modern oral prophylactic antibiotics in colon surgery. Neomycin and erythromycin base were chosen because they are well tolerated by patients, inexpensive, and remain in the bowel lumen (although oral erythromycin does produce measurable serum concentrations). The authors gave 1 g of each antibiotic orally at 1:00, 2:00, and 11:00 PM on the day before surgery, in anticipation of an 8:00 AM operating time; if the surgery was planned for later than 8:00 AM, they made appropriate adjustments in the timing of the doses. Neomycin was selected because of its activity against aerobic coliform bacteria, whereas erythromycin base was chosen because of its activity against anaerobic bacteria. Other studies have confirmed that these two antibiotics in combination are effective in reducing septic complications of colonic surgery.[46] Recently some surgeons have substituted metronidazole (250 to 500 mg) instead of erythromycin to prevent the GI symptoms associated with erythromycin.

Parenteral Antibiotics

The utilization of systemic antibiotics in elective colorectal surgery is prophylactic rather than therapeutic. The goal of the prophylactic use of antibiotics is to prevent potential infectious sequelae rather than treat preexisting sepsis. Surgeons should know the pharmokinetics of the antibiotics selected and be aware that tissue levels of the drugs must be achieved before the operation is begun. Polk and Lopez-Mayer[50] in 1969 set the stage for the preoperative prophylactic use of parenteral antibiotics in colorectal surgery. In their study, patients were randomly assigned to one of two groups. All patients underwent mechanical cleansing of the bowel; then one group received cephaloridine, 1 g, immediately before surgery and two additional doses within 12 hours after the operation, and the other group received a placebo. Only 8% of the patients given the antibiotics developed infections, whereas 30% of the group given placebo had infectious complications.

Edmondson and Rissing[51] demonstrated that the combination of oral neomycin and erythromycin was superior to cephaloridine alone. Slama et al.[52] agreed that the same oral combination was superior to cefamandole, which they noted was inactive against *B. fragilis.* Many studies in which prophylactic parenteral antibiotics were used in colorectal surgery have yielded conflicting results. Significant problems in the experimental design have been found in many of these studies, which leaves the conclusions suspect. In comparisons of certain studies in which patients received intravenous metronidazole and gentamicin or cefamandole or cefoxitin or cefazolin or doxycycline in combination with tinidazole with studies in which patients received only enteral antibiotics effective against anaerobic and aerobic bacteria, there appears to be no advantage to parenteral antibiotics. Thus it is apparent that intravenous antibiotics without oral antibiotics have succeeded in some trials but failed in others.

Oral Plus Intravenous Antibiotics

Clinical trials indicate that oral antibiotics or parenteral antibiotics alone, along with adequate bowel preparation, have demonstrated efficacy in reducing infection in patients undergoing elective procedures of the colon. The question arises, then, Does the combination of an oral plus an intravenous antibiotic reduce the prevalence of wound infections and other septic postoperative complications even more? The theory supporting improved clinical results is based on the concept that the oral antibiotics would suppress the intraluminal bacterial flora and the intravenous antibiotics would achieve high serum and tissue levels against infectious organisms. Condon[53] pointed out that this approach has obvious dual-benefit appeal to clinicians but that it has not been conclusively shown to be superior to other antibiotic regimens now in use. He noted the combination of oral and parenteral antibiotics adds a marginally positive outcome through a decrease in urinary tract infections and other secondary postoperative infections. Because of the current low prevalence of postoperative wound infections, a very large number of patients would be required to complete such a study. It is therefore unlikely that such a study will be done.

Complications of Antibiotic Use

Although prophylactic antibiotics are of proven benefit in reducing postoperative wound infections, use of antibiotics is not without risks. A myriad of adverse reactions can occur with the antibiotics used in colorectal surgery patients: gastrointestinal disturbances, allergic reactions, development of bacterial resistance, organ injury, and hematologic and immunologic abnormalities.

Gastrointestinal disturbances. Gastrointestinal complaints including diarrhea, nausea, and vomiting may arise from use of cephalosporins, penicillins, erythromycin, and metronidazole. Pseudomembranous colitis is an infectious disease of the colon and rectum that is associated with diarrhea and a morphologic identification of yellowish white mucosal plaques. The majority of cases are directly related to antibiotic therapy, most notably, clinidamycin, ampicillin, cephalosporin, and lincomycin.[54] The nidus of this disease is a toxin produced by *C. difficile*. Diagnosis is made on the basis of clinical symptoms and laboratory detection of a fecal toxin and/or analysis of biopsy specimens of plaques during endoscopy. Treatment consists of oral metronidazole or vancomycin. In patients unable to take oral therapy, intravenous metronidazole can be used. Despite adequate therapy and an initial clinical response to the therapy, relapse will occur in up to 20% of patients.

Diarrhea associated with antibiotic use may be caused by alterations in the patient's normal colonic flora. This may be a mild form of the physiologic alterations described previously for pseudomembranous colitis. Antibiotic-associated diarrhea usually resolves when antibiotic therapy is discontinued. Yogurt and lactobacillus capsules have also been recommended as treatment.

ALLERGIC REACTIONS

Hypersensitivity or an allergic reaction can occur with any medication. Penicillin allergy is one of the more common, with hypersensitivity reactions occurring in more than 5% of patients.[55] A 10% incidence of cross-reactivity with cephalosporins and penicillins has been described. Most surgeons will therefore avoid use of a cephalosporin in a patient who has had a significant allergic reaction (anaphylactic symptoms, respiratory insufficiency, or hypotension) to either class of drug. The entire health care team should have a high index of suspicion for any unusual patient symptoms after administration of an antibiotic. Anaphylactic reactions should be treated expeditiously with epinephrine, oxygen, and intravenous fluid. Less serious reactions are managed with discontinuation of the medication. Symptoms may be reduced with antihistamines such as diphenhydramine hydrochloride. More serious symptoms may require stronger anti-inflammatory medications such as steroids. Long-term use of cefamandole and cefotetan, which share a similar side chain, have been associated with bleeding secondary to hypoprothrombinemia. This problem is related to vitamin K metabolism and can be prevented with concomitant administration of vitamin K.

REFERENCES

1. Farber BF, Wenzel RP. Postoperative wound infection rates: Results of prospective statewide surveillance. Am J Surg 140:343, 1980.
2. Cruse PJE, Foord R. The epidemiology of wound infection. A 10-year prospective study of 62,939 wounds. Surg Clin North Am 60:27, 1980.
3. National Research Council Division of Medical Sciences, Ad Hoc Committee of the Committee of Trauma. Postoperative wound infections: The influence of ultraviolet irradiation of the operating room and various other factors. Ann Surg 160(Suppl 2):1, 1964.
4. Woobes TH, Bemelmans BLH, Kuypers HC, Been Thuizen GM, Theeuwes AGM. Risk of postoperative septic complications after abdominal surgical treatment in relation to perioperative blood transfusion. Surg Gynecol Obstet 171:59, 1990.
5. Jensen LS, Andersen A, Fristrup SC, et al. Comparison of one dose versus three doses of prophylactic antibiotics, and the influence of blood transfusion on infectious complications in acute and elective colorectal surgery. Br J Surg 77:513, 1990.
6. Green JW, Wenzel RP. Postoperative wound infection. A controlled study of the increased duration of hospital stay and direct costs of hospitalization. Ann Surg 185:264, 1977.
7. Brachman PS, Dan BB, Haley RW, Hooton TM, Garner JS, Allen JS. Nosocomial infections. Incidence and cost. Surg Clin North Am 60:15, 1980.
8. Le T, Timmcke AE, Gathright JB. Outpatient bowel preparation for elective colon resection [abst]. Dis Colon Rectum 35:P5, 1992.

9. Frazee RC, Roberts J, Symmonds R, et al. Prospective, randomized trial of inpatient vs. out-patient bowel preparation for elective colorectal surgery. Dis Colon Rectum 35:223, 1992.
10. Hares MM, Alexander-Williams J. The effect of bowel preparation on clonic [sic] surgery. World J Surg 6:175, 1982.
11. Beck DE, Harford EJ, DiPalma JA, Brady CE III. Bowel cleansing with polyethylene glycol electrolyte lavage solution. South Med J 78:1414, 1985.
12. Beck DE, Fazio VW. Current preoperative bowel cleansing methods. Results of a survey. Dis Colon Rectum 33:12, 1990.
13. Beck DE. Mechanical bowel cleansing for surgery. Perspect Colon Rectal Surg 7:97, 1994.
14. Nichols RL, Gorbach SL, Condon RE. Alteration of intestinal microflora following preoperative mechanical preparation of the colon. Dis Colon Rectum 14:123, 1981.
15. Bartlett JG, Condon RE, Gorbach SL, et al. Veterans Administration Cooperative Study on Bowel Preparation for Elective Colorectal Operations. Impact of oral antibiotic regimen on colonic flora, wound irrigation cultures and bacteriology of septic complications. Ann Surg 188:249, 1978.
16. Raahave D, Hansen OH, Carstensen HE, et al. Septic wound complications after whole bowel irrigation before colorectal operations. Acta Chir Scand 147:215, 1982.
17. Arabi Y, Dimock F, Burdon DW, et al. Influence of bowel preparation and antimicrobials on colonic microflora. Br J Surg 65:555, 1978.
18. Keighley MRB. A clinical and physiological evaluation for elective colorectal surgery. World J Surg 6:464, 1982.
19. DiPalma JA, Brady CE, Stewart DL, et al. Comparison of colon cleaning methods in preparation for colonoscopy. Gastroenterology 86:856, 1984.
20. Burbige EJ, Bourke E, Tarder G. Effect of preparation for colonoscopy on fluid and electrolyte balance. Gastrointest Endosc 24:286, 1978.
21. Vanner SJ, MacDonald PN, Paterson WG, Prentice RS, DaCosta LR, Beck IT. A randomized prospective trial comparing oral sodium phosphate with standard polyethylene glycol–based lavage solution (GoLytely) in the preparation of patients for colonoscopy [comments]. Am J Gastroenterol 85:422, 1990.
22. Huynh T, Vaner S, Paterson W. Safety profile of 5-h oral sodium regimen for colonoscopy cleansing. Lack of clinically significant hypocalcemia or hypovolemia. Am J Gastroenterology 90:104, 1995.
23. Cohen SM, Wexner SD, Binderow SR, et al. Prospective, randomized, endoscopic-blinded trial comparing precolonoscopic bowel cleansing methods. Dis Colon Rectum 37:689, 1994.
24. Golub RW, Kerner BA, Wise WE Jr, et al. Colonoscopic bowel preparations—which one? A blinded, prospective, randomized trial. Dis Colon Rectum 38:594, 1995.
25. Mikal S. Metabolic effects of preoperative intestinal preparation. Am J Proctol 16:437, 1965.
26. Tadros S, Watters JM. Retroperitoneal perforation of the rectum during barium enema examination. Can J Surg 1:49, 1988.
27. Chung RS, Gurill NJ, Berglund EM. A controlled clinical trial of whole gut lavage as a method of bowel preparation for colonic operations. Am J Surg 137:75, 1979.
28. Crapp AR, Tillotson P, Powis SFA, et al. Preparation of the bowel by whole-gut irrigation. Lancet 2:1239, 1975.
29. Keighley MR, Taylor EW, Hares MM, et al. Influence of oral manitol bowel preparation on colonic microflora and the risk of explosion during endoscopic diathermy. Br J Surg 68:554, 1981.

30. Beck DE, Fazio VW, Jagelman DG. Comparison of oral lavage methods for preoperative colonic cleansing. Dis Colon Rectum 29:699, 1986.
31. Levy EI. Explosions during lower bowel electrosurgery. Am J Surg 88:754, 1954.
32. Taylor EW, Bentley S, Youngs D, et al. Bowel preparation and the safety of colonoscopic polypectomy. Gastroenterology 81:1, 1981.
33. Kirk E. Quantity and composition of human colonic flatus. Gastroenterology 12:782, 1949.
34. Bigard M. Gaucher P, Lassalle C. Fatal colonic explosion during colonoscopic polypectomy. Gastroenterology 77:1307, 1979.
35. La Brody SJ, Augerinos A, Fendick CL, Williams CB, Misiewicz JJ. Potentially explosive colonic concentrations of hydrogen after bowel preparation with mannitol. Lancet 1:634, 1981.
36. Davis GR, Santa Ana CA, Morawski SG, Fordran JS. Development of a lavage solution associated with minimum water and electrolytes absorption or secretion. Gastroenterology 78:991, 1980.
37. DiPalma JA, Brady CE III. Colon cleansing for diagnostic and surgical procedures: Polyethylene glycol electrolyte lavage solution. Am J Gastroenterol 84:1008, 1989.
38. Rhodes JB, Engstrom J, Stone KF. Metoclopramide reduces the distress associated with colon cleansing by an oral electrolyte overload. Gastrointest Endosc 4:162, 1978.
39. Golub RW, Kerner BA, Wise WE, et al. Colonoscopic bowel preparation—which one? A blinded prospective, randomized trial [abst]. Dis Colon Rectum 35:P2, 1992.
40. Brady CE III, DiPalma JA, Beck DE. Colon cleansing with GoLytely. Does biscodyl improve cleansing? Ann Clin Res 19:348, 1987.
41. Pockros PJ, Foroozan P. GoLytely versus standard colonoscopy preparation. Effect on normal colonic mucosal histology. Gastroenterology 88:545, 1984.
42. Smith B. Pathologic changes in the colon produced by anthraquinone purgatives. Dis Colon Rectum 16:455, 1973.
43. Stewart J, Diament RH, Brennan TG. Management of obstructing lesions of the left colon by resection, on-table lavage, and primary anastomosis. Surgery 114:502, 1993.
44. Koruth NM, Krukowski ZH, Youngson GG, et al. Intra-operative colonic irrigation in the management of left-sided large bowel emergencies. Br J Surg 72:708, 1985.
45. Parker MCD, Ashby EC, Nicholls MWN, Dowding CH, Brooks JC. Providone-iodine bowel irrigation before resection of colorectal carcinoma. Ann R Coll Surg Engl 67:227, 1985.
46. Baum ML, Anish DS, Chalmers TC, et al. A survey of clinical trials of antibiotic prophylaxis in colon surgery. Evidence against further use of no-treatment controls. N Engl J Med 305:795, 1981.
47. Polk HC, Ausobsky JR. Preoperative preparation and antibiotic utilization in operations for carcinoma of the colon and rectum. In Spratt JS, ed. Neoplasms of the Colon, Rectum and Anus. Philadelphia: WB Saunders, 1984, p 114.
48. Nichols RL, Condon RE. Preoperative preparation of the colon. Surg Gynecol Obstet 132:323, 1971.
49. Nichols RL, Broido P, Condon RE, et al. Effect of preoperative neomycin-erythromycin intestinal preparation on the incidence of infectious complications following colon surgery. Ann Surg 178:453, 1973.
50. Polk HC, Lopez-Mayor JF. Postoperative wound infection. A prospective study of determinant factors and prevention. Surgery 66:97, 1969.
51. Edmondson HT, Rissing JP. Prophylactic antibiotics in colon surgery. Arch Surg 118:227, 1983.
52. Slama TG, Carey LC, Fass RJ. Comparative efficacy of prophylactic cephalothin and

cefamandole for elective colon surgery. Results of a prospective, randomized, double-blind study. Am J Surg 137:593, 1979.

53. Condon RE. Preoperative bowel preparation. In Fazio VW, ed. Current Therapy in Colon and Rectal Surgery. Toronto: BC Decker, 1990, pp 213-216.
54. Keighley MRB. Antibiotic associated pseudomembranous colitis. Pathogenesis and management. Drugs 20:49, 1980.
55. Wilson RF, Jennings SW. Handbook of Antibiotic Therapy for Surgery Related Infections. Springfield, N.J.: Scientific Therapeutics Information, 1994, pp 92-93.

CHAPTER 3

Anesthesia and Intraoperative Positioning

RICHARD E. KARULF

For the colorectal surgeon who must work deep in the pelvis during abdominal operations or at the limit of instruments during transanal excisions, proper patient positioning and adequate anesthesia make the crucial difference between a procedure that is difficult for the surgeon and uncomfortable for the patient and one in which visualization is excellent and the procedure is painless. Complications during surgery that result because of either improper positioning of the patient or method of anesthesia are a cause of serious concern and a common cause of litigation. Awareness on the part of the operative team of potential hazards may help to prevent these problems and result in a better outcome for the patient.

A patient undergoing colorectal surgery is vulnerable to the same complications as any other patient undergoing anesthesia. This chapter highlights those complications of anesthesia and positioning that are unique to or most common in colorectal surgery.

ANESTHETIC COMPLICATIONS

Common Complications

One of the most common complications of anorectal surgery is postoperative urinary retention because of anal pain. Although not caused by anesthetic agents, the incidence of postoperative retention can be reduced by the anesthesiologist or anesthetist through judicious use of intravenous fluids in the perioperative period and avoiding overdistention of the bladder.[1] Avoiding routine placement of a Foley catheter before surgery or intermittent catheterization after surgery, unless specifically indicated, may also prevent this complication.

Another problem that must be considered before induction of anesthesia is the possibility of adrenal insufficiency. In patients receiving prolonged corticosteroid therapy for inflammatory bowel disease or medical conditions such as obstructive pulmonary disease or rheumatoid arthritis, there may be suppression of the hypothalamic-pituitary-adrenal axis. This alters the patient's ability to mount an endocrine response to stress. Adrenal suppression is related to steroid dose, frequency of dosage, route of administration, and duration of therapy.[2] Treatment with large doses (>40 mg/m^2 of prednisone or its equivalent) for as little as 5 to 7 days can suppress adrenal gland function for longer than a week.[3] With longer duration of steroid administration, adrenal function may not be fully recovered for up to a year or more after cessation of steroid therapy.[4]

To prevent problems, patients who have received glucocorticoids capable of adrenal suppression within 1 year should receive perioperative exogenous steroids to ensure an appropriate endocrine response to operative stress.[5] Recommended regimens, listed below, include 200 to 300 mg/day of hydrocortisone or its equivalent in divided doses, which is equivalent to the response of normal adrenal glands to major stress.[5] This dosage is gradually tapered over 2 to 3 days to maintenance therapy.

Preoperative: Hydrocortisone phosphate, 75 to 100 mg IV, just before the procedure

Day of surgery: Hydrocortisone phosphate, 75 to 100 mg IV, every 8 hours

Postoperative day 1 until oral diet is resumed: Hydrocortisone phosphate IV; taper from 75 to 100 mg every 8 hours to 25 to 50 mg every 12 hours

When taking oral diet: Prednisone, 20 mg/day orally, if the disease is cured or treated; otherwise, resume the preoperative dosage; decrease by 5 mg over 7 to 14 days

Patients who develop perioperative complications or experience additional stress should be given the original perioperative dosage. Few physiologic studies or prospective trials have been conducted to confirm these recommendations.

Few data are available to recommend the dosage of steroids a patient should receive after the initial disease process is surgically cured (e.g., ulcerative colitis) or treated (e.g., removal of all active Crohn's disease). In a recent large survey of colorectal surgeons, the majority of respondents administered 20 mg of prednisone/day. This dose was reduced by 5 mg every 7 to 14 days.[6]

Inadequate steroid levels can lead to adrenal insufficiency. Symptoms of acute adrenal insufficiency include pyrexia, tachycardia, and hypotension. Laboratory abnormalities include hyponatremia, hyperkalemia, elevated urinary sodium concentration, and low urinary potassium level. A major differential diagnosis in the postoperative patient with these signs and symptoms is sepsis. Therefore patients with these findings should undergo adequate evaluation for sepsis along with concomitant empirical administration of corticosteroids (e.g., 100 mg hydrocortisone phosphate IV every 8 hours). If the patient has adrenal insufficiency, this will quickly resolve the problem. If the patient has sepsis, the additional steroids will help the patient cope with the stress of sepsis while other evaluations and treatment are instituted.

A less acute form of adrenal insufficiency may produce fatigue, weight loss, anorexia, arthralgias, watery diarrhea, and dehydration. The alteration in GI motility is related to a disappearance of gut migrating motor complexes.[7] These patients respond well to intravenous hydration and increased steroid dosage.[8]

Local Anesthesia

Use of local anesthesia for minor procedures may lull the surgeon into a false sense of security because of its minimal effect on total body physiology. Many surgeons tend to try to complete a procedure with an unsatisfactory or failing local block by adding intravenous sedation. However, the addition of intravenous sedation to local blockade may mask problems that would otherwise be noted with local anesthesia alone. In addition to the risks associated with the use of local anesthesia, there is an increased chance for technical error as a result of patient movement and lack of relaxation.

The most common use of local anesthesia in colorectal surgery is during anorectal procedures with simple infiltration or an anal block. Although commonly used in office procedures, relaxation of regional muscles is not achieved and exposure may not be so good as with other forms of anesthesia.

Systemic reactions to high blood levels of local anesthetic drugs are attributed to inadvertent intravenous injection, accelerated absorption, or overdosage (Table 3-1). As a general rule, doses of lidocaine, <5 to 7 mg/kg, and bupivacaine, <2 to 4 mg/kg, are safe. The most common cause of systemic reaction to local anesthetic agents is inadvertent intravenous injection. Frequent aspiration during injection should be performed to try to avert this problem.

Clinical features of toxicity are represented by a spectrum of symptoms that range from talkativeness and altered personality in the early stages to confusion, seizures, and coma, with respiratory arrest in its most severe form. Other common symptoms of toxicity include ringing in the ears, dizziness, nystagmus, perioral numbness and tingling, visual disturbances, and muscle twitching.

Table 3-1 Maximum dose of local anesthetic in a healthy 70 kg adult

Solution	Plain solution (mg)	Solution containing epinephrine (mg)
Tetracaine	100	200
Lidocaine	300	500
Mepivacaine	300	500
Prilocaine	600	600
Bupivacaine	175	225

From Raj PP, Winnie AP. Immediate reactions to local anesthetics. In Orkin FK, Cooperman LH, eds. Complications in Anesthesiology. Philadelphia: WB Saunders, 1983, p 59.

Treatment for presumed reaction to high levels of local anesthetic includes administration of intravenous benzodiazepine to increase the seizure threshold and supportive care with intravenous hydration until the local anesthetic agent has been metabolized.

Epinephrine is often added to local anesthetic agents to prolong their effect. Rapid absorption of epinephrine can result in sweating, tachycardia, palpitations, and apprehension. Although these symptoms may be unpleasant, they usually resolve without treatment and do not represent a toxic or allergic response.

Regional Anesthesia

Regional anesthesia has been improved to where it is the preferred form of anesthetic management for anorectal and some abdominal surgery by many surgeons. Regional anesthesia is ideal for outpatient surgery, because the duration of anesthesia can be controlled, with complete pain relief during the procedure and the return of function within a short period. One especially appealing feature of regional anesthesia for colorectal surgery is that patients can protect their own airways, even in the prone position.

Caudal anesthesia. Caudal anesthesia is commonly used for outpatient anorectal and gynecologic surgery. Good anesthesia is produced in an area limited to the perineum, but skeletal muscles remain unaffected. This type of anesthesia is therefore best suited for distal rectal and perianal procedures, in which exposure is not a problem.

The best review article on the incidence of complications is a retrospective review by Dawkins[9] of 350 articles on epidural and caudal anesthesia. The most common complications in this review include severe hypotension (6.3%), failure to find the sacral hiatus (3.1%), dural puncture (1.2%), and blood vessel puncture (0.6%); other rare complications included sepsis (0.2%) and transient paralysis (0.02%).

Epidural anesthesia. Epidural anesthesia is used in anorectal surgery that is anticipated to last beyond the duration of spinal anesthesia effect or are of uncertain duration, or when epidural anesthesia is part of the postoperative pain management plan.

The safety of awake epidural anesthesia for abdominal procedures in both general abdominal and colorectal surgery has been documented.[10,11] Reported benefits of epidural anesthesia in abdominal surgery include preservation of spontaneous respiration and airway reflexes, decreased blood loss, better postoperative pain control, reduced risk for thromboembolism, and more rapid recovery of GI motility.[12] That not all studies concur with the rapid recovery of bowel function may be a result of the frequent combination of general and epidural anesthesia or the addition of narcotics in the postoperative period.[13]

The use of epidural anesthesia for postoperative pain management is gaining widespread popularity. A recent well-controlled study of 100 patients undergoing abdominal surgery with general anesthesia showed a statistically significant improvement in postoperative pain relief when epidural anesthesia was included, compared with conventional postoperative pain management.[14]

Common complications of epidural anesthesia include blood vessel puncture (2.8%), dural puncture (2.5%), backache (2%), and severe hypotension (1.8%); rare complications include toxic reaction (0.2%) and transient paralysis (0.1%).[9] Epidural block in which anesthesia is achieved only on one side of the body has been observed in many patients, but no estimate of incidence is available.

Spinal anesthesia. Spinal anesthesia is often used for anorectal and perineal procedures of limited duration. When used for these indications, there is good relaxation of perianal muscles and therefore good exposure in the majority of cases.

Complications of spinal anesthesia are similar to those of caudal and epidural anesthesia. Spinal headache most often occurs after spinal anesthesia but may occur after epidural anesthesia as well. The cause is thought to be a rent in the dura, with loss of cerebrospinal fluid, which results in a decrease in intracranial pressure. The incidence of spinal headache is related to the size of the spinal needle. With a 22-gauge needle, the incidence of headache is 26%, but with a 26-gauge needle is only 0.4%.[15] Treatment includes positioning the patient flat in bed, hydration, and relief of headache pain with analgesia. In persistent or severe cases, an epidural blood patch has been shown to be 94% to 100% effective.[16]

General Anesthesia

Patients who are unable or unwilling to cooperate with local or regional anesthesia and are considered at good surgical risk may elect general anesthesia for anorectal surgery. General anesthesia is also considered to be the traditional choice for the majority of patients undergoing intra-abdominal colon surgery and virtually all laparoscopic surgery. Traditional contraindications to general anesthesia, such as poor pulmonary function and prohibitive cardiac disease, are well described in other textbooks and not listed here.

A wide range of complications has been attributed to general anesthesia. Common problems include sore throat (19.3%) and hoarseness (2.5%),[17] cardiac complications (hypotension, dysrhythmias, myocardial infarction), and awareness during surgery. Airway-related complications including laryngospasm, bronchospasm, and migration of the endotracheal tube with mainstem intubation and subsequent atelectasis are also common during general anesthesia. Pneumothorax, although not uncommon with traditional general anesthesia, is relatively more common when associated with laparoscopic surgery. Hepatic dysfunction (e.g., hepatitis) is an unusual problem associated with some general anesthetic agents.

Aspiration of gastric contents is a common complication in general and colorectal surgery. The risk for aspiration increases with obesity, bowel obstruction, pregnancy, a full stomach, abnormal gut motility, and factors that lower gastroesophageal junction tone. Common factors that lower tone in the gastroesophageal junction include alcohol, cigarette smoking, some drugs (e.g., theophylline, phentolamine, isoproterenol), and fatty meals. The incidence of "silent," or asymptomatic, aspiration is 6% to 8% but may range as high as 50% with use of the prone, lateral, and Trendelenburg positions.[18,19] Aspiration can be minimized with the use of cuffed endotracheal tubes, cricoid pressure, or awake intubation in patients at high risk and avoidance of head down positions.

Hypothermia is a significant problem because of the heat loss from exposure and loss of temperature autoregulation while under anesthesia. The smaller a person's body mass, the greater the problem of maintaining core temperatures within an acceptable range. Keeping the room warm, use of heating blankets and lamps, placing heat-retaining devices in the anesthesia circuits, and wrapping exposed body parts will all help to preserve core temperature in vulnerable patients.

The use of electrical equipment in the modern operating room is standard. However, complications can result if this equipment is not carefully used. Disconnection of leads from the ECG, displacement of the pulse oximeter, and other loss of monitoring equipment may result in incorrect readings, which could affect patient care. Movement or repositioning of the patient may increase risk for electrical injury and/or burns from defective or improperly grounded electrocautery machines if grounding pads are dislodged. Patient warming devices may burn the patient if not properly monitored. Care must be taken with all of these devices in the perioperative period.

POSITIONING COMPLICATIONS

Although the potential for complications exists, patient positioning is often delegated to residents and other operating room support personnel. After induction of anesthesia, the patient is unable to sense discomfort in the usual manner and protective reflexes are abolished. The entire surgical team must assume responsibility to protect the patient during positioning and throughout the

Table 3-2 Risk of complications based on position

	Supine	Prone	Lithotomy	Lateral decubitus	Trendelenburg
Aspiration	High	High	High	High	High
Alopecia	High	Low	High	Low	Variable
DVT/PE	Low	Low	High	Low	Variable
Soft tissue injury	Low	High	Low	Low	Variable
Compartment syndrome	Low	Low	High	High	Variable
Peroneal nerve injury	Low	Low	High	High	Variable
Ulnar nerve injury	High	High	Variable	Low	Variable
Cervical brachial plexus injury	Low	Low	High	Low	High

DVT, deep venous thrombosis; PE, pulmonary embolism.

course of a long operation. Potential complications based on position are listed in Table 3-2.

One category of possible complications during anesthesia is pressure injuries. Most people shift their weight, roll over, or move to a more comfortable position after they have been lying in one position for a long time. During anesthesia, patients are unable to sense discomfort and unable to move even if they wanted to. Constant pressure on various structures of the body results in ischemic damage and possible local tissue loss. Without proper padding, constant pressure on the skin may result in alopecia or pressure sores.

Damage to soft tissues can develop in a similar manner. Damage to the breasts, genitalia, or other soft tissues is most common in the prone position. Pressure on an unprotected ear can damage the skin and/or cartilage. Compartment syndrome can develop when positioning or restraint straps are too tight or there is pressure on a muscle group within a compartment because of insufficient padding.

The eye is especially vulnerable during anesthesia because the patient is unable to blink or provide protection against injury. Conjunctivitis, corneal abrasion, and ulcer are all possible from lack of tears or contact with foreign objects. The eyes should be adequately lubricated and then taped shut to avert injury. Prolonged pressure on the eye, even with the eye taped shut, could result in vascular thrombosis from increased intraocular pressure. Reports indicate the risk of blindness resulting from central retinal artery occlusion is highest in the prone and lateral decubitus positions.[20]

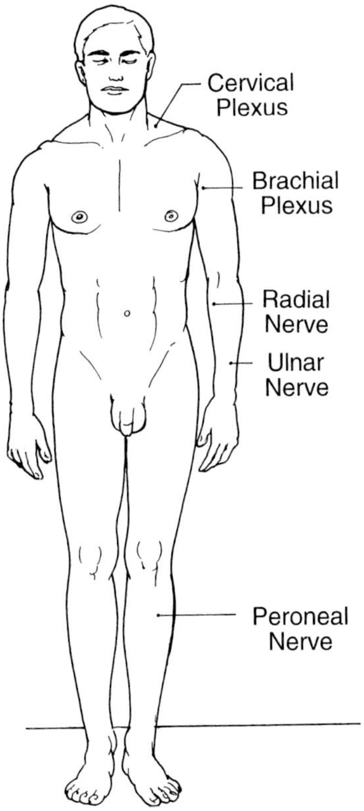

Fig. 3-1 Nerves at risk for injury during positioning for a surgical procedure.

There are two basic mechanisms for peripheral nerve injuries. Prolonged compression of a nerve against a hard surface, such as a peroneal nerve against a stirrup or retractor post in the lithotomy position, can result in nerve injury. Nerves can also be injured by stretching under anesthesia, as is seen in some brachial and cervical plexus injuries. Awareness of the patient's position and nerves that are at risk for potential injury both before and after the drapes are placed is crucial (Fig. 3-1).

The sciatic nerve arises from L4, L5, S1, S2, and S3 spinal nerves. It has a lateral (common peroneal) trunk and a medial (tibial nerve) trunk, which diverge in the popliteal fossa. All the hamstrings except the short head of the biceps femoris are supplied by the medial trunk (Fig. 3-2).

The nerve may be compressed in the gluteal region during anesthesia or operative positioning on a hard edge. Severe hip flexion may accentuate the risk for injury. A significant lesion produces weakness or paralysis of the hamstrings

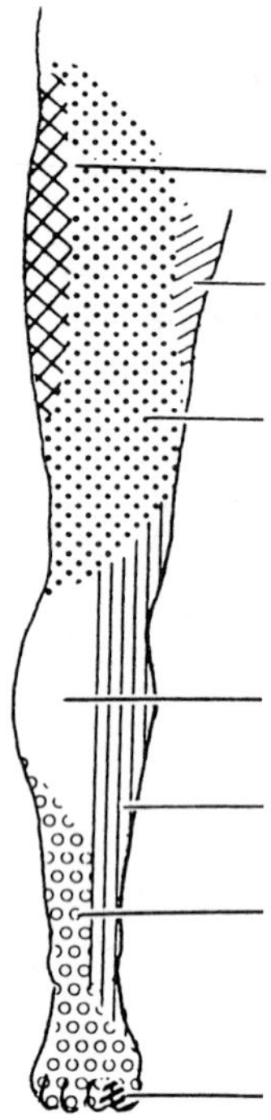

Fig. 3-2 Cutaneous innervation of the anterior aspect of the right leg. (From Dyke PJ, Thomas PK. Peripheral Neuropathy, vol 2, 3rd ed. Philadelphia: WB Saunders, 1993, pp 970–972. With permission.)

and all the muscles below the knee, with sensory loss in the distribution of the tibial and common peroneal nerves (Fig. 3-3). This involves the entire foot except the medial portion, which is supplied by the saphenous nerve (Fig. 3-4). The sensory loss extends to the lower two thirds of the posterolateral aspect of the calf.

After dividing in the lower thigh, the sciatic nerve passes through the popliteal fossa as the tibial nerve and enters the calf deep to the gastrocnemius muscle and divides into the plantar nerves in the foot. This supplies all the calf muscles, small muscles of the foot, and sensation to the sole. Therefore, injury limits plantar flexion, flexion of the toes, and sensation of the sole of the foot.

The sural nerve, which arises from the sciatic nerve and descends to the back of the calf, supplies sensation to the lateral ankle and joint. Compression leads to neuromas in its distribution. The common peroneal nerve arises as a lateral trunk of the sciatic nerve and splits into two branches after it winds around the head of the fibula. The superficial branch supplies the peroneal muscles and supplies sensation to the lateral two thirds of the calf and dorsum of the foot (see Fig. 3-3). The deep branch supplies the extensor muscles in the anterior com-

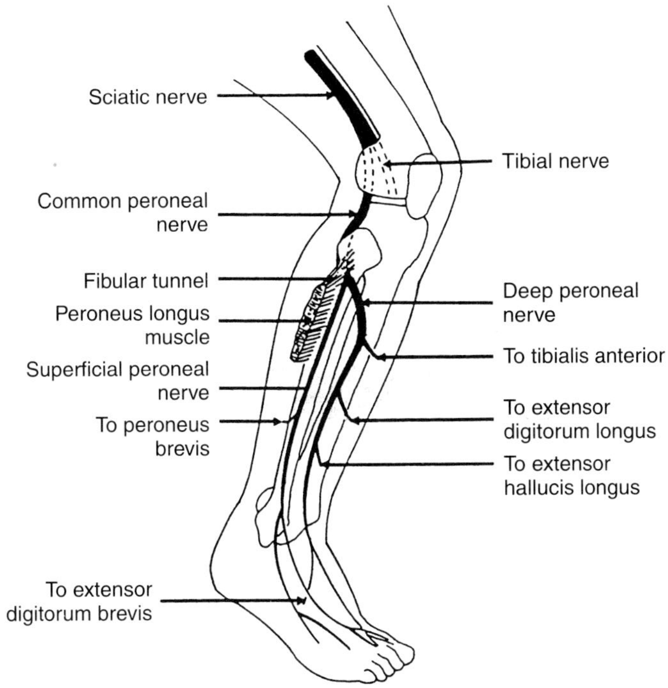

Fig. 3-3 Anterolateral view of the right leg shows the course and branches of the common peroneal nerve. (From Dyke PJ, Thomas PK. Peripheral Neuropathy, vol 2, 3rd ed. Philadelphia: WB Saunders, 1993, pp 970-972. With permission.)

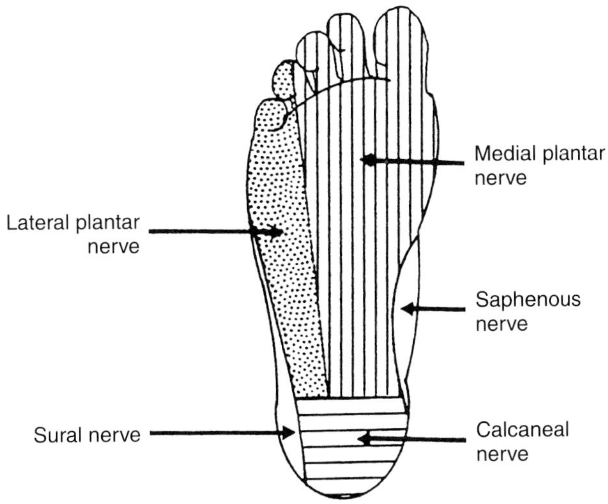

Fig. 3-4 Cutaneous innervation of the sole of the right foot. (From Dyke PJ, Thomas PK. Peripheral Neuropathy, vol 2, 3rd ed. Philadelphia: WB Saunders, 1993, pp 970-972. With permission.)

partment and sensation between the first and second toes. The nerve is subject to compression in stirrups around the head of the fibula.[21-24]

Anterior compartment syndrome with swelling within this confined space has been reported as a consequence of prolonged lithotomy position in stirrups.[25-27] Early recognition of painful muscle weakness, sensory loss, and pain out of proportion to the findings may indicate possible compartment syndrome. Tissue pressure studies and emergency fasciotomy may be required.

The femoral nerve (L2-4) arises within and emerges in the lateral psoas muscle and passes between the psoas and iliacus muscle in the "iliac compartment."[28] It courses deep to the inguinal ligament and supplies the quadriceps muscle and sensation to the anterior thigh. Continuing as a saphenous nerve, it supplies sensation to the medial aspect of the leg below the knee (Fig. 3-5). The nerve is at risk for injury from retractors or hip flexion with compression at the groin. The saphenous nerve may be compressed at the knee. Weakness of the quadriceps, diminished knee reflex, and loss of sensation in its distribution suggest injury to the femoral nerve.

The obturator nerve also rises from L2-4 and descends in the psoas muscle. It

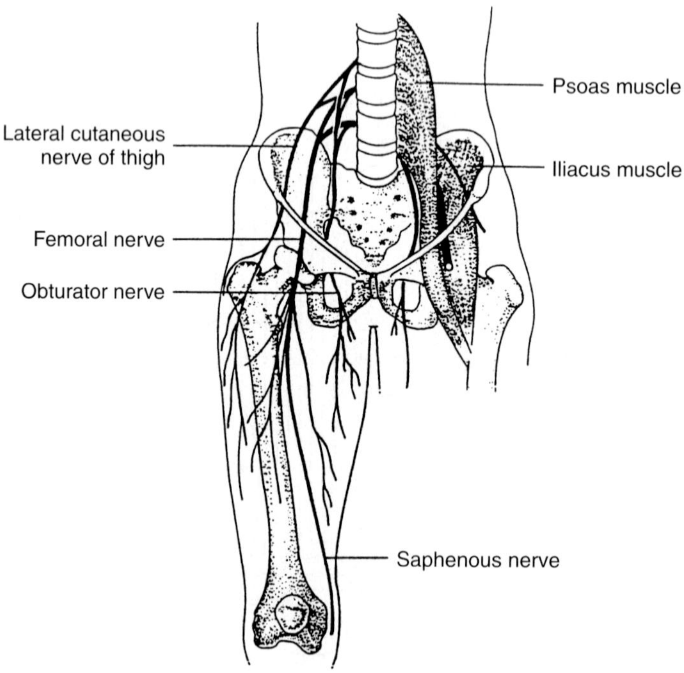

Fig. 3-5 Origins and courses of the lateral cutaneous nerve of the thigh, femoral nerve, and obturator nerve. (From Stewart JD. Focal Peripheral Neuropathies. New York: Elsevier Science, 1987. With permission.)

leaves it medially and crosses the anterior pelvis to the obturator foramen. It supplies the hip abductors and sensation to the medial thigh. It is at risk for injury with direct trauma, retractors, or stretching with hip adduction and external rotation.

The genitofemoral nerve (L1-2) travels on the psoas muscle distally and divides into the genital and femoral branches above the inguinal ligament. The femoral branch supplies sensation in the femoral triangle, and the genital branch is responsible for innervation of the cremaster muscle and sensation to the medial scrotum, labia, and upper inner thigh. Retractors and inguinal compression with positioning lead to this sensory loss.

The lateral cutaneous nerve to the thigh arises from L2-3 and courses from the psoas muscle to split in the lateral aspect of the inguinal ligament. It supplies sensation to the lateral aspect of the thigh, and injury to it may produce burning pain or numbness in that distribution, which generally regress spontaneously but on occasion may need to be injected locally or freed surgically.

Pelvic neuropathies may be minimized by placing the patient in relatively neutral positions, good padding, and avoidance of prolonged surgery. The same principles apply to minimization of DVT.

In the event of injury to a peripheral nerve, the ultimate return of function depends on the degree of nerve injury sustained.[29] Transient ischemic nerve block occurs after short duration of compression of a nerve. It is the mildest form of injury, and full recovery is usual because there is no permanent damage to the nerve fibers or endoneural sheath. *Neurapraxia* is a temporary paralysis or sensory loss. Although there is demyelination of peripheral fibers, the smaller and internal fibers are often spared. With the continuity of the nerve trunk and endoneural sheath preserved, remyelination should occur in 1 to 2 months. Although function may not return for weeks, there is good chance of a full recovery. When the degree of injury is greater, with full disruption of the axons within an intact sheath, the process is called *axonotmesis*. The prognosis for recovery with complete disruption is much worse than when the axons remain intact. Finally, when the entire nerve trunk is severed, the process is called *neurotmesis*. In this case, recovery is unlikely unless there is surgical intervention to suture together the ends of the nerves to assist in regeneration. Obviously, prevention of nerve injuries is preferable to treatment of an injury.

Supine Position

Supine is considered the conventional surgical position for most abdominal operations. Even the best padded operating table will produce problems in this position unless attention is paid to detail. Alopecia, pressure sores, and ulnar nerve injuries can be prevented with careful spot padding and monitoring during anesthesia. Aspiration remains a risk whenever general anesthesia is used.

Lithotomy Position

The lithotomy position is often used for low abdominal, pelvic, and perineal procedures. The use of stirrups creates a potential for peroneal nerve injury, DVT, and subsequent pulmonary embolism. The Trendelenburg position is often used in combination with the lithotomy position. As with the supine position, awareness of the risk for aspiration, improper padding causing alopecia, and pressure on the ulnar nerve must be considered.

Prone Position

The prone or prone-jackknife position is commonly used for anorectal surgery. Care must be taken with this position to avoid pressure on soft tissues (e.g., penis, scrotum, breast) during anesthesia. Patients in the prone position are especially vulnerable under general anesthesia for dislodgment or displacement of the endotracheal tube, resulting in airway compromise. Other risks associated with general anesthesia and patient position (e.g., aspiration, ulnar nerve injury) are increased in this position.

Lateral Decubitus Position

The lateral decubitus position is often used for thoracotomy or thoracoabdominal incisions. In the Sims position, the lower leg is flexed slightly at the knee and the upper leg is flexed both at the hip and at the knee. Use of this position for anything other than anorectal procedures is limited. In the modified Sims position, both legs are drawn up toward the chest and the vertebral column is flexed. This position is often used for administration of regional anesthesia because it widens the interlaminal spaces.[20]

Of the many complications common to anesthesia, several are even more common in the lateral decubitus position. Peroneal nerve injury is possible from pressure of the dependent leg against a poorly padded table. Brachial plexus injuries are caused by both pressure and stretch injuries. Patients are at increased risk for dependent lung aspiration, atelectasis, and other pulmonary complications. Inadequate padding of the face may result in ocular complications including corneal abrasions, ulcers, and blindness from retinal artery thrombosis.[20] Finally, occlusion of the vena cava by abdominal masses has been reported in the lateral decubitus position.[30]

Trendelenburg Position

In the formal description of the Trendelenburg position, the patient lies supine on the operating table with the head tilted lower than the heart and with the feet and lower abdomen higher than the heart. Common usage of the term now implies a head down posture in any position. Complications associated with the Trendelenburg position can therefore be included with those of any individual position if it is used.

The disadvantages of the Trendelenburg position have been well documented. In addition to the increased work of spontaneous ventilation,[31] myocardial oxygen requirements are increased.[32] Both of these factors dictate that the position be used with caution in patients at high risk. The Trendelenburg position produces increased intracranial pressure and therefore reflex hypotension[33] from distention of baroreceptors that stimulate reduction in systolic blood pressure. Reflux of gastric contents is more common in the head down positions.

The relative contraindications to use of the Trendelenburg position are linked to its disadvantages. They include increased intracranial pressure from head injury (due to CNS tumor or other causes), congestive heart failure, pulmonary compromise (as is seen in thoracic trauma or chronic obstructive pulmonary disease), and increased intra-abdominal pressure (as seen in pregnancy, ascites, and obesity).

The Trendelenburg position has limited indications in general surgery. The two chief indications are to distend vessels to assist in vascular access and to shift abdominal viscera out of the pelvis to improve visibility during lower abdominal and pelvic procedures. The Trendelenburg position is specifically not indicated in patients with hypovolemic shock,[33] although it has been used as an adjunct in the treatment of neurogenic shock. In addition to the normal increase in work of ventilation, patients with multiple trauma have frequently sustained injuries to the abdomen and chest, and routine use of the head-down position may interfere with respiratory exchange far more than when the patient is supine.[34] The risk-benefit ratio must be considered before use of the Trendelenburg position in patients at high risk.

CONCLUSION

Patients are vulnerable when they enter the operating room: they lose their protective sensations, reflexes, and ability to move out of uncomfortable positions. The entire operating team is responsible for the safety and protection of patients when they cannot protect themselves. Proper padding of patients and awareness of nerves that are at risk for injury are important to achieve a good outcome. Individualizing the type of anesthesia to the unique needs of the procedure and the state of health of the patient will help minimize risk. The majority of anesthetic and positioning complications can be avoided with careful preparation and diligent monitoring during anesthesia.

REFERENCES

1. Bailey HR, Ferguson JA. Prevention of urinary retention by fluid restriction following anorectal operations. Dis Colon Rectum 19:250-252, 1976.
2. Block GE, Mossa AR. Operative Colorectal Surgery. Philadelphia: WB Saunders, 1994, pp 93-94.
3. Sacla RM, Bennerr WA, Keating RF Jr, Spragye RG. Postoperative adrenal cortical insufficiency: Occurrence in patients previously treated with cortisone. JAMA 152:1509-1515, 1953.
4. Rozein MF. Anesthetic implications of concurrent diseases. In Miller RD, ed. Anesthesia, 2nd ed, vol 1. New York: Churchill Livingston, 1986, pp 255-357.
5. Beigland RM, Gann DS, DeMaria EJ. Pituitary and adrenal. In Schwartz SI, Shires GT, Spencer FC, eds. Principles of Surgery, 5th ed. New York: McGraw-Hill, 1989, pp 1545-1612.
6. Beck DE, Opelka FG. Perioperative steroid usage in colorectal patients: Results of a survey. Dis Colon Rectum (in press).
7. Phillips JD, Stelzner M, Zeng H, Kelley RE, Fonkalsrud EW. Alterations in gastrointestinal motility during postoperative acute corticosteroid withdrawal. Am J Surg 162:251-255, 1991.
8. Stelzner M, Phillips JD, Fonkalsrud EW. Acute ileus from steroid withdrawal simulating intestinal obstruction after surgery for ulcerative colitis. Arch Surg 125:914-917, 1990.
9. Dawkins CJM. Analysis of the complications of extradural and caudal block. Anesthesia 24:554, 1969.
10. Bredtmann RD, Herden HN, Teichmann W, et al. Epidural analgesia in colonic surgery: Results of a randomized prospective study. Br J Surg 77:638-642, 1990.
11. Koltun WA, McKenna KJ, Rung G. Awake epidural anesthesia is effective and safe in the high-risk colectomy patient. Dis Colon Rectum 37:1236-1241, 1994.
12. Koltun WA, McKenna KJ, Rung G. Awake epidural anesthesia is effective and safe in the high-risk colectomy patient. Dis Colon Rectum 37:1236-1241, 1994.
13. Wallin G, Cassuto J, Hogstrom S, Rimback G, Faxen A, Tollesson PO. Failure of epidural anesthesia to prevent postoperative paralytic ileus. Anesthesiology 65:292-297, 1986.
14. Hjortso NC, Neumann P, Frosig F, et al. A controlled study on the effect of epidural anesthesia with local anesthetic and morphine on morbidity after abdominal surgery. Acta Anaesthesiol Scand 29:790-796, 1985.
15. Greene BA. A 26 gauge lumbar puncture needle: Its value in the prophylaxis of headache following spinal analgesia for vaginal delivery. Anesthesiology 11:464-469, 1950.
16. Bart AJ, Wheeler AS. Comparison of epidural saline placement and epidural blood placement in the treatment of post-lumbar-puncture headache. Anesthesiology 48:221-223, 1978.
17. Wolfson B. Minor laryngeal sequelae of endotracheal intubation. Br J Anaesth 30:326, 1958.
18. Berson W, Adriani J. "Silent" regurgitation and aspiration during anesthesia. Anesthesiology 15:644, 1954.
19. Turndorf H, Rodis ID, Clark TS. "Silent" regurgitation during general anesthesia. Anesth Analg 53:700, 1974.
20. Lawson NW. The lateral decubitus position: Anesthetic considerations. In Martin JT, ed. Positioning in Anesthesia and Surgery, 2nd ed. Philadelphia: WB Saunders, 1987, pp 155-179.
21. Dyke PJ, Thomas PK. Peripheral Neuropathy, vol 2, 3rd ed. Philadelphia: WB Saunders, 1993, pp 970-972.
22. Schaumberg HH, Spencer PS, Thomas PK. Disorders of peripheral nerves. Philadelphia: FA Davis, 1983.

23. Berry J, Richardson PM. Common peroneal nerve palsy: A clinical and electrophysiological review. J Neurol Neurosurg Psychiatry 39:1162-1171, 1976.
24. Nivatvongs S. Complications of anorectal and colorectal operations. In Gordon PH, Nivatvongs S, eds. Principles and Practice of Surgery for the Colon, Rectum, and Anus. St. Louis: Quality Medical Publishing, 1992, pp 1003-1021.
25. Lyndon JC, Spielman FJ. Bilateral compartment syndrome following prolonged surgery in the lithotomy position. Anesthesiology 60:236-238, 1984.
26. Masten FA III. Compartment Syndromes. New York: Grune & Stratton, 1980, pp 1-162.
27. Masten FA, Winquist RA, Krugmire RB. Diagnosis and management of compartmental syndromes. J Bone Joint Surg [Am] 62:286-291, 1980.
28. Aichroth P, Rowe-Jones DC. Iliacus compartment compression syndrome. Br J Surg 58: 833-834, 1971.
29. McAlpine FS, Seckel BR. Complications of positioning: The peripheral nervous system. In Martin JT, ed. Positioning in Anesthesia and Surgery, 2nd ed. Philadelphia: WB Saunders, 1987, pp 155-179.
30. Matlatinsky J, Kadlic T. Inferior vena cava occlusion in the left lateral position. Br J Anesth 46;165-167, 1974.
31. Chiang ST, Lyons HA. The effect of postural change on pulmonary compliance. Respir Physiol 1:99-105, 1966.
32. Kubal K, Komatsu T, Sanchala V, et al. Trendelenburg position used during venous cannulation increases myocardial oxygen demand. Anesth Analg 63:239, 1984.
33. Sibbald WJ, Patterson NAM, Holliday RL, et al. The Trendelenburg position: Hemodynamic effects in hypotensive and normotensive patients. Crit Care Med 7:218-224, 1979.
34. Fantini GA, Shires GT III, Shires GT. Management of shock. In Moore EE, Mattox KL, Feliciano DV, eds. Trauma, 2nd ed. Norwalk, Conn.: Appleton & Lange, 1991, p 153.
35. Raj PP, Winnie AP. Immediate reactions to local anesthetics. In Orkin FK, Cooperman LH, eds. Complications in Anesthesiology. Philadelphia: WB Saunders, 1983, pp 51-75.

CHAPTER 4

Sepsis

FRANCIS J. HARFORD

WOUND INFECTIONS

Wound infection depends on three factors: the size and virulence of the bacterial inoculum, local wound environment, and the integrity of the host organism defenses (Fig. 4-1). In 1964 the National Research Council (NRC) devised a wound categorization, based on the extent of the potential contamination of the wound by bacteria,[1] which has been adopted by the American College of Surgeons (Table 4-1).[2]

Haley et al.,[3] in their subsequent Study of the Efficacy of Nosocomial Infection Control (SENIC), identified four independent and additive risk factors for wound infection: operations on the abdomen, operations lasting longer than 2 hours, three or more associated medical diagnoses, and an NRC wound classification of dirty or contaminated.[3] The effect of this stratification of the NRC categories of wounds can be seen in Table 4-2. In a larger, prospective study, Cruse and Foord[4] found that clean wounds had an infection rate of ≤1% and class IV

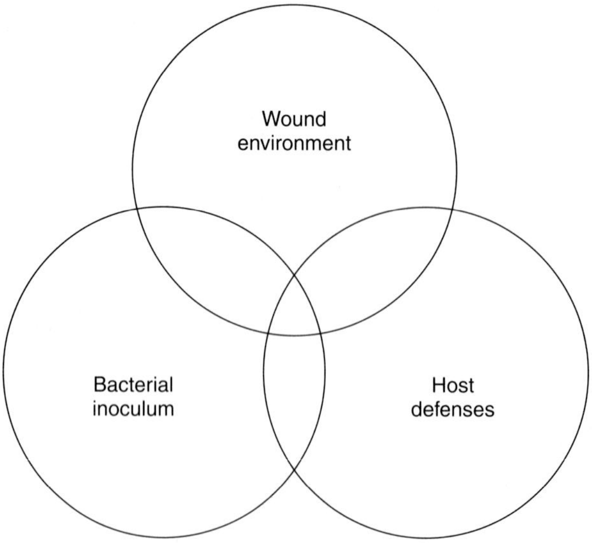

Fig. 4-1 Factors related to wound infections.

wounds had an infection rate as high as 50%. Wounds at high risk of becoming infected should be left open and packed. If quantitative wound bacterial cultures are less than 10^5 colonies per gram of tissue, closure of these open wounds (delayed primary closure) will usually be successful.[5] Although quantitative wound culture is not commonly practiced, most surgeons find that secondary closure is successful if the wound appears lined with healthy granulation tissue without a great deal of exudate. If this is not the case, the wound should be left open to heal by secondary intention. The ideal time for delayed primary closure is on days 4 to 6.[6]

If a wound that has been closed shows signs of erythema, increased tenderness, or drainage, several skin sutures or staples should be removed and any purulent material drained. The entire length of the abscess cavity should be unroofed. The wound may then be packed with saline solution–soaked gauze in a wet-to-dry fashion. If a great deal of drainage accumulates in the wound, dry dressings may

Table 4-1 National Research Council wound classification

Clean	Elective, no accute inflammation or entry into GI, biliary, or respiratory tract
Clean-contaminated	Operation during which the GI, biliary, or respiratory tract is entered in a controlled fashion with minimal contamination
Contaminated	Operation during which there is entry into nonpurulent inflammation, a major break in technique, major spill from a hollow viscus, penetrating trauma less than 4 hours old, or wounds near contaminated skin
Infected	Operations during which purulent infection is encountered

Modified from Coit DG, Sclafani L. Care of the surgical wound, vol 2. In American College of Surgeons. Care of the Surgical Patient. New York: Scientific American, 1990, pp 1-10.

Table 4-2 Rates of wound infection (%) based on National Research Council Wound Classification and SENIC risk factors

SENIC risk factors	Clean	Clean-contaminated	Contaminated	Dirty
0	1.1	0.6	—	—
1	3.9	2.8	4.5	6.7
2	8.4	8.4	8.3	10.9
3	15.8	17.7	11.0	18.8
4	—	—	23.9	27.4

Modified from Haley RW, Culver DH, Morgan WM, et al. Identifying patients at high risk of surgical wound infection. Am J Epidemiol 121:206-215, 1985.

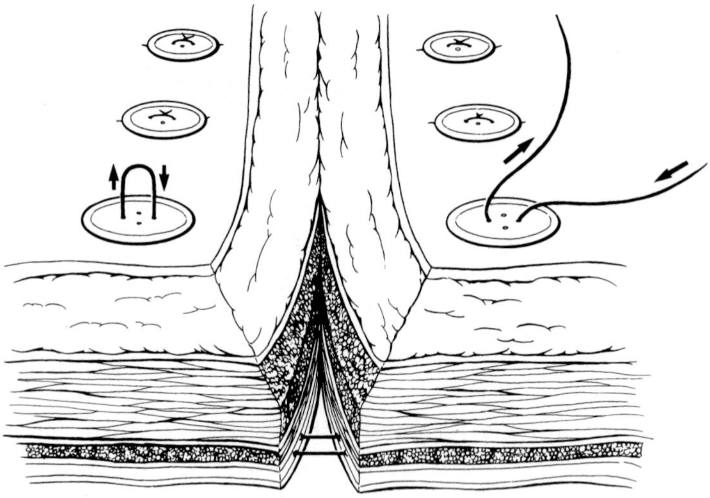

Fig. 4-2 Closure of fascial dehiscence.

be substituted. Antiseptic solutions such as povidone-iodine or Dakin's solution (sodium hypochloride) are commonly used, although much controversy surrounds their use in such wounds.[7-10] Toxicity to fibroblast cultures in animal wounds in vivo has been demonstrated, but it is difficult to translate some of the study results to the human wound. Studies in some wound models have shown that sodium hypochloride in very dilute concentration (0.025% to 0.005%) retains its bacterial activity without interfering with wound healing,[11,12] whereas others show it to be cytotoxic even at these very dilute concentrations.[13] If there is fascial dehiscence of an infected wound, the patient should be taken back to the operating room and the wound should be debrided and closed with retention sutures. I prefer to use the technique described by Maull[14] in which no suture is placed over the top of the wound and it is thus accessible for local care (Fig. 4-2).

If there is diffuse erythema around the wound, one should suspect a streptococcal infection, and the patient should be given parenteral antimicrobial drugs that are effective against streptococci. Sometimes the organism may be recovered from the cellulitic skin by injection and aspiration of sterile saline solution with a needle and syringe. The most important postoperative wound infections are the necrotizing soft tissue infections. These are uncommon in the postoperative period but are disastrous if not recognized early and treated immediately. Lewis[15] has provided a simple and useful classification of these infections based on the primary anatomic location and the main pathologic lesion (see box). In the postoperative setting, a complaint of an unusual amount of incisional pain should arouse suspicion. Erythema and edema of the skin or crepitus may be

CLASSIFICATION OF NECROTIZING SOFT TISSUE INFECTIONS

Spreading focal infections	
Postoperative bacterial synergistic gangrene	Skin and subcutaneous tissue
Idiopathic (Fournier's) scrotal gangrene	Subcutaneous tissue
Diffuse infections	
Monomicrobial necrotizing cellulitis	Skin and subcutaneous tissue
Necrotizing fasciitis	Subcutaneous tissue and superficial fascia
Gram negative synergistic necrotizing cellulitis	Subcutaneous tissue, fascia, and muscle
Clostridial myonecrosis	Muscle

From Lewis RT. Necrotizing soft-tissue infections. Infect Dis Clin North Am 6:693-702, 1992. With permission.

observed. Patients will often have fever, and if the diagnosis is delayed, hypotension may develop. Once the problem is recognized, the patient should be taken back to the operating room for prompt debridement. The general principle is to remove all necrotic tissue while viable skin is preserved if possible. The deep fascia should be opened to inspect the muscle. Tissue should be removed and submitted for histologic analysis, gram staining, and culture. Necrotic fascia is dull gray. Gas produced by the infecting organisms may diffuse beyond the gangrenous fascia, and an incision in the skin should be made over these areas to inspect the fascia (Fig. 4-3). Initial antibiotic therapy should be with a broad-spectrum drug such as penicillin, aminoglycoside, or clindamycin. Therapy can be adjusted when the results of cultures and sensitivity determination are returned. If the infection proves to be a monomicrobial cellulitis or clostridial myonecrosis, it may be treated with penicillin. It is important to check the culture: if only one organism grows but multiple organisms are seen at gram staining, broad-spectrum antibiotics should be continued. Hyperbaric oxygen therapy is effective in clostridial myonecrosis, but its value in other necrotizing infections is unproved.[16]

The most effective strategy for preventing postoperative wound morbidity is to attempt to manipulate the factors we know are operant in the establishment of wound infection (see Fig. 4-1). The host defenses should be optimized by attending to any medical problems the patient may have and providing nutri-

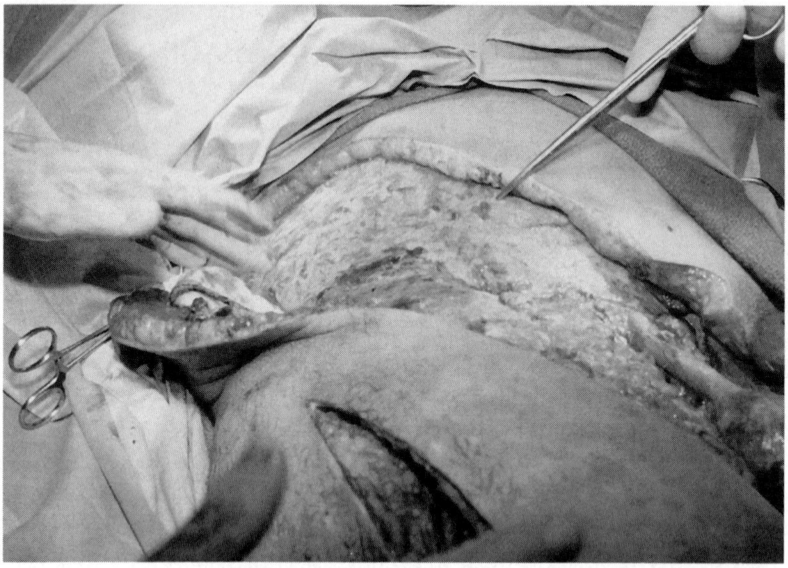

Fig. 4-3 Debridement of the abdominal wall. A lower incision has been made to assess the viability of the distal fascia.

tional replenishment when appropriate. The wound environment should be optimized by careful handling of tissues. Necrotic tissue should be removed from the wound by judicious use of cautery and wound irrigation to remove any devitalized tissue. Antibiotics will make the wound a hostile environment for contaminating bacteria. Efforts should also be made to reduce contamination to the wound during the surgical procedure with mechanical preparation of the bowel and intraluminal antibiotic prophylaxis.

MECHANICAL BOWEL PREPARATION

The inoculum of bacteria in the wound in elective cases can be reduced with bowel preparation. Although the efficacy of mechanical bowel preparation to prevent wound infection has never been prospectively studied in humans, it is rational to expect that decreasing the fecal mass will decrease the potential wound inoculum, to say nothing of improving the aesthetics of the surgery. It should be pointed out, however, that although the total number of bacteria is reduced with mechanical preparation, the concentration of organisms in the residual feces is not affected. Although mechanical preparation with cathartics and enemas is effective, most patients are more comfortable with either a polyethylene glycol lavage solution or Fleet Phospha-Soda oral preparation.[17,18] Additional information about bowel preparation is presented in Chapter 2.

WOUND BARRIERS

Plastic wound drapes have been used to prevent contamination of the wound with endogenous enteric organisms. Adhesive plastic drapes, some impregnated with povidone-iodine, have been used to protect against contamination with skin organisms. Plastic ring drapes have been used to protect the wound edges from abdominal contents as well as desiccation of the tissue. Inasmuch as the majority of wound infections in GI surgery are caused by enteric organisms, plastic ring drapes have been evaluated for use in such procedures. Harrower[19] examined 224 patients undergoing gastrointestinal or biliary operations and used the ring drape in alternating patients. The wound infection rate was 2.4% in patients on whom the drape was used and 15% in the control group. Subsequent studies of similar groups of patients, however, have failed to demonstrate any difference in clinical wound infection.[20-23] In a study of 140 patients undergoing only elective colorectal surgery, the incidence of wound infection in patients with the wound drape was 10% and in those without the drape was 9%.[22] Cultures of the wounds obtained in 85% of the cases showed no evidence that the drape protected the wound from contamination.

ANTIBIOTIC PROPHYLAXIS

It is well established that wound infection is decreased with the use of antibiotics in addition to mechanical preparation, but there is still controversy as to whether oral or parenteral antibiotics, or a combination of the two, are superior. There is agreement that the antibiotics used should be active against the normal flora of the colon and thus must be effective against both aerobic and anaerobic organisms. Nichols et al.[24] introduced the use of oral neomycin and erythromycin base in 1972, and a Veteran's Administration cooperative study[25] published in 1977 demonstrated a significant difference in wound infection with neomycin and erythromycin (9%) compared with mechanical bowel preparation alone (43%). Neomycin plus erythromycin remains the most widely used combination of orally administered agents among North American colon and rectal surgeons.[26] Those who advocate the use of parenteral antibiotics point out that with good mechanical preparation the potential inoculum is low and adequate tissue levels of a parenterally administered antimicrobial agent should be sufficient protection. Indeed, results of several large studies demonstrate that the wound infection rate can be kept within acceptable limits with the use of mechanical preparation along with parenteral antibiotics with activity against both aerobic and anaerobic organisms (Table 4-3).

An increasing number of surgeons are using both oral and parenteral antibiotics,[26] affecting both the concentration of organisms in the stool and the environment of the wound. However, relatively few studies compare use of oral

Table 4-3 Studies of parenteral antibiotics and mechanical cleansing

Author (year)	No. of patients	Antibiotic	Wound infection rate (%)
Periti et al.[27] (1989)	403	Cefoxitin	11.0
		Cefotetan	9.0
Rowe-Jones et al.[28] (1990)	943	Cefotaxime/metronidazole (one dose)	7.1
		Cefotaxime/metronidazole (three doses)	7.3
Andaker et al.[29] (1992)	517	Fosfomycin/metronidazole	2.7
		Doxycycline/metronidazole	6.2
Arnaud et al.[30] (1992)	208	Amoxycillin–clavulanic acid	1.9
		Cefotetan	4.8
Kwok et al.[31] (1993)	164	Amoxycillin–clavulanic acid	7.9
		Cefotaxime/metronidazole	7.9
Hakansson et al.[32] (1993)	567	Cefotaxime	16.0
		Cefotaxime/metronidazole	7.0
Matikainen and Hiltunen[33] (1993)	628	Ceftriaxone/tinidatsole	3.0
		Aminoglycoside/tinidatsole	12.0
AhChong et al.[34] (1994)	128	Ampicillin-sulbactam	9.5
		Gentamicin/metronidazole	10.7

Table 4-4 Studies of oral antibiotics versus oral antibiotics and parenteral antibiotics

Author (year)	No. of patients	Antibiotic	Wound infection rate (%)
Condon et al.[35] (1993)	1082	Neomycin/erythromycin	8.0
		Neomycin/erythromycin + cephalothin	6.0
		Neomycin/erythromycin + cefoxitin	5.0
Coppa et al.[36] (1983)	241	Neomycin/erythromycin	18.0*
		Neomycin/erythromycin + cefoxitin	7.0
Portnoy et al.[37] (1983)	104	Neomycin/erythromycin	27.0*
		Neomycin/erythromycin + cefazolin	4.7
		Neomycin/erythromycin + ticarcillian	2.3
Schoetz et al.[38] (1990)	197	Neomycin/erythromycin	14.6*
		Neomycin/erythromycin + cefoxitin	5.0

*Statistically significant.

antibiotics alone with the combination of oral and parenteral antibiotics (Table 4-4). Most of these studies show a significant reduction in wound infection with the addition of a parenteral agent. The lack of significant difference in wound infection rates in the large study of Condon et al.[35] comparing oral antibiotics alone versus oral and parenteral antibiotic therapy may be the result of the low rate of wound infection with oral antibiotics or the use of a first-generation cephalosporin with a short half-life as the parenteral agent.

INTRA-ABDOMINAL INFECTION

Postoperative intra-abdominal infection should be suspected if the patient exhibits fever or leukocytosis not otherwise explained or has an undue degree of postoperative pain. Physical evaluation is always hampered by the presence of the fresh abdominal incision, which impedes the evaluation of abdominal tenderness or appreciation of an intra-abdominal mass. Fry et al.[39] reported a series of 143 patients with proven intra-abdominal abscess. Localized tenderness was useful in identifying the abscess in only one third of the patients; a palpable mass was felt in only 10%, most on rectal examination. Plain abdominal films were thought to be helpful in only 15% of those patients. Abdominal contrast material–enhanced radiographs can demonstrate compression or displacement of the intestine and help differentiate between intraluminal and extraluminal gas collections, but this is accomplished with much more definition with computed tomography (CT). Contrast-enhanced studies have a definite place in demonstrating suture line dehiscences, but these findings are also usually well demonstrated with CT with enteric contrast material. Ultrasonography is useful in enabling detection of abscesses within or adjacent to specific organs but is less useful as a technique to survey the entire abdomen and pelvis for abnormal fluid or gas collections. There are also technical problems with ultrasonography in the postoperative patient with an open wound, dressings, or drainage tubes. In addition, the intraluminal gas present if the patient has a postoperative ileus also interferes with accurate interpretation in this examination. Imaging with gallium-67– or indium-111–labeled leukocytes enables detection of intra-abdominal abscess, but both isotopes have very limited usefulness in postoperative examination because of lag time between injection of the isotope and acquisition of the scan and false positive results caused by radioisotope localization to the area of surgical dissection. Abdominal and pelvic CT is the procedure of choice in the postoperative evaluation of suspected intra-abdominal or pelvic abscess. Several authors[40-42] have reported sensitivity of CT in excess of 90% for localization of intra-abdominal abscesses. Norwood and Civetta,[43] however, found a sensitivity of 48% and specificity of 64% in their series of 53 critically ill postoperative patients in the surgical intensive care unit. They noted that no true positive scan was obtained before the eighth postoperative day. The high prevalence of false positive studies in the early postoperative period confirms the advisability of diagnostic aspiration of these putative abscesses to determine whether they are merely loculated fluid or true abscess cavities.

Since the first report by Gerzof et al.[44] in 1979 of percutaneous catheter drainage of abdominal abscess with CT or ultrasound guidance, percutaneous drainage has become a mainstay in the treatment of postoperative abscesses. Percutaneous drainage may be accomplished by penetration of the abscess cavity with either ultrasound or CT guidance. The advantage of CT is that the viscera and blood vessels surrounding the mass are visualized. If the mass is contiguous with the abdominal wall, ultrasound is adequate. If CT guidance is used to direct the needle into the cavity, it is sometimes advantageous to complete the procedure under fluoroscopy. Often after diagnostic aspiration of the contents of the cavity, 5 to 10 ml of contrast solution is injected and fluoroscopy is used to define the size and configuration of the cavity and detect any communications with the bowel. At the time of placement of the drainage catheter, contrast medium is injected to ensure that the side holes in the catheter are in the abscess cavity. The cavity is then gently irrigated with saline solution and the catheter is affixed to the skin. If the catheter is in a dependent position, drainage can be left to gravity. If this is not possible, suction may be necessary. If suction is necessary, a sump-type drainage catheter should be used. If drainage is left to gravity, the catheter should be irrigated with saline solution at least once daily to ensure that it remains patent. Clinical signs of sepsis should resolve in 24 to 48 hours of drainage. If they do not, the patient should be scanned again to look for additional abscesses not appreciated on the first study. The original cavity should appear smaller on the repeat study (Fig. 4-4). If it is not, the drain should be manipulated or changed or additional drains placed to ensure adequate drainage. If these maneuvers are not successful and the cavity remains

A

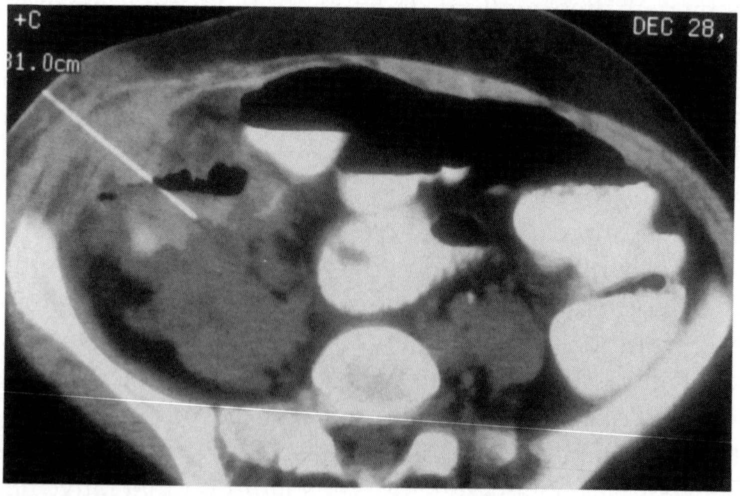

Fig. 4-4 **A,** Needle aspiration of an abdominal abscess.

B

C

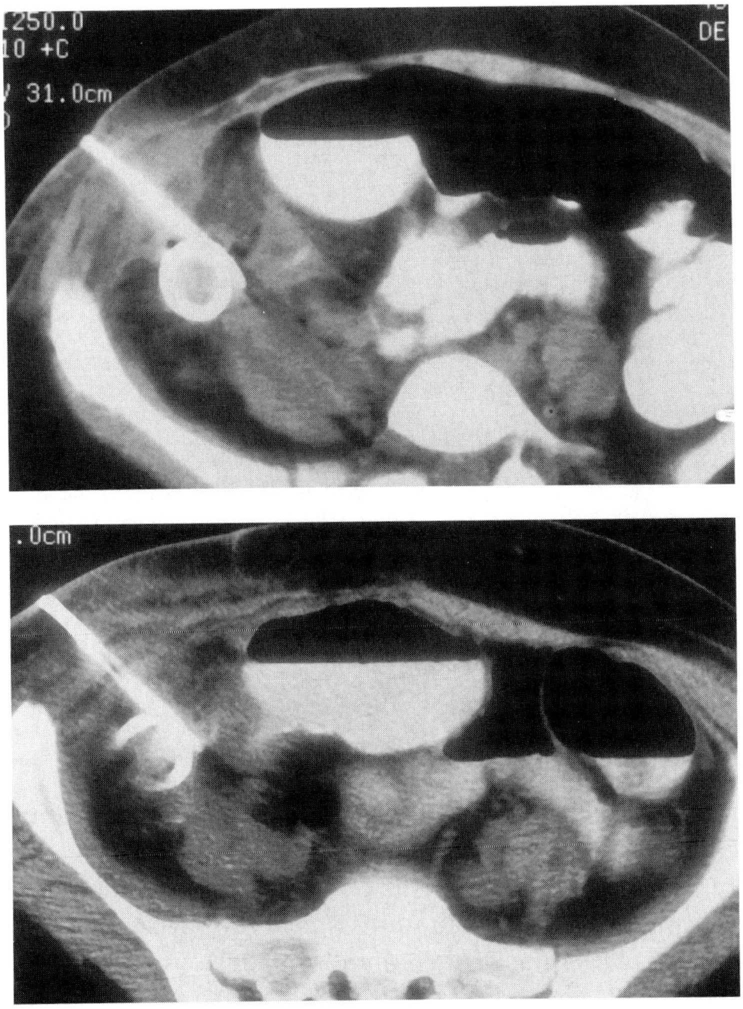

Fig. 4-4, cont'd **B,** Pigtail catheter in place. **C,** Three days later, abscess has decreased in size.

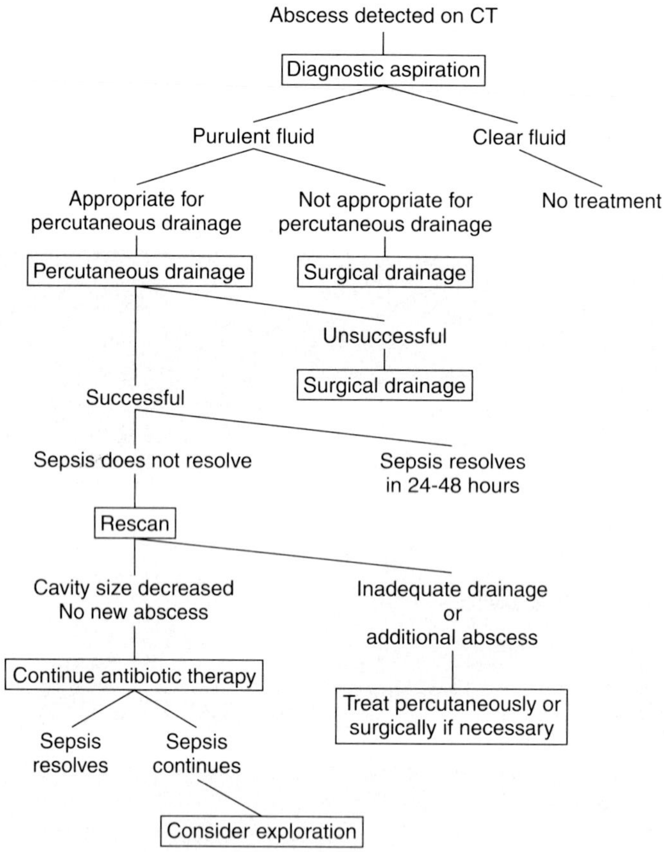

Fig. 4-5 Algorithm for management of abdominal or pelvic abscesses by percutaneous drainage or surgical drainage.

septic, surgical drainage should be instituted. A management schema is outlined in Fig. 4-5.

The only firm contraindication to percutaneous drainage is lack of clear access for the catheter. In some situations, however, success with percutaneous drainage is less likely. Some of the conditions that militate against successful drainage include the following:

No clear access
Interloop abscess
Fungal abscess
Infected hematoma
Necrotic or infected tumor

At times, percutaneous drainage may act as a palliative rather than curative procedure, as in drainage of symptomatic necrotic tumor. Results of several studies of percutaneous and surgical drainage of abdominal or pelvic abscesses

Table 4-5 Drainage of abdominal and pelvic abscesses

Author	Year	No. of abscesses	Success rate (%)
Percutaneous drainage			
Malangoni et al.[45]	1990	18*	61
Lent et al.[46]	1990	54*	57
Hemming et al.[47]	1991	42*	93
Levison and Zeigler[48]	1991	45†	47
Brolin et al.[49]	1991	86*	76
Longo et al.[50]	1993	13†	85
Schechter et al.[51]	1994	44†	87
Surgical drainage			
Malangoni et al.[45]	1990	30*	53
Hemming et al.[47]	1990	41*	88
Levison and Zeigler[48]	1991	46*	54
Longo et al.[50]	1993	32†	84

* Primary and postoperative abscesses.
† Postoperative abscesses.

are presented in Table 4-5. No prospective randomized study has compared percutaneous and surgical drainage. In those studies that report both methods, there were historic controls in the surgical drainage group or the method of drainage was chosen on an individual basis according to the preference of the surgeon. In most studies, the patients were not classified as to the severity of their illness or the appropriateness of one method or the other. In the report by Malangoni et al.,[45] although the success rate for percutaneous and surgical drainage was 61% and 53%, respectively, successful abscess resolution was accomplished in 79% of patients with surgical drainage when percutaneous drainage was unsuccessful. They classified abscesses as simple when there was a single unilocular cavity and complex when a multilocular cavity or multiple abscesses were present, an enteric fistula that communicated with the abscess was demonstrated, or there was neoplasm or tissue necrosis. They found that the rate of successful drainage was comparable between treatments for simple abscesses but that complex abscesses were treated successfully more often by surgical drainage. These techniques are not competitive, but complementary. Fry et al.,[39] in their study of intra-abdominal abscesses, concluded that delay in diagnosis, ineffective drainage, and failure of the host defense mechanisms were the determinates of poor outcome. Pichter and Musher[52] also found that delay in definitive treatment was the main determinant of morbidity and mortality in these patients.

Ercoli et al.[53] reported on 15 of 99 patients undergoing percutaneous drainage of abscesses associated with an enteric fistula. Fourteen were postoperative fistulas. The fistula was recognized at the initial percutaneous drainage in only six patients; the other fistulas were detected with GI or retrograde contrast medium injected through a drainage catheter. In two of the 15 patients, the abscess resolved after one percutaneous drainage; in three, the abscess never resolved; and in 10, the first abscess resolved but recurrent abscesses developed. In eight of these 10 patients, a second percutaneous drainage procedure was successful, and the other two eventually underwent small bowel resection. Abscesses with enteric fistulas in the postoperative period are almost always associated with anastomotic dehiscences. (This subject is discussed in more detail in Chapter 6.)

Antimicrobial treatment of intra-abdominal abscess usually begins before the abscess is drained and the contents cultured. The choice of antimicrobial agents is therefore made on an empiric basis. The Surgical Infection Society in a policy statement has made recommendations for antimicrobial treatment based on the bacteria usually cultured from intra-abdominal infections[54] (Table 4-6). These organisms include facultative gram negative bacilli, aerobic gram negative bacilli, obligate and aerobic organisms, and enterococci or other fecal streptococci found in the bowel flora. The benchmark agents for the treatment of postoperative intra-abdominal abscesses are combinations of an antianaerobe plus an aminoglycoside or aztreonam, or a third-generation cephalosporin, or clindamycin and aztreonam in patients at high risk for renal toxicity. The Surgical Infection Society has endorsed several single agents for treatment of community-acquired

Table 4-6 Microorganisms cultured from abdominal infection sites

Facultative gram negative bacilli	Obligate anaerobes	Facultative gram positive cocci	Aerobic gram negative bacilli
E. coli	*B. fragilis*	Enterococci	*Pseudomonas aeruginosa*
Klebsiella species	*Bacteroides* species	*Staphylococcus* species	
Proteus species	*Fusobacterium* species	*Streptococcus* species	
Enterobacter species	*Clostridium* species		
Morganella morganii	*Peptococcus* species		
Other enteric gram negative species	*Peptostreptococcus* species		
	Lactobacillus species		

From Bohnen JMA, Solomkin JS, Dellinger EP, et al. Guidelines for clinical care: Anti-infective agents for intra-abdominal infection. Arch Surg 127:83-89, 1992. With permission.

infections of mild to moderate severity. These include cefoxitin, cefotetan, cefmetazole, and ticarcillin–clavulanic acid. They recommend imipenem-cilastatin for severe infections.[54] Disadvantages of the combination regimens include the increased costs in equipment and nursing time necessary for administration. The risk for side effects likewise increases when two drugs are used rather than one. In the case of the aminoglycoside, the cost is increased because serum levels must be monitored so that adequate but not toxic doses may be given. Indeed, in some series, failure of combination therapy with aminoglycoside is directly related to failure to obtain adequate therapeutic levels. For all of these reasons, there has been a great deal of interest in the use of single agents. The single agents studied have been cephalosporins with good antianaerobic activity or a combination of a β-lactam antibiotic and a β-lactamase inhibitor such as ampicillin-sulbactam, imipenem-cilastatin, or piperacillin-tazobactam. DiPiro and Cue[55] point out that relatively few good trials have compared single agent with combination regimens for treatment of established intra-abdominal infection, and most excluded patients at high risk for mortality. Most of the authors conclude that they are unable to demonstrate any difference in efficacy of single versus combination therapy. However, the numbers in these trials were relatively small, and subsequently the possibility of a type II statistical error is high. Hackford et al.,[56] in a prospective study, compared 32 patients given imipenem-cilastatin with 25 patients given clindamycin-gentamicin. The failure rate was 17.5 in the imipenem-cilastatin group and 20% in the clindamycin-gentamicin group. There were 13 adverse reactions in the first group, and 10 in the second. They concluded that single-agent therapy was as efficacious as combination therapy. In a larger, multi-institutional study. Malangoni et al.[57] studied 112 patients, most of whom were at high risk for abdominal infections, and compared treatment with cefoxitin plus placebo vs. clindamycin and tobramycin. There were 21 clinical failures. Ten patients receiving cefoxitin-placebo (17%) and 11 patients receiving clindamycin-tobramycin (21%) had recurrence of infection or died. These authors suggested that both treatments were appropriate for antimicrobial therapy of intra-abdominal infections. They also noted that clinical failure is more common in patients at high risk and when antibiotic-resistant organisms were isolated from the initial cultures. Eckhauser et al.,[58] in another multicenter randomized study, compared 117 patients with serious intra-abdominal infections who were prospectively randomized to receive either imipenem-cilastatin or clindamycin and an aminoglycoside. Clinical failure rates were 3.8% and 7.8%, respectively (not statistically significant). Solomkin et al.,[59] in a multicenter trial, reported on 162 patients with established intra-abdominal infections who were randomized to receive either imipenem-cilastatin or clindamycin-tobramycin. Treatment failure occurred in 17.3% and 29.6%, respectively. The difference in outcome resulted primarily from a high failure rate in patients with gram negative bacterial infections who were given clindamycin-tobramycin. It was noted that it took approximately 4 days to achieve therapeutic levels of tobramycin. Polk et al.,[60] in another multicenter trial, studied 331 patients to compare piperacillin-tazobactam with clindamycin-gentamicin. They concluded that piperacillin-tazobactam was as efficacious as the combination therapy. Walker et al.,[61] in a double-blind trial, compared two single agents, ampicillin-sulbactam and cefoxitin, in 197 patients with suspected bacterial intra-abdominal infections. The infections were successfully treated in 86% of the patients receiving ampicillin-sulbactam and 78% of the patients receiving cefoxitin (not significant). There was no difference in the frequency of side effects.

Dougherty et al.[62] studied 341 pediatric and adult patients at six centers who were determined at the time of surgery to have intra-abdominal infections. These patients were randomized to receive ticarcillin-clavulanate potassium or clindamycin-gentamicin with or without ampicillin. Cure rates were 79%, 80%, and 82%, respectively. Most of these patients were moderately ill and relatively young. Drug-induced nephrotoxicity was not observed in either group.

THE ROLE OF ENTEROCOCCUS

On the basis of both experimental and clinical evidence, the importance of the enterococci as pathogenic in surgical infection has been minimized aside from their recognized role as a causative agent in urinary or biliary tract infections. Onderdonk and his co-workers demonstrated that pure cultures of enterococci injected into the peritoneal cavity of laboratory animals did not cause sepsis or abscess formation,[63] and in other models that mixed intra-abdominal infections containing enterococci are adequately treated with appropriate antimicrobial agents that were not active against enterococci.[64,65] Two clinical studies of surgical sepsis have demonstrated that treatment with adequate drainage and debridement plus antibiotics that have no activity against enterococci resulted in the same cure rate whether or not enterococci were present in the infected tissue.[66,67] Horvitz and Von Graevenitz[68] found that the frequency of clinical infections in wounds or tissue growing pure colonies of enterococci was not significantly different from the frequency of clinical infection in a control group of patients with negative cultures. There has, however, been some renewed interest in *Enterococcus* as a pathogen in surgical infections.[69] In a study from the University of Wisconsin, there was an increase in the prevalence of enterococcal bacteremia. Of note, 48% of the patients with enterococcal bacteremia had undergone recent surgery or were trauma or burn victims.[70] In this series, 77% of the infections were considered nosocomial. Dougherty et al.[71] have reported "breakthrough" enterococcal septicemia in surgical patients who were being given broad-spectrum antibiotics. Cephalosporins are widely used in GI surgery, and none of these drugs is effective against enterococci. Feliciano et al.[72] reported secondary infection with enterococci in surgical patients with penetrating abdominal trauma after or during treatment with these drugs. The source of the enterococci in these infections was considered to be endogenous; however, this assumption may not be universally valid. Zervos et al.[73] noted a strain of gentamicin-resistant enterococci in a surveillance study. Using plasmid content as a marker, they were able to make a convincing case that these infections were extrinsically acquired from hospital personnel and other patients.

Current recommendations are to treat *Enterococcus* only if it is isolated as a sole organism at the site of infection or if it is found in the blood either as a sole organism or in association with another organism. Therapy for *Enterococcus*, if it is cultured with other organisms from an intra-abdominal infection, is necessary only if the patient has valvular heart disease or a prosthetic valve, if the *Enterococcus* was cultured previously during a hospitalization, or the infection is nosocomial, especially if there was previous antibiotic therapy. If none of these conditions apply but the patient is not doing well despite adequate drainage and antimicrobial treatment directed against the other isolates, therapy against *Enterococcus* should be instituted. The drugs of choice are ampicillin, piperacillin, and vancomycin. The necessity of the addition of an aminoglycoside to these drugs is controversial. The combination may produce a synergistic effect. Aminoglycoside penetration of the bacterium is facilitated by damage to the cell wall by the other antibiotic. If the infection is polymicrobial, the other isolate should be treated appropriately.

REFERENCES

1. National Academy of Sciences, National Research Council, Division of Medical Sciences, Ad Hoc Committee on Trauma. Postoperative wound infections: The influence of ultraviolet irradiation in the operating room and of various other factors. Ann Surg 160(Suppl 2): 1-96, 1964.
2. Coit DG, Sclafani L. Care of the surgical wound, vol 2. In American College of Surgeons. Care of the Surgical Patient. New York: Scientific American, 1990, pp 1-10.
3. Haley RW, Culver DH, Morgan WM, White JW, Emori TG, Hooton TM. Identifying patients at high risk of surgical wound infection. Am J Epidemiol 121:206-215, 1985.
4. Cruse PJE, Foord R. The epidemiology of wound infection: A ten year prospective study of 62,939 wounds. Surg Clin North Am 60:27-40, 1980.
5. Robson MC, Heggers JP. Bacterial quantification of open wounds. Mil Med 134:19-24, 1969.
6. Lowry KF, Curtis GM. Delayed suture in the management of wounds. Analysis of 721 traumatic wounds illustrating the influence of time interval in wound repair. Am J Surg 1:280-287, 1950.
7. Lineaweaver W, Howard R, Soucy D, McMorris S, et al. Topical antimicrobial toxicity. Arch Surg 120:267-270, 1985.
8. Goldenheim PD. An appraisal of povidone-iodine and wound healing. Postgrad Med J 69(Suppl 3):S97-S105.
9. Viljanto J. Disinfection of surgical wounds without inhibition of normal wound healing. Arch Surg 115:253-256, 1980.

10. Kjolseth D, Frank JM, Barker JH, et al. Comparison of the effects of commonly used wound agents on epithelialization and neovascularization. J Am Coll Surg 179:305-312, 1994.
11. Heggers JP, Sazy JA, Stenberg BD, et al. Bactericidal and wound-healing properties of sodium hypochlorite solutions: The 1991 Lindberg Award. J Burn Care Rehabil 12: 420-424, 1991.
12. McKenna PJ, Lehr GS, Leist P, Welling RE. Antiseptic effectiveness with fibroblast preservation. Ann Plast Surg 27:265-268, 1991.
13. Kozol RA, Gillies C, Elgebaly SA. Effects of sodium hypochlorite (Dakin's solution) on the cells of the wound module. Arch Surg 123:420-423, 1988.
14. Maull KI. Management of high-risk wounds by retention suture closure over buttons. In O'Leary JP, Woltering EA, eds. Techniques for Surgeons. New York: Wiley, 1985, pp 38-40.
15. Lewis RT. Necrotizing soft-tissue infections. Infect Dis Clin North Am 6:693-702, 1992.
16. Eltorai IM, Hart GB, Strauss MB, Montroy R, Juler GL. The role of hyperbaric oxygen in the management of Fournier's gangrene. Int Surg 71:53-58, 1986.
17. Beck DE, Harford FJ, DiPalma JA. Comparison of cleansing methods in preparation for colonic surgery. Dis Colon Rectum 28:491-495, 1985.
18. Cohen SM, Wexner SD, Binderow SR, Nogueras JJ, et al. Prospective, randomized, endoscopic-blinded trial comparing precolonoscopy bowel cleansing methods. Dis Colon Rectum 37:689-696, 1994.
19. Harrower HW. Isolation of incisions into body cavities. Am J Surg 116:824-826, 1968.
20. Maxwell JG, Ford CR, Peterson DE, Richards RC. Abdominal wound infections and plastic drape protectors. Am J Surg 118:844-847, 1969.
21. Williams JA, Oates GD, Brown PP, et al. Abdominal wound infections and plastic wound guards. Br J Surg 59:142-146, 1972.
22. Psaila JV, Wheeler MH, Crosby DL. The role of plastic wound drapes in the prevention of wound infection following abdominal surgery. Br J Surg 64:729-732, 1997.
23. Nystrom PO, Broome A, Hojer H, Ling L. A controlled trial of a plastic wound ring drape to prevent contamination and infection in colorectal surgery. Dis Colon Rectum 27:451-453, 1984.
24. Nichols RL, Condon RE, Gorbach SC, et al. Efficacy of preoperative antimicrobial preparation of the bowel. Ann Surg 176:227-232, 1972.
25. Clarke JS, Condon RE, Bartlett JG, et al. Preoperative oral antibiotics reduce septic complications of colorectal operations: Result of prospective randomized double blinded clinical study. Ann Surg 186:251-258, 1977.
26. Solla JA, Rothenberger DA. Preoperative bowel preparation: A survey of colon and rectal surgeons. Dis Colon Rectum 33:154-159, 1990.
27. Periti P, Mazzei T, Tonelli F, et al. Single dose cefotetan versus multiple dose cefoxitin antimicrobial prophylaxis in colorectal surgery. Dis Colon Rectum 32:121-127, 1989.
28. Rowe-Jones DC, Peel AL, Kingston RD, et al. Single dose cefotaxime plus metronidazole versus three dose cefuroxime plus metronidazole as prophylaxis against wound infection in colorectal surgery: Multicentre prospective randomised study. Br Med J 300:18-22, 1990.
29. Andaker L, Burman LG, Eklund A, et al. Fosfomycin/metronidazole compared with doxycycline/metronidazole for the prophylaxis of infection after elective colorectal surgery. Eur J Surg 158:181-185, 1992.
30. Arnaud JP, Bellissant E, Boissel P, et al. Single-dose amoxycillin–clavulanic acid vs. cefotetan for prophylaxis in elective colorectal surgery: A multicentre, prospective, randomized study. J Hosp Infect 22(Suppl A):23-32, 1992.

31. Kwok SPY, Lau WY, Leung KL, et al. Amoxycillin and clavulanic acid versus cefotaxime and motronidazole as an antibiotic prophylaxis in elective colorectal resectional surgery. Chemotherapy 39:153-139, 1993.
32. Hakansson T, Raahave D, Hansen OH, Pedersen T. Effectiveness of single dose prophylaxis with cefotaxime and metrodidazole compared with three doses of cefotaxime alone in elective colorectal surgery. Eur J Surg 159:177-180, 1993.
33. Matikainen M, Hiltunen M. Parenteral single dose ceftriaxone with tinidatsole versus aminoglycoside with tinidatsole in colorectal surgery: A prospective single-blind randomized multicentre study. Int J Colorect Dis 8:148-150, 1993.
34. AhChong K, Yip AWC, Lee FCW, Chiu KM. Comparison of prophylactic ampicillin/sulbactam with gentamicin and metronidazole in elective colorectal surgery: A randomized study. J Hosp Infect 27:149-154, 1994.
35. Condon RE, Bartlett JG, Greenlee H, et al. Efficacy of oral and systemic antibiotic prophylaxis in colorectal operations. Arch Surg 118:496-502, 1993.
36. Coppa GF, Eng K, Gouge TH, et al. Parenteral and oral antibiotics in elective colon and colorectal surgery. Am J Surg 145:62-65, 1983.
37. Portnoy J, Kagan E, Gordon PH, Mendelson J. Prophylactic antibiotics in elective colorectal surgery. Dis Colon Rectum 26:310-313, 1983.
38. Schoetz DJ, Roberts PL, Roberts PL, et al. Addition of parenteral cefoxitin to regimen of oral antibiotics for elective colorectal operations. Ann Surg 212:209-212, 1990.
39. Fry DE, Garrison RN, Heitch RC, et al. Determinants of death in patients with intra-abdominal abscess. Surgery 8:517-523, 1980.
40. Knochel JQ, Koehler PR, Lee TG, Welch DM. Diagnosis of abdominal abscesses with computed tomography, ultrasound and ^{111}In leukocyte scans. Radiology 137:425-432, 1980.
41. Koehler PR, Moss AA. Diagnosis of intra-abdominal and pelvic abscesses by computerized tomography. JAMA 244:49-52, 1980.
42. Saini S, Kellum JM, O'Leary MP, et al. Improved localization and survival in patients with intra-abdominal abscesses. Am J Surg 145:136-142, 1983.
43. Norwood SH, Civetta JM. Abdominal CT scanning in critically ill surgical patients. Ann Surg 202:166-175, 1985.
44. Gerzof SG, Robbins AH, Birkett DH, et al. Percutaneous catheter drainage of abdominal abscesses guided by ultrasound and computed tomography. AJR 133:1-8, 1979.
45. Malangoni MA, Shumate CR, Thomas HA, Richardson JD. Factors influencing the treatment of intra-abdominal abscesses. Am J Surg 159:167-171, 1990.
46. Lent WM, Goldman MJ, Bizer LS. An objective appraisal of the role of computed tomographic (CT) guided drainage of intra-abdominal abscesses. Am Surg 56:688-690, 1990.
47. Hemming A, Davis NL, Robins RE. Surgical versus percutaneous drainage of intra-abdominal abscesses. Am J Surg 161:593-595, 1991.
48. Levison MA, Zeigler D. Correlation of Apache II score, drainage technique and outcome in postoperative intra-abdominal abscess. Surg Gynecol Obstet 172:89-94, 1991.
49. Brolin RE, Flancbaum L, Ercoli FR, et al. Limitations of percutaneous catheter drainage of abdominal abscesses. Surg Gynecol Obstet 173:203-210, 1991.
50. Longo WE, Milsom JW, Lavery IC, et al. Pelvic abscess after colon and rectal surgery—what is optimal management? Dis Colon Rectum 36:936-941, 1993.
51. Schechter S, Eisenstat TE, Oliver GC, et al. Computerized tomographic scan-guided drainage of intra-abdominal abscesses. Preoperative and postoperative modalities in colon and rectal surgery. Dis Colon Rectum 37:984-988, 1994.

52. Pichter WD, Musher DM. Critical importance of early diagnosis and treatment of intra-abdominal infection. Arch Surg 117:328-333, 1982.
53. Ercoli FR, Milgrim LM, Nosher JL, Brolin RE. Percutaneous catheter drainage of abscesses associated with enteric fistulae. Am Surg January:45-49, 1988.
54. Bohnen JMA, Solomkin JS, Dellinger EP, Bjorneson HS, Page CP. Guidelines for clinical care: Anti-infective agents for intra-abdominal infection. Arch Surg 127:83-89, 1992.
55. DiPiro JT, Cue JI. Single-agent versus combination antibiotic therapy in the management of intraabdominal infections. Pharmacotherapy 14:226-272, 1994.
56. Hackford AW, Tally FP, Reinhold RB, Barza M, Gorbach SL. Prospective study comparing imipenem-cilastatin with clindamycin and gentamicin for the treatment of serious surgical infections. Arch Surg 123:322-326, 1988.
57. Malangoni MA, Condon RE, Spiegel CA. Treatment of intra-abdominal infections is appropriate with single-agent or combination antibiotic therapy. Surgery 98:648-654, 1985.
58. Eckhauser FE, Knol JA, Raper SE, Mulholland MW, Helzerman P. Efficacy of two comparative antibiotic regimens in the treatment of serious intra-abdominal infections: Results of a multicenter study. Clin Ther 14:97-109, 1992.
59. Solomkin JS, Dellinger EP, Christou NV, Busuttil RW. Results of a multicenter trial comparing imipenem/cilastatin to tobramycin/clindamycin for intra-abdominal infections. Ann Surg 212:581-591, 1990.
60. Polk HC, Fink MP, Laverdiere M, Wilson SE, et al. Prospective randomized study of piperacillin/tazobactam therapy of surgically treated intra-abdominal infection. Am Surg 59:598-605, 1993.
61. Walker AP, Nichols RL, Wilson RF, et al. Efficacy of a β-lactamase inhibitor combination for serious intra-abdominal infections. Ann Surg 217:115-121, 1993.
62. Dougherty SH, Sirineki KR, Schauer PR, Fink MP, et al. Ticarcillin/clavulanate compared with clindamycin/gentamicin (with or without ampicillin) for the treatment of intra-abdominal infections in pediatric and adult patients. 61:297-303, 1995.
63. Onderdonk AB, Bartlett JG, Louie T, Sullivan-Seigler N, Gorbach SL. Microbial synergy in experimental intra-abdominal abscess. Infect Immun 13:22-26, 1976.
64. Weinstein WM, Onderdonk AB, Bartlett JG, Louie TJ, Gorbach SL. Antimicrobial therapy of experimental intraabdominal sepsis. J Infect Dis 132:282-286, 1975.
65. Bartlett JG, Louie TJ, Gorbach SL, Onderdonk AB. Therapeutic efficacy of 29 antimicrobial regimens in experimental intraabdominal sepsis. Rev Infect Dis 3:535-541, 1981.
66. Stone HH, Morris ES, Geheber CE, Kolb LD. Clinical comparison of cefotaxime with gentamicin plus clindamycin in the treatment of peritonitis and other soft-tissue infections. Rev Infect Dis 4(Suppl):S439-S443, 1982.
67. Tally FP, McGowan K, Kellum JM, Gorbach SL, O'Donnell TF. A randomized comparison of cefoxitin with or without amikacin and clindamycin plus amikacin in surgical sepsis. Ann Surg 193:318-323, 1981.
68. Horvitz RA, Von Graevenitz A. A clinical study of the role of enterococci as sole agents of wound and tissue infection. Yale J Biol Med 50:391-395, 1977.
69. Barie PS, Christou NV, Dellinger EP, Rout WR, Stone HH, Waymack JP. Pathogenicity of the enterococcus in surgical infections. Ann Surg 212:155-159, 1990.
70. Maki DG, Agger WA. Enterococcal bacteremia: Clinical features, the risk of endocarditis, and management. Medicine 67:248-265, 1988.
71. Dougherty SH, Flohr AB, Simmons RL. "Breakthrough" enterococcal septicemia in surgical patients. Arch Surg 118:232-238, 1983.

72. Feliciano DV, Gentry LO, Bitondo CG, et al. Single agent cephalosporin prophylaxis for penetrating abdominal trauma: Results and comment on the emergence of the enterococcus. Am J Surg 152:674-681, 1986.
73. Zervos MJ, Kauffman Ca, Therasse PM, Bergman AG, et al. Nosocomial infection by gentamicin-resistant *Streptococcus faecalis:* An epidemiologic study. Ann Intern Med 16:687-691, 1987.

CHAPTER 5

Intraoperative Anastomotic Complications

DAVID E. BECK

Colorectal surgery is a technique-oriented specialty, and many of the procedures require an anastomosis to reestablish bowel continuity. Achievement of a successful anastomosis is related to a number of surgical principles, which can be subdivided into patient-related factors and surgeon-related factors.[1,2] Patient-related factors, such as nutritional status, associated medical conditions, or medications, which are not under the control of the surgeon, are discussed in other chapters. Here we focus on anastomotic problems (e.g., leakage, ischemia, stenosis, and hemorrhage) that can be identified and managed during the procedure.

PREANASTOMOTIC CONSIDERATIONS

It is critical that spillage of intraluminal contents be avoided to minimize complications and neoplastic dissemination. Adequate preoperative mechanical and antibiotic bowel preparation (see Chapter 2) helps to reduce potential for spillage but cannot compensate for poor technique. Before the anastomosis is constructed, the bowel ends should be closed off (with tape or noncrushing clamps) to prevent leakage of residual intestinal contents.[3]

Systematic attention to operative details enables orderly progression of the procedure. Important considerations for exposure of the operative field include patient positioning (e.g., Lloyd-Davies position for pelvic surgery), a correctly placed and sized incision, and retraction of the wound edges and viscera. Difficulties with a low pelvic anastomosis are lessened if the midline incision is continued to the pubis and retractors (e.g., St. Mark's retractor) are used. Lighting from overhead lights, a head lamp, or lighted retractors helps to illuminate the operative field.

After completing the appropriate resectional procedure, sufficient proximal and distal mobilization provides tension-free bowel ends for a secure anastomosis. Difficulty in obtaining tension-free bowel occurs more commonly with a left-sided (e.g., colorectal) anastomosis. Additional left colon length is obtained with the following procedures, in order: division of the lateral colonic attachments, division of the splenic flexure, division of the inferior mesenteric artery at its aortic takeoff, and division of the inferior mesenteric vein at the inferior border of the pancreas. If these maneuvers do not provide adequate bowel length, branches of the distal middle colic artery and veins may need to be divided. However, this may compromise the blood supply to the remaining colonic end. If this occurs, the ischemic bowel must be resected and additional vessels divided to provide the required bowel length. In some cases, the middle colic vessels will have to be divided proximally and the blood supply of the residual colon will need to be based on the right, or the ileocolic artery. In most patients, these vessels will provide adequate blood supply to the proximal transverse colon or hepatic flexure, which can be made to reach the rectum with one of two techniques.

One method is to make an opening in the ileal mesentery medial to the ileocolic artery and vein, then bring the proximal transverse colon through this opening to reach the pelvis[4] (Fig. 5-1). Another option is to completely mobilize the right colon and turn it to the right. This rotates the cecal tip to the right middle abdomen (toward the liver), reverses the direction of the colon, and provides enough length for the hepatic flexure to reach the pelvis (Fig. 5-2). This maneuver moves the cecum to an abnormal position, so it is important to remove the appendix. Development of appendicitis would produce confusing signs and symptoms.

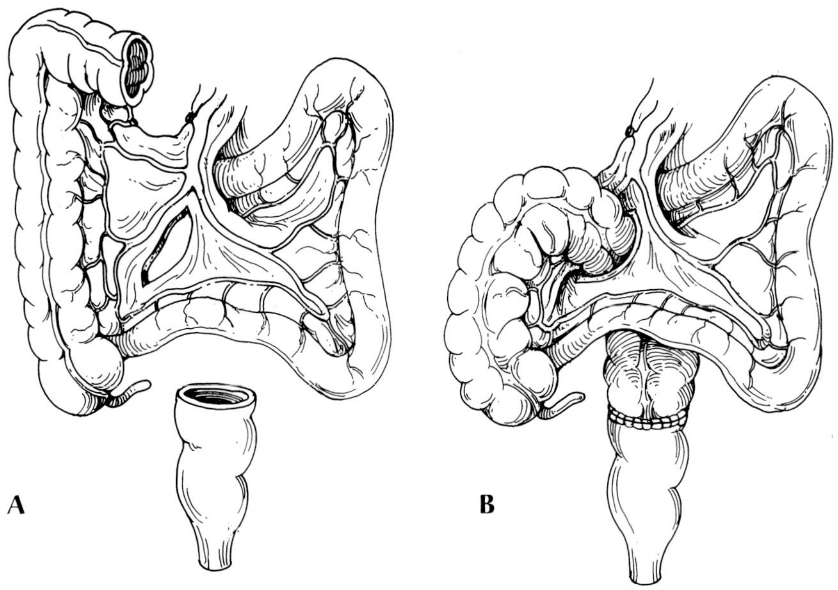

Fig. 5-1 **A**, Opening in mesentery is created medial to the ileocolic artery and vein. **B**, Transverse colon is brought through the ileomesenteric opening to reach the pelvis.

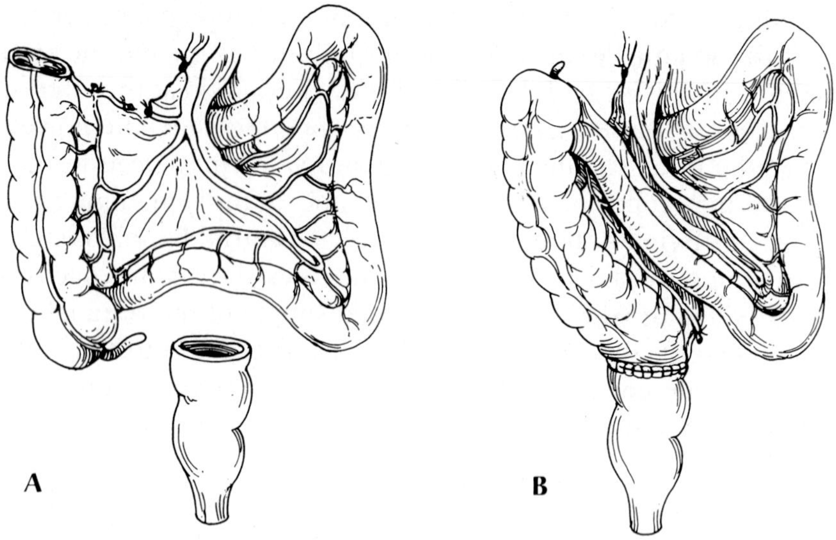

Fig. 5-2 **A**, Right colon is mobilized, right colic vessels are divided, and appendix is removed. **B**, Right colon is turned to allow the hepatic flexure to reach the pelvis.

In addition to a lack of tension, it is also critically important that the anastomotic site have a good blood supply. Before the anastomosis is constructed, the bowel should be routinely checked for viability (normal color and peristalsis and a pulsatile blood supply). Well-perfused bowel and its appendages (e.g., epiploic appendices) will bleed when cut. I frequently divide epiploic appendices at the proximal bowel end intended for the anastomosis to objectively confirm an adequate blood supply.

Finally, bowel used for an anastomosis must not be edematous, irradiated, or ischemic. Appropriate resection should remove ischemic or irradiated bowel. Edema of the residual bowel (e.g., associated with peritonitis) may preclude anastomosis in favor of a diverting stoma.

ANASTOMOTIC TECHNIQUE

Numerous techniques have been described to construct a bowel anastomosis, each with advantages and disadvantages. Suturing has always been used in intestinal surgery. In experiments, suture materials have shown some differences, but few if any differences have been observed in clinical trials. Suture techniques such as the number of layers or use of interrupted rather than running sutures have some clinical differences. An inverting anastomosis is superior to an everting anastomosis. A number of investigators advocate single-layer anastomosis; they believe it causes less narrowing of the lumen because a smaller amount of tissue is strangulated.[5,6] A single layer anastomosis is believed to cause less devascularization, infection, and necrosis, whereas the continuous suture distributes tension more evenly around the lumen.[6,7] In clinical practice, however, technical factors such as the correct placement of sutures, correct suture tension, and secure knots appear to be more important than the experimental findings discussed. Experience, training, clinical judgment, and ability are major factors in a surgeon's choice of anastomotic technique. However, some of the reported experience with suturing merits additional comment.

Extensive experience with a running monofilament suture has been described by Max et al.[7] In a retrospective report of 1000 single-layer, continuous, polypropylene intestinal anastomoses, these authors found this technique quick, simple, economical, and safe. Although an intraoperative leakage rate was not reported, their postoperative leakage rate of 1% with the technique compares favorably with other reports of alternate techniques.[7] Additional aspects of suture techniques are discussed in Chapter 18.

The use of surgical staplers has advantages in certain situations (e.g., the very low colorectal anastomosis), and they have enjoyed widespread clinical usage. These mechanical devices, however, do not compensate for improper or poor technique.

In an early survey of stapler-related complications published in 1981 by the American Society of Colon and Rectal Surgeons (ASCRS), 243 surgeons responded that they had performed 3594 end-to-end anastomoses.[8] Intraoperative complications were reported in 15.1% of patients and included anastomotic leak (9.8%), tear during stapler extraction (1.9%), anvil not extractable (1.2%), complete anastomotic failure that required use of another technique (0.9%), instrument failure (0.8%), and bleeding (0.5%). This report represents surgeons' early experience with the use of staplers, and therefore the results must be evaluated in the proper context. Improvements in the instruments, anastomotic technique, and surgeon experience have resulted in fewer complications.

An early experience with 73 consecutive stapled end-to-end colorectal anastomoses by Gordon and Vasilevsky[9] identified intraoperative complications in 19 patients (26%), which included instrument failure (four patients), incomplete or inadequate doughnuts (five patients), bleeding (three patients), bowel injury associated with use of sizers (one patient), anvil extraction (one patient), anvil insertion (three patients), difficulty with stapler extraction (one patient), and anvil not extractable (one patient). The relatively high prevalence of these problems reflects the early learning curve with stapling instruments and the early developmental nature of the instruments used. Increased experience and technical advancements in instruments have minimized the frequency of these problems.

A recent prospective randomized multicenter study by Dochetry et al.[10] described 652 patients who were randomized to undergo sutured (321 patients) or stapled large bowel anastomosis (331 patients) between 1985 and 1989. In five of the 331 patients (1.5%) randomized to receive a stapled anastomosis, instrument or technical failure occurred. Intraoperative anastomotic testing was not routinely performed, but postoperative leakage was identified radiologically in 14.4% of the sutured and 5.2% of the stapled colorectal anastomoses and was clinically evident in 4.4% of the sutured and 4.5% of the stapled anastomoses.

Proper technique is critical to obtaining a good anastomosis with a circular intraluminal stapler. To minimize problems, the largest diameter stapler that can be accommodated by both bowel ends should be used.[11] As originally described, intraluminal stapling entails use of purse-string sutures to hold the bowel over the stapler cartridge and anvil during staple closure. This purse-string suture can be placed by hand (with a baseball or in-and-out suture technique), with a fenestrated purse-string clamp (Purse String device, Davis & Geck, Wayne, N.J.), or with a stapling device (Purstring 65, U.S. Surgical Corp., Norwalk, Conn.). To work properly, the sutures must be placed correctly (approximately 1 to 2 mm from the bowel ends and 2 to 3 mm apart). If the sutures are placed too close, the bowel will not close tightly around the stapler shaft. This nonconstricting purse-string suture may be corrected by carefully cutting the bowel overlying the suture in two or more places to release additional suture to "bunch up" more of the bowel end. If the sutures are placed too far apart or some sutures tear through the bowel, gaps in the bowel ends will appear when the suture is tightened. This can be repaired with a Pulley stitch[12] (Fig. 5-3). These interrupted 4-0 or 3-0 braided sutures (e.g., silk or braided polyester) hold the purse-string suture to the bowel ends and assist in pulling it tightly around the shaft. Finally, suture placement too near the bowel end results in their tearing through the bowel, whereas placing the sutures too far back from the bowel ends produces an excessive bulk of tissue around the shaft.

If a purse-string clamp is used, it is important that the bowel be divided close to the clamp before the clamp is released. Leaving excess tissue adjacent to the

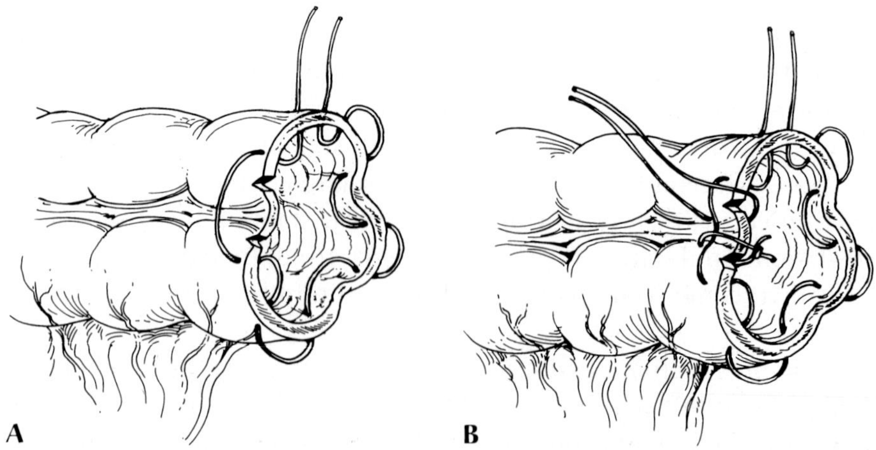

Fig. 5-3 Repair of purse-string suture. **A**, Gap is identified in purse-string suture. **B**, Gap is closed with pulley sutures.

clamp may result in too much tissue at the purse-string, which may prevent the stapler from closing and firing properly. Releasing the clamp before dividing the bowel may result in inadequate tissue to hold the purse-string sutures. Difficulties in using the purse-string clamp low in the pelvis are minimized by use of a double-armed suture (e.g., 2-0 monofilament polypropylene, double-armed TS-9, Davis & Geck). Both needles are placed through the clamp, and the needles can be bent several times during withdrawal to allow the needles to be removed from the clamp in the confined pelvis.

Many surgeons use clamps to hold the bowel ends while placing purse-string sutures or to hold the bowel open to aid placement of the anvil or stapler. Several problems can occur with the use of these clamps. If they are placed too far from the bowel end and too tightly, the bowel wall may be injured, which can result in leakage despite a secure anastomosis. If open-ended clamps (e.g., Babcock clamps) are used, it is possible for the purse-string to go through the end of the clamp, and the clamp or the purse-string suture will have to be cut. Use of solid-end clamps eliminates the chance of this happening. Large clamps increase the difficulty of inserting an anvil in bowel with a diameter close to that of the anvil.

Another method of end-to-end anastomosis involves a double-staple technique.[13,14] With this method a linear staple line is placed across the distal bowel and a circular stapler is inserted into this bowel (through the anus for a left-sided anastomosis). To avoid creating an ischemic area, the trocar of the circular stapler should exit adjacent or as close as possible to the linear staples. The anvil is placed in the proximal bowel and secured with a purse-string suture, as described. When closed and fired, the circular stapler removes a portion of the crossed linear staple line to create the anastomosis. Initially, surgeons expressed concern about these crossing staple lines. However, subsequent experimental and clinical evidence has confirmed the relative safety of this method.[15,16] The double-staple technique is helpful in anastomosis of bowel ends of dissimilar size and in ultralow colorectal or coloanal anastomoses. Other than in these situations, the extra cost of using a stapler rather than purse-string sutures argues for the purse-string.

One serious problem associated with double stapling of the low rectum is the inadvertent creation of a rectovaginal fistula from incorporating the posterior wall of the vagina into the staple lines. Techniques to reduce this occurrence include adequate dissection of the rectum off the posterior vagina, careful visualization of the bowel ends during closure of the stapler, and intravaginal palpation of the posterior vaginal wall before firing the stapler.

A variation of double stapling is triple stapling. In this anastomotic method, an extralinear stapler is used to close the bowel end after placement of the anvil into the proximal bowel. The anvil trocar is then advanced through the closed bowel. This technique has been suggested for use in intracorporeal laparoscopy; however, it is costly and produces another linear suture line that must be incorporated into the final anastomotic staple line. The technique has not gained widespread acceptance because of the relative ease of proximal purse-string suture placements.

Difficulty with anvil insertion in the proximal bowel lumen usually occurs when the stapler is too large for the diameter of the bowel. Experience or the use of sizers allows accurate selection of the correct size of circular stapler. Additional helpful techniques include the use of dilators to overcome bowel spasm, lubrication of the anvil head (with povidone-iodine, saline solution, or blood), and distraction of the bowel ends with three small-ended forceps or clamps. Use of a recently developed low-profile anvil (CDH Ethicon-Endosurgery, Cincinnati) has diminished this occurrence.

Detachable Staplers

For colorectal anastomosis, the circular stapler is usually inserted through the anus. With currently available staplers with detachable heads, the flat stapler shaft may be difficult to pass without trauma through the anal sphincter muscles. Khoury and Opelka[17] recently described a technique to facilitate this maneuver. A Fansler or Chelsey-Eaton anoscope allows gradual, controlled dilation of the sphincter muscles. After removal of the obturator, the stapler shaft can easily be passed through the anoscope (Fig. 5-4). Once through the sphincter, the stapler must be inserted up to the resected end of the rectum. Knowledge of rectal anatomy, adequate mobilization of the posterior rectum, and selection of

A

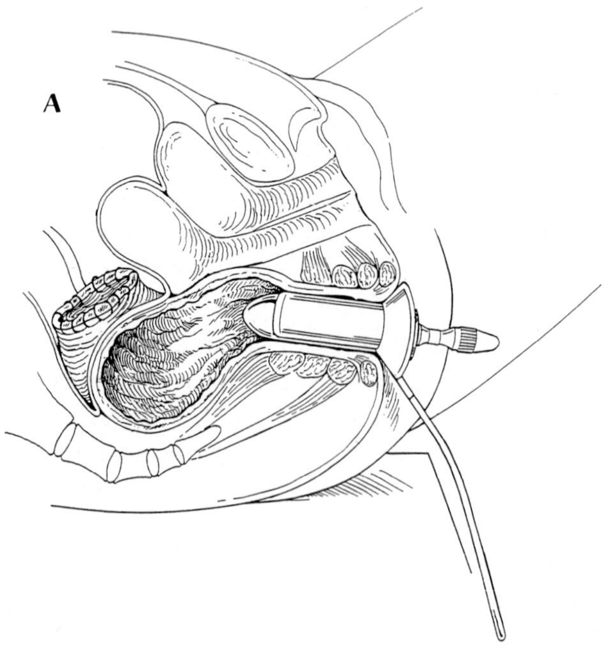

Fig. 5-4 Anoscope-assisted stapler insertion. **A,** Fansler anoscope is inserted after gentle anal dilation.

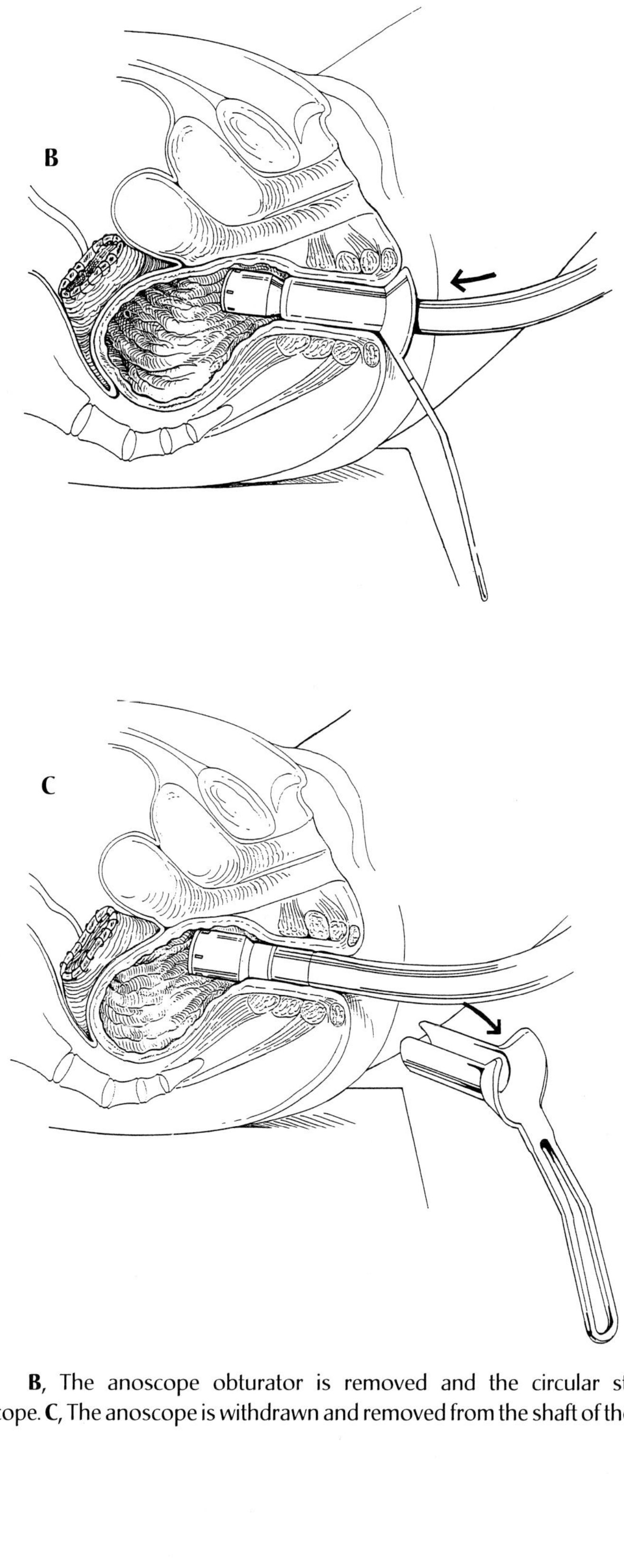

Fig. 5-4, cont'd **B**, The anoscope obturator is removed and the circular stapler is inserted through the anoscope. **C**, The anoscope is withdrawn and removed from the shaft of the stapler.

an appropriate size stapler assist in accomplishing this advancement. Incorrect insertion can tear or split the rectum. Such an injury mandates a very low or coloanal anastomosis to reestablish intestinal continuity. Proctoscopic examination of the rectum ensures an adequate lumen, confirms adequate preparation and mobilization, and assists in identifying the apex of Hartmann's pouch.

Once the stapler is closed and fired, it must be removed. Stapler extraction from the anastomotic area may be aided with a traction stitch. Bowel spasm or stapler misfire may cause extraction difficulty. Gentle traction and careful stapler manipulation usually allow it to be removed. If a misfire results in inability to remove the stapler, it may be necessary to excise and redo the anastomosis.

Inadequate Anastomotic Lumen

Adequate lumenal patency is important for several reasons. Bowel edema occurs in the perioperative period, and a marginal lumen may lead to partial obstruction. The anastomotic lumen can be sized with palpation or visual inspection. The ability to remove the anvil of a circular stapler confirms that the lumen corresponds to the size of the stapler. Distal rectal anastomosis can be evaluated with proctoscopy.

Leakage

The prevalence of anastomotic leakage is difficult to determine accurately. Few studies have reported the frequency of intraoperatively identified anastomotic problems. The frequency of postoperative leakage is described in Chapter 6.

A defective anastomosis can be repaired with several methods. Additional sutures can approximate a small gap, or the anastomosis can be resected and completely redone with a stapler or hand-sewn technique. Another option is to replace purse-string sutures around the defective anastomosis and reinsert a new stapler through the lumen. The purse-string sutures are tightened, which should close the defect and hold the previously placed staples toward the stapler shaft. After closure and firing of the new stapler, the new doughnuts (which should also contain the old staples) are removed with the stapler.[18] If the anastomosis is very low, the defect may also be repaired transanally.

Proximal Protection (Stomas)

For high-risk anastomosis, a proximal diverting stoma is often used. A diverting stoma will not prevent an anastomotic leak but will reduce sepsis-associated morbidity and mortality. A properly constructed loop stoma is almost totally diverting[19]; however, if absolute total diversion is desired, a Prasad-type end-loop stoma may be constructed.[20]

If diversion is needed, we prefer ileostomy over colostomy. A diverting colostomy after colonic resection presents several problems. A colostomy is a larger stoma and, because of its proximal location, the ostomy output is loose or liquid and very odorous. If a significant colonic resection has been performed, the remaining colon length is often insufficient to easily reach the abdominal wall at a preferred stomal location.

A loop ileostomy has several advantages.[21] First, it is easy to construct and close. Since it is usually created in bowel removed from the anastomotic site, tension and blood supply are rarely a problem. Ileostomy output is liquid, has little odor, and unless the mesentery is abnormally shortened, an ileostomy will reach almost any site on the abdominal wall.

Anastomotic Testing

All surgeons test anastomoses in some way. At a minimum, the anastomotic site is inspected and in some cases palpated. Visual inspection of a side-to-side anastomosis may be performed before closing the ends of the bowel. Gentle constriction of the bowel proximal or distal to the anastomosis will confirm a patent lumen and the absence of a gross leak. A more sensitive test can easily be performed in the colorectal anastomosis (which is at higher risk for a leak).

I prefer to test the colorectal anastomosis with intraluminal instillation of a dilute solution of povidone-iodine. After the bowel is occluded above the anastomosis with finger pressure, the testing solution is instilled gently with a bulb syringe inserted into the anus. Any leakage is readily apparent. Irrigation with this dilute povidone-iodine solution also provides antimicrobial and tumoricidal activity.

Some surgeons prefer to test the anastomosis with air. The pelvis is first filled with saline solution, and the distal bowel (containing the anastomosis) is distended with air instilled transanally. Any anastomotic defect will produce air bubbles. With this method, it is often difficult to accurately identify the location of the leak if any blood has mixed with the saline solution. The saline solution must also be removed before any identified leak can be repaired.

A proctoscope can be used to inspect the colorectal anastomosis. Sufficient lumen size is usually confirmed by the lack of stenosis, hemostasis is confirmed, and the bowel can easily be distended with air.

Finally, some surgeons inspect the intraluminal stapler doughnuts. I have not found this to be helpful, because complete doughnuts do not ensure the absence of a leak at the anastomotic site (e.g., a leak resulting from a tear in the bowel or staple lines during stapler removal). Also, an incomplete doughnut may be produced with an intact anastomosis. Intraoperative testing as described is more sensitive and specific.

Anastomotic Hemorrhage

Hemorrhage can occur at both a staple and a suture line. Proper staple height and correct suture tension minimize the frequency of this problem. Techniques to stop hemorrhage include cautery of the bleeding vessels or placement of a suture at the site of bleeding. Excessive cautery is to be avoided, because the staple line has the potential to transfer the electrical energy to adjacent bowel. Reduction or stoppage of bleeding may also be helped by digital compression or instillation of an epinephrine solution (1:100,000 or 1:200,000 μm/ml) into the bowel lumen.

Adherence to established surgical principles and techniques should minimize anastomotic problems. Mechanical devices cannot overcome limitations in experience, skill, or judgment. Intraoperative identification of problems permits their correction with minimal morbidity.

REFERENCES

1. Goligher JC. Surgery of the Anus, Rectum, and Colon, 5th ed. London: Baillière Tindall, 1984.
2. Steichen FM, Ravitch MM. Contemporary stapling instruments and basic mechanical suture techniques. Surg Clin North Am 64:425-440, 1984.
3. Wexner SD, Beck DE. Sepsis prevention in colorectal surgery. In Fielding LP, Goldnerg SM eds. Operative Surgery, 5th ed. London: Butterworth-Heineman, 1993, pp 41-46.
4. Le TH, Gathright JB Jr. Reconstruction of intestinal continuity after extended left colectomy. Dis Colon Rectum 36:197-198, 1993.
5. Gambee LP, Garnjobst W, Hardwisk CE. Ten years' experience with a single layer anastomosis in colon surgery. Am J Surg 92:222-227, 1956.
6. Templeton JL, McKelvey ST. Low colorectal anastomoses. An experimental assessment of two sutured and two stapled techniques. Dis Colon Rectum 28:38-41, 1985.
7. Max E, Sweeney WB, Baily HR, Oommen SC, Butts DR, Smith KW, Zamora LF, Skakun GB. Results of 1,000 single-layer continuous polypropylene intestinal anastomoses. Am J Surg 162:461-467, 1991.
8. Smith LE. Anastomosis with EEA stapler after colonic resection. Dis Colon Rectum 24:236-242, 1981.
9. Gordon PH, Vasilevsky CA. Experience with stapling in rectal surgery. Surg Clin North Am 64:555-566, 1984.
10. Dochetry JG, McGregor JR, Akyol AM, Murray GD, Galloway DJ. Comparison of manually constructed and stapled anastomoses in colorectal surgery. Ann Surg 221:176-184, 1995.
11. Fazio VW. Cancer of the rectum. Sphincter-saving operation: stapling techniques. Surg Clin North Am 68:1367-1382, 1988.
12. Last MD, Fazio VW. The rational use of the purse-string device in constructing anastomoses with the circular stapler. Dis Colon Rectum 28:979-980, 1985.
13. Cohen Z, Myers E, Langer B, Taylor B, Railton RH, Jameson C. Double stapling technique for low anterior resection. Dis Colon Rectum 26:231-235, 1983.
14. Griffen FD, Knight CD. Stapling technique for primary and secondary rectal anastomoses. Surg Clin North Am 64:579-590, 1984.
15. Julian TB, Ravitch MM. Evaluation of the safety of end-to-end (EEA) stapling anastomoses across linear stapled closures. Surg Clin North Am 64:567-578, 1984.

16. Ravitch MM. Varieties of stapled anastomosis in rectal resection. Surg Clin North Am 64:543-554, 1984.
17. Khoury DA, Opelka FG. Anoscopic-assisted insertion of end-to-end anastomosing staplers. Dis Colon Rectum 38:553-554, 1995.
18. Makabeli G, Williams LG. Repair of defective EEA anastomosis. Dis Colon Rectum 27:490-491, 1984.
19. Pearl RK, Abcarian H. Diverting stomas. In MacKeigan JM, Cataldo PA, eds. Intestinal Stomas: Principles, Techniques, and Management. St. Louis: Quality Medical Publishing, 1993, pp 107-126.
20. Prasad ML, Pearl RK, Orsay CP. End-loop ileocolostomy for massive trauma to the right side of the colon. Arch Surg 119:975-976, 1984.
21. Williams NS, Nasmyth DG, Jones D, et al. Defunctioning stomas: A prospective controlled trial comparing loop ileostomy with transverse colostomy. Br J Surg 73:566-570, 1986.

CHAPTER 6

Postoperative Anastomotic Complications

ANTHONY M. VERNAVA III
WALTER E. LONGO

One of the characteristics that distinguishes intestinal operations from other extirpative operations in general surgery is that reconstruction of the alimentary tract is usually necessary and requires that an anastomosis be created. This additional requirement to restore intestinal continuity has associated risks to the patient but has the benefit of avoiding an intestinal stoma when successful. The significant shift from abdominoperineal resection to low anterior resection without permanent colostomy and from proctocolectomy with ileostomy to ileoanal reservoir is a testimony to human ingenuity applied to overcome the need for a permanent stoma.

Essentially, three significant complications can occur that are specifically related to the performance of an anastomosis: hemorrhage, leakage, and stricture. Anastomotic hemorrhage and dehiscence are acute complications that become manifest during the initial postoperative hospitalization, whereas an anastomotic stricture is usually a late complication that is not noted until several weeks to months after surgery.

The technical construction of an intestinal anastomosis can be accomplished in a variety of ways, including hand suturing (single layer, interrupted and continuous, and double layer), stapling, and the Valtrac biofragmentable ring. Use of the circular stapler extends the ability to routinely restore intestinal continuity down to the dentate line and allows creation of an anastomosis in patients in whom a stoma would be required if a hand-sutured anastomosis were the only option available. Recent investigations indicate no significant difference in the risk for anastomotic dehiscence between the two basic techniques.[1-3] The risk for anastomotic stricture is probably higher for circular-stapled coloproctostomy than for hand-sutured anastomosis, although the only study that evaluated this relationship reported no difference.[3] Stricture of anastomoses located above the peritoneal reflection is rare.

ANASTOMOTIC HEMORRHAGE

The risk for anastomotic hemorrhage after a colocolonic or colorectal anastomosis is 0.5% to 1.0%.[4-6] There does not appear to be a difference in risk between stapled and sutured anastomoses, and the risk is not reduced with creation of a two-layer sutured anastomosis.

Most episodes of bleeding from an intestinal anastomosis occur in the early postoperative period and resolve spontaneously. Initial management includes close observation and serial blood cell counts, usually every 6 hours. Clotting studies including PT, PTT, bleeding time, and platelet count should be performed, and when results are abnormal the appropriate blood and blood factor products should be transfused.

When bleeding is significant and persistent, it is important to precisely identify its source and not presume it originates from the anastomosis. Although the anastomosis is the most likely source of bleeding, other possible sites include gastroduodenal ulcers, diverticular disease, and angiodysplasias, among others. Upper GI endoscopy should be performed to exclude an upper alimentary tract source. Rigid or flexible sigmoidoscopy should be performed to evaluate a low colorectal anastomosis. Bleeding from a colorectal, coloanal, or ileoanal anastomosis is confirmed with anoscopy or rigid proctoscopy. Suction cautery will usually control the hemorrhage. Other adjuvants include irrigation with epinephrine solutions or tamponade with a large Foley catheter.

Some clinicians oppose colonoscopy in the early postoperative period with a new colonic anastomosis, but in our experience colonoscopy can be safely performed without undue risk of anastomotic disruption. Gentle enemas should be given before the endoscopy to cleanse the bowel. The procedure should be performed under controlled conditions in either the operating room with the patient under general anesthesia or in the endoscopy suite with the patient well sedated. A large-channel scope should be used to facilitate irrigation and suction of clots. Air insufflation should be minimized, and the endoscopist should avoid torquing the colonoscope or advancing it against pressure. If the bleeding site is identified, an attempt at coagulation can be made.

When bleeding does not spontaneously cease and transfusion of 4 to 6 units of blood has been required, the patient should be taken to the operating room for either oversewing or resection of the anastomosis and re-creation of an anastomosis or end stoma. Hemorrhage from a low colorectal anastomosis can be managed with transanal suture ligation. Lighted anoscopes and/or a headlight are helpful in such cases. Hemorrhage from an intraperitoneal colonic anastomosis is not amenable to transanal ligation and usually requires laparotomy. An initial attempt at identification and coagulation of the bleeding site can be made endoscopically. If this is not possible, laparotomy and oversewing of the entire anastomosis can be performed. Intraoperative colonoscopy can be performed to confirm the cessation of hemorrhage. We do not advocate opening the anastomosis to identify the bleeding site because of bacterial contamination and the risk for postoperative intraperitoneal sepsis. As an alternative, the anastomosis can be resected and either a new anastomosis or end diverting stoma created, dependent on the clinical condition of the patient.

ANASTOMOTIC DEHISCENCE

Prevalence and Causes

Anastomotic leakage is the most feared complication by surgeons who operate on the alimentary tract. There is good reason for this apprehension, because the consequences of anastomotic dehiscence are severe and include a dramatic increase in morbidity and mortality. Indeed, the risk of death from an anastomotic leak was reported as 13 times higher than after an uncomplicated operation.[7] It is no wonder that a number of precautions are taken to improve the chances for good anastomotic healing, including ensuring adequate preoperative patient nutrition, converting emergent to elective operation, full mechanical and antibiotic bowel preparation, and anastomosis of normal noninflamed intestine to normal noninflamed intestine.

A number of factors are responsible for altering the risk for anastomotic failure and include technical factors related to performance of the surgery and intrinsic patient factors.[7-14]

Technical factors	Patient factors
Ischemia at bowel ends	Anemia
Edema at bowel ends	Malnutrition
Tension on anastomosis	High-dose steroid therapy
Poor closure of anastomosis	No bowel preparation
Sepsis, generalized or localized, in area of anastomosis	Critical illness
	Previous irradiation injury of bowel at anastomosis
	Active inflammatory bowel disease at anastomosis
	Bowel obstruction distal to anastomosis

Among the most significant factors that alter the risk for anastomotic dehiscence is the anatomic location of the anastomosis; anastomoses located below the peritoneal reflection are at significantly higher risk of leaking than are those located intraperitoneally.[7,15] The prevalence of intraperitoneal anastomotic dehiscence varies in the literature between 0.5% and 30%[16] but is generally between 2% and 5%.[8,17] The prevalence of clinically significant leakage from anastomoses located below the peritoneal reflection is significantly higher and ranges from 8% to 20%[18-38] (Table 6-1). Indeed, the risk for leakage from an extended low anterior anastomosis located 0 to 6 cm from the anal verge is even higher and has led some authors to advocate routine temporary fecal diversion in such cases.[39] The double-staple anastomotic technique does not appear to

Table 6-1 Complications with the circular stapler

Author	Year	No. of cases	Leaks (%) Identified clinically	Leaks (%) Identified radiologically	Stenosis (%)
Kirkegaard et al.[18]	1980	30	7	17	13
Cade et al.[19]	1981	50	6	NA	4
Cutait et al.[20]	1981	49	12	NA	6
Heald and Leicester[21]	1981	100	13	17	1
Killingback[22]	1981	64	9	NA	14
Goligher[23]	1982	101	3	9	5
Leff et al.[24]	1982	106	8	NA	11
Polglase et al.[25]	1982	19	16	36	30
Vezeridis et al.[26]	1982	58	0	NA	3
Anderberg et al.[27]	1983	34	12	NA	NA
Fegiz et al.[28]	1983	134	16	30	NA
Isbister et al.[29]	1983	88	15	NA	1
Kennedy et al.[30]	1983	236	3	NA	NA
Fazio et al.[31]	1985	85	1	4	NA
McGinn et al.[32]	1985	58	12	24	NA
Gillen and Peel[33]	1986	55	6	24	NA
Antonsen and Kronborg[34]	1987	178	15	NA	8
Zannini et al.[35]	1987	209	9	NA	9
Belli et al.[36]	1988	74	4	NA	3
Malmberg et al.[37]	1988	96	14	NA	NA
Kyzer and Gordon[38]	1992	215	0.4	NA	13

Data from Kyzer S, Gordon PH. Dis Colon Rectum 35:696-706, 1992.

increase the risk for anastomotic leak, which has been reported to be 2.7%.[40] It should be noted that the creation of a proximally diverting stoma to protect a low pelvic or technically inadequate anastomosis does not alter the risk for dehiscence but does ameliorate the septic effects of the leak.[41,42]

Evaluation of the blood supply at the ends of the bowel being used for the anastomosis can include observation,[43] Doppler ultrasound,[44,45] intravenous fluourescein,[45,46] and transmural oximetry measurement.[47] Experimental evidence nicely demonstrates the adverse effect of corticosteroid therapy on anastomotic healing during the critical time period 6 to 20 days after surgery.[48]

Also, it should be noted that the prevalence of anastomotic leakage varies widely, depending on the definition and diagnostic method used. For example, the prevalence of asymptomatic, clinically insignificant leaks identified radiographically with meglumine diatrizoate (Gastrografin, Squibb Diagnostics Division, E.R. Squibb & Sons, Princeton, N.J.) enema has been reported to be three to four times higher than clinically apparent dehiscences.[33,49]

Clinical Presentation

The clinical manifestation of anastomotic dehiscence varies, depending on its location, severity, and whether any adjacent tissue such as omentum or small intestine contain the leak, and hence ranges from failure to thrive to profound sepsis[50]:

Fever
Vague abdominal pain
Intractable diarrhea
Failure to thrive
Intestinal obstruction
Septic shock

Recognition of a significant anastomotic leak may be delayed as the nonspecific symptoms of low-grade sepsis, including elevated temperature, prolonged ileus, diarrhea, malaise, and failure to thrive, can be attributed to recovery from a major operation rather than to major anastomotic failure. Catastrophic anastomotic failure can result in feculent peritonitis with hemodynamic instability and shock. A less severe but still serious leak walled off by adjacent organs and omentum may not be manifested by gross peritonitis but by symptoms such as vague abdominal pain, failure to thrive, temperature elevation, tachycardia, prolonged ileus, diarrhea or obstruction, and multiorgan system failure (e.g., renal failure, hepatic failure manifested as jaundice, acute respiratory distress syndrome). Leukocytosis with a marked left shift to immature cells is a sign of infection. Frequently, extraperitoneal colorectal anastomotic dehiscence is manifested in this fashion. Longo et al.[50] described the initial symptoms in 56 patients with postoperative pelvic abscess that developed after colorectal surgery: 93% had fever, 20% had intractable diarrhea, 14% experienced failure to thrive, 9% had intestinal obstruction, and 4% were in shock. A leak that has subsequently sealed may produce symptoms of abscess. A leak that has been effectively walled off by adjacent organs may become manifest at a later time, with extravasation through the abdominal incision as an enterocutaneous fistula.

Diagnosis

After any intestinal anastomosis, the clinician should have a high index of suspicion when evaluating any unusual signs of sepsis. The symptoms of an anastomotic leak can be subtle and masked by those normally attributed to routine postoperative recovery. A CT scan with intravenous, oral, and rectal contrast material should be obtained in those patients with suspected anastomotic leak and should demonstrate any abscess or extravasation of contrast from the intestine.[51-53] A Gastrografin enema can also be used to evaluate the integrity of a colorectal anastomosis but is less useful for more proximal anastomoses because it becomes too dilute to accurately define the anastomosis. Barium enema should not be used in this circumstance because of the increase in morbidity and mortality associated with barium peritonitis. Indium-labeled leukocyte scans can also be helpful to identify otherwise occult abdominal abscesses.[54]

Management

The specific method of management of an anastomotic dehiscence depends on the manifestation of the leak and the clinical condition of the patient. An anastomotic leak may be silent or can manifest as a leak with or without an abscess, as generalized peritonitis, or as an enterocutaneous or colocutaneous fistula. A management algorithm is presented in Fig. 6-1.[55] The possible manifestations of anastomatic leakage are listed below:

- Asymptomatic
- Sepsis without abscess
- Leak with associated abscess
- Peritonitis
- Enterocutaneous/colocutaneous fistula

The key to successful management is control of sepsis, and proximal fecal diversion may or may not be required. Completely asymptomatic, radiographically discovered anastomotic dehiscences require no therapy. Management options for symptomatic leaks depend on the specific manifestation of the leak and the clinical condition of the patient and range from bowel rest and antibiotic therapy to operative laparotomy with resection of the anastomosis, proximal fecal diversion, and a distal mucous fistula or Hartmann pouch.

Asymptomatic radiographically demonstrated leak. As many as 36% to 49% of patients with a pelvic anastomosis will have a leak that is demonstrated radiographically when Gastrografin enemas are routinely used during the first postoperative week[6,25] (Fig. 6-2). When the patient has no symptoms and is clinically thriving, no intervention is necessary. The leak is of no clinical consequence and will heal spontaneously.

Leak without abscess. For a clinically ill patient with signs of infection and radiographic documentation of an anastomotic leak by Gastrografin enema, without abscess, initial management may include broad-spectrum intravenous antibiotic therapy and bowel rest. The duration of treatment is empiric and depends on the clinical response. An initial treatment period of 7 days is routine. Failure to improve or clinical deterioration mandate surgical intervention. In most patients, this should include resection of the anastomosis, drainage of the space, and creation of a proximal stoma. Diversion without resection has been used in selected patients with good results. Low extraperitoneal anastomotic

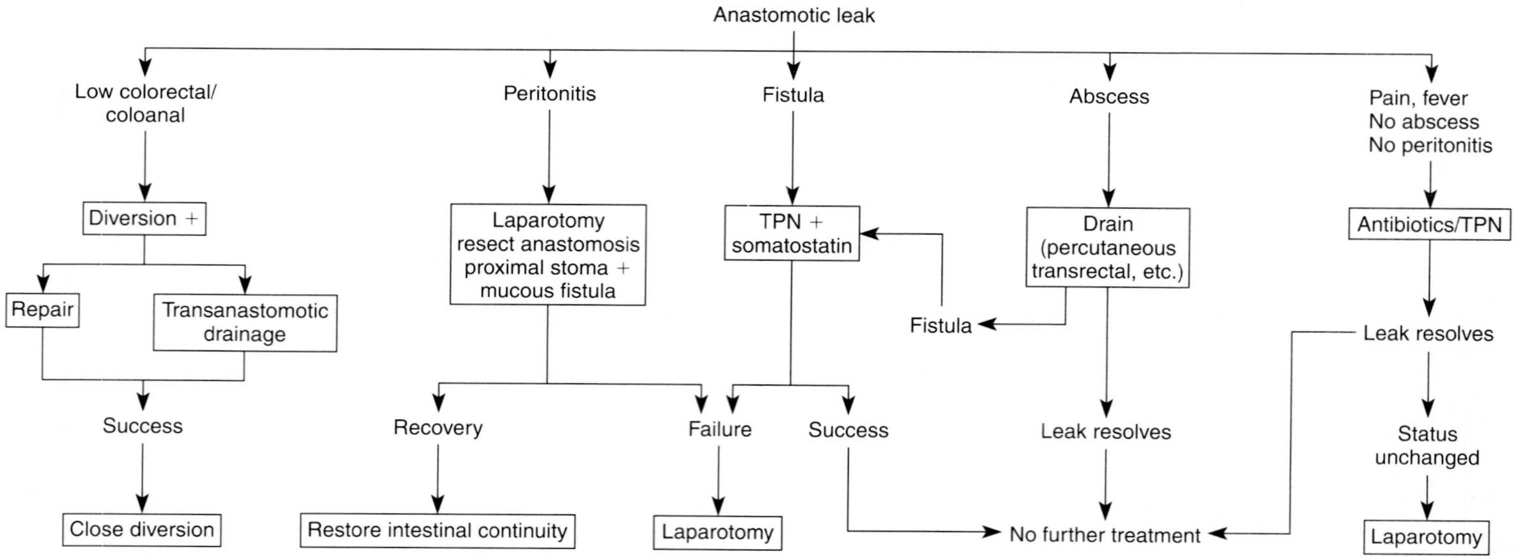

Fig. 6-1 Algorithm for the management of anastomotic dehiscence. (Modified from Church JM. Surgical management of anastomotic leaks and intra-abdominal sepsis. In Rothenberger DA, ed. Colorectal Disease: Challenging Problems. Probl Gen Surg 9:634-640, 1992.)

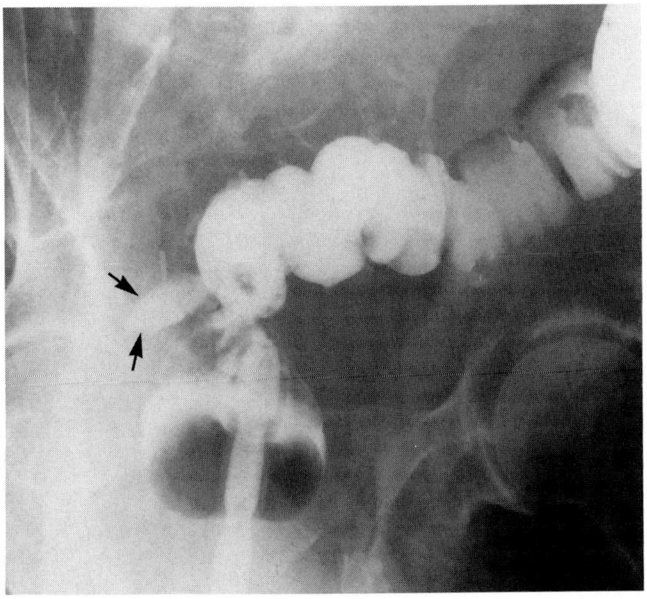

Fig. 6-2 Gastrografin enema demonstrating anastomotic leak *(black arrows)* from colorectal anastomosis (anterior-posterior view).

leaks have been managed with proximal diversion (e.g., loop or end-loop ileostomy). This may be accomplished with laparoscopically assisted techniques, but experience and patient selection are extremely important.

Leak with abscess. In a patient with evidence of low-grade sepsis and documentation of a contained anastomotic leak (Fig. 6-3) and an abdominal or pelvic abscess, drainage of the abscess and broad-spectrum parenteral antibiotic therapy are required. Laparotomy and fecal diversion may or may not be required, depending on whether the sepsis can be controlled. Drainage of either an abdominal or pelvic abscess can be accomplished in a variety of ways, and selection of the specific drainage technique should be based on a clear understanding of the anatomy of the abscess and the precise location of the leak. For this reason, routine CT of the abdomen and pelvis with intravenous, oral, and rectal contrast medium is advocated whenever an anastomotic leak and abscess is suspected (Figs. 6-4 and 6-5). CT is highly sensitive and accurate (95%) in determining the presence of abdominopelvic abscess.[53] For a low colorectal anastomosis, drainage can be accomplished through the anastomosis if the dehiscence is readily apparent at endoscopic examination. The defect can be gently enlarged to allow better drainage, and transrectal drains can be placed in the cavity for irrigation, continuously or at specific intervals. Transvaginal and transperineal drainage

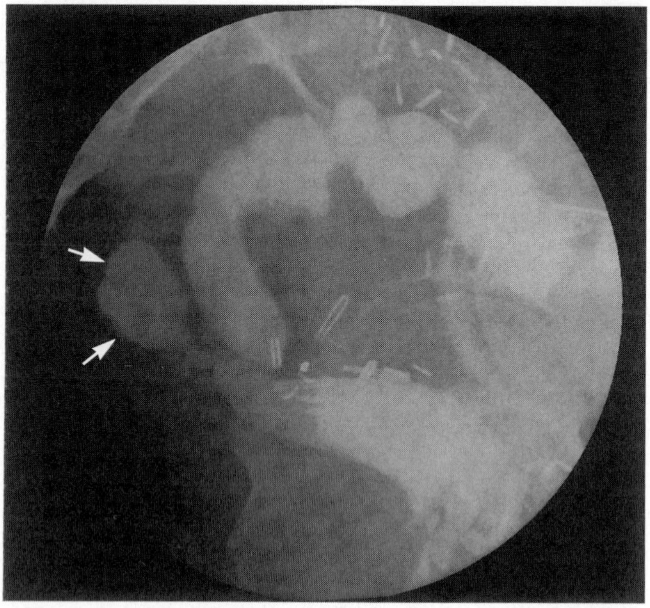

Fig. 6-3 Gastrografin enema demonstrating anastomotic leak with contained abscess *(white arrows)* from colorectal anastomosis (lateral view).

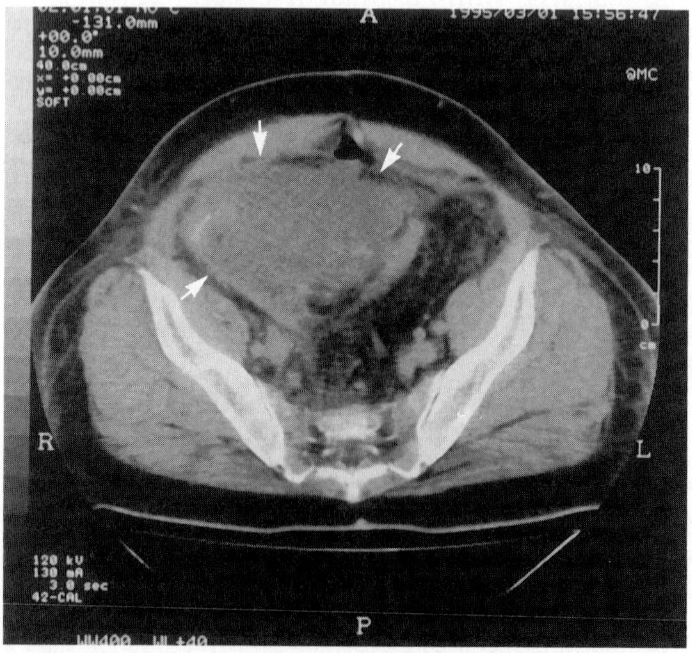

Fig. 6-4 Abdominal CT scan demonstrating large abdominal abscess (*arrows* mark cavity).

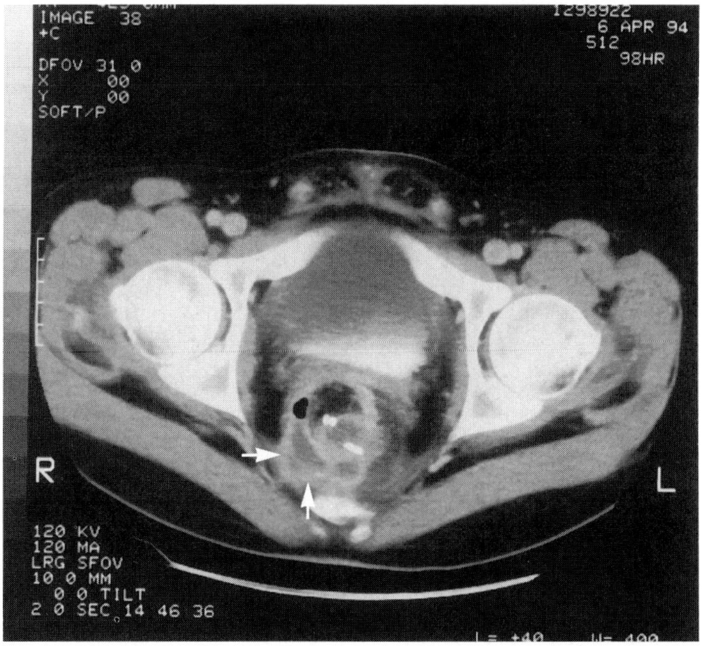

Fig. 6-5 Pelvic CT scan demonstrating abscess *(white arrows)* around Ileoanal pouch anastomosis.

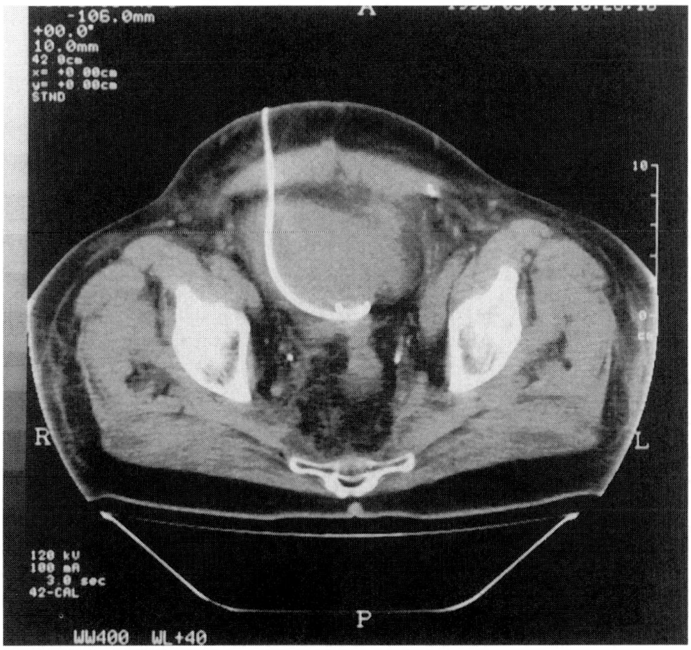

Fig. 6-6 CT scan of patient from Fig. 6-4 with percutaneously guided catheter in abscess cavity.

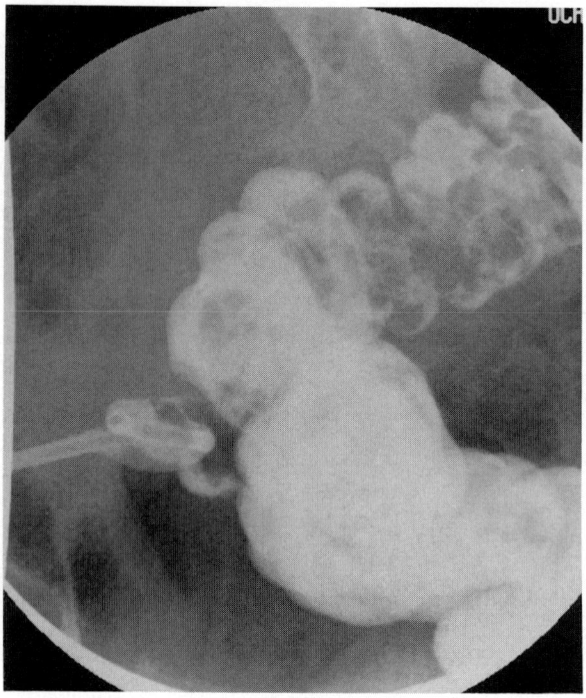

Fig. 6-7 Oblique contrast radiograph demonstrating catheter drainage of small colonic leak.

can also be performed. CT-guided percutaneous drainage is successful in as many as 85% of appropriately selected patients[50,51] (Figs. 6-6 and 6-7).

Peritonitis. Gross peritonitis requires laparotomy, resection of the anastomosis with end colostomy and mucous fistula or Hartmann pouch. Diversion alone without resection of the leaking anastomosis is unacceptable except in patients at highest risk, because of persistent sepsis from the leaking anastomosis. In such cases, wide drainage of the anastomosis should be performed. Repair of the anastomosis, either alone or in combination with a proximal stoma, is unwise and should be avoided because of the certainty of recurrent anastomotic failure in the presence of intra-abdominal sepsis.

Enterocutaneous or colocutaneous fistula. A late manifestation of an unrecognized anastomotic leak is the development of an enterocutaneous fistula. A radiograph and/or CT scan should be obtained to determine the site of the defect in the intestine and whether any undrained collection of pus is present. Any collection of pus should be drained to facilitate closure of the fistula. After control of the sepsis and in the absence of distal bowel obstruction and a foreign body, most enterocutaneous fistulas will close without operative intervention.

FACTORS RESPONSIBLE FOR ANASTOMOTIC STRICTURE

Early	Late
Ischemia	Recurrent neoplasm
Aggressive mesenteric stripping	Recurrent inflammatory bowel disease
Crush injury to bowel ends	Crohn's disease
Localized sepsis	Diverticular disease
Anastomotic leak	Radiation injury
Proximal fecal diversion	

Other important management guidelines include correction of anemia and fluid and electrolyte abnormalities, excellent wound care, and adequate nutrition. Bowel rest and TPN may be necessary to facilitate closure.[56] In some fistulas the use of somatostatin analog can be helpful in nonsurgical closure.[57]

ANASTOMOTIC STRICTURE

Clinically significant anastomotic strictures usually occur with low colorectal anastomoses, but generally not with anastomoses located above the peritoneal reflection, in the absence of Crohn's disease. The reasons for this discrepancy are related to the differences in anastomotic surgical technique and the frequency of use of the circular stapler to close colorectal anastomoses. Definitions of anastomotic strictures vary, but perhaps the best definition is the inability to pass a 19 mm sigmoidoscope through the anastomosis. Circular-stapled coloproctostomies are associated with the highest risk of stricture, and the incidence averages approximately 8% (range, 1% to 13%).[38,58,59] According to Akyol et al.,[3] the risk for stenosis after sutured colorectal anastomosis is the same as for stapled anastomosis. The incidence of stenosis or stricture[63] after the double-staple anastomotic technique for coloproctostomy was recently reported to be 2.7% among 75 patients.[40] The specific cause of stenosis in the majority of cases (see the box) is probably related to tissue ischemia from a crush injury to the ends of the bowel during application of the stapler. Ischemia resulting in stenosis after circular-stapled coloproctostomy may also be caused by aggressive stripping of the mesentery with its blood supply from the edge of the bowel wall.[38] Indeed, Kyzer and Gordon[38] reported a drop in the stenosis rate from 20% to 13% by decreasing the amount of mesentery stripped from the bowel edge. Localized sepsis or infected hematoma in the area of the anastomosis can also be responsible for stricture, and an anastomotic leak may be manifested as an excessive inflammatory response and stricture formation; these patients may

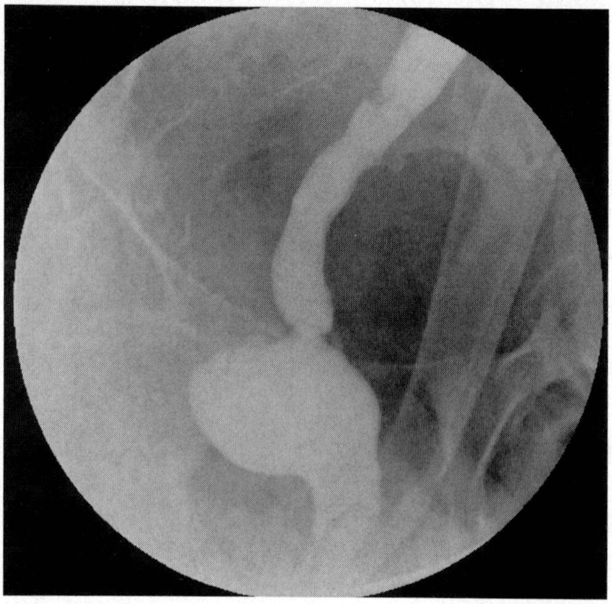

Fig. 6-8 Contrast enema demonstrating colorectal anastomotic stricture.

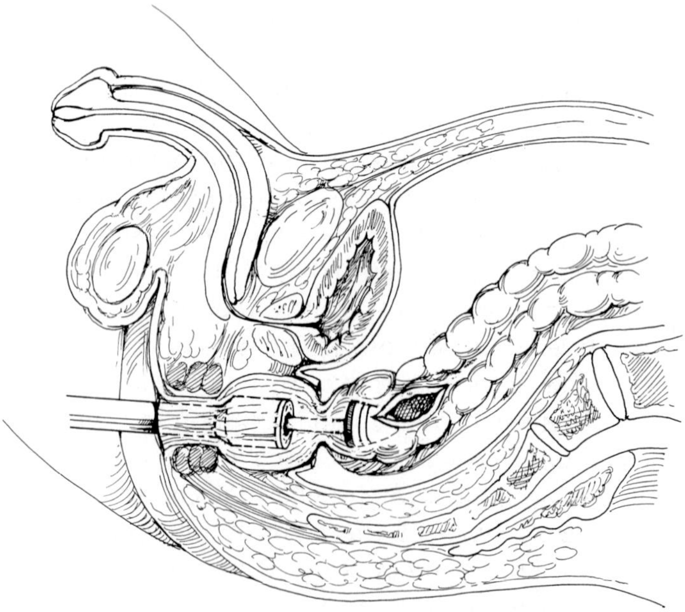

Fig. 6-9 Stapling technique to manage stricture without formal resection. Stapler has been advanced via anus to stricture and connected through stricture to anvil (inserted via proximal colotomy).

have bowel obstruction.[50] Proximal fecal diversion after a colorectal anastomosis may also be responsible for stricture formation by not allowing the passage of stool through the anastomosis, which would dilate it. Radiation intestinal injury can also cause significant anastomotic stricturing, requiring dilation, proctectomy with coloanal anastomosis, or fecal diversion.[60,61]

Strictures that become manifest several months to years after surgery should alert the clinician to the possibility of recurrent disease, either neoplastic or inflammatory bowel disease. Aggressive biopsy of the stricture should be performed to evaluate that possibility. In the event that histopathologic analysis reveals recurrent disease, it should be managed accordingly.

Diagnosis and Treatment

Symptoms of a significant anastomotic stricture consist of obstipation, frequent small bowel movements, alternating constipation and diarrhea, small-caliber bowel movements, and abdominal bloating. A contrast enema or endoscopy can be used to specifically define the stricture (Fig. 6-8).

Asymptomatic strictures are usually best treated conservatively by bulking the stool with a dietary fiber supplement and gentle digital dilation. Alternatively, dilation of the stricture can be performed in the office with a rigid proctosigmoidoscope. Ability to pass a 19 mm proctoscope represents sufficient therapy. More difficult strictures may require operative dilation with Hegar or balloon dilators. Several treatment sessions may be required. Between dilation treatments, the patient should be given a dietary fiber supplement to bulk the stool, which then gently dilates the anastomosis during passage through it. Occasionally a severe stricture may require formal reresection and reanastomosis. A specific technique has been described to manage a severe anastomotic stricture without the need for resection[62] (Fig. 6-9). After laparotomy and adhesiolysis are performed, a colotomy just above the stricture is made and the head of an EEA stapler is placed into the lumen of the bowel. The body of the stapler is then introduced transanally and connected to the head of the stapler, passing the shaft of the stapler through the stricture. The stapler is then closed and fired to create a new anastomosis through the stricture. The stapler is removed transanally, and the colotomy is closed.

CONCLUSION

Adherence to intraoperative techniques, as described in other chapters, minimizes postoperative anastomotic complications. Monitoring, with a high index of suspicion, during the postoperative period is crucial to early identification of problems that may occur. This is important, because early diagnostic evaluation of unusual findings and management aid in minimizing the morbidity associated with anastomotic complications.

REFERENCES

1. Beart RW, Kelly KA. Randomized prospective evaluation of the EEA stapler after anterior colonic resection. Dis Colon Rectum 24:236, 1981.
2. Brennan SS, Pickford IR, Evans M, Pollack AV. Staples or sutures for colonic anastomosis—A controlled clinical trial. Br J Surg 69:722, 1982.
3. Akyol AM, McGregor JR, Galloway OJ, Murray G, George WD. Recurrence of colorectal cancer after sutured and stapled large bowel anastomosis. Br J Surg 78:1297-1300, 1991.
4. Manson PN, Carmen ML, Collar JA, Veidenheimer MC. Anterior resection for adenocarcinoma—Lahey Clinic experience from 1963 through 1969. Am J Surg 131:434-441, 1976.
5. Smith LE. Anastomosis with EEA stapler after anterior colonic resection. Dis Colon Rectum 24:236, 1981.
6. Goligher JC. Surgery of the Anus, Rectum and Colon. London: Baillière Tindall, 1984.
7. Schrock TR, Deveney CW, Dunphy JE. Factors contributing to leakage of colonic anastomoses. Ann Surg 177:513, 1973.
8. Aszodi A, Ponski J. Effects of corticosteroid on the healing bowel anastomosis. Am Surg 10:546, 1984.
9. Haydock DA, Hill GL. Improved wound healing response in surgical patients receiving intravenous nutrition. Br J Surg 74:320, 1987.
10. Jex RK, Van Heerden JA, Wolff BG, et al. Gastrointestinal anastomoses. Factors affecting early complications. Ann Surg 206:138, 1987.
11. Post S, Betzler M, von Ditfurth B, et al. Risks of intestinal anastomoses in Crohn's disease. Ann Surg 213:37, 1991.
12. Jonsson K, Jiborn H, Zederfeldt B. Healing of anastomoses after obstruction of small intestine. Surg Gynecol Obstet 167:324, 1988.
13. Yesilkaya Y, Soyhan N, Sen M, Artas Y. The effects of different suture techniques on collagen metabolism in experimental distal colonic anastomoses. Br J Surg 72:987-989, 1985.
14. Yamakawa T, Snyder Platin C, Sobel S, Morgenstern L. Healing of colonic anastomoses following resection for experimental "diverticulitis." Arch Surg 103:17-20, 1971.
15. Vernava AM, Fitzgerald SD, Longo WE, Kaminski DL. Sutured versus stapled colonic anastomoses: Does method affect outcome? Contemp Surg 43:337-340, 1993.
16. Fielding LP, Stewart-Brown S, Blesovsky L, Kearney G. Anastomotic integrity after operations for large-bowel cancer: A multicenter study. Br Med J 281:411-414, 1980.
17. West of Scotland and Highland Anastomosis Study Group. Suturing or stapling in gastrointestinal surgery: A prospective randomized study. Br J Surg 78:337, 1991.
18. Kirkegaard P, Christianson J, Hjortrup A. Anterior resection for midrectal cancer with the EEA stapling instrument. Am J Surg 140:312-314, 1980.
19. Cade D, Gallagher P, Schofield PF, Rurner L. Complications of anterior resection of the rectum using the EEA stapling device. Br J Surg 68:339-340, 1981.
20. Cutait DE, Cutait R, DaSilva JH, et al. Stapled anastomoses in colorectal surgery. Dis Colon Rectum 24:155-160, 1981.
21. Heald RJ, Leicester RJ. The low stapled anastomoses. Br J Surg 68:333-337, 1981.
22. Killingbeck M. Intrapelvic restorative resection for carcinoma of the large bowel. Hunterian lecture. Ann R Coll Surg Engl 1:1-52, 1981.
23. Goligher JC. The use of circular staplers for the construction of colorectal anastomoses after anterior resection. In Heberer G, Denecke H, eds. Colorectal Surgery. Berlin: Springer-Verlag, 1982, pp 107-113.
24. Leff EI, Hoexter B, Labow SB, Eisenstat TE, Rubin RJ, Salvati IP. The EEA stapler in low colorectal anastomoses: Initial experience. Dis Colon Rectum 25:704-707, 1982.

25. Polglase AL, Cunningham IG, Hughes ESR, Masterson JP. Initial clinical experience with the EEA stapler. Aust N Z J Surg 52:71-75, 1982.
26. Vezeridis M, Evans TJ, Mittelman A, Ledesma EJ. EEA stapler in low anterior anastomosis. Dis Colon Rectum 25:364-367, 1982.
27. Anderberg B, Enblad P, Sjodahl R, Wetterfors J. The EEA stapling device in anterior resection for carcinoma of the rectum. Br J Surg 149:99-103, 1983.
28. Fegiz G, Angelini L, Bezzi M. Rectal cancer: Restorative surgery with the EEA stapling device. Int Surg 68:13-18, 1983.
29. Isbister WH, Beasley SW, Dowle CS. The EEA stapler—A Wellington experience. Coloproctology 6:323-326, 1983.
30. Kennedy HL, Rothenberger DA, Goldberg SM, et al. Colocolostomy and coloproctostomy utilizing the circular intraluminal stapling devices. Dis Colon Rectum 26:145-148, 1983.
31. Fazio VW, Jagelman DG, Lavery IC, McGonagle BA. Evaluation of the proximate ILS circular stapler: A prospective study. Ann Surg 201:108-114, 1985.
32. McGinn FP, Gartell PC, Clifford PC, Brunton FJ. Staples or sutures for low colorectal anastomoses: A prospective randomized trial. Br J Surg 72:603-605, 1985.
33. Gillen P, Peel AL. Comparison of the mortality, morbidity and incidence of local recurrence in patients with rectal cancer treated by either stapled anterior resection or abdominoperineal resection. Br J Surg 73:339-341, 1986.
34. Antonsen HK, Kronborg O. Early complications after low anterior resection for rectal cancer using the EEA stapling device: A prospective trial. Dis Colon Rectum 30:579-583, 1987.
35. Zannini G, Renda A, Lepore R, Coppola L, Landi R, Dantonio M. Mechanical anterior resection for carcinoma of the mid rectum: Long term results. Int Surg 72:18-19, 1987.
36. Belli L, Beati CA, Frangi M, Aseni P, Rondinara GF. Outcome of patients with rectal cancer treated by stapled anterior resection. Br J Surg 75:422-424, 1988.
37. Malmberg M, Graffner H, Ling L, Olsson SA. Recurrence and survival after anterior resection of the rectum using the end to end anastomotic stapler. Surg Gynecol Obstet 163:231-234, 1986.
38. Kyzer S, Gordon PH. Experience with the use of the circular stapler in rectal surgery. Dis Colon Rectum 35:696-706, 1992.
39. Karanjia ND, Corder AP, Holdsworth PJ, Heald RJ. Risk of peritonitis and fatal septicaemia and the need to defunction the low anastomosis. Br J Surg 78:196, 1991.
40. Griffin FD, Knight CD, Whitaker JM. The double stapling technique for low anterior resection. Ann Surg 211:745-752, 1990.
41. Graffner H, Fredlund P, Olsen S, et al. Protective colostomy in low anterior resection of the rectum using the EEA stapling instrument. A randomised study. Dis Colon Rectum 26:87-90, 1983.
42. Fielding LP, Stewart Brown S, Hittinger R, Blesovsky L. Covering stoma for elective anterior resection of the rectum: An outmoded operation. Am J Surg 147:524-530, 1984.
43. Novell JR, Lewis AAM. Preoperative observation of marginal artery bleeding: A predictor of anastomotic leakage. Br J Surg 77:137, 1990.
44. Shepard AP, Reidel GL. Continuous measurement of intestinal mucosal blood flow by laser Doppler velicometry. Am J Physiol 242:G668-G672, 1982.
45. Mann A, Fazio VW, Lucas F. A comparative study of the use of fluorescein and the Doppler device in the determination of intestinal viability. Surg Gynecol Obstet 154:53-55, 1982.
46. Carter M, Fantani G, Sammartano R, et al. Qualitative and quantitative fluorescence for determining intestinal viability. Am J Surg 147:117-123, 1984.

47. Locke R, Hauser CJ, Shoemaker WC. The use of surface oximetry to assess bowel viability. Arch Surg 119:1252-1256, 1984.
48. Furst MB, Stromberg BV, Blatchford GJ, Christensen MA, Thorson AG. Colonic anastomoses: Bursting strength after corticosteroid treatment. Dis Colon Rectum 37:12-15, 1994.
49. Goligher JC. The use of circular staplers for the construction of colorectal anastomoses after anterior resection. In Heberer G, Denecke H, eds. Colorectal Surgery. Berlin: Springer-Verlag, 1982, pp 107-113.
50. Longo WE, Milsom JW, Lavery IC, Church JC, Oakley JR, Fazio VW. Pelvic abscess after colon and rectal surgery—What is appropriate management? Dis Colon Rectum 36:936-941, 1993.
51. Haaga Jr, Weinstein AJ. CT-guided percutaneous aspiration and drainage of abscess. Am J Radiol 135:1187-1194, 1980.
52. Dobrin PB, Gully PH, Greenlee HB, et al. Radiologic diagnosis of an intra-abdominal abscess. Do multiple tests help? Arch Surg 121:41-46 1986.
53. Robbins AH, Pugatch RD, Gerzof SG, et al. Further observations on the medical efficacy of computed tomography of the chest and abdomen. Radiology 137:719-725, 1980.
54. Goldman M, Ambrose NS, Drolc Z, Hawker RJK, McCollum C. Indium-111 labelled leucocytes in the diagnosis of abdominal abscess. Br J Surg 74:184-186, 1987.
55. Church JM. Surgical management of anastomotic leaks and intra-abdominal sepsis. In Rothenberger DA, ed. Colorectal Disease: Challenging Problems. Probl Gen Surg 9:634-640, 1992.
56. Soeters PB, Ebeid AM, Fischer JE. Review of 404 patients with gastrointestinal fistulas: Impact of parenteral nutrition. Ann Surg 190:189, 1979.
57. Nubiola P, Badia JM, Martinez-Rodenas F, et al. Treatment of 27 postoperative enterocutaneous fistulas with the long half-life somatostatin analog SMS 201-995. Ann Surg 210:56, 1989.
58. Rothenberger DA, Finne CO. Radical surgery for early rectal cancer: The case against it. In Simmons R, Udekwu A, eds. Debates in Clinical Surgery. Chicago: Year Book Medical Publishers, 1990.
59. Killingbeck MJ. Indications for local excision of rectal cancer. Br J Surg 72(Suppl):S54-S56, 1985.
60. Gazet JC. Parks' coloanal pull-through anastomosis for severe, complicated radiation proctitis. Dis Colon Rectum 28:110-114, 1985.
61. Cooke SAR, DeMoor NG. The surgical treatment of the radiation-damaged rectum. Br J Surg 68:488-492, 1981.
62. Makabeli G, Williams LG. Repair of defective EEA anastomosis. Dis Colon Rectum 27:490-491, 1984.
63. Ross AHM. Rectal stricture resection using the EEA Autostapler. Br J Surg 67:281-282, 1980.

CHAPTER 7

Urologic Complications of Colorectal Surgery

MARTHA B. ROACH
D. SCOTT DONALDSON

URETHRAL INJURIES

Urologists agree that the most common reason for an intraoperative call to the operating room is to place a urethral catheter. The essentials of catheter placement include adequate lubrication, cephalad extension of the penis in males, and slow constant pressure on the catheter. The balloon should be inflated only when the entire catheter is in the penis and when clear urine return is established. Most standard catheter kits contain a 16 or 18 Fr catheter. Should one fail to pass either of these, one should attempt to pass an 18 Fr catheter coudé. If it is impossible to pass a catheter coudé, a urologist should be consulted. Inflation of a catheter balloon in the posterior urethra or creation of a false passage in the urethra could require cystoscopy or suprapubic catheterization.

Urethral catheterization has become somewhat more complicated with the introduction of artificial urinary sphincters and penile prosthesis. A penile prosthesis provides minimal difficulty with adequate lubrication of the catheter and cephalad extension of the penis. A urinary sphincter device, however, requires a working knowledge of its mechanics (Fig. 7-1). Ideally, the sphincter should be deflated before a well-lubricated catheter is placed. There are several different types of sphincters, each with different mechanisms. The patient is the expert regarding his or her sphincter and can explain and activate it. Should a question arise concerning the function of an artificial device, a urologist should be consulted. A catheter should never be placed if the sphincter cuff is activated, because sphincter erosion into the urethra will result.

Urethral surgical injuries are associated with extensive rectal neoplasms or inflammatory conditions that destroy surgical planes. Typically, urethral injuries are identified at surgery because of the previously placed indwelling catheter. The catheter serves as an excellent landmark and guide and is mandatory in extensive pelvic operations. Injuries not identified at surgery will become manifest postoperatively as urinary extravasation through the perineal wound or rectum. A retrograde urethrogram will confirm the diagnosis. Treatment options vary

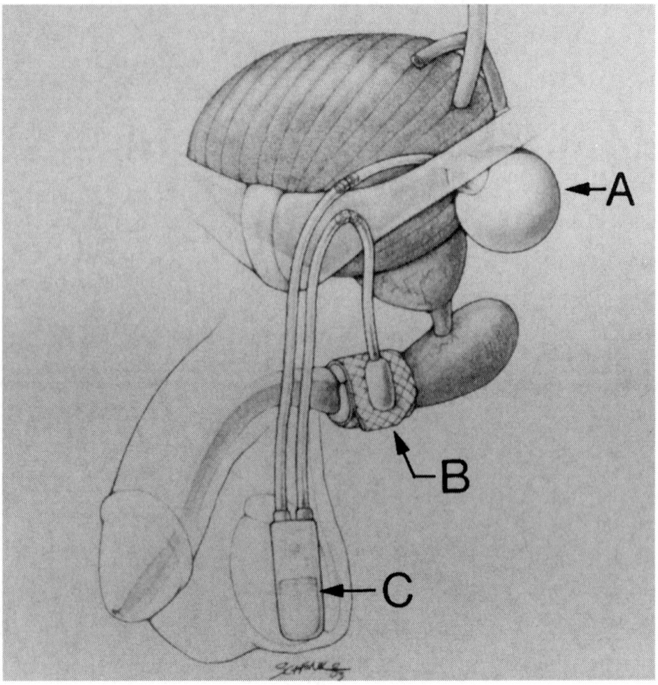

Fig. 7-1 Artificial urinary sphincter (AVS-800, American Medical Systems, Minnetonka, Minn.). *A*, reservoir; *B*, cuff; *C*, pump.

with the extent of injury. Small, incidental injuries identified intraoperatively may be treated by primary closure with 5-0 interrupted absorbable sutures and urethral catheterization for 3 weeks.[1] More extensive injuries require suprapubic catheterization and delayed imaging and reconstruction.[2] There are many descriptions of rectourethral fistula closure. Turner-Warwick[2] described an abdominal approach with interposition of omentum. Others have described a perineal approach in which the rectum and sphincters are divided posteriorly, the fistula is closed in layers, and the rectum is reconstructed.[3] Transrectal mucosal advancements with and without fecal diversion have also been described.[4,5] Rectourethral fistulas and Crohn's disease with rectal sparing may be treated with a rectal advancement flap.[4] The approach taken must allow for adequate fistula excision, layered closure, and mucosal advancement over the fistulous tract. If the pelvis has been irradiated, the gracilis muscle can be rotated through a subcutaneous tunnel and interposed between the rectum and urethra.[6] Rotation of the rectal fistula laterally to bring it to a different level of the urethra may also aid fistula closure. After surgery, the urinary stream should be diverted for 3 to 4 weeks with a Foley catheter and suprapubic cystostomy.

Prostatic and seminal vesicle injuries have been described in case reports in both the surgical and urologic literature.[7] These conditions are manifested as perineal drainage. A retrograde urethrogram is diagnostic. This condition is treated with urethral catheterization for 1 month.[8] If this fails, a York-Mason type of repair should be performed.[9] The fistulous tract must be excised, and the urethral and rectal mucosa must be free of tethering. The urethral and rectal mucosa are closed, and muscle or omental tissue is interposed.

To summarize, adequate lubrication is the key to successful urethral catheterization, suprapubic catheter drainage is required with most urethral injuries, and a retrograde urethrogram is the best test to identify a urethral injury.

URETERAL INJURIES

Ureteral injury is the most common intraoperative urologic complication. The prevalence of ureteral injury has been reported to range from 1% to 10%. In a review of 24 patients from Parkland Hospital, 12.5% of ureteral injuries occurred during colon surgery.[10] As with all complications, early identification is the key to controlling morbidity. A review of 30 ureteral injuries demonstrated that only 23% were identified intraoperatively.[11] Ureteral stents have been proposed as a mechanism to prevent ureteral injury. Stents, however, do not prevent injury. Ureteral stents do improve intraoperative identification of the ureter and ureteral injuries.[12] Large pelvic masses or severe inflammatory conditions are excellent opportunities to use ureteral stents. Stents may be placed preoperatively with a cystoscope or intraoperatively through a cystotomy, as previously described.[13] The most important aspects in avoiding injury are adequate anatomic knowledge and careful dissection.

Ureteral injuries occur in three typical locations: at the takeoff of the inferior mesenteric artery, where the uterine vessels cross the pelvic brim, and between the lateral rectal ligaments (Fig. 7-2). The ureter courses retroperitoneally anterior to the psoas muscle. It crosses the iliac vessels and enters the pelvis at the level of the bifurcation of the internal and external iliac arteries. Abdominal masses, including abscesses, adenopathy, or tumor, will distort and laterally displace the ureteral course. The right ureter is adjacent to the cecum, terminal ileum, and appendix; the left ureter is related to the descending and sigmoid colon and their mesenteric vessels.

The ureter tends to adhere to the peritoneum during its reflection rather than stay adherent to underlying tissue. The ureter may often be identified by its peristaltic response to light touch. Studies of both the surgical and gynecologic literature revealed that preoperative urologic evaluation of the genitourinary system with intravenous pyelography does not aid in prevention of ureteral injury.[14,15]

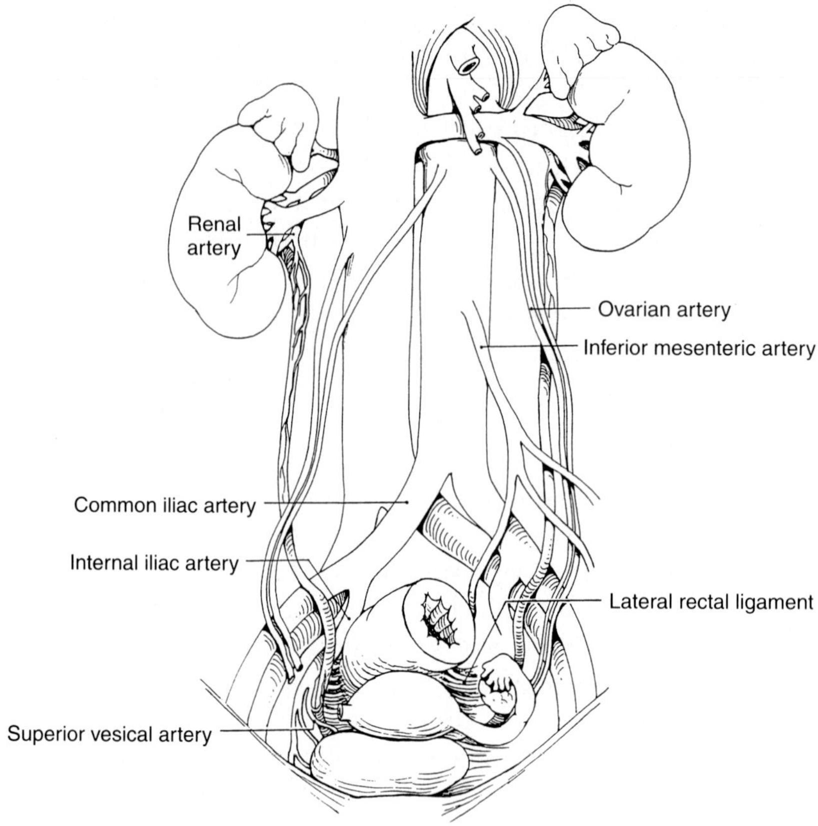

Fig. 7-2 Anatomy of the ureter.

Types of Injuries

Types of injuries include devascularization, crush, transection, and avulsion. Injuries identified intraoperatively may often be treated with primary reanastomosis. Ureteral injury with fever, flank pain, or persistent urinary drainage from the wound is the most debilitating.

Devascularization. Devascularization injuries result from the sacrifice of segmental ureteral blood supply. Arteries that contribute blood supply include the aorta and renal, gonadal, inferior mesenteric, and iliac vessels. The midportion of the ureter has the poorest blood supply and thus is most prone to vascular injury. Dissection should always be lateral to the abdominal ureter, because the blood supply is medial. Dissection in the pelvis should be medially approached, because the blood supply is lateral. Vascular compromise injuries will become manifest postoperatively as a fistula or stricture (Figs. 7-3 and 7-4).

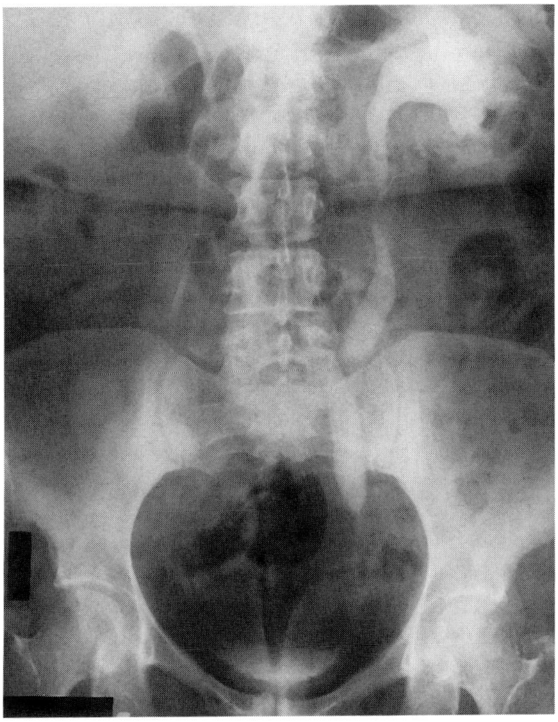

Fig. 7-3 Intravenous pyelogram demonstrates ureteral stricture inferior to the pelvic brim.

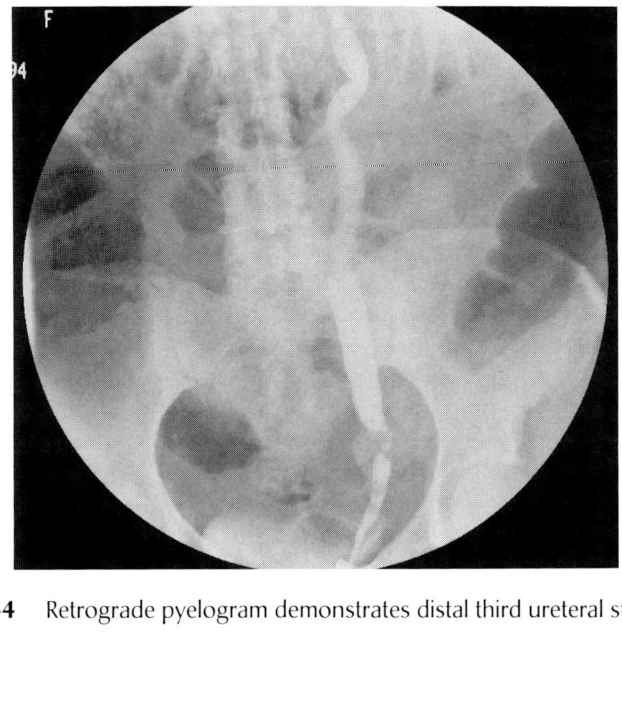

Fig. 7-4 Retrograde pyelogram demonstrates distal third ureteral stricture.

Intraoperatively, a devacularized ureter may appear discolored, may lack peristalsis, or will not bleed at the transected site. Repair must include debridement of the ureteral edges and primary reanastomosis of spatulated ends.

Ligation or crush injury. Ligation and crush injuries, if identified intraoperatively, may be treated with release of the clamp or ligature followed by ureteral catheterization for 5 to 7 days.[16] If the injury is not identified until the postoperative period, retrograde stent placement may be attempted. If this fails, a percutaneous nephrostomy tube must be placed to preserve renal function. Untreated crush injuries may lead to ureteral strictures and chronic renal obstruction.

Transection. Transection injuries, when promptly identified, and with adequate length, may be repaired primarily with spatulated ends. If a section of ureter is removed, a more sophisticated repair is required.

Diagnosis

If a question of ureteral injury develops intraoperatively, there are techniques to aid the diagnosis. Methylene blue may be injected intravenously, which will be seen extravasating and may stain a devascularized ureter transmurally. Fluid boluses with furosemide (Lasix) may be given to produce prompt diuresis, causing bulging and peristalsis of the ureter. Intravenous pyelography may be performed in the operating room to further aid diagnosis.

After surgery, intravenous pyelography is the best test to identify ureteral injury. If there is a question of injury or for further delineation of the site of injury, retrograde pyelography is indicated. If there is incomplete obstruction, a double-J stent may be placed retrograde. If this fails, the kidney must be percutaneously drained and delayed definitive repair planned.

Repair of the Injured Ureter

Distal third of the ureter. The procedure of choice for lower-third injuries is ureteroneocystotomy. The ureter is mobilized proximally, the bladder is opened, and a clamp is passed through the bladder mucosa, thus creating a new orifice. The ureter is then tunneled submucosally to the site of ureteral entry into the bladder. A stent may be placed intraoperatively. The psoas hitch is the procedure to perform if it is impossible to mobilize an adequate length of ureter to reimplant into the bladder. The superior bladder pedicle, on the contralateral side of the injury, may be released and the bladder rotated and advanced onto the psoas muscle. The posterior bladder is then attached to the psoas muscle. The ureter may then be reanastomosed without tension (Fig. 7-5).

The Boari flap is highly reliable to replace extensive loss of the distal ureter. A flap of bladder is raised as a rectangle and then tapered into a tube, and the distalmost portion is anastomosed to the ureter (Fig. 7-6). This neoconduit is

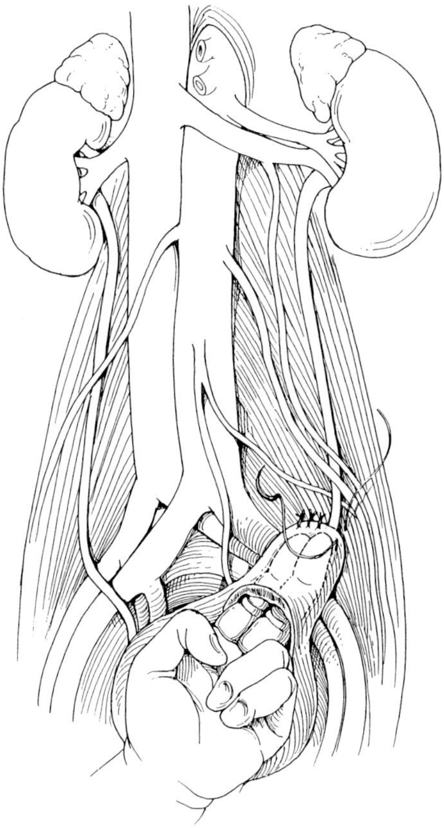

Fig. 7-5 Psoas bladder hitch. Mobilized bladder is anchored to psoas muscle and the ureter is reimplanted.

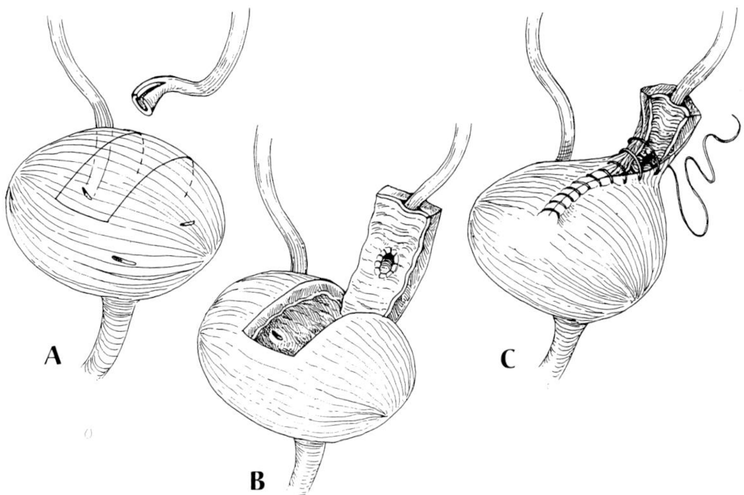

Fig. 7-6 Boari or bladder flap procedure. **A,** Creation of tapered bladder flap, based posteriorly. **B,** Submucosal ureteral reimplantation. **C,** Closure of bladder flap.

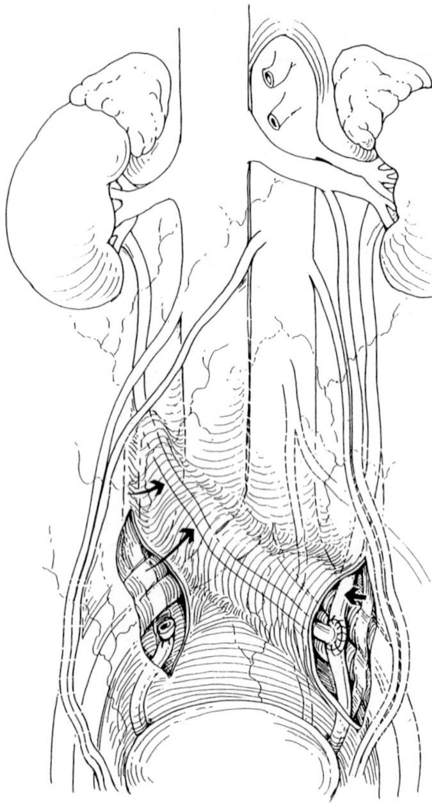

Fig. 7-7 Right-to-left transureteroureterostomy. Note retroperitoneal tunnel anterior to the great vessels.

closed in two layers and a stent is placed in the ureteral anastomosis. There are reports of this flap spanning 18 cm.[17] Finally, transureteroureterostomy is an effective method to replace the ureter in carefully selected patients[18] (Fig. 7-7). This technique is used when the lower ureter is damaged and the psoas hitch or Boari flap procedures are not possible. The damaged ureter is passed through a retroperitoneal tunnel anterior to the great vessels and reanastomosed to the contralateral ureter. Great care must be taken not to compromise the ureter's segmental blood supply. The gonadal vessels may be mobilized with the ureter if necessary. The donor ureter is then spatulated and anastomosed with 45-degree angulation. A stent need not be placed unless the tissue has been compromised with radiation, chemotherapy, or extensive infection. As always, the ureter should be handled gently. The greatest risk of this operation is transforming a unilateral ureteral injury into a bilateral problem.

A

B

C

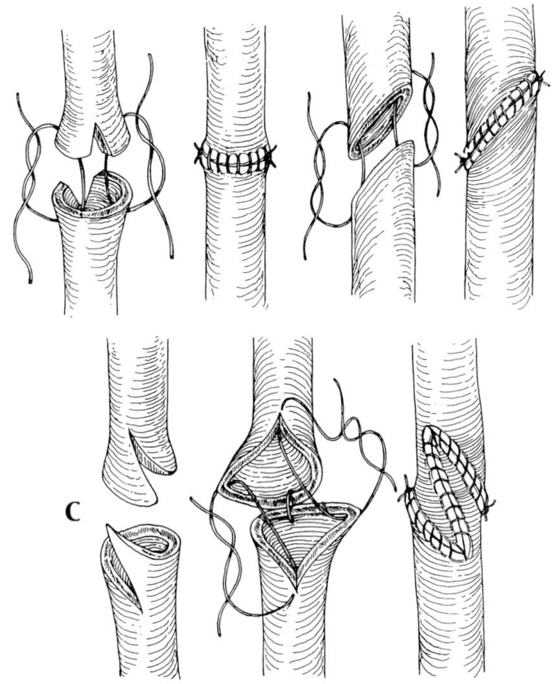

Fig. 7-8 Ureteroureterostomy. Ureteral margins are spatulated and running locked sutures are placed. **A**, Horizontal anastomosis. **B**, Oblique anastomosis. **C**, Zigzag anastomosis.

Middle portion of the ureter. The preferred technique for midureteral repair is ureteroureterostomy. The ureteral ends are spatulated and closed with running absorbable 5-0 sutures (Fig. 7-8). A ureteral stent should be placed and the anastomotic site drained.

Proximal third of the ureter. Proximal third ureteral injuries are the most challenging. Complete ureteral replacement with ileum has been well described since the 1950s. A segment of ileum, approximately 25 cm, is mobilized. The ileum is then passed through the mesocolon to the retroperitoneal position.[19] The proximal anastomosis is made to the remnant ureter at the level of the renal pelvis. The proximal ileum is not tapered. The distal ileum is trimmed of redundant tissue and anastomosed widely to the bladder (Fig. 7-9).

Renal transplantation has aided in development of the technique of renal autotransplantation. The affected kidney is carefully removed and immediately chilled in iced Ringer's solution. The artery is perfused with the solution until venous effluent is clear. The kidney may then be autotransplanted into the iliac

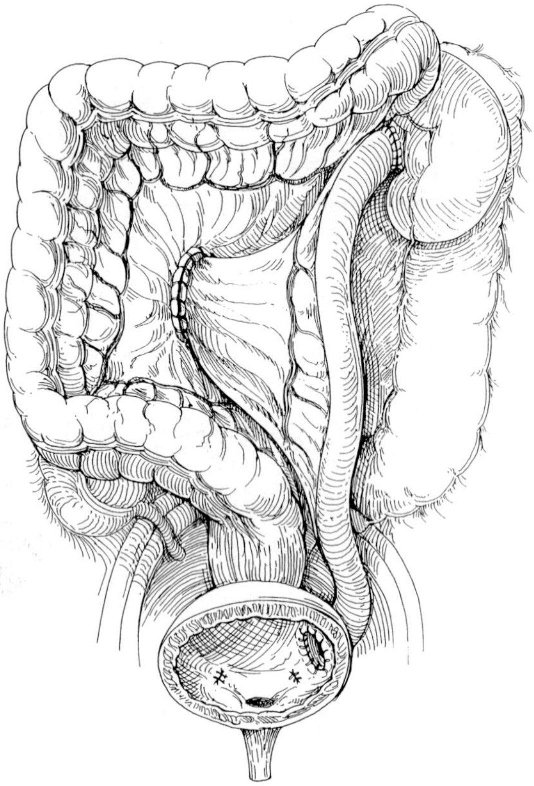

Fig. 7-9 Ureteral replacement with ileum. Left colon is retracted medially, and ileum is brought through a hiatus in the colonic mesentary. Ileal ureter is in retroperitoneal position.

fossa. The artery and vein are anastomosed to the iliac or other available vessels, and the ureter is anastomosed to the bladder with a technique chosen on the basis of the amount of ureter available.

BLADDER INJURY

Bladder injuries have long been recognized as both a part of colorectal disease and a complication of colon surgery. The very intimate relationship between the rectum, sigmoid colon, and bladder predisposes the bladder to injury during surgery of extensive inflammatory or neoplastic conditions. An extensive review of 2000 abdominal perineal resections by Lapides and Tank[20] revealed the frequency of bladder injury to be less than 5%.

Injuries recognized intraoperatively typically may be closed primarily with few long-term complications. Those injuries not recognized immediately will demonstrate evidence of enterovesicular fistulas or persistent perineal drainage.

The delineation of the injury may be difficult to demonstrate. A colovesical fistula may be successfully demonstrated on a CT scan obtained with contrast material in the bladder.[21] However, a recent study cited CT performed with oral contrast material only as the best diagnostic test.[22] A CT scan would demonstrate a urinoma or abscess, either of which portend fistula formation. Many authors agree that a lower GI barium study, cystoscopy, or cystography with lateral views may also be helpful.

Repair of a bladder injury depends on the site of the injury. A cystotomy in the anterior surface of the bladder may easily be closed with two layers of absorbable suture with a watertight method. The bladder should be drained with a urethral catheter for 5 to 7 days. The prevesicle space should also be drained perioperatively.

Injury to the posterior bladder requires a much more conservative approach. The surgeon must be concerned about and assess the patency and integrity of the ureters. If the tear is small, the bladder may be closed primarily. However, if there is any question, the bladder should be opened anteriorly and the posterior tear closed from the interior. At this time the patency of the ureters may be assessed. The ureters should efflux clear urine bilaterally. Indigo carmine or methylene blue, along with furosemide, may be given intravenously to better identify efflux. Ureteral stents may be passed retrograde to assess patency. If the distal ureter is damaged, it must be repaired as previously described.

Vesicoperineal fistulas are identified by urine drainage from the perineal wound. A cystogram will enable clear diagnosis of this condition. Small fistulas in nonirradiated tissue and without previous chemotherapy may close with urethral drainage of urine alone. Most authors believe the patient should undergo suprapubic catheter drainage for a minimum of 6 weeks. If there is a history of radiation cystitis, the bladder should be drained suprapubicly for up to 6 months before surgical repair.

Enterovesical fistulas that develop postoperatively typically are associated with abscess formation[10] (Fig. 7-10). Symptoms include pneumaturia, fecaluria, and persistent urinary tract infections. Attempts to culture the urine may be unsuccessful, because the culture will continue to grow multiple organisms and may be discarded as a contaminated specimen. Prompt surgical intervention, drainage of the abscess, excision of the fistulous tract, closure of the bladder, and diversion of the fecal stream are required. We believe the fistulous edges of the bladder should be trimmed and the bladder closed with a watertight method. The bladder should then be drained for 10 days.

RENAL INJURY

Direct renal injury is rare in colorectal surgery. McAninch et al.[23] have reported that 90% of renal injuries can be managed without nephrectomy. Although this

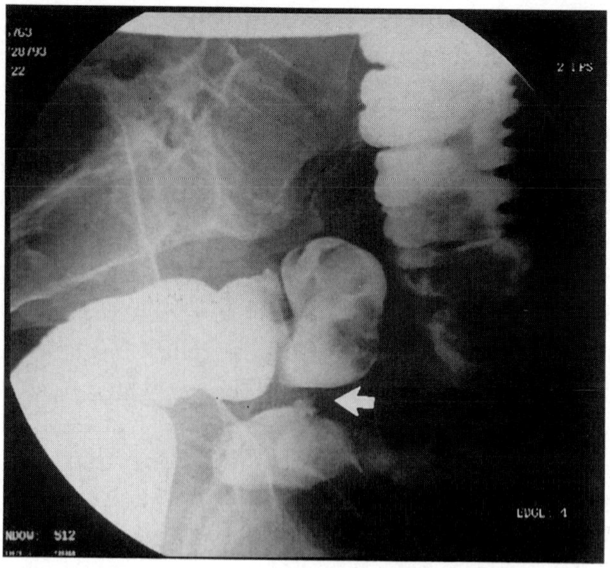

Fig. 7-10 Enterovesical fistula *(arrow)*.

work does not address iatrogenic injuries, the principle of renal salvage must be adhered to. Every attempt to evaluate the extent of injury and assessment of the entire genitourinary tract must be made before repair. The literature is full of anomalous solitary kidneys that were removed, necessitating dialysis or transplantation.[24,25] Pelvic kidneys have an anomalous blood supply that generally arises from multiple arteries along the aorta and iliac vessels. Ten percent are solitary,[26] and they may easily be mistaken for a pelvic mass because they are not reniform but discoid. An intraoperative intravenous pyelogram will provide evidence of both the renal injury and the function of the contralateral kidney. Simple palpation of the unaffected kidney does not delineate function. An intraoperative angiogram may be obtained to assess renal artery integrity. If caliceal injury is suspected, intravenous indigo carmine may be injected to delineate the extent of injury.

Once the injury has been well defined, formal repair may be planned. Minor renal lacerations or penetrating injuries may be repaired primarily with absorbable sutures and buttressed with fat, omentum, or hemostatic materials. All necrotic tissue should be debrided until the renal parenchyma bleeds; the bleeding should then be controlled with suture ligation of individual vessels. If a major salvage procedure is undertaken, such as partial nephrectomy, extraperitoneal drainage of the renal bed must be adequate. Nephrostomy tubes may be necessary with ureteropelvic reanastomosis or heminephrectomy. If a major vascular injury occurs and the patient's intraoperative condition allows, every attempt to reestablish vascular integrity should be made.

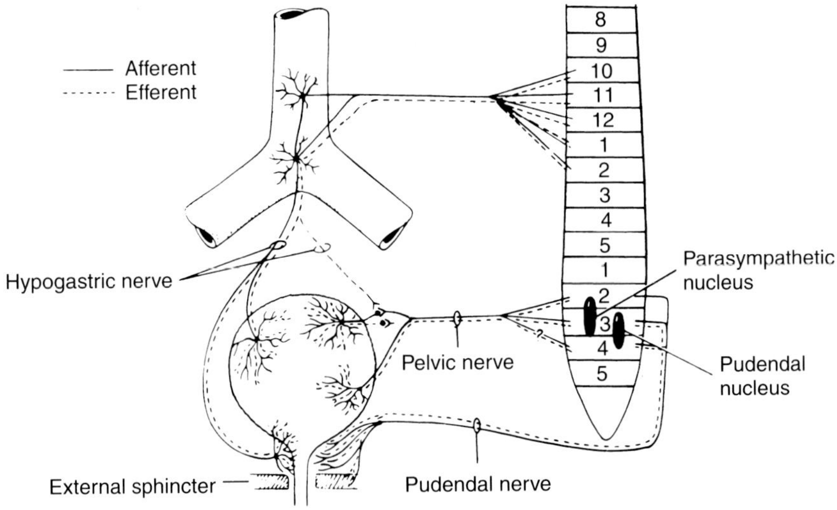

Fig. 7-11 Innervation of the lower urinary tract.

ARTIFICIAL DEVICES

Since the introduction of the artificial urinary sphincter in 1972 (American Medical Systems, Minnetonka, Minn.) and subsequently the inflatable penile prosthesis, thousands of these devices have been implanted worldwide. The penile prosthesis has one to three components, whereas the artificial sphincter has three components. The three component systems include a reservoir, pump, cuff or prosthesis, and interconnecting tubing. These devices are silicon and are usually filled with radiopaque fluid. After surgery a capsule will form around each component. The reservoir is typically found suprapubically in the space of Retzius. The pump is located in the right hemiscrotum. Every attempt should be made to avoid entering this capsule or exposing it to infectious material. If injury to any portion of the device is suspected, a radiograph will confirm extravasation of fluid. If any component becomes contaminated, it should be irrigated vigorously and the capsule closed. Every attempt to salvage these devices should be made unless the patient's condition warrants removal. The fate of these devices should be discussed with the patient before surgery.

BLADDER DYSFUNCTION

To completely understand the potential effects of colorectal surgery on the urinary tract, a detailed description of the basic neuroanatomy of the urinary tract is necessary. The lower urinary tract innervation has three basic levels of input. The parasympathetic nerve supply, which causes the bladder to contract, exits the spinal cord at the S2 to S4 level (Fig. 7-11). It sends a presynaptic fiber via the pelvic nerve[27] to synapse on the bladder peripherally and provide parasympathetic innervation. The preponderance of these nerve fibers are lateral to the superior rectum bilaterally.

The sympathetic nerve supply to the bladder arises at the level of L2 to L4 and sends a presynaptic fiber to the sympathetic ganglion, which is adjacent to the spinal cord. A synapse occurs in the sympathetic ganglion, and a postsynaptic fiber is sent to the bladder. This postsynaptic, sympathetic fiber provides relaxation of the bladder body and contraction of the bladder neck. The overall affect of the sympathetic nervous system on the bladder is to improve storage of urine.

The somatic motor innervation to the striated pelvic floor musculature exits at the S2 to S4 cord level and travels through the pudendal nerve to the striated sphincter.[28]

The parasympathetic nerve supply to the bladder is the component of innervation that is most often injured during colorectal surgery, by transection of the nerve supply or neuropraxia. The most common bladder injury is detrusor areflexia or a poorly contractile bladder body. More peripheral injuries end in pudendal nerve weakening and result in a week striated sphincter muscle and a poorly contractile bladder. Rarely is the sympathetic nerve supply to the bladder damaged in colorectal surgery.

Should urinary retention occur postoperatively, a multifactorial approach should be taken initially. Any anticholinergic medication, epidural anesthesia, central narcotic anesthesia, prolonged bed rest, and alpha$_1$ agonist medications can contribute to urinary retention. In addition, myotonic injury of the bladder body secondary to overdistention intraoperatively or perioperatively can also cause urinary retention.

In the immediate perioperative period, Foley catheter drainage of the bladder for 4 or 5 days is optimal treatment. After the initial perioperative period, clean intermittent catheterization with a 12 to 14 Fr Foley catheter should be instituted every 4 to 6 hours. Administration of any drugs that may contribute to urine retention should be minimized if possible.

Any patient with urinary retention that continues longer than 6 weeks after surgery should undergo formal urodynamic studies to better discern the nature of the injury (Fig. 7-12). The patient is placed in the upright position on a toilet seat, in front of a fluoroscope. The basic urodynamic tests involve measurement of postvoid residual bladder capacity, perineal EMG studies, complex uroflometry, urethral pressure profile, complex cystometrogram, bladder compliance measurements and abdominal pressure subtraction. A computer analysis of the relationship between abdominal pressure, bladder pressure, and sphincter function is obtained. A typical urodynamic study is demonstrated in Fig. 7-13.

If the bladder dysfunction is caused by transection of the innervation bilaterally, the patient will most likely require clean intermittent catheterization indefinitely. No drugs have been consistently proven to improve bladder function

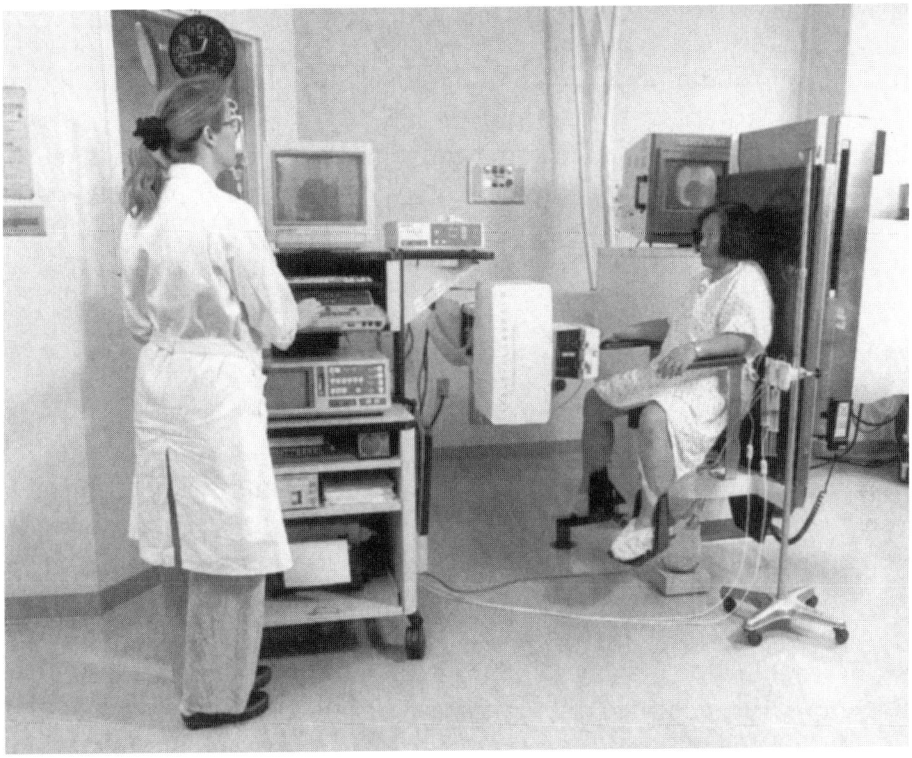

Fig. 7-12 Fluorodynamic study. (Courtesy Liebel-Flarsheim Hydra Vision Systems, Cincinnati, Ohio.)

A

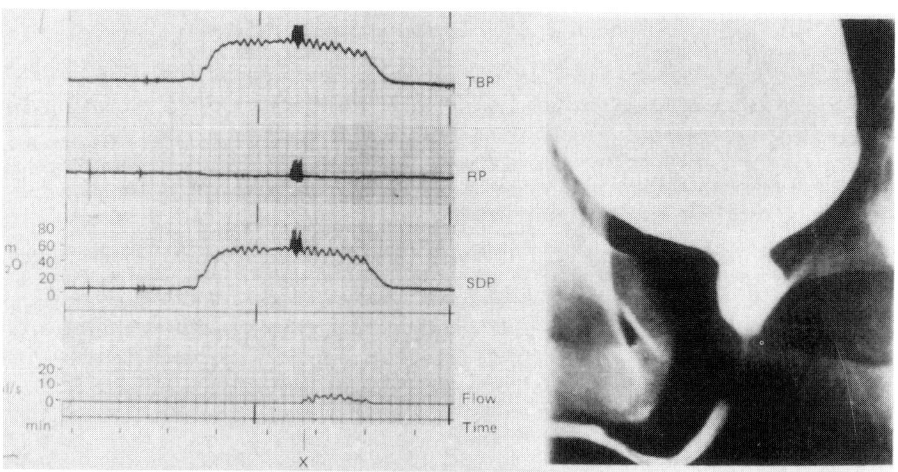

B

Fig. 7-13 **A**, EMG tracing shows abdominal and bladder pressures. **B**, Cystogram.

after such an injury. With a unilateral injury or neuropraxia, some bladder function may return after surgery. Myotonic injuries should improve over time, and drug effects should completely improve over time. Bladder infections and overdistention should be minimized, because both of these complications will delay return of complete bladder function.

In examination of the male patient, the effect of the prostate gland should not be underestimated. All male patients should undergo prostate gland examination, prostate-specific antigen should be measured, and expressed prostatic secretion should be analyzed to rule out low-grade chronic prostatitis as a potential cause of urinary retention.

SEXUAL DYSFUNCTION

Sexual dysfunction has long been associated with rectal surgery in both men and women. Women experience dyspareunia more often with ileorectal anastomosis than with ileostomy (50% versus 10%) for inflammatory bowel disease.[29] The psychologic effect of a stoma has been thought to account for a lower marriage rate among patients with a stoma and a lower rate of premarital sexual activity.[29]

Sexual dysfunction in men is a different phenomenon because of the intimate relationship of the rectum to the nerves responsible for sexual function. Patients undergoing low anterior resection experience ejaculatory absence (60%), erectile impotence (17%), and varying degrees of both (23%).[30] Abdominoperineal resection is associated with sexual dysfunction rates in 50% to 100% of patients.[31-33] Some patients have both impotence and retrograde ejaculation; others have impotence alone, retrograde ejaculation alone, or anejaculation.

Sexual dysfunction can be understood as a failure of erection or a failure to ejaculate. Erection is parasympathetically mediated and is governed by impulses that travel along the nervi ergentes (S1 to S5). These preganglionic fibers enter the pelvic plexus and are joined by sympathetic fibers (T10 to L4) from the hypogastric plexus. The pelvic plexus is adherent to the pelvic wall by surrounding tissue and is usually well removed from the surgical planes.[31] The pelvic plexus then courses inferior and medial to innervate the seminal vesicles, prostate gland, corpora cavernosa, rectum, and sphincter muscles[34] (Fig. 7-14). In general, parasympathetic damage will result in loss of erectile reflex and impotence. Damage to sympathetic pathways in the hypogastric plexus will result in retrograde ejaculation, whereas damage to the mesenteric plexus will cause anejaculation. However, because of the complexity of these nerve plexi, mixed lesions are often seen.

Treatment of erectile dysfunction must be adjusted for the individual patient. Retrograde ejaculation in a patient who wants to father a child can be treated with sympathomimetic agents. If this fails, postejaculatory semen can be collected

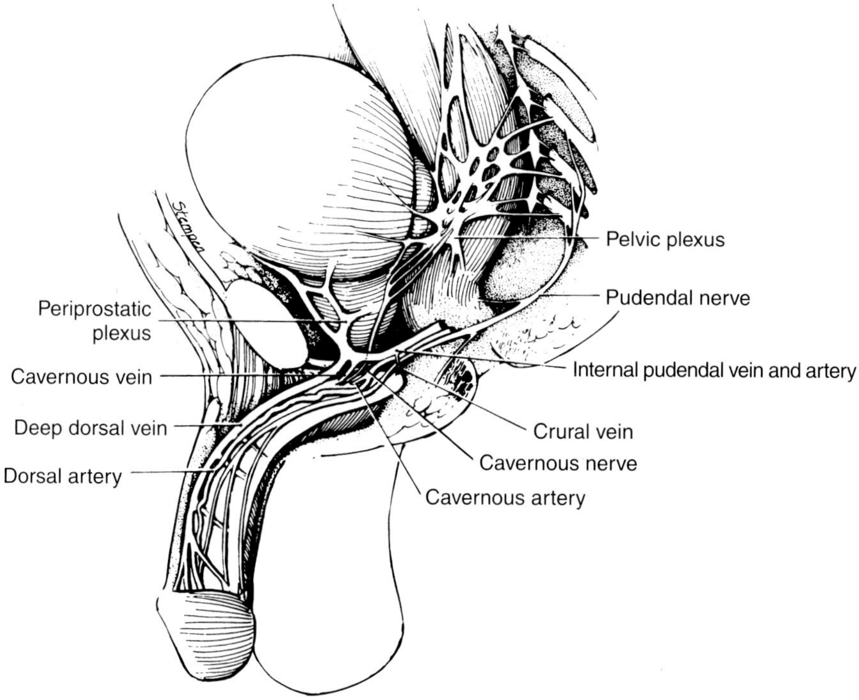

Fig. 7-14 Innervation of the penis. (From Lue TF, Carroll PR, Moore C. The treatment of impotence in cancer patients. In Devita VJ, Hellmans, Rosenberg SA, eds. Important Advances in Oncology, 1989. Philadelphia: JB Lippincott, 1989, pp 193-203. With permission.)

from the bladder and used successfully in artificial insemination. Electroejaculation is possible for a patient with anejaculation. If a patient is completely impotent, treatment options include intracavernous pharmacotherapy, penile vacuum devices, and penile prosthesis. It is important to counsel these men that there are solutions to sexual dysfunction and that most men and their partners are satisfied with the results.[35]

REFERENCES

1. Tank E, Ernest C, et al. Urinary tract complication of anorectal surgery. Am J Surg 123:118-122, 1977.
2. Turner-Warwick R. The use of pedicle grafts in the repair of urinary tract fistulae. Br J Urol 44:644-656, 1972.
3. Mason AY. The place of local resection in the treatment of rectal carcinoma. Proc R Soc Med 63:1259-1262, 1970.
4. Fazio VW, Jones IT, Jagelman DG, et al. Rectourethral fistulas in Crohn's disease. Surg Gynecol Obstet 164:148-150, 1987.

5. Parks AG, Motson RW. Perianal repair of rectoprostatic fistula. Br J Surg 70:725-726, 1983.
6. Ryan JA Jr, Beebe HG, Gibbons RP. Gracilis muscle flap for closure of rectourethral fistula. J Urol 122:124-125, 1979.
7. Mason AY, Kilpatrick FR. Rectoprostatic and rectourethral fistulae. Proc R Soc Med 66:245-246, 1973.
8. Anderson A, Bergdahil. Urological complications following abdominoperineal resection of the rectum. Arch Surg 111:969-971, 1976.
9. Kilpatrick FR, Mason AY. Post-operative recto-prostatic fistula. Br J Urol 41:649-654, 1969.
10. Bright TC III, Peters PC. Ureteral injuries secondary to operative procedures. Report of 24 cases. Urology 9:22-26, 1977.
11. Carlton CE. Injuries of the kidney and ureter. In Harrison JH, Gittees RF, Perlmutter AD, et al., eds. Campbell's Urology, 4th ed. Philadelphia: WB Saunders, 1978, p 896.
12. Leff EI, Groff W, Rubin RJ, et al. Use of ureteral catheters in colonic and rectal surgery. Dis Colon Rectum 25:457-460, 1982.
13. Pennington EE, Ray JE. Intraoperative ureteral catheterization in pelvic and abdominal operations. South Med J 70:179-180, 1977.
14. Kramhoft J, Kronborg O, Backer OG, et al. Urologic complications after operations for anorectal cancer, with an evaluation of preoperative intravenous pyelography. Dis Colon Rectum 18:2,118-122, 1975.
15. Sack RA. The value of intravenous urography prior to abdominal hysterectomy for gynecologic disease. Am J Obstet Gynecol 134:208-212, 1979.
16. Beahrs JR, Beahrs OH, Beahrs MM, et al. Urinary tract complications with rectal surgery. Ann Surg 187:542-548, 1978.
17. Kelami A, Fiedler U, Schmidt V, et al. Replacement of the ureter using the urinary bladder. Urol Res 1:161-165, 1973.
18. Boxer RJ, Johnson SF. Ureteral substitution. Urology 12:269-278, 1978.
19. Pearse HD, Barry JM, Fuchs EF. Intraoperative consultation for the ureter. Urol Clin North Am 12:423-443, 1985.
20. Lapides J, Tank ES. Urinary complications following abdominal perineal resection. Cancer 28:230-235, 1971.
21. Goldman SM, Fishman EK, Gatewood OM, et al. CT in the diagnosis of enterovesical fistulae. Am J Roentgenol 144:1229-1233, 1985.
22. Jarrett TN, Vaughan ED. Accuracy of CT in the diagnosis of colovesicle fistula secondary to diverticular disease. J Urol 153:44-46, 1995.
23. McAninch JW, Carroll PR, Klosterman PW, et al. Renal reconstruction after injury. J Urol 145:932-937, 1991.
24. Granat M, Gordon T, Issaq E, et al. Accidental puncture of pelvic kidney: A rare complication of culdocentesis. Am J Obstet Gynecol 138:233-235, 1980.
25. Zusmer N, Maturo V, Stern M. Pelvic kidney masquerading as an adnexal mass. Rev Interam Radiol 5:95-96, 1980.
26. Perlmutter AD, Retik AB, Bauer SB. Anomalies of the upper urinary tract. In Harrison JH, Gittees RF, Perlmutter AD, et al., eds. Campbell's Urology, 4th ed. Philadelphia: WB Saunders, 1979, pp 1309-1398.
27. el-Badawi A, Shenk EA. A new theory of the innervation of bladder musculature. I. Morphology of the intrinsic vesicle innervation apparatus. J Urol 99:585-587, 1968.
28. Gosling J. The structure of the bladder and urethra in relation to function. Urol Clinic North Am 6:31-38, 1979.

29. Brouillette JN, Pryor E, Fox TA Jr. Evaluation of sexual dysfunction in the female following rectal resection and intestinal stoma. Dis Colon Rectum 24:96-102, 1981.
30. de Bernardinis G, Tuscano D, Negro P, et al. Sexual dysfunction in males following extensive colorectal surgery. Int Surg 66:133-135, 1981.
31. Yeager ES, Van Heerden JA. Sexual dysfunction following proctocolectomy and abdominoperineal resection. Ann Surg 191:169-170, 1980.
32. Fazio VW, Fletcher J, Montague D. Prospective study of the effect of resection of the rectum on male sexual function. World J Surg 4:149-152, 1980.
33. Bernstein WC, Bernstein EF. Sexual dysfunction following radical surgery for cancer of the rectum. Dis Colon Rectum 9:328-332, 1966.
34. Gerstenberg TC, et al. Bladder function after abdominal perineal resection of the rectum for anorectal cancer: Urodynamic investigation before and after operation in a consecutive series. Ann Surg 191:81-86, 1980.
35. Gruner OP, Naas R, Fretheim B, Gjone E. Marital status and sexual adjustment after colectomy. Results in 178 patients operated on for ulcerative colitis. Scand J Gastroenterol 12:193-197, 1977.

CHAPTER 8

General Postoperative Complications

MICHAEL J. STAMOS
CHARLES P. THEUER
CHARLES N. HEADRICK

The success of an operative procedure depends in large part on minimizing postoperative complications. Complications may be related to the primary disease, the operation itself, or to organ systems other than that affected by the primary surgical disease.

Many postoperative complications may be anticipated and measures instituted to prevent them. Often they can be controlled with careful attention to operative technique. Complications that do occur can be minimized with early diagnosis and appropriate treatment. In this chapter, we emphasize methods of prevention, diagnosis, and treatment of common complications of colorectal surgery, including atelectasis, hemorrhage, bowel obstruction, deep venous thrombosis (DVT), and fistulas. Common problems associated with outpatient anorectal surgery and management of patients with retained foreign bodies are discussed.

ATELECTASIS

Postoperative atelectasis is common and may complicate as many as 60% of laparotomies in patients whose pulmonary status is not compromised, when preventive measures are not instituted perioperatively.[1,2] Patients with preexisting lung disease are at even higher risk. Although atelectasis is more common after upper abdominal procedures, colorectal surgery can be complicated by atelectasis in approximately one of three cases.[3]

Atelectasis is caused by alveolar collapse, the mechanism of which is easily understood. The functional residual capacity (FRC) is the volume of air remaining in the lungs after expiration. The closing volume is the volume of lung below which alveolar collapse occurs. When the FRC is less than the closing volume, alveolar collapse ensues. Hence, factors that either increase the closing volume (e.g., bronchitis, mucosal edema from cigarette smoking) or decrease FRC (e.g., obesity, advanced age, anesthesia) predispose to atelectasis.

Patients with clinically significant postoperative atelectasis have pulmonary symptoms including cough, dyspnea, and pleuritic chest pain and systemic signs of fever and tachycardia. Symptoms commonly occur within the first 48 hours of surgery, and atelectasis is the most common cause of fever during this period. Although CT is the most sensitive means to detect atelectasis, a plain chest radiograph is most commonly used for diagnosis and typically shows lower lobe findings that range from subsegmental collapse to lobar collapse. Major atelectasis is accompanied by relative hypoxemia as measured by arterial blood gas levels or pulse oximetry. While usually not a highly morbid complication, atelectasis may lengthen the hospital stay, predispose to retained secretions and bacterial infection, and if severe or complicated may necessitate mechanical ventilation.

Prevention of postoperative atelectasis should be part of the perioperative plan for every patient. Significant risk factors for atelectasis are present in patients with an ASA score of more than 2, upper abdominal surgery, residual intraperitoneal sepsis, age greater than 60 years, obesity, and in those undergoing colorectal or gastroduodenal surgery.[3] Preoperative hospital stay longer than 4 days and a significant duration of surgery also increase the incidence of clinically significant atelectasis.[3]

Risk factors should be modified when possible. Obese patients should attempt to lose weight, and smokers should be counseled to stop for at least 4 weeks before surgery. Incentive spirometry, intermittent positive pressure breathing, resistance breathing, and deep breathing exercises all reduce postoperative pulmonary complications to approximately 20% and can shorten hospital stay.[2,4,5] It must be stressed that deep breathing exercises and incentive spirometry should begin before the operation. Ambulation should begin as early as possible after surgery, and pain management should be designed to allow maximal diaphragmatic function. Systemic, epidural, and intrapleural narcotics and nerve blocks are useful adjuncts in this regard. Once atelectasis has occurred, treatment includes the same measures used for prevention, and occasionally bronchoscopy. Antibiotics should be reserved for complicating bacterial infection (e.g., pneumonia).

SMALL BOWEL OBSTRUCTION

Small bowel obstruction is a frequent cause of postoperative morbidity and even mortality. Adhesions account for the vast majority of postoperative bowel obstructions and are a peritoneal cavity response to injury. Fibrinous adhesions form in the peritoneal cavity after surgery in response to inflammation and ischemia.[6] If not absorbed, these adhesions become organized by the invasion of fibroblasts, and capillaries sprout to form permanent fibrous adhesions. Factors that impair the peritoneal cavity's ability to absorb early fibrinous adhesions include tissue ischemia, infection, inflammation and granulomas from starch powder contamination.[7,8] Patients with bowel obstruction demonstrate one or more of four cardinal symptoms: vomiting, intestinal distention, pain, and obstipation. If these symptoms occur in the postoperative period, one must consider the possibility of small bowel obstruction. The pain of a simple small obstruction is central and colicky and may be synchronous with episodes of borborygmus. In postoperative patients who do not have external hernias, adhesions are the most likely cause of bowel obstruction. The differential diagnosis includes ileus, radiation enteritis, intra-abdominal abscess, malignancy, hernia (internal or external), volvulus, intussusception, inflammatory bowel disease, and anastomotic edema.

Plain radiographs are most frequently used for diagnosis of small bowel obstruction, and upright views typically show dilated loops of small bowel with air-fluid levels (Fig. 8-1). The absence of colonic air is highly suggestive of a complete bowel obstruction. Identification of a complete bowel obstruction on plain radiographs is important because most patients with complete bowel obstruction will require surgery.[9] All patients with small bowel obstruction should be treated by intestinal decompression and given intravenous fluid. The adequacy of rehydration should be assessed by monitoring urine output. Patients with coexisting medical problems may require invasive hemodynamic monitoring.

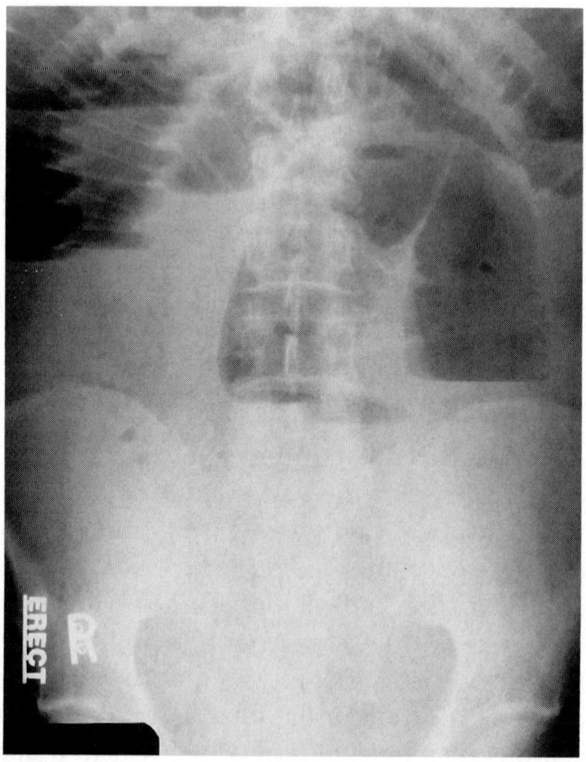

Fig. 8-1 Upright radiograph of abdomen of patient with a partial small bowel obstruction demonstrates multiple air-fluid levels.

Nasogastric or nasoenteric suction may be used for intestinal decompression. Nasogastric tubes minimize the amount of swallowed air and help prevent further intestinal distention. Long tubes may be passed through the pylorus into the small bowel and theoretically decompress dilated loops of bowel to facilitate relief of the obstruction. Long tubes that cannot be advanced through the pylorus at the bedside can be placed with fluoroscopic guidance or at endoscopy.[10-12] Long tubes may be more useful to resolve complete or partial small bowel obstruction.[10] Long tube therapy, however, has not gained widespread use because of difficulties in tube placement, doubts about its effectiveness compared with that of nasogastric suction, and concerns that long tube decompression may mask symptoms of bowel strangulation.[9]

The key decision in managing postoperative small bowel obstruction is when to abandon conservative treatment. In approximately one of 10 patients with small bowel obstruction secondary to postoperative adhesions, strangulated bowel will develop.[13,14] In a large review of cases of small bowel obstruction, the presence of peritoneal signs, a markedly elevated white blood cell count ($>18.0 \times 10^9$/L), and hypoactive or absent bowel sounds were the only signs or symptoms significantly associated with strangulation.[13] Patients with nonviable bowel often have at least one classic sign of compromised bowel such as fever, leukocytosis, tachycardia, and localized abdominal tenderness. Each of these signs, however, is also frequently seen in simple small bowel obstruction and therefore is a poor predictor of intestinal strangulation. In addition, most patients with nonviable bowel do not have peritoneal signs, a markedly elevated white blood cell count, or silent abdomen.[15] Base deficit is the most common laboratory abnormality in patients with strangulated bowel obstruction, but it also is too nonspecific to reliably predict strangulated small bowel obstruction.[15]

Early small bowel obstruction (within the first 30 postoperative days) presents an even greater diagnostic and therapeutic dilemma. Intestinal distention, obstipation, vomiting, and pain may result from postoperative ileus, although small bowel obstruction is more likely in a patient with a temporary return of bowel activity in whom signs of obstruction subsequently develop. As many as one of four patients with small bowel obstruction in the early postoperative period has nonspecific findings on plain radiographs.[16] In addition, upper GI studies with small bowel followthrough views will show a point of obstruction in only three of four patients.[16] While strangulation occurs less frequently than in late small bowel obstruction, it is poorly predicted from clinical symptoms, and experienced clinicians failed to recognize bowel compromise in one third of cases of strangulated small bowel in one study.[15]

The inability to diagnose strangulated small bowel obstruction at presentation emphasizes the importance of serial abdominal examinations in patient management. Patients with worsening clinical signs, acidosis, increasing leukocytosis, or fever require operative intervention. Patients in whom evidence of high-grade or complete bowel obstruction remains after 24 to 48 hours of observation should be operated on as well. In patients with a partial small bowel obstruction or early postoperative small bowel obstruction, longer nonoperative management frequently is allowed, because often the obstruction resolves and bowel strangulation occurs infrequently.[15]

Patients who are taken to the operating room with small bowel obstruction should receive broad-spectrum intravenous antibiotics. Antibiotics may serve to prevent the translocation of bacteria through the bowel wall and also minimize the consequences of contamination from inadvertent or purposeful enterotomy. Preoperative optimization of concurrent medical problems and volume resuscitation are also critical in ensuring a successful operation.

A midline incision is used by most surgeons. This incision incorporates the old scar but also permits attempts to incise virgin abdominal wall to facilitate entrance into the peritoneal cavity. In most cases of small bowel obstruction, a single adhesive band can be identified as the cause, and simple lysis will suffice. The bowel can be gently milked retrograde and evacuated with a functioning nasogastric tube to facilitate abdominal closure, if necessary. Some surgeons choose to free the entire small bowel, although the benefit of this has not been proved.

Management of postoperative bowel obstruction in patients with a prior history of cancer requires careful judgment. In nearly one third of these patients, the obstruction is from a benign and surgically correctable cause.[17] These patients benefit from surgical intervention if conservative management fails. Some patients with malignant bowel obstruction also may benefit from surgical intervention. In a series of patients with advanced, unresectable, recurrent colorectal cancer with bowel obstruction, normal bowel function was restored in 63%, and 57% were discharged from the hospital.[15] Most patients underwent some type of bypass procedure. Overall, however, the prognosis with malignant postoperative bowel obstruction remains poor. Patients who appear terminally ill and those with carcinomatosis who have ascites or a palpable abdominal mass do not benefit from exploratory laparotomy.[19] However, a draining gastrostomy tube offers some degree of palliation in this subset of patients with unresolved obstruction.

Prevention of small bowel obstruction begins at surgery. Gentle tissue handling to avoid enterotomy, ischemia, and serosal tears and minimizing the presence of foreign bodies (including glove powder and sutures) are important. Mechanical means to prevent obstruction from adhesions include plication and long tube stenting. Plication procedures attempt to maintain the bowel in a kink-free orientation so that adhesions form in a controlled manner. The original Noble procedure is seldom used today because of the time required to perform it and the frequent complications and mortality associated with it.[20] Transmesenteric small bowel plication is used occasionally.[20,21] Long tube stenting has been reported frequently in the literature and is the most popular method of prophylaxis at this time. It is advocated for patients with extensive adhesions in whom a recurrence can be expected, because they are prone to adhesion formation. The long tube can be placed via gastrostomy, enterostomy, or cecostomy and passed through the length of the intestine.[20] It is usually removed after 7 to 10 days, although it may be left in place indefinitely in cases of carcinomatosis in which efforts to bypass, resect, or construct stomas are pointless.[22] Follow-up is limited, and it is unclear whether long tube stenting reduces the likelihood of small bowel obstruction over the short or long term.

POSTOPERATIVE HEMORRHAGE

Postoperative hemorrhage is a dangerous complication that, if overlooked, can result in significant patient morbidity and mortality. The abdomen and pelvis represent large potential spaces for fluid accumulation. Inattention to hemostasis before closure may allow bleeding from a small arterial or venous source to cause exsanguination. Intra-abdominal hematomas may contribute to abscess formation.

At surgery, clamps, clips, suture ligation, and cautery are essential to attain hemostasis from specific bleeding points. Diffuse oozing may require the use of chemical agents. Sponges or pledgets of gelatin foam (Gelfoam), oxidized regenerated cellulose (Surgicel), or micronized collagen (Avitene) can be used to apply pressure against the wound surface and form a matrix for clot formation. Gelatin foam and cellulose pledgets soaked in bovine thrombin have intrinsic hemostatic function. Thrombin can also be sprayed onto surfaces in conjunction with cryoprecipitate to produce a hemostatic fibrin glue. Refractory bleeding may require temporary packing. Tamponade of presacral bleeding after abdominoperineal or low anterior resection can be accomplished with a Foley catheter, laparotomy packs, or a titanium thumbtack. Postoperative hemorrhage may be easy to recognize if drains are placed before closure, although the lack of output can also be misleading because drains often fail to function in the presence of active hemorrhage because of blood clot obstruction.

The primary physiologic compensation for acute blood loss occurs through the sympathetic autonomic nervous system. Adrenergic signals augment venous return by constricting small veins and venules and preserve blood flow to critical organs by constricting arterioles that serve tissues that are able to withstand warm ischemia (skin, fat, and muscle). The conservation of salt and water by the kidney is also stimulated by adrenergic nerves and intrinsic renal mechanisms.

Mild acute blood loss is characterized by cutaneous vasoconstriction and sweat gland output (producing cool, clammy skin) and decreased capillary refill of >2 seconds. Tachycardia and orthostatic hypotension occur. Greater degrees of blood loss cause oliguria, mental status changes, and overt hypotension. Coexisting medical conditions may mask these clinical signs. For example, a hypertensive patient with acute blood loss may have a "normal" heart rate if he or she is taking a beta blocker or may have "normal" blood pressure with significant blood loss if the baseline pressure was elevated. It is important to note that acute hemorrhage does not immediately reduce the hematocrit level. Serial hematocrit measurements will, however, show a precipitous decline after fluid resuscitation and will confirm the diagnosis of hemorrhage.

Treatment includes immediate isotonic crystalloid fluid infusion through large-bore peripheral or central vein catheters and obtaining blood for crossmatching. Blood should be given if the patient remains hemodynamically unstable after infusion of 30 ml/kg of crystalloid solution. The adequacy of volume replacement is assessed by means of urinary output (0.5 to 1 ml/kg/hr) and central venous pressure measurements. Blood should be transfused to keep the hematocrit level >0.30 in patients with coexisting cardiopulmonary disease. Healthier patients can tolerate a much lower hematocrit level (e.g., 0.20 to 0.24). The possibility of GI hemorrhage should always be considered in the differential diagnosis, and placement of a nasogastric tube should be considered and rectal examination performed. A patient with a clear chest radiograph and no evidence of external or GI bleeding after laparotomy most likely has bleeding into the peritoneum or retroperitoneum.

Every patient with major postoperative blood loss should be evaluated for medical hemostasis. Blood should be tested for platelet count, PT, and partial thromboplastin time (PTT). If test results are abnormal, analysis of fibrinogen and fibrin degradation product may be useful to identify a cause for the failure of medical hemostasis. The differential diagnosis includes liver failure, vitamin K deficiency, a congenital factor deficiency not recognized before surgery, disseminated intravascular coagulation, fibrinolysis, or a reaction to blood transfusion. Unless the patient's condition is markedly unstable, medical management to correct coagulopathies should precede repeat surgery.

Patients with hemodynamic instability and a falling hematocrit level despite fluid resuscitation and normal clotting mechanisms will need to undergo careful exploratory surgery to restore hemostasis. Most bleeding in postoperative patients will abate, however, without surgical intervention. The decision of whether to perform repeat surgery in a hemodynamically stable patient with evidence of potential ongoing bleeding requires experienced clinical judgment.

DEEP VEIN THROMBOSIS

Thrombosis of the veins of the lower extremities is an all too common complication of abdominal and pelvic surgery. In the absence of preventive measures, approximately 30% of patients undergoing general surgical procedures of moderate severity and with no significant associated risk factors can be expected to develop DVT detectable by phlebography.[23,24] Although many of these thrombi are asymptomatic and isolated to the calf area, approximately 25% extend into the larger proximal veins, where they may potentially break free and migrate to produce clinically obvious pulmonary emboli that can produce potentially fatal events. Many patients with DVT subsequently have postphlebitic syndrome, including brawny edema, venous stasis ulcers, and even venous claudication.[23]

In 1975, Dalen and Alpert[25] estimated that 630,000 cases of symptomatic pulmonary emboli occurred in the United States, with an estimated 200,000 deaths directly attributable. Given the difficulty in establishing the diagnosis and the relatively low rate of autopsy performed in the United States, these estimates are no doubt low. In addition, there is little if any evidence to suggest that the prevalence has decreased in the past two decades. It is therefore obvious that DVT is a major problem. Although in the vast majority of patients undergoing colon and rectal surgical procedures perioperative DVT does not develop, the prevalence still is significant. Risk factors are numerous (see the box) and include

RISK FACTORS FOR DVT*

Clinical	Operative
Age >40 years	Duration of surgery >1 hour
Age >70 years	Pelvic surgery
Previous DVT, pulmonary embolism	Major orthopedic surgery
Malignancy	General (versus regional) anesthesia
Obesity	Use of stirrups (lithotomy position)
Congestive heart failure, cardiomyopathy	
History of stroke or myocardial infarction	
Extensive lower extremity trauma	
Estrogen use (high dose)	
Pelvic fracture, hip fracture	
Paraplegia, quadriplegia	
Prolonged immobility	
Hypercoagulable state	
Varicose veins	
Sepsis	
Polycythemia rubra vera	
Inflammatory bowel disease	
Dehydration	
Postpartum state	
Preoperative hospitalization >5 days	

Data compiled from references 23, 24, 26, 27, 40.
*Risks are cumulative.

age >40 years, duration of surgery >60 minutes, malignancy, previous DVT or pulmonary emboli, and pelvic surgery with associated trauma to the iliac veins.[23,24,26,27] In patients at moderate risk undergoing intra-abdominal procedures, DVT will develop in 10% to 40% and fatal pulmonary emboli in 0.1% to 0.4%.[24,26] In high-risk patients or procedures, these complications can be expected in 50% and 1% to 5% of patients, respectively.[26]

Although these statistics are staggering, considering the number of patients who undergo moderate- and high-risk procedures each year, equally important is the recognition that of the patients who ultimately die of pulmonary emboli, the majority do not survive the first hour after the event. Clearly, prevention of DVT is preferable to treatment, and the only remaining issues are deciding which patients to administer prophylaxis to and which form of prophylaxis to use.

Prevention

Prevention of DVT may be accomplished with pharmacologic or nonpharmacologic means. Pharmacologic options include administration of subcutaneous heparin, low-dose aspirin, warfarin, low-molecular-weight heparin, dextran, as well as numerous other agents. Heparin administered subcutaneously at a dose of 5000 U bid has obtained the most widespread use and popularity in the United States, with proved efficacy and low morbidity.[28]

Bleeding complications related to subcutaneous heparin use occur in about 2% of patients, and most are minor (e.g., wound hematomas).[28] Heparin-induced thrombocytopenia occurs rarely[29]; a decrease in platelet count to $<100 \times 10^9$/L should alert the clinician to the possibility, and the heparin should be discontinued.

Dextran, low-molecular-weight heparin, and other heparin admixtures have not gained wide popularity in the United States, because they are frequently unavailable and their cost is relatively prohibitive, although they may have an enhanced safety profile and/or efficacy.[27,30] Warfarin therapy is preferred in patients at very high risk, although dextran may be equally efficacious.[31] Another option is low-dose heparin combined with sequential compression stockings.[32]

Nonpharmacologic measures include graduated elastic stockings and sequential compression stockings. Graduated elastic stockings are appropriate for low-risk procedures or perhaps for patients at low risk who are undergoing moderate-risk procedures. Sequential compression stockings have a proved efficacy comparable to pharmacologic prophylaxis for patients at low and moderate risk. Their use requires attention by the clinician, however, because compliance and improper use can be a problem.[33] They are contraindicated in patients with significant peripheral vascular disease.

Diagnosis

Deep venous thrombosis may occur despite these or other preventive measures or in the absence of prophylaxis. The diagnosis frequently requires a high index of suspicion, because the vast majority of these thrombi are clinically occult. It is inappropriate to ignore subtle findings simply because the patient is otherwise ready for discharge or ambulatory, because a significant percentage of fatal pulmonary emboli occur after the patient is discharged. Classic findings including calf swelling and discomfort, distal venous engorgement, and pain on passive dorsiflexion of the foot (Homan's sign) are important but are present in a minority of patients with a confirmed diagnosis of a DVT. Alternatively, the clinical suspicion of DVT requires confirmation with an objective diagnostic test, because a thrombosis is found in only 50% of suspected cases.[23]

Duplex scanning with or without color flow Doppler imaging has replaced phlebography (venography) as the initial diagnostic test of choice. In experienced hands, this test has a sensitivity >98% and a specificity approaching 100% for proximal, symptomatic DVT.[34,35] Its sensitivity suffers a bit in evaluation for calf thrombi, but the specificity remains high.[36,37] If a distal DVT is suspected, duplex Doppler examination should be repeated in 7 to 10 days.[38] Visualization of a thrombus is often possible, but the most sensitive and reliable finding is relative noncompressibility of the vein.[23,24,38] Iodine 125–labeled fibrinogen nuclear scintigraphy, once a widely used and reported test, is no longer available in the United States because of concerns about transmission of infectious agents. This test was quite sensitive for calf thrombi but had poor sensitivity for proximal DVT and required 24 to 48 hours for results.

Impedance plethysmography measures electrical impedance with the use of two calf electrodes. Changes in venous volume can be detected, because impedance is decreased as the leg becomes engorged with blood. Application of a thigh tourniquet and subsequent release should show a characteristic decrease and subsequent increase in impedance in the absence of a DVT. Impedance plethysmography produces results inferior to those with compression ultrasonography.[39]

Phlebograpy remains the standard diagnostic modality for DVT, but the associated morbidity (pain, phlebitis) and relatively high cost should limit its use to delineate required noninvasive examinations. Other studies currently under investigation that show promise include magnetic resonance venography, radiolabeled monoclonal antibody to cross-linked fibrin, and plasma D-dimer levels.[24]

Treatment

Treatment of DVT is aimed primarily at prevention of pulmonary embolism and secondarily at restoration of venous patency and valvular function and prevention of postembolic pulmonary hypertension.[23,24]

Heparin therapy should be instituted expeditiously in all patients with confirmed DVT and should be considered in patients with suspected DVT, particularly if a pulmonary embolism is likely to have occurred. Failure to provide adequate anticoagulation therapy in a patient with a proximal DVT or pulmonary embolism within the first 24 hours after diagnosis dramatically increases (as much as 15 times) subsequent morbidity.[40] Contraindications to the use of heparin include recent CNS or ophthalmologic surgery or hemorrhage, active bleeding (e.g., GI bleeding), and malignant hypertension. In these patients, vena caval interruption (e.g., Greenfield filter) should be performed promptly.

Heparin therapy should be titrated to the activated PTT, with a therapeutic goal of one and one half to two and one half times control value. Daily doses of heparin frequently exceed 30,000 to 40,000 U/day, with continuous intravenous infusion or subcutaneous injections, although risk of embolism is higher with the subcutaneous route in patients at high risk.[40] Intermittent intravenous injections may have equal efficacy but are associated with significantly more episodes of serious bleeding as a side effect.[41] The duration of heparin therapy is controversial. Most authors recommend therapy for 5 to 7 days,[23] with administration of oral anticoagulation (warfarin) therapy beginning after 1 to 3 days of heparin therapy. An overlap period is necessary even in the presence of a therapeutic PT because of a potential early thrombogenic effect of warfarin.[23] Prolongation of PT to one and one half to two times control value is effective and has an acceptable safety profile. More recently, attempts at standardizing PT have resulted in reporting the values as an international normalized ratio (INR) with a value between 2.0 and 3.0 the recommended goal.[24] Warfarin therapy should be continued for 3 months, with consideration of longer therapy in patients with hypercoagulable states,[40] including malignancy, and in patients with recurrent DVT or pulmonary embolism.[23]

Occasionally DVT will progress locally and impair arterial circulation in the affected extremity and lead to phlegmasia cerulea dolens, a limb- and potentially life-threatening complication. Surgical intervention may be necessary, with iliofemoral thrombectomy to restore adequate flow to save the extremity.[24]

Thrombolytic therapy with tissue plasminogen activator (tPA) or streptokinase has received attention in the treatment of DVT. Although early restoration of venous patency and possible preservation of valve function may be improved compared with conventional therapy, a twofold to fourfold increase in bleeding complications, including intracranial sites, has tempered the early enthusiasm.[42]

GASTROINTESTINAL FISTULA

Few if any complications are as distressing to the surgeon as GI fistula formation in a postoperative patient. The mere presence of enteric or fecal contents draining from a surgical wound or drain (or occasionally from the vagina) implies failure on the part of the surgeon associated with technical misadventure, poor patient preparation, or poor judgment. Clearly this conclusion is not always valid, although frequently alterations in management can be identified that might have prevented the complication.

A GI fistula is an abnormal communication between the GI tract and the skin or another hollow organ. In colorectal surgery the presence of a fistula in the postoperative period almost always implies an anastomotic complication. Alternative causes include inadvertent enterotomy during lysis of adhesions, retractor injuries with resultant bowel ischemia, mesenteric injuries, deserosalization with unrecognized injury to the underlying bowel wall, and injury to the bowel during closure of the abdominal wall. The enterocutaneous fistula easiest to recognize and deal with is one that is captured by a drain placed during surgery. Indeed, this may even be a predictable complication, because evidence suggests that the use of drains in the perianastomotic area may increase leak rates and hence fistula formation.[43,44] This can be a desired objective, by converting an anastomotic leak and abscess into a well-captured enterocutaneous or colocutaneous fistula. In the absence of ischemia or total disruption of the anastomosis, these fistulas can be expected to close, usually in the early postoperative period (<30 days). Attention to maintenance of drain patency and assurance that no associated abscess exists will ensure a good clinical outcome. Many fistulas do not manifest in such a benign fashion, and even the presence and use of drains do not guarantee capture of an anastomotic leak.

Mortality from enterocutaneous fistulas has decreased from the 40% to 50% seen before 1960 to 10% to 20% in most later series. Two factors currently account for most deaths: sepsis and extensive malignancy. The value of total parenteral nutrition (TPN) in this improvement seen is debatable.[45,46] Improved postoperative care, including effective antibiotic usage, ventilatory support, aggressive correction of electrolyte imbalances, and improved monitoring are at least equally important.[45] One fact is clear: without control of accompanying sepsis, fistula closure and even patient survival is unlikely.[47]

After diagnosis or suspicion of a GI fistula, an evaluation for sepsis should closely follow resuscitation of the patient. "Soft signs" of sepsis may include relative oliguria (third spacing), hyperglycemia, and tachycardia. More obvious signs include fever, hypotension, leukocytosis, and peritoneal signs.

In the presence of diffuse peritonitis, surgical intervention with diversion should be only briefly delayed for resuscitative efforts. If the patient lacks evidence of peritonitis but demonstrates evidence of sepsis, resuscitation should be accompanied by placement of a nasogastric tube, administration of broad-spectrum antibiotics, and examination for the source of sepsis. Potential extra-abdominal sources must not be ignored, and evaluation for urinary tract infections, pneumonia, phlebitis, and wound infection should precede a search for an intra-abdominal source of sepsis.[47] If findings are unrevealing or equivocal, an ultrasound or CT scan of the abdomen and pelvis should be performed. If the above diagnostic regimen fails to reveal a possible source and the patient continues to show unequivocal, worsening sepsis despite appropriate broad-spectrum antibiotic therapy, consideration should be given to exploratory laparotomy. If, however, an intra-abdominal or pelvic abscess is detected, drainage is indicated. Radiologically guided percutaneous drainage may have distinct advantages over other techniques, although extraperitoneal and transrectal drainage are appropriate alternatives. Transperitoneal drainage should be reserved for patients undergoing laparotomy because of diffuse peritonitis or abscesses not amenable to other techniques. Failure to control sepsis is responsible for most deaths resulting from enterocutaneous fistulas; thus abdominal exploration and proximal enteric diversion should be considered if sepsis continues despite the above measures.

Once sepsis is controlled, the additional challenges in managing enterocutaneous fistulas are wound and skin care, nutritional support, and electrolyte and fluid maintenance. Colocutaneous fistulas rarely present such problems, because their output typically is low (<500 ml per 24 hr) with relatively innocuous contents. Small bowel fistulas, particularly proximal jejunal fistulas, can be taxing, with high-output fluid losses rich in destructive pancreatic enzymes and bile. An experienced enterostomal therapy nurse can and should be an integral part of the team (when available) to prevent potentially disastrous skin loss. Electrolyte measurements in high-output fistulas should be liberally performed and replacement fluid adjusted on the basis of actual losses. Nutritional support usually consists of TPN delivered through a central vein. Some patients with low-output fistulas, including many colocutaneous fistulas, can be given an elemental diet administered orally or through a feeding tube.

Over the past decade, somatostatin and somatostatin analog (octreotide acetate) have been introduced and received significant attention in the treatment of GI fistulas. Somatostatin, a GI hormone, is a potent inhibitor of GI endocrine and exocrine secretions. Native somatostatin has a short half-life, requiring continuous intravenous infusion, and is associated with secondary hyperglycemia because it inhibits insulin secretion. Somatostatin analog has a half-life of 8 hours, less effect on insulin secretion, and similar effects on decreasing the volume and enzyme content of GI secretions. Although investigations continue, the effects of somatostatin on GI fistulas are to diminish fistula output, hasten closure, and reduce morbidity. No evidence suggests that somatostatin will increase the closure rate of fistulas over that seen with standard conservative treatment (70% to 85%).[41,48,49]

Several causes have been identified as preventing "spontaneous" fistula closure. These include distal bowel obstruction, an adjacent abscess, inflammatory bowel disease, presence of a foreign body, radiation damage, malignancy at the site of fistulization, and epithelialization of the fistula tract. The best method for evaluating a fistula—determining its location and length and often the presence or absence of local abscess, as well as ruling out distal obstruction—is to obtain a fluoroscopic image of the fistula, preferably with the surgeon present. Imaging of the fistula is often complemented by barium contrast studies and other GI contrast material–enhanced studies. Although radiation damage, inflammatory bowel disease, the presence of a foreign body, and malignant fistulization all predict failure of conservative management to elicit closure of fistulas, this therapy may have significant positive effect on the patient's medical and metabolic condition and may allow intra-abdominal inflammation to subside and a less "hostile" abdominal environment to develop before surgical intervention.

COMPLICATIONS OF AMBULATORY ANORECTAL SURGERY

Among the many changes in our health care delivery system in the past decade, one of the most dramatic has been a decrease in the average hospital stay of surgical patients. This change has been particularly evident in the case of anorectal surgery. Procedures that once were believed to require a 4- or 5-day hospital stay currently are being performed in most centers as same-day surgery. Given the current economic climate, the pressure to continue this trend is clearly in place.

Critical to the success of this approach is appropriate patient and procedure selection and, equally important, appropriate patient eduction and patient expectation. A knowledgeable and cooperative anesthesiologist is also crucial, because urinary retention and inadequate early pain control are two of the principal reasons for unplanned admissions.

Urinary Retention

Postoperative urinary retention is a complex and poorly understood problem with a frequency of 0.5% to 30.0% or higher in modern series.[50,51] The underlying mechanism is presumed to be neural, given the common innervation of the anal sphincter mechanism and urethral sphincter from the sacral nerves and pelvic parasympathetic nerves. Numerous factors have been implicated in the development of urinary retention, including patient and health care giver anxiety, poor control of pain, excess intravenous fluid administration, male sex, and the use of spinal anesthesia.[50,52,53] The use of pharmacologic agents, including bethanechol chloride, is not of value in prevention or treatment in routine cases.[54] Liberal intraoperative use of perianal anesthetic or analgesic, limitation of intravenous fluids to <250 ml perioperatively, and lack of insistence on voiding before discharge are all reasonable means to avert this potential complication.[50] Some patient education about urinary retention, however, is warranted, because appropriate therapy (intermittent sterile catheterization) will prevent troublesome or even permanent voiding difficulties. A return trip to the surgical suite or the emergency department or the use of home health care nurses should be readily available to the patient but are seldom necessary.

Postoperative Pain

Pain after outpatient anorectal surgery is virtually universal. Controlling the pain is crucial to the success of both the procedure and the planned at-home convalescence. For many patients, the simple reassurance that the physician is available for questions or problems will go far to prevent problems; for others, including those who undergo apparently simple, straightforward procedures, relief without resorting to parenteral narcotics is seemingly impossible. Both patient and procedure selection for ambulatory management are crucial.

Postoperative pain therefore can be a normal expectation after successful surgery but may also indicate the onset of a complication. Complications that may manifest as postoperative pain include fecal impaction, development of an anal fissure, unresolved perianal or perirectal sepsis, and development of perianal or perirectal sepsis. Pain that persists after the surgical procedure is most commonly the result of inadequate analgesia. The use of intraoperative or perioperative local injections of long-acting anesthetic or analgesic agents may minimize this problem. In addition, appropriate prescription of narcotics and careful avoidance of constipation postoperatively are of great importance. Patients who habitually use narcotics because of chronic pain will have problems with "normal" postoperative pain and may be more appropriately selected for a brief inpatient stay. Pain that worsens or develops after the first 48 to 72 hours after surgery is most commonly caused by fecal impaction. This can frequently be diagnosed or strongly suspected during a phone conversation with the patient who has constant pressure that progresses to unremitting pain, occasionally resulting in a vasovagal reaction and complaints of weakness, orthostasis, or both. A coexistent history of low frequency or absence of bowel movements since surgery will help confirm the diagnosis.

Treatment of true fecal impaction is difficult for the patient to accomplish, although a warm tap water or mineral oil enema may be effective. Magnesium citrate or senna (Senokot) tablets are an alternative. Evaluation in the emergency department, when necessary, should be performed by an experienced examiner, because unnecessarily aggressive attempts at rectal examination will be neither productive nor appreciated by the patient. Gentle digital examination with a well-lubricated fifth digit may be attempted, but if the patient has extreme pain, a lubricated cotton swab[52] or a well-lubricated small red rubber catheter may be inserted to confirm the diagnosis. Advantages of the red rubber catheter include the ability to then administer an enema to alleviate the impaction. Avoiding impaction is the best approach, and adequate postoperative instructions about the liberal use of stool softeners or mineral oil, adequate bulking agents, and hydration are essential in the early postoperative period.[55] Sitz baths and patient reassurance are equally important.

Infection

It may seem surprising, given the large number of enteric bacteria in the vicinity, but infection after anorectal surgery is uncommon. This is most likely the result of good local blood supply and spontaneous drainage through the freshly created surgical wounds in the event of subacute infection. Indeed, the fairly frequent occurrence of fever in the postoperative period and the observation that many anal and perianal wounds (particularly when closed primarily) do not heal by primary intention indicates that spontaneous drainage may be common. Despite these facts, disastrous anorectal sepsis can occur postoperatively, and suspicion of sepsis is a frequent cause for physician concern. The symptoms of local sepsis include constant unremitting pain, fever, and often disturbances in urination or inability to urinate.[56] With the possible exception of fever, these are the same symptoms that accompany fecal impaction. For this reason, if the concern is significant, physician examination is mandatory, and if doubt persists, an examination with the patient under anesthesia is indicated. Broad-spectrum intravenous antibiotic administration and wide debridement are the mainstays of therapy on confirmation of perianal or perirectal sepsis.

Bleeding

A small amount of bleeding after anorectal surgery is common, and if the patient is forewarned and reassured, typically this is satisfactory to avert unnecessary phone calls. Massive bleeding within the first 48 hours is usually the result of a technical error, with incomplete ligation of a vascular pedicle or an unligated open vessel not recognized because of distention of the rectum from retractors. Alternatively, a slipped ligature may be responsible for acute massive bleeding. The diagnosis is usually obvious, although one may have concern about a more proximal, unrelated site of bleeding. Surgical intervention with adequate anesthesia is essential to appropriate management in these patients.

Delayed hemorrhage is usually caused by the sloughing of previously placed ligatures resulting from trauma from defecation or from local suppuration. Unrecognized coagulopathy or ingestion of medications that alter coagulation may contribute. Observation in a hospital setting is mandatory for these patients, although most bleeding will subside spontaneously. The patient should be given nothing by mouth, and appropriate resuscitative measures should be available including appropriate blood products. If bleeding continues, examination with the patient under anesthesia, with an attempt at ligation of the bleeding site, should be undertaken. More minor bleeding is usually of little concern to the physician but may cause great concern and anxiety for the patient. Early reevaluation of persistent nuisance bleeding should be considered for this reason. Often a simple, gentle examination in the office, with chemical cauterization or electrocauterization if necessary, is adequate. Alternatively, injection of an epinephrine solution may suffice.

RETAINED OPERATIVE FOREIGN BODIES

In any complex surgical procedure there is the potential for items to be unknowingly left in body cavities. To minimize this risk, current standards require that

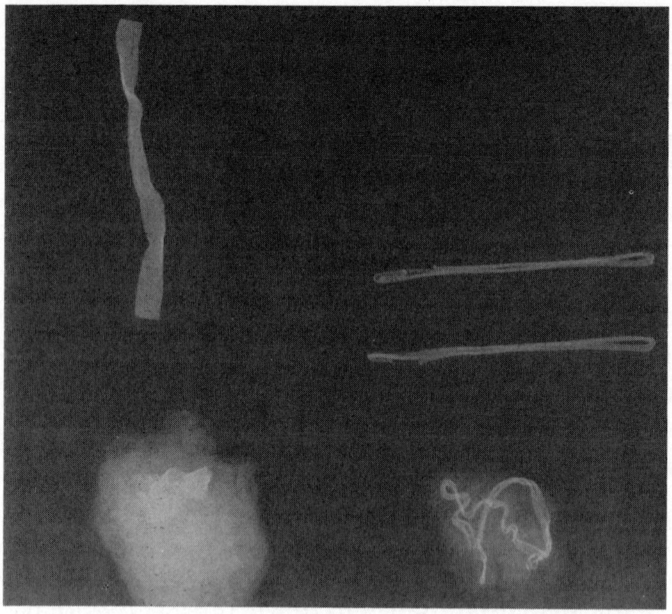

Fig. 8-2 Radiograph demonstrating radiopaque markers. *Left to right:* Laparotomy sponge, Ray-tec sponge. The upper image is flattened, whereas the lower image demonstrates the radiologic view when the item is crumpled.

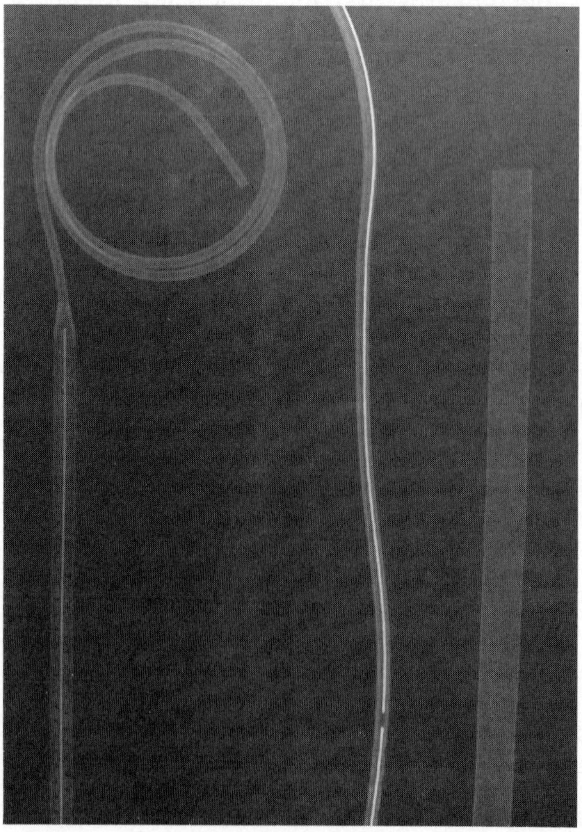

Fig. 8-3 Radiograph of *(left to right)* Jackson-Pratt drain, Penrose drain, nasogastric tube.

all sponges, needles, surgical instruments, equipment, and items small enough to be misplaced be counted before the procedure and one or two times after completion of the procedure to confirm that all items are accounted for. These activities are usually performed and documented by the operating room nurses and technicians; however, the surgeon is ultimately responsible and should conduct each operation so as to minimize the risk of misplaced foreign bodies. In accordance with this goal, most surgeons avoid using small Ray-tec sponges in the abdomen and avoid placing laparotomy sponges in areas that are hard to visualize. If sponges must be used to pack areas, the sponge marker should be left in an obvious area or a clamp or ring may be attached to the sponge. Most important is a thorough exploration of the entire operative field, which should be performed routinely before closing the incision. Items used during the operation that have the potential to be easily lost should be radiopaque or contain a radiopaque marker (e.g., Ray-tec sponges and Silastic drains). Figs. 8-2 and 8-3 demonstrate the radiologic view of several common surgical items. Plain radiographs are often the best study to identify the radiopaque markers incorporated into these items; the markers may be much less obvious on studies such as CT scans (Figs. 8-4 and 8-5).

If an instrument, sponge, or needle count is not correct, several actions are indicated. All sponge wrappers and suture packages should be counted to confirm the accuracy of the original count. The entire operating room and especially the trash bags and floor under the operating table should be searched for the misplaced item. Simultaneously, the surgeon should inspect the operative field thoroughly for the missing item. If the missing item cannot be located, a radiograph of the entire operative field should be obtained before closure of the body cavity to identify any radiopaque object and minimize the morbidity of locating the missing item. Because of the potential for human error, a "correct" instrument, needle, or sponge count does not absolutely exclude the presence of a foreign body. Therefore each member of the team must maintain a high index of suspicion.

A sponge or other foreign body left in a body cavity can present or be identified in a number of ways. The foreign body may be seen on a radiograph obtained for other reasons, or the patient may develop symptoms that lead to the need for radiographs or an exploratory procedure. Symptoms may be infectious (fever, elevated white cell count, wound infection or abscess) or inflammatory (ileus, tenderness, mass effect). For any postoperative patient with unusual or unexplained symptoms, radiographs should be included in the evaluation.

Finding a retained foreign body is usually an indication for an urgent exploratory procedure. The exception may be an asymptomatic patient with a retained small needle. The morbidity associated with localizing and removing a small needle must be weighed against the potential risk of leaving it alone, and the patient can assist in this decision. Review of the biplanar radiographs

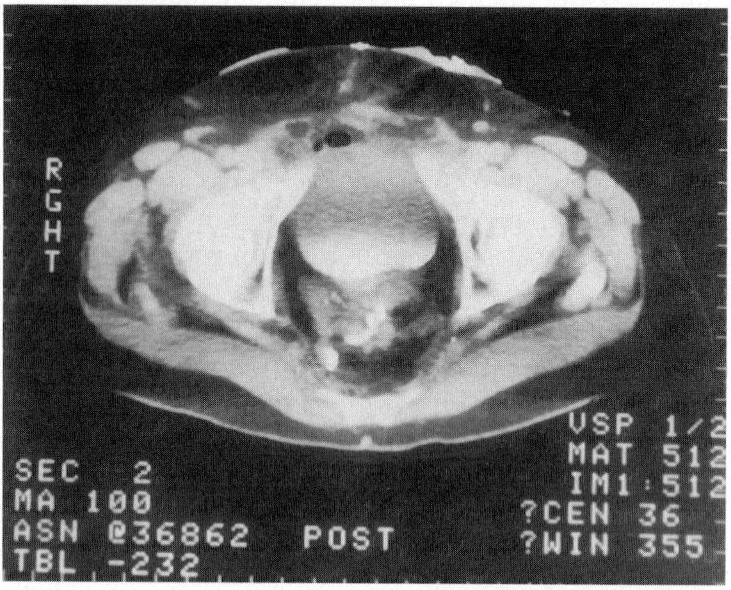

Fig. 8-4 CT scan of patient with a retained Ray-tec sponge. Image is the inferior cut of the study. The upper edge of the Ray-tec marker is demonstrated as white dots lines between the bladder (filled with contrast) and the sacrum.

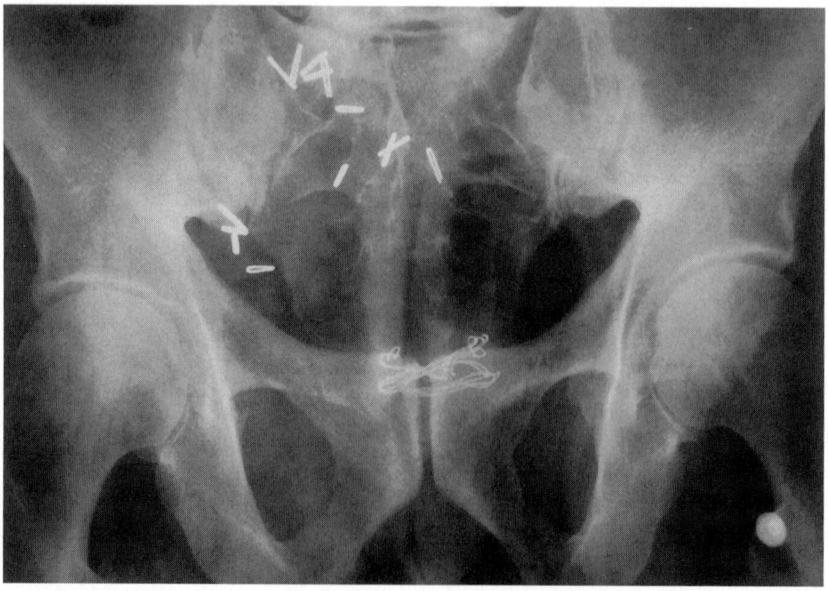

Fig. 8-5 Pelvic radiograph of patient in Fig. 8-4 clearly demonstrating Ray-tec marker in pelvis.

may assist in localizing the retained item, and early identification will minimize the morbidity associated with the object's removal. Retention of operative foreign bodies is uncommon, and a surgical team that adheres to careful practices should avert its occurrence.

REFERENCES

1. Dubin HG. Perioperative respiratory management. Probl Gen Surg 5:309-329, 1988.
2. Roukema JA, Cavol EJ, Prins JG. The prevention of pulmonary complications after upper abdominal surgery in patients with noncompromised pulmonary status. Arch Surg 123:30-34, 1988.
3. Hall JC, Javala RA, Hall JL, et al. A multivariate analysis of the risk of pulmonary complications after laparotomy. Chest 99:973-927, 1991.
4. Celli BR, Rodriguez KS, Snider GL. A controlled trial of intermittent positive pressure breathing, incentive spirometry, and deep breathing exercises in preventing pulmonary complications after abdominal surgery. Am Rev Respir Dis 130:12-15, 1984.
5. Jung R, Wright J, Nasser R, Rosoff L. Comparison of three methods of respiratory care following upper abdominal surgery. Chest 78:31-35, 1980.
6. Buckman RF, Woods M, Sargent L, Gervin AS. A uniting pathogenetic mechanism in the etiology of intraperitoneal adhesions. J Surg Res 20:1-5, 1976.
7. Jagelman DG, Ellis H. Starch and intraperitoneal adhesion formation. Br J Surg 60:111-114, 1973.
8. Cooke SAR, Hamilton DG. The significance of starch powder contamination in the etiology of peritoneal adhesions. Br J Surg 64:410-412, 1977.
9. Hofsteeter SR. Acute adhesive obstruction of the small intestine. Surg Gynecol Obstet 152: 141-144, 1981.
10. Wolfson PJ, Bauer JJ, Gelernt IM, et al. Use of the long tube in the management of patients with small intestinal obstruction due to adhesions. Arch Surg 120:1001-1006, 1985.
11. Gowen GF. Endoscopic decompression in partial small bowel obstruction. Am J Surg 149: 252-257, 1985.
12. Peetz DJ, Gamelli RL, Pilcher DB. Intestinal intubation in acute mechanical small bowel obstruction. Arch Surg 117:334, 1982.
13. Bizer LS, Liebling RW, Deland HM, Gliedman ML. Small bowel obstruction. Surgery 89:407-414, 1981.
14. Sevor D, Feign E, Szold A, et al. How conservatively can postoperative small bowel obstruction be treated? Am J Surg 165:121-126, 1993.
15. Sarr MG, Bulkley GB, Zuidema GD. Preoperative recognized intestinal strangulation obstruction. Am J Surg 145:176-182, 1982.
16. Pickleman J, Lee RM. The management of patients with suspected early postoperative small bowel obstruction. Ann Surg 210:216-219, 1989.
17. Butler JA, Cameron B, Morrow M, et al. Small bowel obstruction in patients with a prior history of cancer. Am J Surg 162:624-627, 1991.
18. Lau PWK, Lorentz TG. Results of surgery for malignant bowel obstruction in advanced unresectable, recurrent, colorectal cancer. Dis Colon Rectum 36:61-64, 1993.
19. van Ooijen B, van der Burg M, Planting AS, et al. Surgical treatment or gastric drainage only for intestinal obstruction in patients with carcinoma of the ovary or peritoneal carcinomatosis of other origin. Surg Gynecol Obstet 176:469-474, 1993.

20. Close MB, Christensen NM. Transmesenteric small bowel plication or intraluminal stenting. Am J Surg 138:89-96, 1979.
21. Childs WA, Phillips RB. Experience with intestinal plication and a proposed modification. Ann Surg 152:258-265, 1960.
22. McCarthy JD. A strategy for intestinal obstruction of peritoneal carcinomatosis. Arch Surg 121:1081-1082, 1986.
23. Cross J. Perioperative venous thromboembolism. Probl Gen Surg 5:330-354, 1988.
24. Weinmann EE, Salzman EW. Deep-vein thrombosis. N Engl J Med 24:1630-1641, 1994.
25. Dalen JE, Alpert JS. Natural history of pulmonary embolism. Prog Cardiovasc Dis 17:257-270, 1975.
26. Wheeler HB, Anderson FA Jr. Prophylaxis against venous thromboembolism in surgical patients. Am J Surg 161:507-512, 1991.
27. Silver D. An overview of venous thromboembolism prophylaxis. Am J Surg 161:537-540, 1991.
28. Collins R, Scrimgeour A, Yusuf S, et al. Reduction in fatal pulmonary embolism and venous thrombosis by perioperative administration of subcutaneous heparin: Overview of results of randomized trials in general, orthopedic, and urologic surgery. N Engl J Med 318:1162-1173, 1988.
29. Silver D, Kapsch N, Edmund KM, et al. Heparin-induced thrombocytopenia, thrombosis and hemorrhage. Ann Surg 198:301-306, 1983.
30. Hirsh J. Rationale for development of low-molecular weight heparins and their clinical potential in the prevention of postoperative venous thrombosis. Am J Surg 161:512-518, 1991.
31. Conti S, Daschbach M. Venous thromboembolism prophylaxis. Arch Surg 117:1036-1040, 1982.
32. Hull RD, Raskob GE, Hirsh J. Prophylaxis of venous thromboembolism: An overview. Chest 89(Suppl):374S-383S, 1986.
33. Comerota AJ, Katz ML, White JV. Why does prophylaxis with external pneumatic compression for deep vein thrombosis fail? Am J Surg 164:265-268, 1992.
34. Lensing AWA, Prandoni P, Brandjes D, et al. Detection of deep-vein thrombosis by real-time B-mode ultrasonography. N Engl J Med 320:342-345, 1989.
35. Elias A, Le Corff G, Bouvier JL, et al. Value of real time B mode ultrasound imaging in the diagnosis of deep vein thrombosis of the lower limbs. Int Angiol 6:175-182, 1987.
36. White RH, McGahan JP, Daschbach MM, et al. Diagnosis of deep-vein thrombosis using duplex ultrasound. Ann Intern Med 111:297-304, 1989.
37. Baxter GM, Duffy P, Partridge E. Colour flow imaging of calf vein thrombosis. Clin Radiol 46:198-201, 1992.
38. Cronan JJ, Dorfman GS, Scola FH, et al. Deep venous thrombosis: Ultrasound assessment using vein compression. Radiology 162:191-194, 1987.
39. Heijboer H, Buller HR, Lensing AWA, et al. A comparison of real-time compression ultrasonography with impedance plethysmography for the diagnosis of deep-vein thrombosis in symptomatic outpatients. N Engl J Med 329:1365-1369, 1993.
40. Hull RD, Raskob GE, Hirsh J, et al. Continuous intravenous heparin compared with intermittent subcutaneous heparin in the initial treatment of proximal-vein thrombosis. N Engl J Med 315:1109-1114, 1986.
41. Spiliotis J, Brian D, Gouttebel MC, et al. Treatment of fistulas of the gastrointestinal tract with total parenteral nutrition and octreotide in patients with carcinoma. Surg Gynecol Obstet 176:575-580, 1993.

42. Levine MN, Goldhaber SZ, Califf RM, et al. Hemorrhagic complications of thrombolytic therapy in the treatment of myocardial infarction and venous thromboembolism. Chest 102(Suppl):364S-373S, 1992.
43. Smith SRG, Connolly JC, Crane PW, et al. The effect of surgical drainage materials on colonic healing. Br J Surg 69:153-155, 1982.
44. Duthie HL. Current concepts: Drainage of the abdomen. N Engl J Med 287:1081-1083, 1972.
45. Soeters PB, Ebeid AM, Fischer JE. Review of 404 patients with gastrointestinal fistulas. Ann Surg 190:189-202, 1979.
46. Rose D, Yarborough MF, Canizaro PC, et al. One hundred and fourteen fistulas of the gastrointestinal tract treated with total parenteral nutrition. Surg Gynecol Obstet 163:345-350, 1986.
47. Rubelowsky J, Machiedo GW. Reoperative versus conservative management for gastrointestinal fistulas. Surg Clin North Am 71:147-157, 1991.
48. Borison DI, Bloom AD, Pritchard TJ. Treatment of enterocutaneous and colocutaneous fistulas with early surgery or somatostatin analog. Dis Colon Rectum 35:635-639, 1992.
49. Torres AJ, Landa JI, Mereno-Azcoita M, et al. Somatostatin in the management of gastrointestinal fistulas. Arch Surg 127:97-100, 1992.
50. Hoff SD, Bailey HR, Butts DR, et al. Ambulatory surgical hemorrhoidectomy: A solution to postoperative urinary retention. Dis Colon Rectum 37:1242-1244, 1994.
51. Nivatvongs S. Complications of anorectal and colorectal operations. In Gordon PH, Nivatvongs S, eds. Principles and Practice of Surgery for the Colon, Rectum, and Anus. St. Louis: Quality Medical Publishing, 1992, pp 999-1021.
52. Bevans DW, Westbrook KC, Thompson BW, et al. Perirectal abscess: A potentially fatal illness. Am J Surg 126:765-768, 1973.
53. Bleday R, Pena JP, Rothenberger DA, et al. Symptomatic hemorrhoids: Current incidence and complications of operative therapy. Dis Colon Rectum 35:477-481, 1992.
54. Corman ML. Management of postoperative constipation in anorectal surgery. Dis Colon Rectum 22:149-151, 1979.
55. Bowers FJ, Hartmann R, Khanduja K, et al. Urecholine prophylaxis for urinary retention in anorectal surgery. Dis Colon Rectum 30:41-42, 1987.
56. Fleischer M, Marini CP, Statman R, et al. Local anesthesia is superior to spinal anesthesia for anorectal surgical procedures. Am Surg 11:812-815, 1994.

PART II

SPECIFIC COMPLICATIONS

CHAPTER 9

Transanal Endoscopy

FRANK G. OPELKA

Endoscopy is commonly used to evaluate the GI tract. Endoscopy of the lower GI tract may include colonoscopy, flexible sigmoidoscopy, rigid proctoscopy, and anoscopy. Colonoscopy is commonly used to diagnose and treat colonic conditions and has significant advantages over other examinations such as lower GI barium studies. Colonoscopy allows direct inspection of the mucosal surface to identify and treat polyps, neoplasias, vascular lesions, and inflammatory bowel diseases. The procedure is invasive, but complications are infrequent. The major complications that can arise during either diagnostic or therapeutic colonoscopy include hemorrhage, perforation, and postpolypectomy coagulation syndrome; minor complications include problems related to mechanical bowel preparation, intravenous medications, cardiorespiratory effects, and infections.[1] Flexible sigmoidoscopy, rigid proctoscopy, and anoscopy are more commonly performed and are associated with fewer complications. This chapter reviews the complications of endoscopy of the colon and rectum.

MINOR COMPLICATIONS

Colorectal Preparations

To achieve an accurate examination, the colon must be cleansed of as much feces and particulate matter as possible. Despite years of intestinal surgery and endoscopy, no method of mechanical cleansing of the bowel has pleased both physicians and patients. Often the preparations are intolerable for patient consumption, which limits compliance and impairs bowel preparation. Finding a tolerable cleansing agent remains a problem for patients receiving colonoscopy. Bowel preparation, which in the past required several days, can now be accomplished in 2 to 3 hours with a lavage that provides adequate preparation for surgery or endoscopic review. Bowel preparation on the evening before or on the day of the examination can be safely performed on an outpatient basis.[2]

Preparations currently used for colonoscopy include whole-gut irrigation with mannitol, saline solution lavage, or balanced electrolyte solutions with polyethylene glycol (PEG-lavage; GoLytely or NuLytely, Braintree Laboratories, Braintree, Mass., or CoLyte, Reed and Carnrick, Piscataway, N.J.) and cathartics such as oral sodium phosphate (Phospho-soda, C.B. Fleet, Lynchburg, Va.).[3] Whole-gut lavage requires large volumes over a short period of time. During administration of these preparations, patients may experience nausea, vomiting, intestinal cramps, or chills. Mannitol lavage effectively cleanses the colon, but colonic bacteria metabolize mannitol, which creates explosive hydrogen gases. Several reports of explosions during colonoscopic electrocautery and use of bowel preparations containing mannitol have limited its usefulness.[4] Providers who continue to use mannitol dilute the hydrogen gases during the examination by infusing CO_2 through the colonoscope. Recently, orally administered sodium phosphate preparations have been reported to be equally as effective as saline solution or PEG-lavage preparations while limiting the volume consumed and improving patient compliance.[5] Their use, however, is contraindicated in patients with cardiac or renal insufficiency. (For additional information on complications of mechanical bowel preparation, see Chapter 2.)

The cleansing requirements for sigmoidoscopy are less stringent than for colonoscopy. Most providers use two small-volume hypertonic enemas (e.g., Fleet enemas). These should be administered just before the examination to remove the stool from the distal bowel that would impair the examination. Administration of enemas too soon before the procedure allows more proximal stool to move to the distal bowel. The most common potential problems related to this type of enema include chemical proctitis and mechanical injury to the anus or rectum. Injuries caused by enema tips usually occur on the anterior rectal wall.[6] The use of soft, flexible, lubricated enema tips minimizes the potential for this type of injury. (For management of rectal perforations, see Chapter 28.) Chemically induced proctitis is usually self-limiting can be managed with bowel rest and administration of steroid enemas. Overdosage with sodium phosphate enemas can result in hypocalcemia, hyperphosphatemia, hypernatremia, hypernatremic dehydration, and acidosis.

Intravenous Sedation

Conscious sedation during endoscopy reduces patient symptoms associated with the procedure. However, conscious sedation can produce respiratory depression, hypotension, tachycardia, or bradycardia.[7] Severe hypotension and hypoxia associated with sedation can lead to myocardial infarction. Endoscopists can prevent excessive sedation by carefully titrating the level of sedation throughout the procedure. In patients in whom conscious sedation is used, monitoring of pulse, blood pressure, and pulse oximetry is necessary. Hemodynamic depression requires that intravenous fluid be administered for resuscitation. Respiratory depression responds to patient stimulation, supplemental oxygen, and reversal of sedation, if necessary. Naloxone (Narcan; 0.4 mg intravenously and 0.4 mg intramuscularly) will reverse the narcotic effects. Flumazenil (Romazicon; 0.2 to 1.0 mg intravenously), a benzodiazepine-receptor antagonist, will reverse sedation from midazolam. Vasovagal episodes that occur during induction of anesthesia represent excess sedation. Similar episodes that occur during the course of endoscopy more frequently develop from vasovagal reactions resulting from colonic distention. Clinical support can be provided with intravenous fluids and simultaneous decompression of the colon of all excessive gaseous distention. Extensive stretching of the colon and its mesentery during insertion of the scope may also induce the vasovagal reflex. All colonoscopic loops should be removed to assist in resolution of the vasovagal episode.

Narcotic (meperidine) and sedative hypnotic (diazepam or midazolam) agents are most frequently used for conscious sedation during intestinal endoscopy. Titration of these agents allows endoscopy of the entire colon with minimal patient discomfort. Use of sedative hypnotic agents potentiates the narcotic effect and permits reduction of narcotic dosage and complications. An additional feature of sedative hypnotics is their amnestic properties, which impair the patient's memory of a difficult or painful procedure. Midazolam has several advantages over diazepam: superficial phlebitis caused by the rapid infusion of diazepam occurs rarely[1]; midazolam's shorter half-life allows prompt recovery from sedation; and it is effective at doses half those of diazepam.

Cardiorespiratory Effects

Cardiorespiratory effects can result from medication, mechanical forces, or physiologic responses associated with the stress of endoscopy. Intraluminal distention or bowel traction can produce a vasovagal response, which may reflect a decrease in venous return. Abdominal distention, external abdominal pressure, or direct intra-abdominal pressure from the scope leads to elevation of the diaphragm. This pressure decreases pulmonary compliance and ventilation and adds to the respiratory depression associated with conscious sedation.

INFECTIOUS COMPLICATIONS

Infectious complications of colonoscopy are caused by transmission of disease from patient to patient (infection control) or from patient to examiner and from bacteremia related to the procedure. Present recommendations suggest limiting patient-to-patient transmission with mechanical cleansing of the endoscopic equipment, and 30-minute submersion in glutaraldehyde solution provides protection from tuberculosis. This protection is used to extrapolate similar protection from HIV infection and hepatitis. Patient-to-examiner transmission can be prevented with proper facial, eye, and hand protection. Most endoscopy rooms are equipped with splashguards or goggles, disposable aprons, and gloves.

Lower GI tract endoscopy may cause bacteremia, but only five cases of endocarditis have been associated with these procedures.[8,9] These reported cases are poorly documented and have minimal clinical implications. Despite this low risk, instrumentation of the lower GI tract with resultant bacteremia has led the American Heart Association to recommend antibiotic treatment for patients at high risk. Factors associated with high risk for bacteremia are listed below:

Prosthetic heart valves
Congenital cardiac malformations
Rheumatic and other acquired valvular dysfunction
Surgically constructed systemic pulmonary shunts
Idiopathic hypertrophic subaortic stenosis
Mitral valve prolapse with insufficiency
Previous history of endocarditis
Vascular prosthesis

Risks of antibiotic therapy include allergic reaction, anaphylaxis, and antibiotic-induced colitis. Clinical judgment suggests that the risks of antibiotic complications be weighed against the risks for bacteremia and endocarditis. Although the risk for endocarditis is extremely low compared with the risks of antibiotic complications, the complications associated with endocarditis are significant in certain risk groups. The mortality rate for infective endocarditis in a patient with a valvular prosthesis is 44%.[10] Thus selective use of antibiotics limits the risks associated with antimicrobial agents and may prevent endocarditis in high-risk groups.

MAJOR COMPLICATIONS

Hemorrhage

The prevalence of hemorrhage after colonoscopy ranges from 0.05% to 3.0%.[11,12] Hemorrhage occurs most commonly with therapeutic endoscopy (0.20% to 3.0%) but can occur with diagnostic procedures (0.05% to 0.1%).[11,13] Hemorrhage is most frequently associated with intraluminal bleeding, but bleeding can arise from extraluminal sources such as mesenteric lacerations associated with stretching during instrument manipulation. Intraperitoneal hemorrhage from splenic injury and rupture has also been reported after colonoscopy.[14,15]

Intraluminal hemorrhage can occur during or immediately after the examination. Delayed bleeding occurs within 2 to 15 days of the procedure. Hemorrhage after snare excision or hot biopsy of a polyp is related to the technical aspects of the procedure. Inadequate cautery or improper snare technique prevents proper coagulation of the polyp vasculature and leads to bleeding. If bleeding occurs during or immediately after an examination, initial treatment includes washing the bleeding site with epinephrine-saline solution (1:1000 in saline solution). If the bleeding continues, the site may require additional coagulation. Reencirclement of bleeding polyp stalks with the snare may stop the hemorrhage. Judicious use of further electrocautery is important to prevent full-thickness intestinal injury at a site already treated with electrocautery.

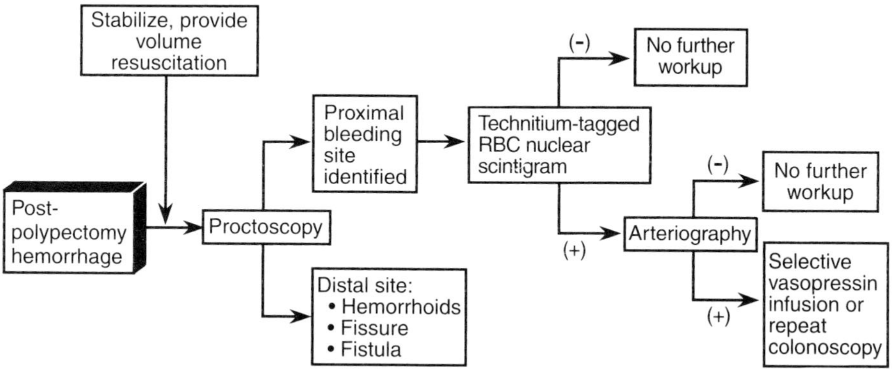

Fig. 9-1 Algorithm for management of postpolypectomy bleeding.

Delayed hemorrhage occurs when the eschar from the polyp site separates prematurely from the coagulation bed, leading to hematochezia. Delayed bleeding occurs within 2 to 15 days after the procedure, typically within the first 7 to 10 days. The bleeding may be massive, and in-hospital fluid resuscitation and observation may be necessary. Minimal hemorrhage ceases spontaneously with fluid resuscitation and intestinal rest. Moderate bleeding may require repeat colonoscopy to identify and treat the bleeding site. Clinically, it is difficult to determine whether the hemorrhage has ceased, because hematochezia may continue for several hours afterward. Nuclear scintigraphy with tagged red blood cell scans is useful to establish whether the bleeding persists and further treatment is necessary. In cases of severe hemorrhage or persistent bleeding, angiography may be required to identify the location of the bleeding and for treatment with selective arterial vasopressin infusion. The management of postpolypectomy bleeding is summarized in Fig. 9-1.

Colonoscopic Perforation

Perforation, the most frequent major complication of diagnostic colonoscopy, occurs in 0.06% to 0.8% of diagnostic procedures.[11,16-18] The endoscopist may immediately identify the perforation during the procedure when free air in the peritoneal cavity or extraluminal adipose tissue is noted. When the perforation is not seen during the examination, the index of suspicion increases if the patient complains of abdominal pain or distention. Supine and erect abdominal radiographs may display the presence of free air within the peritoneal cavity.

Delayed manifestation occurs with small intraperitoneal or retroperitoneal perforations. Symptoms of delayed perforations arise after the patient has returned home. Opelka et al.[19] reported that in 58% of patients with perforations after colonoscopy, symptoms were noted within 24 hours and included fever, persistent abdominal pain, distention, nausea, or vomiting. Retroperitoneal perforations may dissect along the root of the mesentery, which allows the pneumoretroperitoneum to extend along the aorta into the chest and cervical area and create pneumomediastinum and cervical subcutaneous emphysema. Retroperitoneal air may be identified on abdominal radiographs outlining the psoas muscle or in the perirectal soft tissue.

Perforations result from mechanical forces during colonoscopic insertion or from barotrauma during colonic insufflation. Mechanical forces that cause perforations include forceful instrument insertion, endoscopic torquing with creation or withdrawal of an alpha loop, slide-by insertion technique, and insertion of a sigmoid splinting instrument. Mechanical perforations also result from a direct injury at the colonoscopic tip or from colonic stretching or bowing by the endoscope at sites remote from the distal end of the scope. Most mechanical perforations occur in the rectosigmoid colon and may result from fixation of the rectum or sigmoid colon from surgical adhesions or other inflammatory conditions within the pelvis.[11] Colon disease that contributes to rectosigmoid fixation includes ulcerated or friable tumors, stricture, inflammatory bowel disease, and diverticulitis. The endoscopist who encounters excessive resistance during insertion or torquing of the scope should withdraw the instrument and inspect the colon carefully to ensure that it remains intact.

Colonic insufflation is essential in introducing the scope and examining the lumen of the colon. Excessive insufflation causes significant abdominal pain and discomfort and increases the difficulty of the examination. The endoscopist should limit air insufflation to the minimum required for safe endoscope insertion and adequate inspection of the colon. Cadaver studies reveal that the cecum is most susceptible to pneumatic perforations, followed by the transverse colon, sigmoid colon, and rectum.[16] The injuries begin with serosal linear tears from luminal distention and progress to full-thickness perforation. Clinical examinations that involve intraluminal pressures and simple diverticular rupture during colonoscopy have not revealed a predisposition to pneumatic rupture. Perforation is more probably associated with endoscopy in patients with acute diverticulitis.

The right colon and cecum are predisposed to barotrauma because the colonic wall is thin and the cecal diameter is large. According to Laplace's law, wall tension is directly related to the radius of a cylinder (e.g., colon lumen). Thus, as the cecum distends during insufflation, the wall tension of the colon increases until the serosa tears and perforations occur.

A rare electrocautery-related problem is colonic explosion. Hydrogen and methane produced by colonic bacteria are cumbustible and potentially explosive. Explosion of colonic gas has occurred during anal surgery, colonic surgery on unprepared bowel, proctosigmoidoscopic polypectomy, and colonoscopic polypectomy.[20] Recommendations to avoid this rare problem include avoidance of the use of mannitol preparation, CO_2 insufflation, air insufflation, and antibiotic therapy.

Perforations during therapeutic colonoscopy occur from thermal or electrical injury when electrocautery or laser is used. Transmural injuries can also occur when colonoscopic instruments inserted through the endoscope directly perforate the bowel. The reported prevalence of therapeutic perforations varies from 0.5% to 3.0%. The injury can extend full thickness or remain limited to the colon wall without perforation. In several reports, patients with colonic electrocautery injuries have had postpolypectomy coagulation syndrome.[17,21] The injury is a transmural burn with serositis overlying the electrocautery site. These limited injuries cause abdominal pain and tenderness, as well as fever, nausea, and vomiting. Abdominal radiographs do not show any evidence of perforation. Often these injuries are difficult to distinguish from frank perforations. In the absence of diffuse peritonitis, treatment entails intravenous antibiotic therapy, intestinal rest, and frequent examination. Progressive symptoms during treatment suggest more extensive injury and require urgent laparotomy.

Electrocautery creates transmural injury when the current proves excessive for the coagulation technique used. These techniques include fulguration, hot biopsy forceps, and snare excision. Wadas and Sanowski[22] noted that perforations from hot biopsy forceps occurred in the right colon, where the coagulation injury quickly extended through the thin colon wall. Full-thickness injuries from coagulation are related to the current density, which is directly related to intensity, duration, and diameter of the application of the electric current. Current density is inversely related to the diameter of tissue involved. Hot biopsy forceps limit the diameter of current application; excessive current duration or intensity, however, can lead to full-thickness injury. Snare electrocautery forceps are tightened during the process of tissue coagulation, which decreases the application diameter of current and sharply increases the current density. This can lead to transmural coagulation and perforation.

Perforations are not always evident immediately after polypectomy. The patient may remain symptom free or localized peritonitis may develop slowly over the next 4 to 12 hours. Localized peritonitis or asymptomatic perforations do not necessitate urgent surgical therapy. Nonsurgical treatment with intestinal rest, intravenous fluids, and antibiotics limits the peritonitis and allows the perforation to seal. Several series have reported that in one third of patients, perforation was treated successfully without surgery.[19,23] If the colon has no underlying disease and the mechanical bowel preparation was adequate, spontaneous healing progresses with resolution of abdominal symptoms over the next 24 to 48 hours. The constellation of symptoms (fever, localized pain and tenderness, and elevated white blood cell count) after polypectomy that responds to nonsurgical management (bowel rest, intravenous hydration, and antibiotic therapy) has been termed postpolypectomy syndrome. Successful management

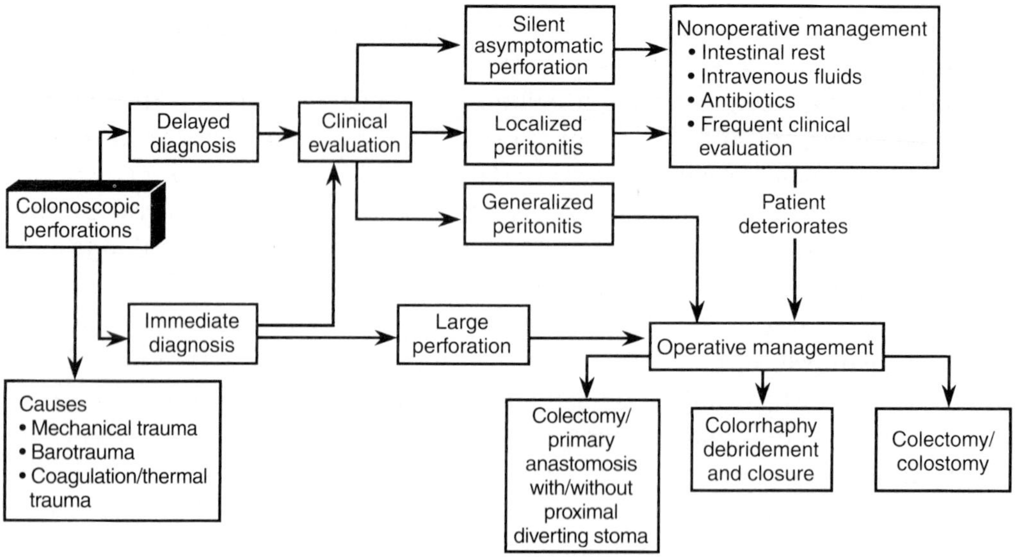

Fig. 9-2 Algorithm for management of colonoscopic perforations.

requires close observation, experience, and judgment. Any patient who fails to respond to nonsurgical treatment should undergo laparotomy.

Perforations recognized during colonoscopy usually represent injuries from barotrauma or are mechanical injuries. These are often larger than electrocautery injuries, do not spontaneously seal, and increase the risk of prolonged peritoneal soilage. Associated colon disease contributes to poor healing and may influence the decision for surgery. Immediate laparotomy with repair or resection of the perforated colon limits further morbidity or mortality. Colorrhaphy is reserved for limited injuries with no significant underlying colon disease. Debridement and closure of the perforation in patients with a mechanically cleansed bowel limits complications associated with bowel resection. Colectomy with creation of a primary anastomosis removes perforated bowel and associated colon disease. Bowel resection and colostomy is useful in patients with significant peritoneal soilage, when surgery must be delayed, and when the underlying colon disease prevents creation of a primary anastomosis.

Colonoscopic perforations arise from various types of injuries. Prevention of these injuries relies on training, experience, and caution. Treatment of colonoscopic perforations depends on the mechanism of injury, size of the perforation, delay in diagnosis, adequacy of the bowel preparation, associated colon disease, and the underlying medical condition of the patient. Nonsurgical management may be considered for small perforations; large perforations with fecal soilage demand urgent surgical intervention. The management of colonoscopic perforations is summarized in Fig. 9-2.

Proctoscopic Perforations

Proctoscopic perforations are rare but serious complications of intestinal endoscopy.[24] Nelson et al.[25] reported only three perforations in 16,325 proctoscopic examinations. The injury most commonly occurs when the bowel wall has been weakened by disease such as colitis, rectal tumor, or constricting lesion. The line of force during insertion guides the scope to the anterior rectal wall, where the usual site of injury is between the peritoneal reflection and the rectosigmoid junction.[26] The perforation is usually recognized as the scope enters the peritoneal cavity or the endoscopist encounters the perirectal fat or local bleeding.[24] Significant rectal trauma with rectal perforation requires surgical treatment. Most authors believe that delayed treatment increases mortality from 8% to 20%.[27] Major morbidity and mortality are associated with nonmechanical cleansing of the proximal colon. Treatment involves resection of associated disease, repair of the perforation site, rectal washout, pelvic drainage, and a diverting colostomy[28] (see Chapter 28).

CONCLUSION

Training, experience, and conservative technique help to minimize complications associated with endoscopic procedures of the colorectum. Prompt recognition and appropriate management of complications help to minimize morbidity.

REFERENCES

1. Rogers BHG, Silvis SE, Nebel OT, et al. Complications of flexible fiberoptic colonoscopy and polypectomy. Gastrointest Endosc 22:73-77, 1975.
2. Le TH, Timmcke AE, Gathright JB, et al. Outpatient bowel preparation for elective colon resection. J Am Coll Surg (submitted for publication).
3. Beck DE. Mechanical bowel cleansing for surgery. Perspect Colon Rectal Surg 7:97-114, 1994.
4. Bigard MA, Gaucher P, Lassalle C. Fatal colonic explosion during colonoscopic polypectomy. Gastroenterology 77:1307-1310, 1979.
5. Marshall JB, Pineda JJ, Barthel JS, et al. Prospective, randomized trial comparing sodium phosphate solution with polyethylene glycol–electrolyte lavage for colonoscopy preparation. Gastrointest Endosc 39:631-634, 1993.
6. Hool GJ, Bokey EL, Pheils MT. Enema-nozzle injury of the rectum. Med J Aust 1:364, 381, 1980.
7. Corman ML. Colon and Rectal Surgery, 2nd ed. Philadelphia: JP Lippincott, 1989.
8. Meyer GW. Prophylaxis of infective endocarditis during gastrointestinal procedures: Report of a survey. Gastrointest Endosc 25:1-2, 1979.
9. Rumfield W, Wallace G, Scott BB. Bacterial endocarditis after endoscopy [letter]. Lancet 2:1083, 1980.
10. Rosen L, Abel M, Gordon PH, et al. Practice parameters for antibiotic prophylaxis—Supporting documentation. Dis Colon Rectum 35:278-285, 1992.
11. Habr-Gama A, Waye JD. Complications and hazards of gastrointestinal endoscopy. World J Surg 13:193-201, 1989.

12. Peleman RR, Kinzie JL, Desai TK, et al. Colonoscopic polypectomy. Gastroenterol Clin North Am 17:851-858, 1988.
13. Gibbs D, Opelka FG, Beck DE, et al. Postpolypectomy hemorrhage. Dis Colon Rectum (submitted for publication).
14. Heath B, Rogers A, Taylor A, et al. Splenic rupture: An unusual complication of colonoscopy. Am J Gastroenterol 89:449-450, 1994.
15. Telmos AJ, Mittal VK. Splenic rupture following colonoscopy [letter]. JAMA 237:2718, 1977.
16. Kavin H, Sinicrope F, Esker AH. Management of perforation of the colon at colonoscopy. Am J Gastroenterol 87:161-167, 1992.
17. Christie JP, Marrazzo J III. "Mini-Perforation" of the colon—Not all postpolypectomy perforations require laparotomy. Dis Colon Rectum 34:132-135, 1991.
18. Macrae FA, Tan KG, Williams CB. Towards safer colonoscopy: A report on the complications of 5000 diagnostic or therapeutic colonoscopies. Gut 24:376-383, 1983.
19. Opelka FG, McGinity JM, Timmcke AE, et al. Management of colonoscopic perforations. Dis Colon Rectum (submitted for publication).
20. Bigard M, Gaucher P, Lassalle C. Fatal colonic explosion during colonoscopic polypectomy. Gastroenterology 77:1307-1310, 1979.
21. Waye JD. The postpolypectomy coagulation syndrome. Gastrointest Endosc 27:184, 1981.
22. Wadas DD, Sanowski RA. Complications of the hot biopsy forceps technique. Gastrointest Endosc 34:32-37, 1988.
23. Nivatvongs S. Complications in colonoscopic polypectomy: Lessons to learn from an experience of 1576 polyps. Am Surg 54:61-63, 1988.
24. Goligher JC. Injuries of the rectum and colon. In Goligher JC, ed. Surgery of the Anus Rectum and Colon, 4th ed. London: Baillière Tindall, 1980, pp 916-917.
25. Nelson RL, Abcarian H, Prasad ML. Iatrogenic perforation of the colon and rectum. Dis Colon Rectum 25:305, 1982.
26. Befeler D. Proctoscopic perforation of the large bowel. Dis Colon Rectum 10:376, 1967.
27. Andresen AFR. Perforations from proctoscopy. Gastroenterology 9:32-43, 1947.
28. Beck DE, Opelka FG. Pelvic and perineal trauma. Perspect Colon Rectal Surg 6:134-156, 1993.

CHAPTER 10

Laparoscopic Surgery

DAVID E. BECK

Laparoscopy is used increasingly in colorectal surgery and, like other invasive procedures, has associated complications. The rapid adoption of this technology by general surgeons and surgical subspecialists (e.g., colorectal surgeons) and use of new procedures have produced a unique situation. Surgeons adopted this new technology without the benefit of traditional training gained in residency and fellowships. An interim lack of organized progressive experience in colorectal laparoscopic surgery and the challenges of advanced procedures have contributed to complications. Complications are inversely related to the operating surgeon's experience, and several reports document a higher complication rate during a surgeon's early laparoscopic experience.[1-4] Laparoscopic colorectal surgical procedures are more difficult than are other advanced laparoscopic procedures. Colorectal procedures require extensive mobilization of a large hollow organ with ligation of numerous large blood vessels. Laparoscopic intestinal surgery involves extraction of a large specimen and restoration of bowel continuity.[3] Complications of laparoscopic procedures can be categorized as those related to trocars, the pneumoperitoneum, and the procedure itself.

TROCAR-RELATED COMPLICATIONS

Although relatively safe, the placement and use of trocars and pneumoperitoneum needles (e.g., Veress needles) can cause complications. During trocar and needle insertion, every organ and structure in the abdomen is at risk for injury. A trocar injury to the bladder usually is manifested by pneumaturia, hematuria, and occasionally by ballooning of the urinary drainage bag.[3] Injury to solid organs and major vascular structures is usually accompanied by hemorrhage. Many reports and presentations have documented these injuries, but their prevalence is low. Mintz[5] reported a prevalence of 0.05% in a survey of more than 99,000 procedures. Several extensive reviews of diagnostic laparoscopic procedures described a morbidity of 0.15% to 0.6% and a mortality of 0.04% to 0.13%.[6] Intraoperative identification of an injury is important to minimize associated morbidity.

The use of a Veress needle to establish a pneumoperitoneum has the potential to injure organs, blood vessels, or bowel. The small diameter of this needle and its spring-loaded cover limit complications. Knowledge of vascular anatomy (e.g., the location of the epigastric arteries) is helpful to avoid abdominal wall vascular injuries. Methods such as aspiration after needle placement, the saline solution drop test, and pressure monitoring during gas insufflation also help minimize complications. Improper placement of a Veress needle leads to insufflation in the preperitoneal space or possible intestinal insufflation. One study found that in 1.5% of patients, perioperative abdominal radiographs documented air insufflation of an intestinal loop as a result of the use of a Veress needle.[7]

To eliminate the potential complications from use of a Veress needle and the initial trocar insertion, some surgeons insert the first trocar with an open, or Hasson, laparoscopic technique.[8] The open technique, however, has associated complications such as avulsion of adhesions. Comparison of complications with the open versus a closed technique has shown fewer complications with the open method, but scant prospective randomized data are available.[9]

The major risk from trocars is related to their initial insertion. Because this is often a blind procedure, organs that are adherent to the abdominal wall may be inadvertently injured. Additional trocars, inserted under direct vision with the laparoscopic camera placed through the initial trocar, have a lower potential for injury. Bleeding can result from injury to abdominal wall vessels such as the epigastric artery or vein. In most cases, bleeding can be stopped with compression, but transfusion or ligation may be required. Abdominal wall nerve injury is minimized by avoidance of areas of the abdomen where major nerve trunks are located (e.g., inguinal area, medial and superior to the iliac spine, and close to the ribs). Transection of nerves will cause an area of anesthesia distal to the transected nerve trunk, whereas nerve trunk injuries may produce causalgia.

Most trocar-related injuries result from technical problems such as inappropriate placement; inadequate skin incision, which necessitates increased insertion force; extraperitoneal location of the trocar, usually from failure to penetrate a loose peritoneal layer; excessive depth of insertion, usually from excessive force; and faulty instruments.[10] An adequate pneumoperitoneum moves the abdominal wall away from the intraperitoneal organs and lessens the chances of organ injury.

Trocar site hernias occur rarely and are related to the location and size of the trocar (or cannula) wound. Hernias occur more frequently if the cannulas are placed through the linea alba than through the rectus muscle. With small cannulas, the reported frequency is 1 in 5000 to 10,000 cases.[11] The instruments used in laparoscopic colorectal procedures require larger cannulas (10 to 33 mm). With these larger trocars, the incidence of trocar site hernia is 0.1% to 0.3%.[12] To minimize the occurrence of a hernia, the fascia on all trocar wounds 10 mm or larger requires closure.[13] Devices to assist in trocar site closure (e.g.,

Endo-Judge, Ethicon, Cincinnati, Ohio) are now available, and their routine use may reduce this complication.

Wound infection at trocar sites is also uncommon, with a reported frequency of 0.1% to 3.0%.[12] Most of these infections have been associated with intra-abdominal contamination (e.g., ruptured appendix) or with specimen removal (e.g., appendix or gallbladder). These small, deep wounds, if not appropriately managed, have the potential to progress to necrotizing fasciitis, an uncommon but potentially lethal complication. Inasmuch as many patients who undergo laparoscopy are discharged from the hospital in the early postoperative period, it is important that they be instructed about the signs and symptoms of wound infection. Development of wound erythema, drainage, or increasing pain should prompt the patient to seek medical attention. Any suspected wound infection requires exploration (opening), debridement, and drainage of fluid collection.

PNEUMOPERITONEUM-RELATED COMPLICATIONS

A carbon dioxide pneumoperitoneum results in several physiologic changes, including alterations in acid-base balance, pulmonary mechanics, and cardiopulmonary physiology.[3] Transperitoneal absorption of CO_2 results in elevation of arterial PCO_2, and in all patients end-tidal CO_2 should be continuously monitored. Although in most patients intraperitoneal CO_2 can be managed by increasing the ventilation rate, in patients with cardiovascular disease hypercarbia and acidemia may develop. Treatment of severe hypercarbia and acidosis requires prompt evacuation of the intraperitoneal CO_2 and mechanical hyperventilation.[14-16]

Hemodynamic and pulmonary complications resulting from increased intra-abdominal pressure have also been described.[17,18] The magnitude of these alterations is related to the amount of intra-abdominal pressure, baseline hemodynamic function, and volume status. It is recommended that the intra-abdominal pressure be kept lower than 15 mm Hg to minimize these effects. The increased intra-abdominal pressure used in laparoscopy also raises the diaphragm and decreases pulmonary compliance. This can be compensated for by increasing the ventilator inflation pressure.[17-19] Severe bradycardia can occur during the intraperitoneal insufflation of CO_2, because peritoneal distention increases vagal tone. Careful monitoring will identify these changes, and appropriate measures can be instituted.

Subcutaneous emphysema results from failure of an insufflating Veress needle to reach the peritoneal cavity or from CO_2 being forced into the abdominal wall during accidental withdrawal of trocars and their subsequent placement. Minimal subcutaneous emphysema will resolve spontaneously. The presence of significant subcutaneous gas may lead to pneumothorax or pneumomediastinum, which require prompt diagnosis and treatment. A large volume of sequestrated CO_2 can also overwhelm the endogenous clearance mechanisms and lead to hypercarbia and acidosis.[20]

The high flow and volume of gas used to obtain and maintain the pneumoperitoneum causes additional problems. The temperature of CO_2 used to inflate the abdomen is generally 16° to 17° C when it comes in contact with the peritoneum.[3] Prolonged exposure (more than 3 to 4 hours) to unheated gas leads to hypothermia. A core temperature below 32° C is associated with serious complications such as hypotension, cardiac arrhythmias, and clotting disorders. Hypothermia is minimized with the use of air or water warming blankets; warming of intravenous fluids, irrigating fluids, and anesthesia gases; and limiting laparoscopic operating time. An extremely rare and potentially lethal complication is a gas embolus. Direct injection of CO_2 into a blood vessel results in the characteristic "mill wheel" murmur, which requires initiation of treatment (administration of 100% oxygen, placement of the patient in the left lateral head-down position, and attempted aspiration of gas from the ventricle).[21]

A potential secondary problem associated with a pneumoperitoneum is venous oozing. The increased intra-abdominal pressure of the pneumoperitoneum acts to compress or tamponade small veins. Thus during the procedure hemorrhage may not be observed, but after release of the pneumoperitoneum small divided vessels may ooze. This may explain the drop in hematocrit value occasionally seen after laparoscopic surgery. To minimize this problem, surgeons have either lowered the pneumoperitoneum pressure used during the operation or they make a special effort to observe the intra-abdominal cavity for evidence of venous hemorrhage at the completion of the procedure with a lowered pneumoperitoneal pressure.

PROCEDURE-RELATED COMPLICATIONS

Complications related to the procedure can occur early (during the procedure) or late (after the procedure). The frequency of intraoperative complications is 14% to 17%, and of postoperative complications is 8% to 33%.[1] A summary of complications in the larger published laparoscopic bowel surgery series is presented in Table 10-1. Early complications include conversion to an open procedure, organ injury, and hemorrhage.

Conversion to an open procedure is not necessarily a complication but an indicator of good surgical judgment. Reasons for converting to an open procedure include unclear anatomy, excessive operating time, intraoperative complications (e.g., hemorrhage or organ injury), or inability to complete the procedure (e.g., because of the presence of adhesions or abscesses). The reported rates of conversion are 8% to 50%. The large range reflects differences in patient selection, surgeon experience, and definition of what constitutes conversion. Most studies have documented that operations that must be converted result in more frequent complications, higher costs, and longer postoperative hospital stay.

Table 10-1 Complications after laparoscopic colorectal procedures

Author	Year	No. of patients	Morbidity (%)	Mortality (%)
Franklin et al.[22]	1993	19	16	0
Quattlebaum et al.[23]	1993	20	30	0
Scoggin et al.[24]	1993	20	20	0
Peters and Bartels[25]	1993	24	13	0
Musser et al.[26]	1994	24	28	0
Senagore et al.[27]	1993	38	15	0
Puente et al.[28]	1994	38	24	2.0
Monson et al.[29]	1992	40	15	2.5
Phillips et al.[30]	1992	51	8	2.0
Zucker et al.[31]	1994	65	6	0
Guillou[32]	1993	70	17	5.1
Cohen and Wexner[33]	1994	100	22	0

Injury to organs can occur from trocars, laser energy, electrocautery, or trauma from instruments. Lasers are used in gynecologic procedures to vaporize endometriomas but add little to laparoscopic colorectal procedures. Laparoscopy results in loss of the surgeon's tactile ability, which is accentuated by the use of a noncontact laser. Use of a laser adds operative time and expense to the procedure, requires additional protective equipment, and offers no proven benefit in the majority of colorectal procedures.[34] In addition, several of the lethal complications resulting from laparoscopic procedures occurred after laser injuries to the portal vein and vena cava.[1] For these reasons, most colorectal laparoscopic surgeons use scissors or electrocautery and rarely use a laser.

The electrosurgical instruments used in laparoscopy are associated with a significant portion of laparoscopic complications. Injuries caused by energy transfer outside the visual field often go unrecognized. Injuries can also occur because of defective insulation on the active electrode, capacity coupling, or direct coupling of the active electrode and metal instruments or the electrode and the laparoscope.[3,35] The insulation on both disposable and reusable electrosurgical instruments should be inspected and checked before use and on a regular basis. Capacitance coupling is prevented by the use of metal cannulas that disperse the current through the abdominal wall or modern plastic cannulas, which do not store current.

An unrecognized thermal bowel injury may progress to a transmural perforation and become manifest hours to days after the injury. Symptoms of this type of injury usually include an ileus, signs of peritoneal irritation, fever, and leukocytosis.[3] These injuries are minimized by ensuring that the active electrodes come in contact with only the intended tissue. A bowel electrocautery injury is managed by imbrication of small injuries and resection and closure of more extensive burns. It is often best to manage these significant injuries with the abdomen open.

Hemorrhage, if minor, can be managed with laparoscopic techniques such as occlusion with a laparoscopic clamp followed by placement of a ligaclip or Endo Loop ligation. Electrocautery is useful for small vessels only. Bipolar cautery is preferred by some surgeons. Major hemorrhage is appropriately managed by expeditiously opening the abdomen.

Ureteral injury is the most common urologic complication during laparoscopic surgery.[36] Knowledge of pelvic anatomy as seen laparoscopically and good operative technique are essential to avert this complication. Exposing and visualizing the ureter at all times during the procedure minimizes the potential for injury. Electrocoagulation in the vicinity of the ureter should be avoided to prevent thermal injury. A preoperative CT scan or intravenous pyelogram is obtained by some surgeons to confirm the location of the ureter and identify medical deviation associated with inflammatory or neoplastic conditions.[37] Stent placement with standard visable or infrared fiberoptic (Gabriel Medical, Lafayette, La.) ureteral catheters or use of a laparoscopic Doppler probe may be helpful in difficult cases.[3] Injured ureters identified during laparoscopy have been repaired laparoscopically. The technique involves mobilizing the ureter, placing stents antegrade or retrograde, and suturing the injury with a 4-0 chromic catgut.[3] More extensive repairs such as ureteroureterostomy or ureterocyctostomy are best accomplished after a laparotomy (see Chapter 7). Unrecognized urinary tract injuries usually result in fever, abdominal and flank pain, leukocytosis, and peritoneal signs. Aggressive examination will enable identification of the cause of the injury, which can be managed with a multispecialty approach.

Inability to locate intraluminal lesions such as polyps or small tumors remains a problem with laparoscopy. Several reports have documented that the intended lesion was missed at colectomy. Techniques to improve intraoperative identification of the target lesion include preoperatively tattooing the colon near the lesion, preoperative radiologic verification of lesion location, and intraoperative colonoscopy.[3,38]

Laparoscopic procedures are relatively time consuming, so it is imperative that patients be positioned correctly. Adequate padding of extremities and pressure areas is necessary to prevent pressure injuries. Special attention to the elbows and knees is important to prevent injury to the ulnar and perineal nerves. Sequential compression stockings minimize the venous pooling in the lower extremities associated with operative procedures and the use of a pneumoperitoneum. The operating table is frequently moved and repositioned to assist the surgeon in intra-abdominal retraction and exposure during laparoscopy. To prevent the patient from slipping while in extreme positions, the patient must be secured to the operating table with the use of a bean bag or adhesive tape.

Late complications of laparoscopic colorectal surgery result from an anastomotic leak or contamination. All patients having elective surgery should undergo full mechanical and antibiotic bowel preparation.[39] Patients having left colon operations should also undergo rectal irrigation after induction of anesthesia. Some authors have used intraoperative colonoscopy to confirm a clean and decompressed colon before a resection.[22,38] Multiple technical maneuvers used to minimize contamination include wound protectors, specimen bags, and bowel occlusion devices or clamps. Current techniques of performing an intracorporeal anastomosis have a higher potential for contamination. The experience to date has demonstrated equivalent leak rates after comparable open and laparoscopic procedures.

Of special concern is the potential for metastatic tumor recurrence or dissemination to trocar sites. The reports currently available are anecdotal; prospective controlled trials have not been completed.[40-45] Factors to consider include the presence of ascites in some of the case reports. Experience from the gynecology literature documents the problem of tumor implantation in patients with carcinoma of the ovary associated with ascites.[44] Some reports have involved patients with late stage disseminated tumors; however, others occurring after small potentially curable colon cancers suggest violation of well-accepted cancer principles or risks related to the laparoscopic technique or pneumoperitoneum.[22,40-43] From 1993 to 1995, more than 30 cases of port or extraction site recurrence have been reported.[44-55] The stage of these primary tumors has varied from Dukes stages A to D, and the time of presentation has ranged from 1 to 26 months. Although the frequency of this complication appears higher than that observed with open surgery, the true prevalence is not known. Until the results of large prospective trials are available, some authors recommend irrigation of trocar sites with sterile water, and others have refrained from using laparoscopic techniques in patients with potentially curable cancer outside of institutional review board–approved protocols.

With any developmental technology and new procedures, complications will occur. Appropriate training and experience, as well as care and objective review of results, should minimize morbidity in colorectal laparoscopic surgery.

REFERENCES

1. Beck DE, Opelka FG. Complications of laparoscopy. In Wexner SD, Jager RM, eds. Laparoscopy. New York: Churchill Livingston, 1995, pp 267-271.
2. See WA, Cooper CS, Fisher RJ. Predictors of laparoscopic complications after formal training in laparoscopic surgery. JAMA 270:2689-2692, 1993.
3. Ramos R. Complications of laparoscopic colon surgery: Prevention and management. Semin Colon Rectal Surg 5:239-243, 1994.

4. Deziel DJ, Millikan KW, Economou SG, Doolas A, Ko S, Airan MC. Complications of laparoscopic cholecystectomy: A national survey of 4,292 hospitals and an analysis of 77,604, cases. Am J Surg 165:9-14, 1993.
5. Mintz M. Risks and prophylaxis in laparoscopy: A survey of 100,000 cases. J Reprod Med 18:269-272, 1977.
6. Lightdale CJ. Indications, contraindications and complications of laparoscopy. In Sivak M, ed. Gastroenterologic Endoscopy. Philadelphia: WB Saunders, 1987, pp 1039-1044.
7. Reich H. Laparoscopic bowel injury. Surg Laparosc Endosc 2:74-78, 1992.
8. Hasson HM. Window for open laparoscopy. Am J Obstet Gynecol 137:869-870, 1980.
9. Hasson HM. Open laparoscopy versus closed laparoscopy: A comparison of complication rates. Adv Planned Parenthood 13:41-50, 1978.
10. Borten M. Complications of trocar insertion. In Fredman EA, ed. Laparoscopic Complications: Prevention and Management. Philadelphia: BC Decker, 1986, pp 286-295.
11. Kadar N, Reich H, Liu CY, Manko GF, Gimpleson R. Incisional hernias after major laparoscopic gynecologic procedures. Am J Obstet Gynecol 168:1493-1495, 1993.
12. Crist WD, Gadacz RT. Complications of laparoscopic surgery. Surg Clin North Am 3:269-270, 1993.
13. McMurrick PJ, Polglase AL. Early incisional hernia after use of the 12 mm port for laparoscopic surgery. Aust N Z J Surg 63:574-575, 1993.
14. Hall D, Goldstein A, Tynan E, Braunstein L. Profound hypercarbia late in the course of laparoscopic cholecystectomy: Detection by continuous capnometry. Anesthesiology 79: 173-174, 1993.
15. Hodgson C, McClelland RM, Newton JR. Some effects of the peritoneal insufflation of carbon dioxide at laparoscopy. Anaesthesia 25:382-390, 1970.
16. Fitzgerald SD, Andrus CH, Baudendistel LJ, Dohms TE, Kaminski DL. Hypercarbia during carbon dioxide pneumoperitoneum. Am J Surg 163:186-190, 1992.
17. Safran DB, Orlando R III. Physiologic effects of pneumoperitoneum. Am J Surg 167:281-286, 1994.
18. Wittgen CM, Andrus CH, Fitzgerald SD, Baudendistel LJ, Dohms TE, Kominski DL. Analysis of hemodynamic and ventilatory effects of laparoscopic cholecystectomy. Arch Surg 126:997-1000, 1991.
19. Nord HJ. Complications of laparoscopy. Endoscopy 24:693-700, 1992.
20. Kent RB III. Subcutaneous emphysema and hypercarbia following laparoscopic cholecystectomy. Arch Surg 126:1154-1156, 1991.
21. Au-Yeung P. Gas embolism during attempted laparoscopic vagotomy [letter]. Anaesthesia 47:817, 1992.
22. Franklin M Jr, Ramous R, Rosenthal D, Schuessler W. Laparoscopic colonic procedures. World Surg 17:51-56, 1993.
23. Quattlebaum JK, Dorsey FH, Usher CH. Laparoscopically assisted colectomy. Surg Laparosc Endosc 3:81-37, 1993.
24. Scoggin SD, Frazee RC, Snyder SK, Hendricks JC, Roberts JW, Symmonds RE, Smith RW. Laparoscopic-assisted bowel surgery. Dis Colon Rectum 36:747-750, 1993.
25. Peters WR, Bartels TL. Minimally invasive colectomy: Are the potential benefits realized? Dis Colon Rectum 36:751-756, 1993.
26. Musser DJ, Boorse RC, Madera F, Reed JG III. Laparoscopic colectomy: At what cost? Surg Laparosc Endosc 4:1-5, 1994.
27. Senagore AJ, Luchfield MA, MacKeigan JM, Mazier WP. Open colectomy versus laparoscopic colectomy: Are there differences? Am Surg 59:549-554, 1993.

28. Puente I, Sosa JL, Sleeman D, Desal U, Tranakas N, Hartman R. Laparoscopic assisted colorectal surgery. J Laparoendosc Surg 4:1-7, 1994.
29. Monson JRT, Darzi A, Carey PD, Guillou PJ. Prospective evaluation of laparoscopic-assisted colectomy in an unselected group of patients. Lancet 340:831-833, 1992.
30. Phillips EH, Franklin M, Carroll BJ, et al. Laparoscopic colectomy. Ann Surg 16:703-707, 1992.
31. Zucker KA, Pitcherd E, Martin BT. Laparoscopic colon resection. Surg Endosc 8:12-18, 1994.
32. Guillou P. Laparoscopic surgery for diseases of the colon and rectum: Quo vadis? Surg Endosc 8:669-671, 1993.
33. Cohen SM, Wexner SD. Laparoscopic right hemicolectomy. Surg Rounds 17:627-635, 1994.
34. Hunter JG. Laser or electrocautery for laparoscopic cholecystectomy? Am J Surg 161:345-349, 1991.
35. Voyles CR, Tucker RD. Education and engineering solutions for potential problems with laparoscopic monopolar electrosurgery. Am J Surg 164:57-62, 1992.
36. Evans RM, Hulbert JC, Reddy PK. Complications of laparoscopy. Semin Urol 10:164-168, 1992.
37. Grainger DA, Soderstrom RM, Schiff SF, Glickman MG, DeCherney AH, Diamond MP. Ureteral injuries at laparoscopy: Insights into diagnosis, management and prevention. Obstet Gynecol 75:839-843, 1990.
38. Beck DE. Colonoscopy and laparoscopy. In Jager RM, Wexner SD, eds. Laparoscopic Colorectal Surgery. New York: Churchill Livingstone, 1995, pp 143-148.
39. Beck DE. Mechanical bowel cleansing for surgery. Perspect Colon Rectal Surg 7:97-114, 1994.
40. Fusco MA, Paluzzi MW. Abdominal wall recurrence after laparoscopic assisted colectomy for adenocarcinoma of the colon. Dis Colon Rectum 36:858-861, 1993.
41. Fermor B, Umpleby HC, Lever JV, Symes MO, Williamson RC. Proliferative and metastatic potential of exfoliated colorectal cancer cells. J Natl Cancer Inst 76:347-349, 1986.
42. Walsh DC, Wattchow DA, Wilson TG. Subcutaneous metastases after laparoscopic resection of malignancy. Aust N Z J Surg 63:563-565, 1993.
43. Wexner SD, Cohen SM, Johansen OB, Nogueras JJ, Jagelman DG. Laparoscopic colorectal surgery: A prospective assessment and current perspective. Br J Surg 80:1602-1605, 1993.
44. Gleeson NC, Nicosia SV, Mark JE, Hoffman MS, Cavanagh D. Abdominal wall metastases from ovarian cancer after laparoscopy. Am J Obstet Gynecol 169:522-523, 1993.
45. Alexander RJT, Jacques BC, Mitchel KG. Laparoscopically assisted colectomy and wound recurrence. Lancet 341:249, 1993.
46. O'Rourke N, Price PM, Kelly S, Sikora K. Tumor inoculation during laparoscopy. Lancet 342:368, 1993.
47. Guillou PJ, Darzi A, Monson JRT. Experience with laparoscopic colorectal surgery for malignant disease. Surg Oncol 2(Suppl 1):43-49, 1993.
48. Nduka CC, Monson JRT, Menzies-Gow N, Darzi A. Abdominal wall metastases following laparoscopy. Br J Surg 81:648-662, 1994.
49. Berends FJ, Kazemier G, Bonjer HJ, Lange JF. Subcutaneous metasases after laparoscopic colectomy. Lancet 344:58, 1994.
50. Ramous JM, Gupta S, Anthone GJ, Ortega AE, et al. Laparoscopy and colon cancer: Is the port site at risk? A preliminary report. Arch Surg 129:897-900, 1994.

51. Jacquet P, Averbach AM, Jacquet N. Abdominal wall metastases and peritoneal carcinomatous after laparoscopic-assisted colectomy for colon cancer. Eur J Surg Oncol (in press).
52. Drouard F, Passone-Szerzyna H. Les greffer neoplasiques sur les sites de trocarts en chirurgie par laparoscopie des cancers coliques. Presented at the 96th French Congress of Surgery. Paris: October 3-5, 1994.
53. Cirocco WC, Schwartzman A, Golub RW. Abdominal wall recurrence after laparoscopic colectomy for colon cancer. Surgery 116:842-846, 1994.
54. Wexner SD, Cohen SM. Port site metastases after laparoscopic colorectal surgery for cure of malignancy. Br J Surg 82:295-298, 1995.
55. Jacquet P, Averbach AN, Stephens AD, Sugarbaker PH. Cancer recurrence following laparoscopic colectomy: Report of two cases of patients treated with heated intraperitoneal chemotherapy. Dis Colon Rectum 38:1110-1114, 1995.

CHAPTER 11

Hemorrhoidal Surgery

KEMOL I. DEEN
W. DOUGLAS WONG

In 1814, Thomas Copeland,[1] in a treatise on anorectal diseases, reported on three cases of hemorrhoidectomy. The operation was successful in only one patient; one died of pelvic sepsis; and hemorrhoids recurred in the third patient. Patients experienced obstructed defecation for up to 1 week after the procedure, presumably from edema of the pedicles, which were not excised but encircled and left to become ischemic and detach spontaneously. Subsequently in 1882, Whitehead[2] described amputation of hemorrhoids. Later, Milligan et al.[3] described their technique of open hemorrhoidectomy, which is now widely practiced in the United Kingdom and continental Europe. It was only around the middle of the twentieth century that the closed method of hemorrhoidectomy was described by Ferguson and Heaton.[4] Death was a dreaded and not uncommon complication of hemorrhoidal surgery in the early part of this century. Today, neither death nor overwhelming pelvic sepsis are considered common sequelae of hemorrhoidectomy. Indeed, it is unusual for patients to spend more than 24 to 48 hours in the hospital after hemorrhoidal surgery, and many operations are performed on an outpatient basis.

The occurrence of hemorrhoidal disease may be declining.[5] Furthermore, several nonsurgical options are available for treatment of symptomatic hemorrhoids that may, to some extent, have an effect on the prevalence of complications after hemorrhoidectomy. Most important, careful patient selection, attention to detail, and a sound understanding of anal canal anatomy remain key factors in minimizing complications after this procedure. In this chapter, the complications of hemorrhoidal surgery are empirically classified as early, intermediate, and late. Where appropriate, we present a review of the literature and discuss prevention and management of these complications.

EARLY COMPLICATIONS

Postoperative Pain

The anoderm has a rich supply of sensory nerves.[6] Pain may arise chiefly from involvement of anoderm below the dentate line. Although the true mechanism remains unclear, common belief is that posthemorrhoidectomy pain reflexly induces spasm of the urethral and anal sphincter muscles. Spasm of the urethral sphincter may lead to voiding difficulty, and anal sphincter spasm causes difficulty in evacuation. Both result in increased patient anxiety and reduced confidence. Control of pain is essential to ensure uneventful recovery after surgery. Several methods of pain control have been described. Local infiltration of the anal sphincters and the surrounding anoderm are popular either as the sole method of pain control or in combination with other methods.[7] Local anesthetic agents such as 0.25% bupivacaine solution may provide analgesia for up to 8 hours after surgery. Infiltration analgesia with NSAIDs such as toradol (Ketorolac) has been reported to provide effective pain control in patients undergoing in-office hemorrhoidectomy.[8] Other reported techniques include parenteral opiate analgesics administered as either a bolus or continuous infusion.[9] At home, warm sitz baths may also be helpful in alleviating pain. Warm baths reduce resting anal pressure, probably by relieving anal sphincter spasm.[10]

Hemorrhage

Hemorrhage in the recovery room is the result of an error of technique and is invariably caused by either a missed or a slipped ligature. Occasionally bleeding may continue undetected, with blood accumulating in a capacious rectum. The first signs of this complication may be pallor, tachycardia, and hypotension, which may require resuscitation with intravenous fluid and blood transfusion. The patient must be returned to the operating room and the bleeding arrested either with diathermy coagulation or suture transfixation of the bleeding site. Historically, some have advocated methods such as wound packing[11] and direct pressure at the bleeding site.[12] It must be remembered, however, that packing alone may provide a false sense of security because of little evidence of external bleeding, while progressive retrograde accumulation of blood leads to deterioration in the patient's condition.

Urinary Retention

The cause of urinary retention after hemorrhoidal surgery is multifactorial. Postoperative pain is the chief cause of urethral sphincter spasm. Spinal anesthesia has been associated with urinary retention.[13] Injudicious use of intravenous fluids may result in bladder distention with voiding difficulty after surgery.[14] Anal packing has been associated with urinary retention, probably from direct pressure on the bladder outflow track. Opiate analgesics may lead to transient detrusor weakness and consequently retention of urine.[15] Occasionally in elderly men, obstructive uropathy may progress to acute retention of urine after hemorrhoidal surgery.

The reported frequency of retention of urine has been as high as 50%.[16] A recent review of our experience disclosed a 17% prevalence of urinary retention.[17]

More recent evidence suggests that nonsteroidal analgesia combined with early ambulation may help prevent this complication. In a series of 100 hemorrhoidal excisions performed as an office procedure, Richman[8] reported only two cases of acute retention.

Before surgery, it is important to ensure an empty bladder in patients. During surgery, minimization of use of IV fluids will help maintain a reasonably empty bladder. Anal packing should be avoided. Furthermore, control of postoperative pain may have a key role in preventing voiding difficulty. If catheterization becomes necessary, intermittent catheterization under sterile conditions is the option of choice. However, if indwelling catheters are used, as in some patients with prostatic enlargement, small-diameter Silastic catheters are recommended. Appropriate urologic referral should be sought for patients with symptoms of bladder outflow obstruction.

Urinary Tract Infection

Infection of the urinary tract may result from either stasis of urine or instrumentation of the urinary tract. Data from our institution indicate a 3% prevalence of urinary tract infection as a complication of hemorrhoidal surgery.[17] Urine culture is required before appropriate antibiotic therapy is undertaken.

INTERMEDIATE COMPLICATIONS

Complications that characteristically occur from a few days to the first 2 to 3 weeks after surgery have been classified as intermediate. Specifically, delayed hemorrhage and constipation complicated by fecal impaction may occur during this time. Septic complications have been reported but are extremely rare.

Delayed Hemorrhage

Hemorrhage may occur from about the end of the first week to the third week after surgery. It usually is caused by secondary infection at the operation site and is the result of disruption of blood vessel thrombi in the hemorrhoidal pedicle. Bleeding may be from either a specific site or from multiple sites. Rosen et al.[18] have reported a 0.8% incidence of hemorrhage after hemorrhoidal excision. The reported frequency at our institution is approximately 2.5%. Hemorrhage occurred between the seventh and sixteenth postoperative days.[17] In our opinion, this complication is unpredictable and hence cannot be prevented. If it does occur, mild episodes should be treated expectantly with simultaneous withdrawal of any predisposing risk factors, particularly aspirin therapy. If bleeding is severe, a clotting profile should be performed and any deficiencies corrected. In the study by Rosen et al.,[18] 37% of patients with delayed hemorrhage after hemorrhoidectomy were receiving anticoagulant therapy. If surgical intervention becomes necessary, this must be performed in the operating room with the aid of proper lighting. It is important to perform proctoscopy and evacuate accumulated blood clots, which may help to accurately localize the bleeding site and prevent tenesmus during the recovery period. Electrocoagulation of a bleeding site may be all that is required. In some situations, suture transfixion of the bleeding pedicle may be required; in others, debridement of contaminated areas followed by a continuous oversew of the wound edges may help arrest hemorrhage. Furthermore, it must be remembered that patients with persistent intermittent bleeding after hemorrhoidal surgery may have a more proximal source of bleeding, and the proximal colon should be examined.

Constipation and Fecal Impaction

Impaction of feces is a distressing complication of hemorrhoidectomy. Pain at the operation site combined with the patient's fear of pain from defecating after surgery often lead to fecal impaction. Hence, in addition to adequate analgesia, it is important to allay any doubts or fears patients may have about evacuation after operation. Sufficient hydration will help maintain a soft stool. Some have advocated the use of bulking agents and laxatives to facilitate evacuation during this period.[19] Topical anesthetic gels before a bowel movement may help minimize pain and discomfort during evacuation. Where fecal impaction is identified early, simple irrigating enemas may help clear the anorectum of impacted feces. In the extreme situation in which identification of fecal impaction has been delayed, manual disimpaction with the patient under general anesthesia may be necessary.

Infection

The anorectum harbors an abundance of potentially pathogenic bacterial microorganisms. Despite this, infective complications after hemorrhoidectomy are unusually low. Local immunologic mechanisms may be responsible for the low rates of infection. Bacteremia and sepsis have also been documented after hemorrhoidectomy, but abscess formation is particularly rare. The reticuloendothelial system of the liver is thought to cleanse that organ of pathogenic bacteria; however, isolated liver abscesses have been reported as a rare occurrence after hemorrhoidectomy.[20] A high index of suspicion is required to identify this complication in patients with postoperative fever. Early diagnosis with the aid of ultrasound or CT will enable treatment with parenteral antibiotics, percutaneous drainage, or both. Occult infection in the perianal area may be another cause of fever.[17] Septic foci not evident clinically may be identified with anorectal ultrasound.[21] A focal collection, if identified, will require conventional drainage.

Not uncommonly, a few days after closed hemorrhoidectomy, inspection of the perianal wound may reveal partial wound dehiscence with some sloughing around the wound edges.

LATE COMPLICATIONS

Anal Stenosis

Anal stenosis results from overenthusiastic hemorrhoidal surgery. There is the risk of excessive stripping of anal mucosa, which may leave inadequate bridges of anoderm for healing to occur without stenosis. Secondary hemorrhoids should not be an issue but should be treated with either submucosal hemorrhoidectomy[22] or conservative methods such as sclerotherapy or rubber band ligation at a subsequent visit. In the mildest cases, the stenosis may simply be a web that disappears with graduated anal dilation in the office. Moderate anal stenosis may also be treated with four-quadrant incisions in the band of fibrotic tissue followed by regular anal dilation.[23] In more severe cases, surgical intervention may be required to relieve stenosis. Surgical correction of anal stenosis may be accomplished by one of several plastic operations involving skin flaps and subcutaneous tissue. The most common and probably easiest procedure is the Y-V advancement flap.[24] Correction of anal stenosis may also be undertaken with use of diamond-shaped flaps of skin and subcutaneous fat,[25] and extreme stenosis may require circumferential excision of scar tissue and bilateral rotation flaps (S flaps).[26] These flap techniques are discussed in Chapter 14.

Mucosal Ectropion (Whitehead Deformity)

Muscosal ectropion with the classic Whitehead deformity is commonly seen after the type of procedure described by Whitehead.[2] Persistent mucous discharge and perianal irritation may result. This operation entails making a circumferential incision at the level of the dentate line of the anal canal, elevating a flap of anal mucosa, and performing a submucosal hemorrhoidal excision. Redundant mucosa is then excised, and the anal canal is reconstructed with sutures. Currently this procedure is not widely performed.

Fecal Incontinence

Incontinence of feces results chiefly from damage to the internal anal sphincter during hemorrhoidectomy.[27] The internal anal sphincter is a thin, whitish, smooth muscle composed of circular fibers and is located just beneath the anal mucosa. It is almost always absent at the anal verge because its inferior limit is a few millimeters proximal to it. During surgery, the hemorrhoidal column should be lifted off the internal anal sphincter, which must be identified before excision of hemorrhoidal tissue. It is important to document the state of continence in these patients before surgery. Soiling and fecal leakage are the chief impairments of continence that result from internal anal sphincter damage. Once damaged, it is almost impossible to repair the internal anal sphincter. Treatment for soiling and leakage should include bulking agents and slowing agents (e.g., loperamide) and consideration of biofeedback therapy.

Anal Fistula

Fistula in ano is an uncommon complication of hemorrhoidectomy and is thought to occur more commonly after the closed procedure.[28] The fistula is usually a simple submucosal track that may be treated by simple unroofing.

Anal Tags and Pruritus Ani

Anal skin tags after hemorrhoidal excision are not uncommon. Patients may become aware of their presence when performing routine ablution. Invariably, these are edematous areas of anoderm that generally resolve spontaneously some weeks after surgery. Simple reassurance may help allay patients' concerns about recurrence. Occasionally a skin tag may be associated with pruritus ani. Simple excision of the skin tag in the office after administration of local anesthetic will alleviate symptoms.

Pruritus ani commonly results from leakage of anal canal mucus, which leads to irritation and sometimes maceration of the perianal skin. Beware of the rare sensitizing side effect of topical lidocaine.[29] Occasionally pruritus ani may occur for no obvious reason after hemorrhoidal excision. In such situations, patients should be advised to observe meticulous personal hygiene and reduce their intake of caffeine and alcohol, which predispose some individuals to this condition.[30]

Emergency Versus Elective Hemorrhoidal Surgery

Hemorrhoidal excision as an urgent procedure is now standard treatment for prolapsed thrombosed hemorrhoids and is relatively safe in experienced hands.[31] The chief risk is anal stenosis. Portal pyemia is a theoretical possibility. In a comparison of elective versus emergency hemorrhoidal surgery in 704 patients, Eu et al.[32] found no significant differences in the frequency of postoperative hemorrhage, anal stenosis, impairment of continence, and recurrent hemorrhoids.

HEMORRHOIDAL SURGERY IN SPECIAL SITUATIONS

Crohn's Disease

There is little doubt that hemorrhoidal surgery may be associated with a greater complication rate when there is coexistent Crohn's disease. Contrary to earlier belief, hemorrhoidectomy is not absolutely contraindicated in patients with perianal Crohn's disease.[33] It is advisable, however, to operate when the disease is quiescent.

Immunocompromise

Patients with malignancy who may be receiving chemotherapy may sometimes require treatment for hemorrhoids. These patients often have suboptimal blood cell counts and are prone to infective complications. Those with granulocyte defects are at particular risk for infection after any type of anorectal surgery.[34] In some cases, it is possible to stimulate granulocyte production with parenteral agents. Excision may be required in some instances simply to exclude a leukemic deposit in a perianal nodule that appears as a hemorrhoid and should be performed after administration of appropriate parenteral antibiotics, which should be continued for as long as 1 week.[35] Ideally, hemorrhoidal excision should be postponed in these patients until disease is either quiescent or hematologic indices have improved (e.g., after cessation of chemotherapy).

Anorectal Varices

Beware of anorectal varices! Unlike hemorrhoids, varices result from portal venous hypertension. Differentiation from hemorrhoids is essential because excision of varices may result in venous bleeding that may be difficult to control. A history of anal bleeding in a patient with cirrhosis should arouse suspicion of the possibility of variceal disease. Varices may be present in the rectum or anal canal or at the anal verge.[36] A definitive diagnosis may be made with the aid of duplex Doppler ultrasonography of the anorectum.[37] If bleeding complicates inadvertent excision of varices, they should be oversewn with a continuous suture technique.

Postpartum Hemorrhoids

Postpartum hemorrhoids that are refractory to conservative measures may require surgical treatment. Hemorrhoidectomy in this situation is safe, with a low prevalence of complications. Furthermore, it minimizes recovery time. Although it has been customary to deal with the largest hemorrhoidal mass first, we prefer to begin with the smallest hemorrhoids to preserve as much anoderm as possible from the outset.

Complications Associated With Adjunctive Procedures

Hemorrhoids have been associated with a higher than normal basal pressure, which has been attributed to internal anal sphincter hypertonia. Several procedures have therefore been undertaken to try to concomitantly reduce internal sphincter tone. The Lord procedure[38] involves anal dilation, but this is associated with anal sphincter disruption when performed too vigorously and is not recommended.[39,40] Lateral internal anal sphincterotomy has also been performed to reduce internal sphincter tone and consequently, high resting anal pressure.[41] However, its validity in hemorrhoidal disease alone must be questioned after recent evidence that high basal pressure in patients with hemorrhoids is chiefly the result of intrahemorrhoidal hypertension rather than true internal anal sphincter hypertonia.[42] In our experience, 20% of patients undergoing hemorrhoidal excision may have a concomitant fissure in ano.[17] These patients should be subject to conservative sphincterotomy to minimize the risk for incontinence.

Recurrence of Hemorrhoids

Recurrence after surgical hemorrhoidectomy is lower (about 2%) than after injection sclerotherapy or rubber band ligation.[43] If hemorrhoids do recur, they commonly do so 2 to 3 years after hemorrhoidectomy. It is possible that limited (one- or two-column) hemorrhoidectomy rather than three-column hemorrhoidectomy will result in a greater frequency of recurrent disease, but this requires further evaluation.

Because straining at stools is felt to be an etiologic factor in hemorrhoidal disease, many providers feel that adoption of a high-fiber diet may reduce the development of recurrent hemorrhoidal disease.

Laser Hemorrhoidectomy

Laser hemorrhoidectomy has been described as being more effective or less painful. Wang et al.[14] reported a randomized trial comparing Nd:YAG laser hemorrhoidectomy to a closed technique in 88 patients. Overall complications were similar, but prolonged wound healing was noted in the laser-treated group. Senagore et al.[45] conducted a similar prospective randomized trial and found no advantage with the use of the laser. Based on available evidence, the Standards of Practice Task Force of the American Society of Colon and Rectal Surgeons produced the following statement:

> No controlled trials have yet been completed to demonstrate superiority or even equivalence of the laser to more traditional treatment methods. Isolated reports suggest that the laser can be used with success, but there is as yet no reason to believe that results will be superior to current techniques.

The expense and potential operating room hazards of the laser equipment militate against use of this technology. Until convincing evidence is obtained, laser hemorrhoidectomy remains a technique in search of validation.[46]

CONCLUSION

In view of the newly defined nature of hemorrhoids as vascular cushions[46,47] that subserve an important sensory role and aid complete closure of the anal canal, the recent trend has been toward a more conservative approach to hemorrhoidectomy. It may not be important to perform a standard three-column hemorrhoidectomy in all patients with hemorrhoidal disease, as was once advocated. The benefits are shorter hospital stay and possibly a lowered prevalence of complications. Postoperative analgesia is vital in preventing early complications. In addition, patients must be informed of the possibility of recurrent symptoms and potential complications of this procedure.

REFERENCES

1. Copeland T. Haemorrhoidal excrescence. In Observation on the Principal Diseases of the Rectum and Anus. 2nd ed. London, 1814, pp 147-155.
2. Whitehead W. The surgical treatment of haemorrhoids. Br Med J 1:148-150, 1882.
3. Milligan ETC, Morgan CN, Nanton LE, Officer R. Surgical anatomy of the anal canal and the operative treatment of haemorrhoids. Lancet 2:1119-1124, 1937.
4. Ferguson JA, Heaton JR. Closed hemorrhoidectomy. Dis Colon Rectum 2:176-179, 1959.
5. Johanson JF, Sonnenberg A. Temporal changes in the occurrence of haemorrhoids in the United States and England. Dis Colon Rectum 34:585-591, 1991.
6. Duthie HL, Gairns FW. Sensory nerve endings and sensation in the anal canal of man. Br J Surg 47:585-595, 1960.
7. Chester JF, Stanford JB, Gazet JC. Analgesic benefit of locally injected bupivacaine after hemorrhoidectomy. Dis Colon Rectum 33:487-489, 1990.
8. Richman IM. Use of toradol in anorectal surgery. Dis Colon Rectum 36:295-296, 1993.
9. Goldstein ET, Williamson PK, Larach SW. Subcutaneous morphine pump for postop hemorrhoidectomy pain management. Dis Colon Rectum 36:439-446, 1993.
10. Shafik A. Role of warm water bath in anorectal conditions: The "thermosphincteric reflex." J Clin Gastroenterol 16:304-308, 1993.
11. Walker GL, Nigro ND. Postoperative anorectal hemorrhage. Surg Clin North Am 39:1655-1660, 1959.
12. Goligher JC. Surgery of the anus, rectum and colon. London: Baillière-Tindall, 1975, pp 158-162.
13. Petros JG, Bradley TM. Factors influencing postoperative urinary retention in patients undergoing surgery for benign anorectal disease. Am J Surg 159:374-376, 1990.
14. Bailey HR, Ferguson JA. Prevention of urinary retention by fluid restriction following anorectal operations. Dis Colon Rectum 19:250-252, 1976.
15. Hodsman NB, Kenny GN, McArdle CS. Patient controlled analgesia and urinary retention. Br J Surg 75:212, 1988.
16. Salvati EP. Urinary retention in anorectal and colonic surgery. Am J Surg 94:114, 1957.
17. Bleday R, Pena JP, Rothenberger DA, Goldberg SM, Buls JG. Symptomatic hemorrhoids: Current incidence and complications of operative therapy. Dis Colon Rectum 35:477-481, 1992.
18. Rosen L, Sipe P, Stasik JJ, Riether RD, Trimpi HD. Outcome of delayed hemorrhage following surgical hemorrhoidectomy. Dis Colon Rectum 37:288-289, 1994.
19. Corman ML. Management of postoperative constipation in anorectal surgery. Dis Colon Rectum 22:149, 1979.
20. Parikh SR, Molinelli B, Dailey TH. Liver abscess after hemorrhoidectomy: Report of two cases. Dis Colon Rectum 37:185-189, 1994.
21. Cataldo P, Senagore A, Luchtefeld MA. Intrarectal ultrasound in the evaluation of perirectal abscesses. Dis Colon Rectum 36:554-558, 1993.
22. Parks AG. The surgical treatment of haemorrhoids. Br J Surg 43:337-351, 1956.
23. Rothenberger DA, Velasco AL. Complications of anal surgery. In Mazier PW, Levien DH, Luchtefeld MA, Senagore AJ, eds. Surgery of the Colon, Rectum and Anus. Philadelphia: WB Saunders, 1995, pp 345-348.
24. Gingold BS, Arvanitis M. Y-V anoplasty for treatment of anal stricture. Surg Gynecol Obstet 162:241-244, 1986.
25. Caplin DA, Kodner IJ. Repair of anal stricture and mucosal ectropion by simple flap procedures. Dis Colon Rectum 29:92-94, 1986.

26. Ferguson JA. Repair of "Whitehead deformity" of the anus. Surg Gynecol Obstet 108:115-116, 1959.
27. Anal continence after haemorrhoidectomy. Lancet 11:696, 1982.
28. Corman ML. Complications of hemorrhoid and fissure surgery. In Ferrari BT, Ray JE, Gathright JB, eds. Complications of Colon and Rectal Surgery. Philadelphia: WB Saunders, 1985, pp 91-100.
29. Handfield-Jones SE, Cronin E. Contact sensitivity to lignocaine. Clin Exp Dermatol 18:342-343, 1993.
30. Daniel GL, Longo WE, Vernava AM III. Pruritus ani: Causes and concerns. Dis Colon Rectum. 37:670-674, 1994.
31. Mazier WP. Emergency hemorrhoidectomy: A worthwhile procedure. Dis Colon Rectum 15:200-205, 1972.
32. Eu KW, Seow-Choen F, Goh HS. Comparison of emergency and elective haemorrhoidectomy. Br J Surg 81:308-310, 1994.
33. Wolkomir AF, Luchtefeld MA. Surgery for symptomatic hemorrhoids and anal fissures in Crohn's disease. Dis Colon Rectum 36:545-547, 1993.
34. Heden P, Yeomans A, Davitt M, Peters CA, Pastuszek E, Cobb S. Efficacy of chlorhexidine gluconate use in the prevention of perirectal infections in patients with acute leukemia. Oncol Nurs Forum 18:1207-1213, 1991.
35. Milsom JW. Hemorrhoidal disease In Beck D, Wexner SD, eds. Fundamentals of Anorectal Surgery. New York: McGraw-Hill, 1992, pp 192-214.
36. Hosking SW, Smart HL, Johnson AG, Triger DR. Anorectal varices, haemorrhoids and portal hypertension. Lancet 1:349-352, 1989.
37. Lee SH. Transrectal ultrasound in the diagnosis of anorectal varices. Clin Radiol 49:69-70, 1994.
38. Lord PH. A new regimen for the treatment of haemorrhoids. Proc R Soc Med 61:935-936, 1968.
39. Speakman CT, Burnett SJ, Kamm MA, Bartram CI. Sphincter injury after anal dilatation demonstrated by anal endosonography. Br J Surg 78:1429-1430, 1991.
40. MacDonald A, Smith A, McNeill AD, Finlay IG. Manual dilatation of the anus. Br J Surg 79:1381-1382, 1992.
41. Hiltunen KM, Matikainen M. Anal dilatation, lateral subcutaneous sphincterotomy and haemorrhoidectomy for the treatment of second and third degree haemorrhoids: A prospective randomised study. Int Surg 77:261-263, 1992.
42. Sun WM, Read NW, Shorthouse AJ. Hypertensive anal cushions as a cause of the high anal canal pressures in patients with haemorrhoids. Br J Surg 77:458-462, 1990.
43. Bernstein WC. What are hemorrhoids and what is their relationship to the portal venous system? Dis Colon Rectum 26:829-834, 1983.
44. Wang JY, Chang-Chien CR, Chen JS, Lai CR, Tang R. The role of lasers in hemorrhoidectomy. Dis Colon Rectum 34:78-82, 1991.
45. Senagore A, Mazier WP, Luchtefeld MA, MacKeigan J, Wengert T. Treatment of advanced hemorrhoidal disease: A prospective, randomized comparison of cold scalpel vs. contact Nd:YAG laser. Dis Colon Rectum 36:1042-1049, 1993.
46. Milsom JW. Hemorrhoidal disease. In Beck DE, Wexner SD, eds. Fundamentals of Anorectal Surgery. New York: McGraw-Hill, 1992, pp 192-214.
47. Thomson WHF. The nature of haemorrhoids. Br J Surg 62:542-552, 1975.

CHAPTER 12

Nonoperative Treatment of Hemorrhoidal Disease

SERGIO W. LARACH
THOMAS E. CATALDO
DAVID E. BECK

Hemorrhoids are normal anatomic structures of the anal canal that can, for various reasons, cause significant morbidity and symptoms. Treatments are many and varied, some dating back to biblical times. Modern therapy includes identification and correction of GI tract dysfunction, minimization of symptoms, and in some patients correction of anal abnormalities (excision of excess hemorrhoidal tissue and prevention of slippage or prolapse).[1] Treatment can be surgical or nonsurgical. The surgical techniques include tissue fixation and major tissue excision (excisional surgery with or without laser) and physiologic alteration of the anal canal (Lord dilation, lateral internal sphincterotomy; see Chapter 11). Nonsurgical techniques and their associated complications are discussed here.

DIETARY MODIFICATIONS

Dietary modification is a mainstay for any therapy for hemorrhoidal disease. If the patient is constipated and is straining, a diet high in fiber (usually at least 20 to 30 g/day) is recommended, striving for a soft stool that is easy to pass. Moesgaard et al.[2] performed a prospective double-blind trial that demonstrated that psyllium fiber, when added to the diet of patients with anal bleeding and pain with defecation, improved symptoms over a 6-week period. Patients with diarrhea and hemorrhoidal disease, after an evaluation of the underlying cause of their loose stools, receive dietary manipulation with fiber and antidiarrheal agents as indicated.

It is extremely rare for dietary fiber to cause serious complications. An allergic reaction to the active or inactive ingredients is exceptionally rare. The most common problem is noncompliance because of problems with taste or symptoms of bloating and crampy abdominal pain. Fiber products currently available are listed in Table 12-1. Manufacturers have improved the taste of

Table 12-1 Fiber products

Type of fiber	Trade name	Manufacturer
Bran		
Psyllium	Metamucil	Procter & Gamble, Cincinnati, Ohio
	Konsyl	Konsyl Pharmaceuticals, Ft. Worth, Texas
Methylcellulose	Citrucel	Marion Merrell Dow Pharmaceuticals, Cincinnati, Ohio
Calcium polycarbophil	FiberCon	Lederle Laboratories, American Cyanamid, Pearl River, N.Y.
	Konsyl Fiber Tablets	Konsyl Pharmaceuticals, Ft. Worth, Texas

these products with flavoring and sweeteners but usually with the result of higher cost and less fiber per unit volume. The different fiber sources used in the major products may produce variable effects in different patients. It is advisable, therefore, to try different products if one does not produce the desired results.

TOPICAL MEDICATIONS AND MEASURES

Temperature

Sitz baths are used to soothe the acutely painful anal area. Dodi et al.[3] demonstrated a significant reduction in anal pressure in patients with anorectal disorders after soaking in warm (40° C) water. It is important that patients not spend too much time soaking, because prolonged exposure to water can lead to edema of the perineal skin and subsequent pruritus. Some patients prefer application of ice packs to the anal area. If contact is not prolonged, this option is acceptable if it reduces the patient's symptoms.

Lubricants and Medications

The pharmaceutical industry has been active in promoting multiple products such as creams, foams, and suppositories. One percent hydrocortisone may have some effect in reducing the symptoms caused by pruritus associated with hemorrhoidal disease. Suppositories, after insertion, lodge in the lower rectum rather than in the anal canal where hemorrhoids are located. Aside from providing a little lubrication of stool, they have little or no pharmacologic rationale in the management of hemorrhoidal disease. Ointments have the potential to cause or exacerbate pruritus ani and, except for those that contain a topical anesthetic (e.g., pramoxine hydrochloride 1%), offer little benefit except to thrombosed external hemorrhoids. Effective marketing and the intermittent nature of hemorrhoidal symptoms explain the large volume of these products purchased in the United States.

TISSUE FIXATION

Sclerotherapy is one of the oldest forms of therapy. The goal is to cause scarring and thereby fixation and eventual shrinkage of hemorrhoidal tissue. Sclerotherapy works by obliterating the vascularity of the hemorrhoids, fixing them to the adjacent anorectal muscularis propria to prevent prolapse. In 1869, John Morgan described injection of iron persulphate into external hemorrhoids.[4] Since then, various substances have been used. Quinine and urea (5% solution), phenol (5% in almond oil), and sodium tetradecyl sulfate (1% to 3% solution) are the agents currently used. Most practitioners inject 3 to 5 ml of the sclerosing solution into the submucosa of each hemorrhoidal bundle, 1 cm or more above the dentate line, with a 25-gauge spinal needle or a specialized hemorrhoid (Gabriel) needle. Pain occurs if the needle is inserted too deep, causing spasm of the sphincter muscle, or too distal in the anal canal so that sclerosant irritates the sensitive somatic nerves distal to the dentate line.[1]

Contraindications to sclerotherapy include inflammatory bowel disease, portal hypertension, immunocompromised state, presence of anorectal infection, and prolapsed thrombosed hemorrhoids.[1]

Complications of sclerotherapy are related to incorrect placement or excess injection of sclerosing agent. The most frequent problem is superficial sloughing of the hemorrhoidal mucosa. This generally will heal with expectant management. Excessive sloughing may lead to scarring and stricture. Sclerotherapy may also precipitate thrombosis of an adjacent hemorrhoidal complex. If the thrombosis is severe, it may require excision. Most hemorrhoids, however, can be managed with sitz baths, a high-fiber diet, and local measures. Because of the potential for scarring and stricture, repetitive use of sclerotherapy is not recommended.

More unusual complications of sclerotherapy are abscess or oleoma. An oleoma represents a granulomatous reaction to an oil-based sclerosant.[4]

TISSUE FIXATION WITH TISSUE DESTRUCTION

Banding

Rubber band ligation was originally described by Blaisdell[5] in 1958 and refined and popularized by Barron in 1963.[6] Placement of a tight rubber band around excess hemorrhoidal tissue constricts the blood supply to the contained tissue, which sloughs over 5 to 7 days. This leaves a small ulcer that heals, fixing the tissue to the underlying muscle. Because of its simplicity, safety, and effectiveness, it is currently the most widely used technique in the United States for treating first-, second-, and some third-degree internal hemorrhoids. The technique entails using a Barron or McGivney type of hemorrhoid ligator and a modified Allis clamp or a McGown type of suction ligator to draw the upper portion of an internal hemorrhoid into the barrel of the device. Firing the device places a preloaded elastic rubber band around the hemorrhoid. Some providers preload two bands on the applicator to ensure tissue constriction and guard against slippage and breakage.[1]

Complications are infrequent (<2%) with rubber band ligation[1] and vary from transient vasovagal response on placement of the bands to anal pain or rarely to pelvic sepsis. The vasovagal response to banding includes diaphoresis, bradycardia, nausea, and mild hypotension. Reassuring the patient, elevating his or her feet, and applying a cold compress to the patient's forehead are frequently all that is necessary. The symptoms should resolve in 10 to 15 minutes.

Pain occurs as a result of incorporation of somatically enervated tissue into the band. This can occur if the band is placed too close to the dentate line or if internal sphincter muscle is included within the band (i.e., too much tissue in the band). In this case, the pain is acute in onset at the time of banding. Mild pain can be managed with analgesics such as propoxyphene napsylate and acetaminophen or injection of a local anesthetic (e.g., 1% lidocaine hydrochloride). More intense pain is best managed by removal of the band. This is facilitated by hooked scissors or a hooked cutting probe. Most patients will require injection of local anesthetic during removal of the band. Pain and swelling that develop several hours after banding may be caused by edema and thrombosis that develop distal to the banded area. These can usually be managed with conservative measures.

Not infrequently, younger patients with good anal tone may experience mild to severe anismus. Also, fear of pain may cause patients to delay defecation as long as possible. This can lead to harder stools that are more difficult to pass. For these reasons, patients should be carefully counseled as to what to expect after banding. Fecal impaction is best avoided by limiting narcotic use, using stool softeners, and maintaining adequate hydration.

Secondary thrombosis of external hemorrhoids may occur. Reported prevalence varies from 2% to 11%.[7] As with spontaneous thrombosis, mild symptoms can be treated with topical preparations and sitz baths; more severe thrombosis may require excision of the hemorrhoids.

Urinary retention is not common with rubber band ligation. When it does occur, onset is shortly after banding and often resolves spontaneously or may require one-time catheterization. Urinary difficulty or retention that develops days after the procedure may herald pelvic sepsis.

Delayed hemorrhage may also occur, most commonly 7 to 10 days after the procedure as the banded tissue sloughs. Patients should be cautioned that a small amount of bleeding may occur, which can usually be managed expectantly. Major bleeding is very rare.[7] Rothberg et al.[8] reported a rate of 0.5% in 600 patients. Significant bleeding demands immediate attention and may require suture ligation in the operating room.

The most serious complication is postbanding sepsis, believed to be related to necrosis from the banded tissue allowing adjacent soft tissue to become infected.[1] First reported in 1980, it is associated with fever, perineal or pelvic pain or both, and difficulty in urinating.[9,10] Development of these symptoms after banding mandates urgent evaluation. This may require an anesthetic to adequately evaluate the perineum. Large doses of broad-spectrum antibiotics to include clostridial coverage are indicated for empiric treatment to reduce the risk of potentially fatal sepsis. Surgical debridement and removal of the bands is reasonable, and in cases of overwhelming infection, a diverting colostomy may also be required.

Photocoagulation

Photocoagulation involves infrared radiation, generated by a tungsten-halogen lamp, focused on the hemorrhoidal tissue from a gold-plated reflector housing through a solid quartz glass light guide (Redfield Corp., Montvale, N.J.) with technology similar to that of laser devices.[1] The infrared coagulator light penetrates tissue to the submucosal level and is converted to heat, leading to inflammation, destruction, and eventual scarring of the treated area.[11] The tip of the instrument is applied to the base of the hemorrhoid and a 1.0- to 1.5-second pulse of energy is delivered. This produces an immediate area of coagulation 3 to 4 mm^2 in diameter. This area ulcerates and eventually scars over the subsequent 2 weeks. Three or four applications are applied to the base of each treated hemorrhoid. Most authors recommend treating only one or two bundles per visit. Additional treatment, if necessary, can be performed every 3 to 4 weeks.

Complications of this technique have been infrequent. Pain can occur if the energy is inappropriately delivered to the anoderm rather than the base of the hemorrhoid (Fig. 12-1). Excessive application can also lead to bleeding. Most authors report a considerably lower prevalence of bleeding with photocoagulation compared with banding.

Ulcer formation is an expected result of both rubber band ligation and infrared coagulation. The resultant scarring creates fixation. However, large ulcers may rarely be associated with fissure formation and persistent complaints.

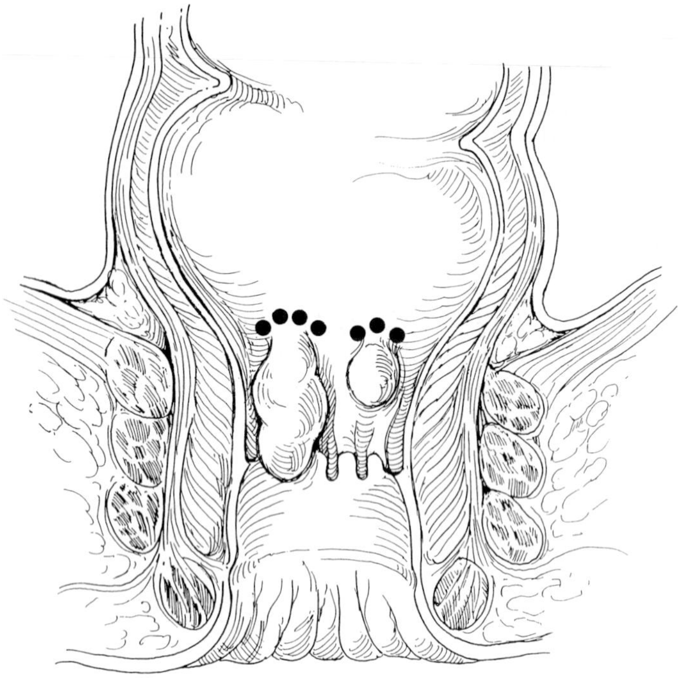

Fig. 12-1 Recommended photocoagulation sites.

Cryosurgery

Cryotherapy is based on rapid freezing and thawing of tissue, which, in theory, causes analgesia and tissue destruction. The "ice ball" that forms around the cryoprobe depicts the extent of tissue destruction. Although initial reports were optimistic, subsequent experience has demonstrated significant problems. After therapy, patients experienced significant pain and a profuse foul discharge from the treatment sites. Healing frequently took 6 weeks or more.[12] The expensive, cumbersome equipment and significant side effects have led to almost total abandonment of this technique.

Electrocoagulation

Bipolar diathermy uses a bipolar radiation frequency electric current to generate a coagulum of tissue at the end of a cautery-tipped applicator (Circon ACMI, Stamford, Conn.). Patient grounding is not necessary, and a 2-second pulse is applied to the base of each hemorrhoid. Yang et al.[13] used bipolar electrocautery in 25 patients in a prospective controlled trial. Ulcerations occurred in 6 patients (24%) and caused some minor rectal pain and self-limited fever. Prolonged pain lasting more than 1 day after therapy occurred in 1 patient (4%), and uncontrolled bleeding developed in two (8%). In another study of 51 patients, fissures were seen in two patients (4%).[14] The expense of the equipment and lack of results superior to those with other available methods has limited widespread acceptance of this technique.

Direct current therapy uses a special probe (Ultroid; Microvasive, Watertown, Mass.) to deliver an electrical current (up to 16 mA) to the internal hemorrhoid. The technique entails delivering the current for up to 10 minutes to each hemorrhoid. In the randomized study of 25 patients by Yang et al.,[13] the procedure had to be terminated in 5 patients (20%) because of pain, four patients (16%) had prolonged pain after the procedure, and 1 patient (4%) had uncontrolled bleeding. The length of time required for treatment and the equivocal results have again limited adoption of this method.

Laser Surgery

The use of laser is more accurately a surgical technique. Its attributes and complications are discussed in Chapter 11.

CONCLUSION

Nonsurgical therapy of hemorrhoidal diseases is safe and effective in the vast majority of patients. Grade 1 and 2 hemorrhoids are best treated initially with fiber or dietary modification that produces good results and minimal to no risk of complication. Topical preparations offer only transient relief of symptoms but no therapeutic efficacy. For persistent complaints, photocoagulation is effective for bleeding and pain, with little or no complication. For higher grade disease, infrared coagulation may not relieve prolapse. Rubber band ligation remains the standard of nonsurgical therapy, especially for grade 3 hemorrhoids. However, although rare, it is more frequently associated with bleeding and discomfort, as well as the rare risk of significant sepsis.

REFERENCES

1. Milsom JW. Hemorrhoidal disease. In Beck DE, Wexner SD. Fundamentals of Anorectal Surgery. New York: McGraw-Hill, 1992, pp 192-214.
2. Moesgaard F, Nielson ML, Hansen JB, et al. High fiber diet reduces bleeding and pain in patients with hemorrhoids. Dis Colon Rectum 25:454-456, 1982.
3. Dodi G, Bogoni F, Infantino A, et al. Hot or cold in anal pain? A study of the changes in internal sphincter pressure profiles. Dis Colon Rectum 29:248-251, 1986.
4. Gabriel WB. The principles and practice of rectal surgery. London: Lewis, 1963, p 131.
5. Blaisdell PC. Prevention of massive hemorrhage secondary to hemorrhoidectomy. Surg Gynecol Obstet 106:485-488, 1958.
6. Barron J. Office ligation treatment of hemorrhoids. Dis Colon Rectum 6:109-113, 1963.
7. Corman ML, Veidenheimer MC. The new hemorrhoidectomy. Surg Clin North Am 53: 417-422, 1973.
8. Rothberg R, Rubin R, Eisenstat T, et al. Rubber band ligation hemorrhoidectomy: Long-term results. Am Surg 49:167, 1993.

9. O'Hara VS. Fatal clostridial infection following hemorrhoidal banding. Dis Colon Rectum 23:570-571, 1980.
10. Russell TR, Donahue JH. Hemorrhoidal banding: A warning. Dis Colon Rectum 28:291-293, 1985.
11. O'Connor JJ. Infrared coagulation of hemorrhoids. Pract Gastroenterol 10:8-14, 1986.
12. Goligher JC. Cryosurgery of hemorrhoids. Dis Colon Rectum 19:213-218, 1976.
13. Yang R, Migkovsky B, Peicher J, et al. Randomized, prospective trial of direct current versus bipolar electrocoagulation for bleeding internal hemorrhoids. Gastrointest Endosc 39:766-769, 1993.
14. Dennison A, Whiston J, Rooney S, et al. A randomized comparison of infrared photocoagulation with bipolar diathermy for outpatient treatment of hemorrhoids. Dis Colon Rectum 33:32-34, 1990.

CHAPTER 13

Surgery for Abscess and Fistula

CAROL-ANN VASILEVSKY

Abscesses and fistulas are intimately related, and surgical procedures to correct these conditions can be extremely challenging. Therapeutic options for abscesses include incision and drainage and catheter drainage, and for fistulas are fistulotomy, fistulectomy, advancement flaps, and seton placement. The major complications of these procedures are incontinence and recurrence. In this chapter, each of these problems is discussed, as well as the special concerns associated with anorectal Crohn's disease and rectovaginal fistulas.

INCONTINENCE

Abscess and fistula surgery provides a challenge to the surgeon because continence must be preserved while the suppurative process is eradicated.

Incision and Drainage

Incontinence may result after incision and drainage of an abscess either from iatrogenic damage to the sphincter or inappropriate wound care. Continence may also be compromised if the superficial external sphincter is inadvertently divided during drainage of a perianal or deep postanal abscess in a patient with preoperative borderline continence. Drainage of a supralevator abscess may lead to incontinence if the puborectalis muscle is inappropriately divided.[1] Prolonged packing of a drained abscess may impair continence by preventing the development of granulation tissue and promoting the formation of excess scar tissue.[2]

Fistulotomy

Continence disorders after fistulotomy have been reported in as many as 52% of patients.[3] Patients most at risk for impaired continence after fistulotomy include elderly persons, who may have already weakened sphincters; women with anterior fistulas, especially those with previous episiotomies; and those with complicated fistulas with high internal openings. Patients with diarrhea associated with inflammatory bowel disease, especially Crohn's disease, are also at risk. The potential for incontinence is directly related to the degree of preoperative control. Another variable is the wound healing process after fistulotomy. A large amount of scar tissue, as might occur with complicated fistulas with multiple extensions, can render the anus unable to properly close, resulting in intermittent leakage of gas and stool.[4] Posterior fistula wounds have also been associated with a greater degree of incontinence because of their more circuitous routes.[3]

Primary Fistulotomy

Performance of a fistulotomy at the time of abscess drainage is controversial. Although advocated to decrease recurrence rates, it may also result in unnecessary division of sphincter muscle in acutely inflamed tissue and thus inadvertently in incontinence.[5,6] Fucini[7] reported a 17% rate of minor incontinence of gas, and Schouten and van Vroonhoven[8] reported a 39% rate of continence disturbances in a prospective randomized trial.

Fistulectomy

The use of fistulectomy in the treatment of fistulas is a controversial issue. It is generally accepted that fistulectomy should not be performed because it creates larger wounds that take longer to heal.[9] A greater separation of the muscle ends occurs,[5] and there is a greater risk of injuring or excising underlying muscle,[10] all of which increase the potential for incontinence. Schouten and van Vroonhoven[8] found that fistulectomy, whether primary or secondary, was associated with a clinically significant disturbance in anal function.

Rectal Advancement Flap

To minimize the loss of control associated with other techniques, the rectal advancement flap has been promoted. The technique offers the following advantages: no muscle is divided, there is no resulting deformity of the anal canal, there is less associated discomfort, and the wound may heal faster. The technique involves coring out of the fistula tract, excision of the primary opening, and closure of the muscular defect with a rectal advancement flap[11] (Fig. 13-1). Excellent results have been reported with respect to continence and recurrence rates,[10,11] although Aguilar et al.[12] observed disturbances in continence to gas and liquid stool in 7% and 6% of patients, respectively.

Seton

Because patients with high internal openings are at risk for development of impaired continence when the lay-open technique is used, a staged approach with seton placement has been advocated. A seton may be any foreign substance inserted into the fistula tract to encircle the sphincter muscles. Materials commonly used include Silastic catheters, vascular loops, rubber bands, Penrose drains, and heavy silk thread. A seton has three major effects: (1) it acts as a

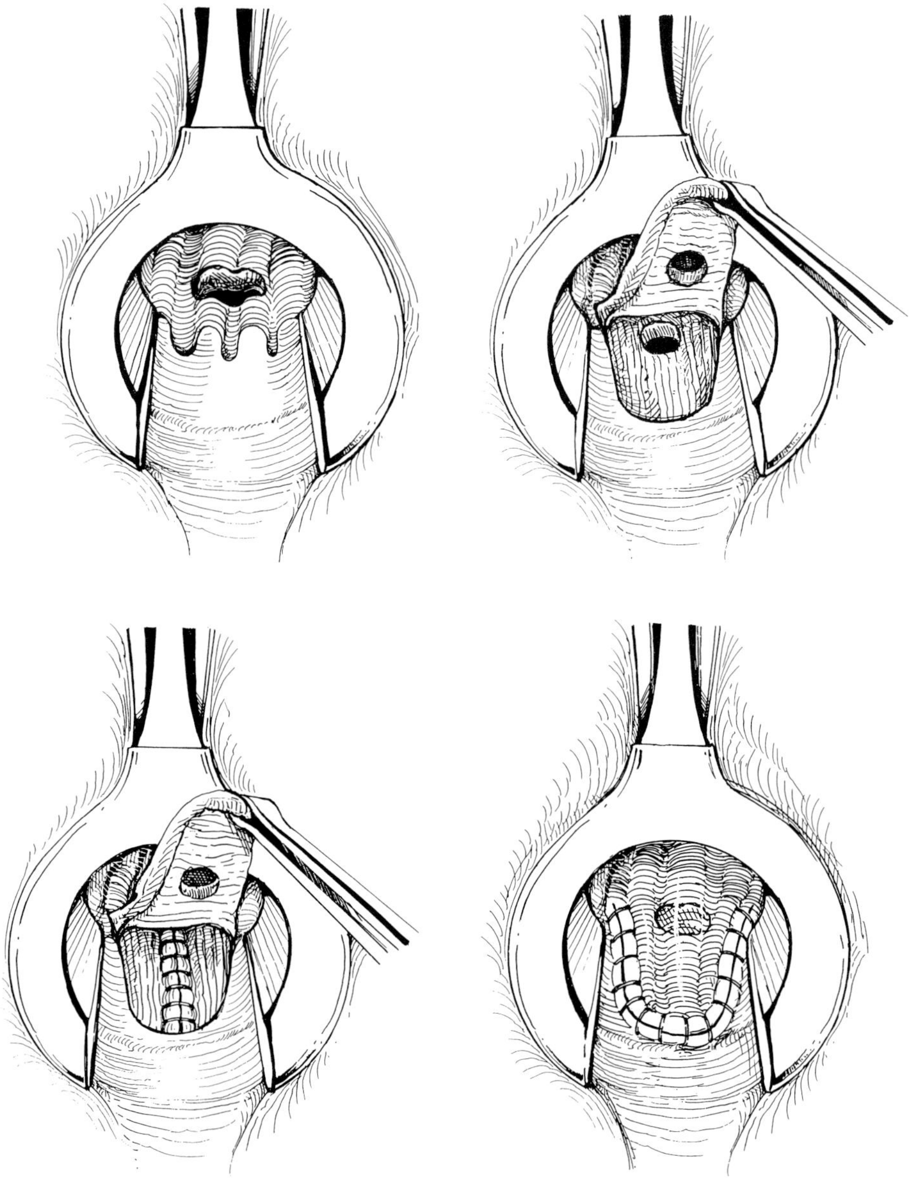

Fig. 13-1 Advancement flap repair. **A**, Internal fistulous opening in rectovaginal septum demonstrated by anal retractor. **B**, Fistula tract is cored out and flap of mucosa, submucosa, and internal sphincter is elevated. **C**, Internal opening is closed and internal sphincter plicated. **D**, The distal end of the flap is excised and the flap is sutured into place to cover the closure of the internal opening.

drain; (2) it promotes fibrosis around a complex anal fistula; and (3) it delineates the amount of muscle beneath the fistula tract. Setons may be useful in the treatment of a high anterior fistula in a female patient. Primary fistulotomy in this situation can lead to frank incontinence because there is a tenuous external sphincter muscle and absent puborectalis muscle. As part of a staged fistulotomy, the proximal portion of the sphincter muscle is divided, leaving the seton to mark the site of the remaining tract, converting a high fistula to a low fistula. Once the proximal portion has healed, the remaining low fistulous tract may be divided. Ramanujam et al.[13] reported excellent results with this technique, but Van Tets and Kuijpers[3] failed to demonstrate an improved functional result. MacLeod et al.[14] described minor control problems in 58% of patients, and major fecal incontinence has been reported in 6.7%[4] after a review of several series. This is especially true of anterior fistulas in women in which a seton has been placed.

RECURRENCE

Incision and Drainage

Ischiorectal and intersphincteric abscesses are associated with development of recurrent abscesses or fistulas in as many as 89% of patients.[8,15,16] In addition, recurrent disease is more likely in patients with a history of previous abscess drainage,[8,15,16] perhaps because the natural barriers to infection have been destroyed.[17]

Reasons for recurrence of anorectal infections include missed infection in adjacent anatomic spaces, the presence of an undiagnosed fistula at abscess drainage, and failure to completely drain the abscess.[18]

The mainstay of treatment of an acute anorectal abscess is incision and drainage. After this treatment, 34% to 60% of patients will have no further anorectal suppuration.[8,15,19]

Catheter Drainage

An adjunct to simple incision and drainage is the use of a mushroom catheter for abscess drainage.[20] Several technical features are important[21]: the stab incision should be made as close to the anus as possible. The diameter and length of the catheter should correspond to those of the abscess cavity. A catheter that is too narrow or too short may be dislodged or fall into the wound. The skin may seal over the catheter and a second incision will be required to retrieve it or to drain a recurrent abscess. The timing of catheter removal depends on the size of the original abscess cavity, the amount of granulation tissue around the catheter, and the amount of drainage.

Primary Fistulotomy

The frequency of a fistula being overlooked during abscess drainage ranges from 18% to 95%.* The prevalence of recurrent abscess or fistula may be decreased substantially to 1.8% with primary fistulotomy.[24] Detection of a primary opening at abscess drainage may not be possible, however, because of the presence of acute inflammation. Failure to detect an internal opening has been reported in as many as 66% of patients.[25] Attempts to search for the true internal opening may result in creation of false passages or openings, with subsequent persistent infection.[6] The debate as to whether primary fistulotomy should be performed is ongoing. A recent prospective study advocated a conservative approach in the treatment of anorectal abscess, reserving fistulotomy for a second-stage procedure if necessary.[8]

Recurrence of abscess after fistulotomy usually results from the failure to identify a primary opening or recognize lateral or upward extensions of a fistula.[23,26,27] Complex fistulas are more likely to recur because an unsuspected anatomic extension may have been present at fistulotomy.[2,26] Premature closure of the fistulotomy wound can result in recurrence[27] but can be obviated by marsupialization of the wound and diligent postoperative care to avoid bridging and pocketing of the wound. A recent study suggests epithelialization of the fistula tract from internal or external openings rather than chronic infection of an anal gland as the cause of persistent anal fistula.[28]

Advancement Flap

If an advancement flap has been used in the repair of a fistula, care must be taken to avoid necrosis or retraction of the flap, which may result in recurrent or persistent fistula. These postoperative problems are reduced if the base of the advancement flap is twice the width of the apex and is advanced without tension, which encourages a good blood supply. Differences of opinion exist as to whether the flap should consist of full-thickness rectal wall or mucosa and submucosa.[10] Lewis and Bartolo,[29] however, advocated use of full-thickness rectal wall to prevent ischemic necrosis.

Extra-anal Causes

Because diagnosis and therapy of recurrent anorectal abscesses and fistulas create problems for the surgeon, it is important to consider extra-anal disease if the usual causes of recurrence have been ruled out. Hidradenitis suppurativa and downward extension of a pilonidal abscess should be considered.[5] A prospective review of recurrent anorectal abscesses by Chrabot et al.[22] reported hidra-

*References 4,7,8,19,22,23.

denitis in one third of patients with recurrent abscesses. In addition, the possibility of Crohn's disease should be suspected.

ANORECTAL CROHN'S DISEASE

Abscess

The traditional approach to anorectal complications of Crohn's disease has been to avert surgery whenever possible except when an abscess must be drained. Proper drainage must be performed by excision of the overlying skin as medial as possible with a small incision to avoid creation of a long fistulous tract. Recurrent abscesses occurred in as many as 90% of patients in one study and required 3 to 20 repeated drainage procedures.[30] For this reason, drainage with small mushroom catheters[31] or setons has been advocated to encourage continued drainage of pus and to avoid reaccumulation in a closed space. Pritchard et al.[31] compared incision and drainage with catheter drainage and found that recurrence of abscess after the two methods was 56% and 45%, respectively. A trend toward an increased need for subsequent proctectomy to control symptoms and delayed healing of the resulting perineal wound was demonstrated after incision and drainage.[31]

Fistula

Anal fistulas are the most difficult anorectal complications of Crohn's disease to manage. They are the most common perianal manifestations, occurring in 6% to 34% of patients.[32] Surgical treatment of fistulas is associated with poor and delayed wound healing and with the risk of sphincter injury. Alexander-Williams and Buchmann[33] stated that "incontinence is likely to be the result of aggressive surgeons, not of aggressive disease." A conservative approach has therefore been advocated, especially inasmuch as 38% of such fistulas heal spontaneously without any surgical intervention.[34] Although fistulas may occur in as many as 73% of patients after previous abscess drainage,[32] it is imperative that primary fistulotomy not be performed, because of the high risk for creating false passages and injuring the sphincter mechanism. Asymptomatic fistulas require no surgical treatment. Low fistulas with simple tracts can be managed with the standard lay-open method. Outcome is successful in 78% to 93% of procedures.[3,30,32,35-38] On the other hand, Allan and Keighley[39] reported a poor outcome, with healing in only 8% of cases.

Delayed Healing

Fistulotomy in Crohn's disease has been associated with prolonged healing time.[40] Factors associated with delayed healing are rectal involvement[25,28,41]; anorectal complications, especially strictures[35]; and the presence or absence of an internal opening.[38] Successful healing has occurred in patients with a classic internal opening at the dentate line and those without rectal involvement[38] although Halme and Sainio[40] found that delayed healing occurred in 80% of cases despite a normal rectum and Van Dongen and Lubbers[42] found no difference in healing even in the presence of rectal involvement.

Incontinence

Incontinence is a dreaded complication of fistula surgery, especially in Crohn's disease. It is interesting that incontinence has been reported in patients with proctitis who have not undergone anal surgery.[42] A patient with severe rectal involvement and a simple low fistula is not a candidate for fistulotomy. Division of any sphincter muscle in this situation will most certainly lead to frank incontinence because the noncompliant rectum acts as a conduit rather than a reservoir. Continence problems have been reported in 25% of patients after incision and drainage of an abscess during which the sphincter mechanism was not touched.[42] Although low fistulas can be successfully treated with the traditional lay-open technique without resulting incontinence, Allan and Keighley[39] reported a 50% frequency of major fecal incontinence, and minor incontinence has been described in 33% of cases.[40] It is thought that diarrhea from either associated intestinal involvement or multiple previous small bowel resections is important in control disorders in these patients.[32,40,42] Appropriate medical therapy should be used in both cases to remedy the diarrhea.

Complex fistulas with high rectal openings must be managed conservatively, because impaired continence will result if the sphincter muscle is divided. Eradication of the fistula in this situation is not possible because of the complexity of the tracts. Thus seton placement has been advocated to promote continued drainage, limit recurrent suppuration and preserve sphincter function.[43] Rectal advancement flaps have been used in the absence of severe rectal disease.[44]

Recurrence

The importance of quiescent intestinal disease for successful outcome of local fistula surgery has been emphasized by several authors.[35,41,45] Although spontaneous healing of perianal fistulas has been observed after intestinal resection, fistula recurrence has been reported in 35% of patients with activation of disease.[41] Resection of intestinal disease is thus advocated for the improvement of intestinal symptoms rather than perianal disease.[46] In this context, proximal fecal diversion has been suggested as an option to ameliorate severe perianal disease. Improvement is temporary, however, because fistulas will become reactivated after restoration of intestinal continuity.[46]

As would be expected, complicated fistulas are more likely to recur, because one is reluctant to divide sphincter muscle. The use of long-term indwelling setons as drains is therefore recommended.[43] The use of a rectal advancement flap has been successful; however, breakdown is possible because of sepsis.[44] In patients with mild proctitis, a 20% success rate has been reported.[44] The presence of a protective stoma in this situation does not guarantee success, however; failure has been reported in 55% of cases.[44] A covering stoma may be beneficial in the patient who has undergone multiple unsuccessful repairs.[44] Finally, it is important to stress that many fistulas require repeat fistulotomy to achieve complete healing.[40]

RECTOVAGINAL FISTULA

Rectovaginal fistula, although less common than other fistulas, occurs in 5% to 15% of women with Crohn's disease.[47,48] In contrast to other fistulas, this type rarely heals spontaneously.[34] It was once thought that the presence of a rectovaginal fistula was an indication for proctectomy. The trend, however, is now toward rectal preservation[45] and more aggressive local therapy in selected patients with quiescent rectal disease.[47] Despite the pessimism with which repair of rectovaginal fistulas is regarded, high success rates ranging from 75% to 92%[47,49,50] have been reported in selected patients with the flap advancement repair method. Factors associated with poor outcome include anorectal complications such as stenosis, fissure, or fistula[51]; an internal opening greater than 2 cm from the dentate line; persistent or undrained sepsis in the rectovaginal septum[50]; and active small bowel Crohn's disease.[51] Factors not indicative of failure include previous failed repair, steroid therapy, and active proctitis.[52] Fecal diversion in addition to local repair with rectal involvement has been advocated by some authors[53] but not others.[47]

A modified transvaginal approach has also been advocated that adheres to the technical details outlined for the rectal advancement flap but, in addition, involves the interposition of the levator ani.[54] This muscle is used to support the rectovaginal septum and separate the suture lines to minimize the chance for recurrence. A covering stoma is thought to be an essential component of this method of repair which has enjoyed a 93% success rate.[54] The recurrence of a rectovaginal fistula after repair may coincide with recrudescence of disease activity elsewhere in the bowel. A failure rate of 30% to 40%[44,53,54] has been reported, with proctectomy ultimately required in 20%.[55]

Rectovaginal fistulas constitute fewer than 5% of anorectal fistulas. Obstetric injury is the most common cause[56-62]; other causes of low rectovaginal fistulas include perianal or Bartholin's gland infection, rectal or vaginal surgery, and inflammatory bowel disease.[56] Radiation proctitis may be followed by ulceration of the anterior rectal wall and eventual progression to rectovaginal fistula. Rectovaginal fistulas may occur as a complication of leukemia or other malignancies.[56]

These low fistulas may be repaired through a vaginal, perineal, or endorectal approach. The rectal advancement flap is the most popular procedure, with success rates ranging from 78% to 100%.[56-59] This technique is effective because it allows the interposition of intact healthy tissue to the high-pressure zone of the rectum, a criterion not fulfilled with transvaginal repairs.[58]

Recurrence

Recurrence rates of 0% to 13% have been reported after rectal flap advancement repairs.[56] This is usually ascribed to postoperative wound infection that results in necrosis of the flap.[50] Attention to technique is important for a successful outcome. In particular, several technical points ensure success.[56] The flap must be designed so that its base is twice the width of the apex to ensure good vascularity. The flap should be mobilized 4 cm proximal to the fistula. The internal sphincter should be mobilized laterally on both sides, then reapproximated without tension to close the opening. Multiple previous repairs are correlated with failure.[56] This may be from decreased blood supply available to the flap as a result of scarring.[60] A more complex repair designed to bring in well-vascularized tissue is subsequently necessary for a successful outcome.[60]

Another local approach, excision of the fistula with a layer closure, can be performed transvaginally or transanally. Care must be taken to avoid excess tension on the suture line. Direct apposition of the vaginal and rectal suture lines without intervening tissue may result in recurrence.[61] For these reasons, a transperineal approach has been advocated.

Incontinence

Wise et al.[57] reported a 17.5% rate of incontinence after the flap advancement repair, with 71% incontinence of gas or liquid stool in 71% of patients and of solid stool in 20%. Only one patient had been incontinent before surgery. This underscores the need to manometrically evaluate those patients who may benefit from sphincter reconstruction in addition to the advancement flap procedure.

Incontinence inevitably results from performance of fistulotomy and drainage by laying open the entire tract, because a significant portion of the sphincter mechanism is transected.[62] This procedure is therefore not advocated. In one study, all patients subsequently became incontinent and required further surgery to repair the damage.[63]

Other complications that have been reported after flap advancement repair and transvaginal or perineal approaches include urinary infection or retention, bleeding, vulvar hematomas, and cellulitis.[56]

Early complications that have been associated with fistula and abscess surgery include urinary retention, hemorrhage, fecal impaction, and thrombosed hemorrhoids.[2] Late complications include bleeding, pain, pruritus, and poor wound healing.[2]

REFERENCES

1. Seow-Choew F, Nicholls RJ. Anal fistula. Br J Surg 79:197-205, 1992.
2. Mazier WP. The treatment and care of anal fistulas: A study of 1000 patients. Dis Colon Rectum 14:134-144, 1971.
3. Van Tets WF, Kuijpers HC. Continence disorders after anal fistulotomy. Dis Colon Rectum 37:1194-1197, 1994.
4. Pearl RK, Andrews JR, Orsay CP, Weisman RI, Prasad ML, Nelson RL, Cintron JR, Abcarian

H. Role of the seton in management of anorectal fistulas. Dis Colon Rectum 36:573-579, 1993.

5. Gordon PH. Anorectal abscesses and fistula-in-ano. In Gordon PH, Nivatvongs S, eds. Principles and Practice of Surgery for the Colon, Rectum, and Anus. St. Louis: Quality Medical Publishing, 1992, pp 221-265.
6. Lockhart-Muminary HE. Symposium: Anorectal problems. Treatment of abscess. Dis Colon Rectum 18:650-651, 1975.
7. Fucini C. One stage treatment of anal abscesses and fistulas: A clinical appraisal on the basis of two different classifications. Int J Colorect Dis 6:12-16, 1991.
8. Schouten WR, van Vroonhoven TJMV. Treatment of anorectal abscess with or without primary fistulectomy: Results of a prospective randomized trial. Dis Colon Rectum 34:60-63, 1991.
9. Kronberg O. To lay open or excise a fistula-in-ano. Br J Surg 72:970, 1985.
10. Fazio VW. Complex anal fistulae. Gastroenterol Clin North Am 16:93-114, 1987.
11. Shemesh EI, Kodner IJ, Fry RD, Neufeld DM. Endorectal sliding flap repair of complicated anterior anoperineal fistulas. Dis Colon Rectum 31:22-24, 1988.
12. Aguilar PS, Plasencia G, Hardy TJ, Hartmann RF, Stewart WRC. Mucosal advancement in the treatment of anal fistula. Dis Colon Rectum 28:496-498, 1985.
13. Ramanujam PS, Prasad ML, Abcarian H. The role of seton in fistulotomy of the anus. Surg Gynecol Obstet 157:419-422, 1983.
14. MacLeod CAH, Balcos EG, Buls JG, Goldberg SM. Seton management of anorectal fistulas: A study of incontinence. Dis Colon Rectum 33:10, 1990.
15. Vasilevsky CA, Gordon PH. The incidence of recurrent abscesses or fistula-in-ano following anorectal suppuration. Dis Colon Rectum 27:126-130, 1984.
16. Buchan R, Grace RH. Anorectal suppuration: The results of treatment and factors influencing the recurrence rate. Br J Surg 60:537-540, 1973.
17. Bevans DW, Westbrook KC, Thompson BW, Caldwell FT. Perirectal abscess: A potentially fatal illness. Am J Surg 26:765-768, 1973.
18. Abcarian H. Surgical management of recurrent anorectal abscesses. Contemp Surg 21:85-91, 1982.
19. Scoma JA, Salvati EP, Rubin RJ. Incidence of fistulas subsequent to anal abscesses. Dis Colon Rectum 17:357-359, 1974.
20. Beck DE, Fazio VW, Lavery IC, Jagelman DG, Weakley FL. Catheter drainage of ischiorectal abscesses. South Med J 89:444-446, 1988.
21. Vasilevsky CA. Fistula-in-ano and abscess. In Beck DE, Wexner SD, eds. Fundamentals of Anorectal Surgery. New York: McGraw-Hill, 1992, pp 131-144.
22. Chrabot CM, Prasad ML, Abcarian H. Recurrent anorectal abscesses. Dis Colon Rectum 27:126-130, 1984.
23. McElwain JW, Maclean D, Alexander RM, Hoexter B, Guthrie JF. Anorectal problems: Experience with primary fistulotomy for anorectal abscess, a report of 1000 cases. Dis Colon Rectum 18:646-649, 1975.
24. Ramanujam PS, Prasad ML, Abcarian H, Tan AB. Perianal abscesses and fistulas. Dis Colon Rectum 27:593-594, 1984.
25. Read DR, Abcarian H. A prospective study of 474 patients with anorectal abscesses. Dis Colon Rectum 22:566-569, 1979.
26. Vasilevsky CA, Gordon PH. Results of treatment of fistula-in-ano. Dis Colon Rectum 28: 225-231, 1984.
27. Rosen L. Anorectal abscess-fistulae. Surg Clin North Am 74:1293-1308, 1994.

28. Lunniss PJ, Sheffreld JP, Talbot IC, Thomson JPS, Phillips RKS. Persistence of idopathic anal fistula may be related to epithelialization. Br J Surg 82:32-33, 1995.
29. Lewis P, Bartolo DCC. Treatment of trans-sphincteric fistulae by full thickness anorectal advancement flaps. Br J Surg 77:1187-1189, 1990.
30. Sohn N, Korelitz BI, Weinstein MA. Anorectal Crohn's disease: Definitive surgery for fistulas and recurrent abscesses. Am J Surg 139:394-397, 1980.
31. Pritchard TJ, Schoetz DJ, Roberts PL, Murray JJ, Coller JA, Veidenheimer MC. Perirectal abscess in Crohn's disease: Drainage and outcome. Dis Colon Rectum 33:933-937, 1990.
32. Williams JG, Rothenberger DA, Nemer FD, Goldberg SM. Fistula-in-ano in Crohn's disease. Results of aggressive surgical treatment. Dis Colon Rectum 34:378-384, 1991.
33. Alexander-Williams J, Buchmann P. Perianal Crohn's disease. World J Surg 4:203-208, 1980.
34. Buchmann P, Keighley MRB, Allan RN, Thompson H, Alexander-Williams J. Natural history of perianal Crohn's disease: Ten year follow-up. A plea for conservatism. Am J Surg 140:642-644, 1980.
35. Morrison JG, Gathright JB, Ray JE, Ferrari BJ, Hicks TC, Timmcke AE. Surgical management of anorectal fistulas in Crohn's disease. Dis Colon Rectum 32:492-496, 1989.
36. Hobbiss JH, Schofield PF. Management of perianal Crohn's disease. J R Soc Med 75: 414-417, 1982.
37. Bernard D, Morgan S, Tasse D. Selective surgical management of Crohn's disease of the anus. Can J Surg 29:318-321, 1986.
38. Levien DH, Surrell J, Mazier WP. Surgical treatment of anorectal fistula in patients with Crohn's disease. Surg Gynecol Obstet 169:133-136, 1989.
39. Allan A, Keighley MRB. Management of perianal Crohn's disease. World J Surg 12:198-202, 1988.
40. Halme L, Sainio P. Factors related to frequency, type and outcome of anal fistulas in Crohn's disease. Dis Colon Rectum 38:55-59, 1995.
41. Hellers G, Bergstrand O, Ewerth S, Holmstrom B. Occurrence and outcome after primary treatment of anal fistulae in Crohn's disease. Gut 21:525-527, 1980.
42. Van Dongen LM, Lubbers GJC. Perianal fistulas in Crohn's disease. Arch Surg 121:1187-1190, 1986.
43. White RA, Eisenstat TE, Rubin RJ, Salvati EP. Seton management of complex anorectal fistulas in patients with Crohn's disease. Dis Colon Rectum 33:587-589, 1990.
44. Jones IJ, Fazio VW, Jagelman DG. The use of transanal rectal advancement flaps in the management of fistulas involving the anorectum. Dis Colon Rectum 30:919-923, 1987.
45. Wolff BE, Culp CE, Beart RW, Istrup DM, Ready RL. Anorectal Crohn's disease: A long-term perspective. Dis Colon Rectum 28:709-711, 1985.
46. McLeod RS. Management of fistula-in-ano: 1990 Roussel lecture. Can J Surg 34:581-585, 1991.
47. Radcliffe AG, Ritchie JK, Hawley PR, Lennard-Jones JG, Northover JMA. Anovaginal and rectovaginal fistulas in Crohn's disease. Dis Colon Rectum 31:94-99, 1988.
48. Francois Y, Descos L, Vignal J. Conservative treatment of low rectovaginal fistulas in Crohn's disease. Int J Colorect Dis 5:12-14, 1990.
49. Bandy LC, Addison A, Pinker RT. Surgical management of rectovaginal fistulas in Crohn's disease. Am J Obstet Gynecol 147:359-363, 1983.
50. Kodner IJ, Mazor A, Shemesh GI, Fry RD, Fleshman JW, Birnbaum EH. Endorectal advancement flap repair of rectovaginal and other complicated anorectal fistulas. Surgery 114:682-690, 1993.

51. Morrison JG, Gathright JB, Ray JE, Ferrari BJ, Hicks TC, Timmcke AE. Results of operation for rectovaginal fistula in Crohn's disease. Dis Colon Rectum 32:497-499, 1989.
52. Bauer JJ, Sher ME, Jaffin H, Present D, Gelernt I. Transvaginal approach for repair of rectovaginal fistulae complicating Crohn's disease. Ann Surg 213:151-158, 1991.
53. Crim RW, Fazio VW, Lavery IC. Rectal advancement flap repair in Crohn's patients: Factors predictive of failure. Dis Colon Rectum 33:P3, 1990.
54. Sher ME, Bauer TJ, Gelernt I. Surgical repair of rectovaginal fistulas in patients with Crohn's disease: Trans-vaginal approach. Dis Colon Rectum 34:641-648, 1991.
55. Pescatori M, Interisano A, Basso L, Arcana F, Buffatti P, Di Bella F, Doldi A, Forcheri V, Gaetini R, Pera A, Mattana C, Prantera C, Pulvirenti A, Segre D, Simi M, Tonelli F. Management of perianal Crohn's disease: Results of a multicenter study in Italy. Dis Colon Rectum 38:121-124, 1995.
56. Lowry AC. Rectovaginal fistulas. In Beck DE, Wexner SD, eds. Fundamentals of Anorectal Surgery. New York: McGraw-Hill, 1992, pp 145-156.
57. Wise WE, Aguilar PS, Padmanabhan A, Meesig DM, Arnold MW, Stewart WRC. Surgical treatment of low rectovaginal fistulas. Dis Colon Rectum 34:271-274, 1991.
58. Greenwald JC, Hoexter B. Repair of rectovaginal fistulas. Surg Gynecol Obstet 146:443-445, 1978.
59. Russell TR, Gallagher DM. Low rectovaginal fistulas. Approach and treatment. Am J Surg 134:1378, 1977.
60. Stone JM, Goldberg SM. The endorectal advancement flap procedure. Int J Colorect Dis 5:232-235, 1990.
61. Buls JG, Rothenberger DA. Anal and rectovaginal fistulas: Repair of the low fistula. In Kodner IJ, Fry RD, Roe JP, eds. Colon, Rectal and Anal Surgery: Current Techniques and Controversies. St. Louis: CV Mosby, 1985, pp 63-75.
62. Senagore A. Treatment of acquired anovaginal and rectovaginal fistulas. Semin Colon Rectal Surg 1:219-223, 1990.
63. Belt RL, Belt RL Jr. Repair of anorectal vaginal fistula utilizing segmental advancement of the internal sphincter muscle. Dis Colon Rectum 12:99-104, 1969.

CHAPTER 14

Surgery for Chronic Anal Fissure and Stenosis

ANTHONY J. SENAGORE

COMPLICATIONS OF SURGERY FOR CHRONIC ANAL FISSURE

Anal fissure is a common anorectal condition in otherwise healthy persons that typically causes them to seek medical attention because of painful rectal bleeding. The pain frequently is severe and may last from minutes to hours after defecation. Although not life-threatening, the discomfort and inconvenience warrant therapeutic intervention. The majority of early, superficial fissures respond to conservative therapy consisting of anal ointments and dietary fiber supplementation and are not the subject of this discussion. Conversely, once the fissure develops scarred, rolled edges, frequently in association with a sentinel tag and hypertrophic anal papilla, conservative therapy offers little hope for cure.

If surgical intervention is required because of chronic anal fissure, the three options are controlled manual anal dilation, lateral internal anal sphincterotomy (open or closed), and fissurectomy followed by flap advancement. Each procedure requires a local, regional, or general anesthetic. The goal of the first two procedures is mechanical reduction of the increased tone of the internal anal sphincter, which is pathognomonic for anal fissure.[1,2] A number of studies have documented marked increases in internal anal sphincter tone, pressure overshoots after defecation, and the association of successful and persistent reduction in anal resting tone with successful therapy.[3-7] The rationale for flap advancement is based on the successful management of other chronic wounds with wound coverage with well-vascularized normal tissue. Although each procedure has its proponents, the goal of therapy for this benign clinical problem should be highly successful management with virtually no complications. The following discussion reviews clinical experience with the various techniques and methods of minimizing complication rates during the surgical management of anal stenosis.

The first to propose anal sphincter stretch for the treatment of fissure was Recamier in 1838,[8] and this technique was popularized by the independent work of Lord[9] and Goligher.[10] The technique involves manual dilation of the anal canal, with the patient under general anesthesia, by insertion of four to eight fingers, depending on the surgeon.[11-14] Manual dilation produces temporary sphincter paralysis and associated relaxation of the internal and external sphincters, which results in fissure healing.[14] Acute complications are rare; however, failed healing of fissures ranges from 5% to 56% with this technique.[11-14] In addition, the procedure requires a general anesthetic and is associated with major incontinence in as many as 7% of patients and minor incontinence in as many as 20%.[13,15] The degree of sphincter injury possible with this technique is corroborated by recent ultrasound evidence of a mean loss of 153 degrees of internal anal sphincter continuity in 11 patients who became incontinent after this treatment.[16] There does not appear to be a clear consensus in the literature with regard to averting incontinence after manual dilation, although it would appear wise to limit dilation to six fingers. In general, it is difficult to recommend this technique when there are alternative procedures that can be performed in the office setting with local anesthesia with similar if not superior results and a lower risk for incontinence.

Eisenhammer[17] was the first to describe fissurectomy and internal anal sphincterotomy for the management of chronic anal fissure, although he recommended a posterior approach. The importance of not incising the subcutaneous external anal sphincter was stressed to prevent formation of a "keyhole" deformity. Although his technique provided excellent pain relief, it was associated with prolonged healing time and a high incidence of fecal soiling as a result of the large, insensate fissurectomy scar.[17] It is also likely that division of a portion of the external anal sphincter contributed to incontinence. Notaras[18] subsequently modified the technique to minimize the size of the wound and associated morbidity with his description of a subcutaneous approach to internal anal sphincterotomy. This variation became popular because of its high success rate, ease of performance with local anesthesia, and minimal complications. More recent experience with various forms of internal anal sphincterotomy has confirmed these conclusions (Table 14-1).

The reported complications associated with internal anal sphincterotomy include bleeding (0.3% to 0.8%), abscess (0% to 2.3%), failed healing (2% to 6%), and impaired continence (early, 11% to 25%; late, 4% to 35%).[17-23,26,27] The most frequent source of postoperative hemorrhage after internal anal sphincterotomy is a lacerated hemorrhoidal vessel, which is usually evident during the procedure. Simple suture transfixion of the hemorrhoidal pedicle immediately proximal to the sphincterotomy acts to ligate the vessel and tamponade the anoderm on the muscle remnant, which controls the bleeding.

Postoperative abscess is usually the result of an unrecognized laceration of the rectal mucosa by the scalpel blade or scissors during sphincterotomy. The result is an intersphincteric abscess and fistula, which can be easily managed in the office setting with fistulotomy with local anesthesia. If the rectal mucosal

Table 14-1 Outcomes of surgical management of anal fissures

Author	Technique (n)	Abscess	Bleeding	Recurrence (%)	Incontinence* (%)
Weaver et al.[11]	MDA (59)	0	0	5.0	0
	LIS (39)	0	0	5.0	5.0
Jensen et al.[12]	MDA (28)	0	0	28.0	39.0
	LIS (30)	0	0	3.0	3.0
MacDonald et al.[13]	MDA (46)	0	0	56.0	24.0
Marby et al.[15]	MDA (78)	0	10.0	10.0	0
	LIS (78)	1.0	1.0	27.0	0
Bell[19]	LIS (56)	NA	NA	2.0	NA
Notaras[20]	LIS (82)	0	0	10.0	10.0
Abcarian[21]	LIS (150)	1.3	0	1.3	0
	Fissurectomy (150)	0	0	1.3	5.0
Keighley at al.[22]	LIS (71)	3.0	3.0	25.0	1.4
Khubchandani and Reed[23]	LIS (1355)	0	0	2.3	35.0
Hsu and MacKeigan[24]	LIS (89)	1.0	0	5.6	0
	Y-V (247)	0.4	0.4	7.2	0
Leong and Seow-Choen[25]	LIS (20)	0	0	0	0
	Flap (20)	0	0	0	15.0

LIS = lateral internal anal sphincterotomy; MDA = manual dilation of the anus; NA = data not available.
*Incontinence of gas or of liquid or solid stool.

laceration is identified during sphincterotomy, the easiest method of management is to convert the closed technique to an open sphincterotomy. This adds minimal morbidity to the procedure and averts the potential problem of a closed space infection. Alternatively, the defect can be sutured when recognized, which still carries the risk of failed closure and abscess formation.

Failed healing is the result of an inadequate internal anal sphincterotomy or an unrecognized associated anodermal scar (when the closed technique is used). Both of these problems indicate inadequate reduction of the elevated internal anal sphincter tone, which perpetuates the fissure.[26] The majority of these patients will respond to a repeated internal anal sphincterotomy, which can be performed at the same location or on the opposite side. The problem of recurrence or failed healing can be minimized with careful digital palpation of the internal anal sphincter after performance of the sphincterotomy to ensure that all fibrous bands have been divided. Often the few remaining strands can be broken down with digital pressure alone.

Anal incontinence is a troubling complication of management of anal fissure. The majority of patients with anal incontinence after anal sphincterotomy experience only temporary difficulty in distinguishing flatus from stool or incontinence of flatus. It should be remembered, however, that the prevalence and degree of anal incontinence is directly related to the extent of sphincterotomy. The prevalence is particularly high in series in which bilateral anal sphincterotomies were performed or the entire length and thickness of the internal anal sphincter was divided.[27] The net result of these extensive sphincterotomies is significant reduction in resting anal tone, which accounts for the incontinence. It is sufficient therapy for the fissure if internal anal sphincterotomy is limited to division of the distal half to two thirds of the internal anal sphincter and approximately 50% of its thickness. Again, manual palpation of the sphincter after sphincterotomy is sufficient to convince the surgeon that all offending cicatricial fibers have been divided.

Y-V anoplasty was reported by Samson and Stewart[28] as a management technique for chronic anal fissure. The technique relies on the theory that chronic wounds can be successfully healed by providing vascularized epithelial coverage of the fissure, with resultant primary healing. A drawback of this technique is its failure to address the hypertonicity of the internal anal sphincter. Although a variety of different flap types have been described, the most frequently used is Y-V anoplasty, which requires elevation of a V-shaped flap with a length-to-breadth ratio of less than 3:1[25,28] (Fig. 14-1). The proponents of this technique believe that postoperative pain and wound care requirements are lessened. Samson and Stewart[28] reported on 2072 patients with a 0.5% frequency of recurrent fissures and a flap slough rate of 2.4%. However, Hsu and MacKeigan[24] found that flap closure required longer operative time and hospitalization and resulted in a higher prevalence of urinary retention compared with lateral internal anal sphincterotomy. The key to reducing complications of flap closure of anal fissures is careful hemostasis, which reduces the risk for hematoma formation and flap loss or infection. Attention must be paid to the design of the flap, in particular the length-to-width ratio, to ensure adequate vascularity.

COMPLICATIONS OF SURGERY FOR ANAL STENOSIS

Acquired anal stenosis can be a late sequela of a variety of anorectal surgical procedures. It has been reported to occur after 5% to 10% of radical hemorrhoidectomies and after fissurectomy, radiation injury, and Moh's chemosurgery.[25,29] The cause of these strictures is excessive removal of the anodermal lining of the anal canal and thus is generally preventable. In cases of severe, symptomatic anal stenosis, a variety of flaps can be used to resurface the anal

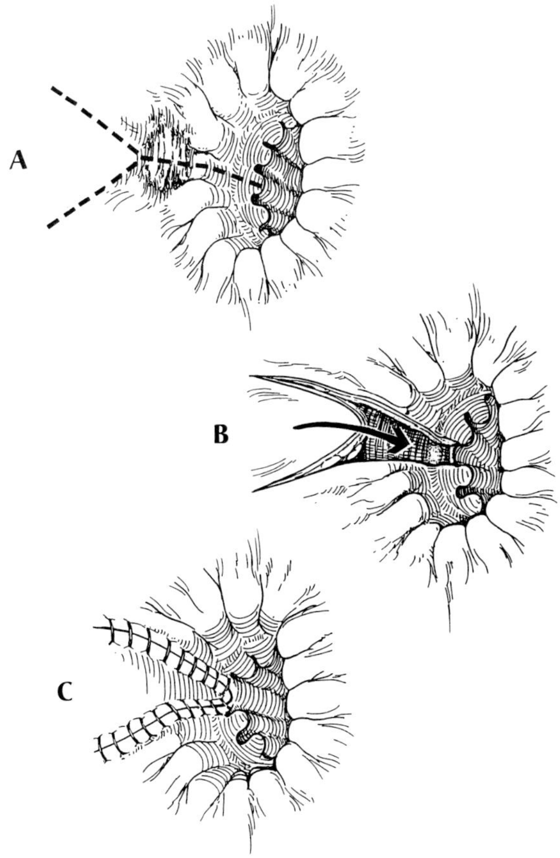

Fig. 14-1 Y-V anoplasty. **A**, Y-shaped incision is made. **B**, V-shaped flap is mobilized. **C**, Flap is advanced to the top of the defect and sutured in place.

canal and expand its circumference. The key to success with any of these flaps is that they be carefully designed to maintain vascularity and that subflap hematoma formation is averted to minimize the risk for infection and flap pressure.

Patients should undergo complete mechanical and oral antibiotic bowel preparation before surgery. In addition, a broad-spectrum prophylactic parenteral antibiotic should be given perioperatively. After surgery, bowel activity should be restricted for a day or two with use of a full liquid diet; after this period, patients should be allowed a regular diet and given fiber supplements and laxatives to avert constipation. One final, important factor is the limitation of patient activity for several weeks so that flap motion is minimal, to allow neovascularization to occur.

Anal S-plasty (Fig. 14-2) was first proposed by Ferguson[30] as a method to correct Whitehead deformities in 13 patients. Later Corman et al.[31] modified the procedure for use in the management of anal stenosis. The key to the success of this approach is development of large, full-thickness skin flaps with a base-to-length ratio >1.0. Ferguson recommended a base of 7 to 10 cm and maintenance of a thin layer of fat globules on the deep aspect of the flap so that adequate vascularity can be ensured. He further cautioned against overzealous hemostasis on the flap itself so as not to impair blood flow. The flaps are then rotated toward the anal canal so that the anodermal defect can be resurfaced. The flaps are sutured in place, and the remaining semilunar defect is sutured to allow its primary healing. It is wise to use a closed suction drain beneath the flap to avert seroma or hematoma formation.

For less severe anal strictures that require less skin coverage, the Y-V anoplasty is an excellent alternative because it is simpler to perform and is less traumatic for the patient. This technique was initially described by Penn[32] in 1948. Again, successful healing of the flap requires a length-to-base ratio <3.0. Gingold and Arvanitis[33] presented a series of 14 patients. Thirteen healed within 14 days with no episodes of infection or hematoma formation. Five patients sloughed a small portion of the flap tip but required no additional treatment. Experiences reported by other authors support the low rate (10% to 25%) of tip necrosis and

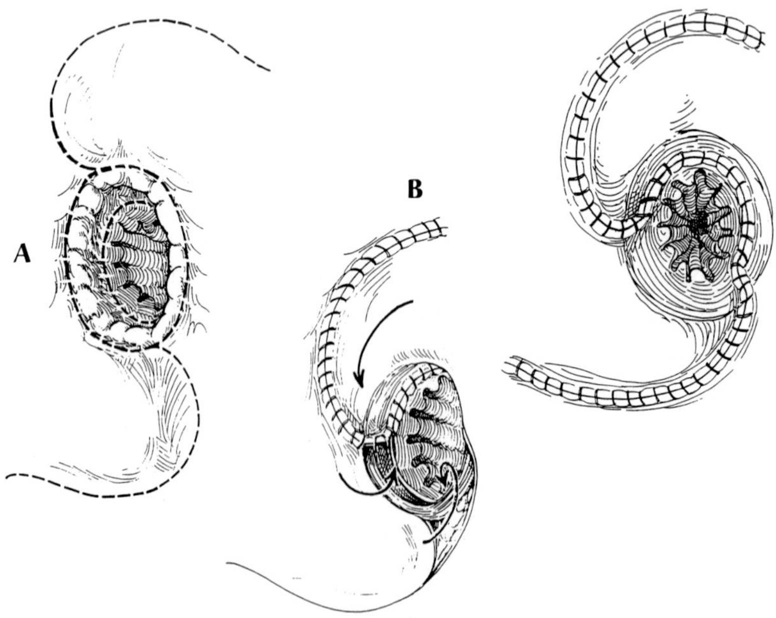

Fig. 14-2 Anal S-plasty. **A,** Ectropion is excised and S-shaped incisions are created. **B** and **C,** Flaps are rotated to close the defects and sutured in place.

the high rate (85% to 92%) of stenosis relief associated with this technique.[34,35] It must be remembered, however, that Y-V advancement flaps limit how much anal resurfacing can be accomplished.

Other uses for the Y-V advancement flap have been advocated. Rosen[36] used it to treat anal stenosis and ectropion (Fig. 14-3). The blood supply for this flap is based on perforating vessels in the subcutaneous fat. The Y-V advancement flap is well suited for covering the lower anal canal but has limited application for stenosis above the dentate line.

Other techniques of flap formation have been suggested. Christensen et al.[37] proposed the use of "house" advancement pedicle flaps. We prefer the house flap because it is easy to construct, can cover as much as 25% of the anal circumference, and permits primary closure of the donor site (Fig. 14-4). If additional coverage is needed, two, three, or four flaps may be used. Caplin and Kodner[38] recommended the use of the diamond flap for many of the same reasons (Fig. 14-5).

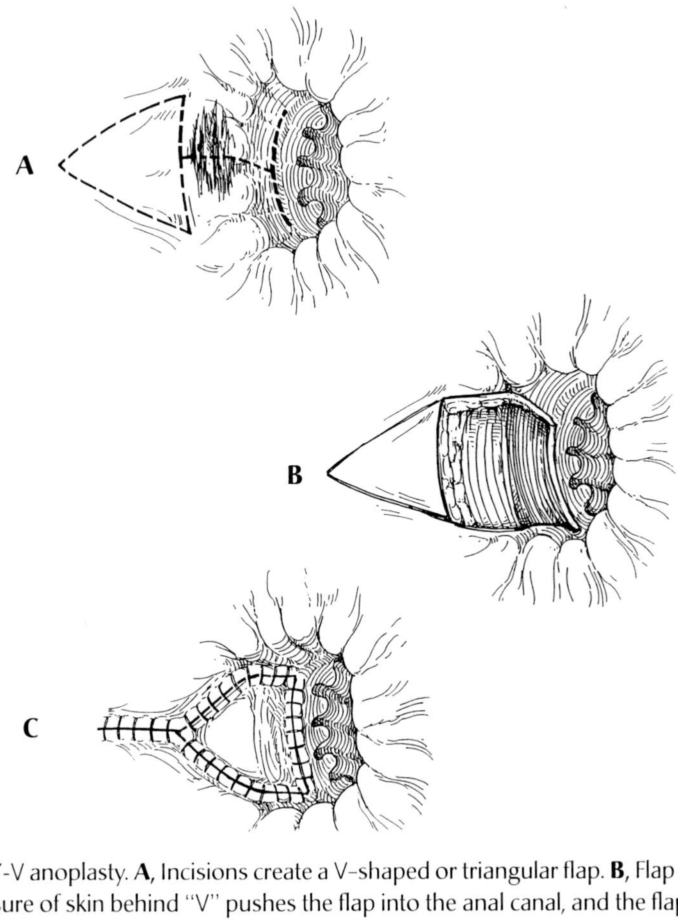

Fig. 14-3 Y-V anoplasty. **A**, Incisions create a V-shaped or triangular flap. **B**, Flap is advanced to close defect. **C**, Closure of skin behind "V" pushes the flap into the anal canal, and the flap is sutured in place.

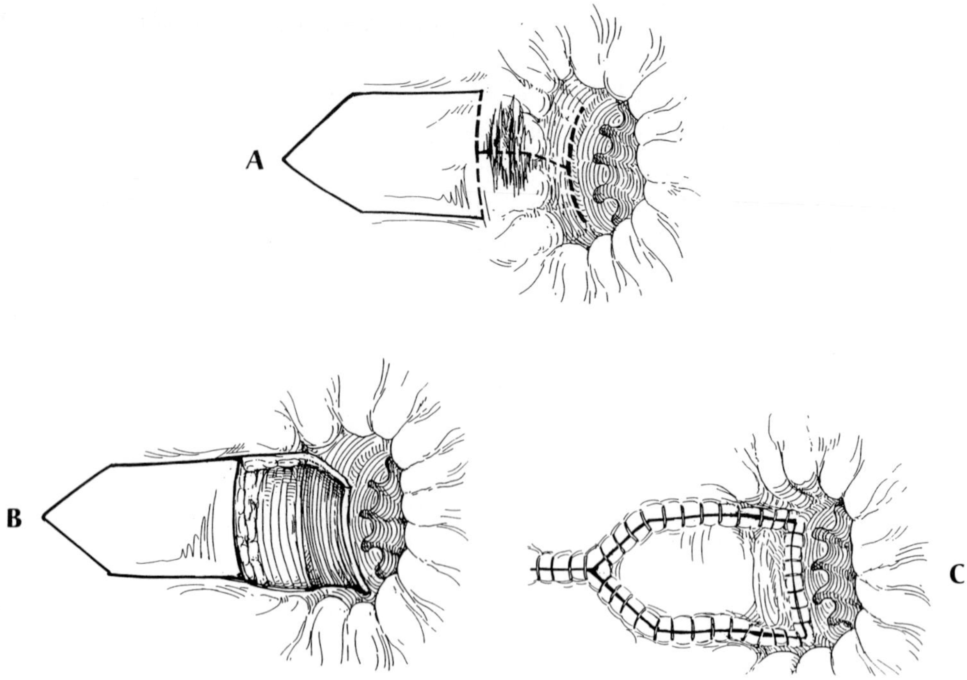

Fig. 14-4 House advancement flap. **A**, House-shaped flap is created. **B**, The flap is advanced into the anal canal and **C**, sutured in place.

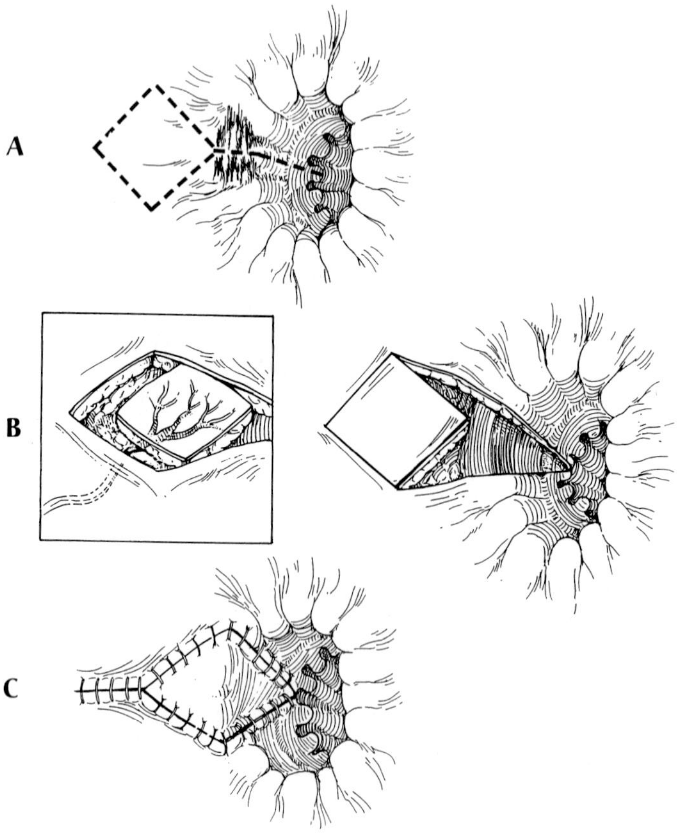

Fig. 14-5 Diamond flap. **A**, Diamond-shaped flap is created. **B**, The flap is advanced into the anal canal to fill the defect. (Inset demonstrates perforating subcutaneous blood supply.) **C**, Flap is sutured in place.

CONCLUSION

The key to minimizing complications of surgery for anal fissure and stricture lies in careful attention to technique. To minimize the risk of anal incontinence, the most serious complication of this procedure, surgical correction should involve as little disruption of the internal anal sphincter as necessary to provide relief of hypertonicity and/or associated scar. The key to successful surgery for anal stricture is a flap of adequate size to correct the stenosis without jeopardizing its vascularity. Attention to these principles will improve surgical results and minimize morbidity from these procedures.

REFERENCES

1. Abcarian H, Lakshmanan S, Read DR, Roccaforte P. The role of internal sphincter in chronic anal fissures. Dis Colon Rectum 25:525-528, 1982.
2. Cerdán FJ, Buiz de León A, Azpiroz F, Martin J, Balibrea JL. Anal sphincteric pressure in fissure-in-ano before and after lateral internal sphincterotomy. Dis Colon Rectum 25:198-201, 1982.
3. Hancock BD. The internal sphincter and anal fissure. Br J Surg 64:92-95, 1977.
4. Nothmann BJ, Schuster MM. Internal anal sphincter derangement with anal fissures. Gastroenterology 67:216-220, 1974.
5. Graham-Stewart CW, Greenwood RK, Lloyd-Davies RW. A review of 50 patients with fissure in ano. Surg Gynecol Obstet 113:445-448, 1961.
6. Chowcat NL, Araujo JGC, Boulos PB. Internal sphincterotomy for chronic anal fissure: Long term effects on anal pressure. Br J Surg 73:915-916, 1986.
7. McNamara MJ, Percy JP, Fielding IR. A manometric study of anal fissure treated by subcutaneous lateral internal sphincterotomy. Ann Surg 211:235-238, 1990.
8. Recamier JCA. Extension, massage et percussion cadencée dans le traitment des contractures musculaires. Rev Med 1:74-89, 1838.
9. Lord PH. Diverse methods of managing hemorrhoids: Dilatation. Dis Colon Rectum 16: 180-183, 1973.
10. Goligher JC. An elevation of internal sphincterotomy and simple sphincter stretching in the treatment of fissure-in-ano. Surg Clin North Am 42:1299-1304, 1965.
11. Weaver RM, Ambrose NS, Alexander-Williams J, Keighley MRB. Manual dilatation of the anus vs. lateral subcutaneous sphincterotomy in the treatment of chronic fissure-in-ano: Results of a prospective, randomized, clinical trial. Dis Colon Rectum 30:420-423, 1987.
12. Jensen SL, Lund F, Nielsen OV, Tange G. Lateral subcutaneous sphincterotomy versus anal dilatation in the treatment of fissure in ano in outpatients: A prospective randomized study. Br Med J 289:528-530, 1984.
13. MacDonald A, Smith A, McNeill AD, Finlay IG. Manual dilatation of the anus. Br J Surg 79:1381-1382, 1992.
14. Ortiz H, Marti J, Jaurrieta E, Masdevall C, Ferrer J, Sitges A. Lord's procedure: A critical study of its basic principle. Br J Surg 65:281-284, 1978.
15. Marby M, Alexander-Williams J, Buchmann P, Arabi Y, Kappas A, Minervini S, Gatehouse D, Keighley MRB. A randomized controlled trial to compare anal dilatation with lateral subcutaneous sphincterotomy for anal fissure. Dis Colon Rectum 22:308-311, 1979.
16. Speakman CTM, Burnett SJD, Kamm MA, Bartram CI. Sphincter injury after anal dilatation demonstrated by anal endosonography. Br J Surg 78:1429-1430, 1991.
17. Eisenhammer S. Surgical correction of chronic internal anal (sphincteric) contracture. S Afr Med J 25:486, 1951.

18. Notaras MJ. The treatment of anal fissure by lateral subcutaneous internal sphincterotomy: A technique and results. Br J Surg 58:96-100, 1971.
19. Bell GA. Lateral internal sphincterotomy in chronic anal fissure: A surgical technique. Am Surg 46:572-575, 1980.
20. Notaras MJ. Anal fissure and stenosis. Surg Clin North Am 68:1427-1440, 1988.
21. Abcarian H. Surgical correction of chronic anal fissure: Results of lateral internal sphincterotomy vs. fissurectomy–midline sphincterotomy. Dis Colon Rectum 23:31-36, 1980.
22. Keighley MRB, Greca F, Nevah E, Hares M, Alexander-Williams J. Treatment of anal fissure by lateral subcutaneous sphincterotomy should be under general anaesthesia. Br J Surg 68:400-401, 1981.
23. Khubchandani IT, Reed JF. Sequelae of internal sphincterotomy for chronic fissure in ano. Br J Surg 76:431-434, 1989.
24. Hsu TC, MacKeigan JM. Surgical treatment of chronic anal fissure: A retrospective study of 1753 cases. Dis Colon Rectum 27:475-478, 1984.
25. Leong AFPK, Seow-Choen F. Lateral sphincterotomy compared with anal advancement flap for chronic anal fissure. Dis Colon Rectum 38:69-71, 1995.
26. Bode WE, Culp CE, Spencer RJ, Beart RW. Fissurectomy with superficial midline sphincterotomy: A viable alternative for the surgical correction of chronic fissure/ulcer-in-ano. Dis Colon Rectum 27:93-105, 1984.
27. Lewis TH, Corman ML, Prager ED, Robertson WG. Long-term results of open and closed sphincterotomy for anal fissure. Dis Colon Rectum 31:368-371, 1988.
28. Samson RB, Stewart WR. Sliding skin grafts in the treatment of anal fissure. Dis Colon Rectum 13:372-375, 1970.
29. Oh C, Albanese C. S-plasty for various anal lesions. Am J Surg 163:606-608, 1992.
30. Ferguson JA. Repair of "Whitehead deformity" of the anus. Surg Gynecol Obstet 108:115-116, 1959.
31. Corman ML, Veidenheimer MC, Coller JA. Anoplasty for anal stricture. Surg Clin North Am 56:727-731, 1976.
32. Penn JA. A case of anal reconstruction by means of local skin flaps. Br J Plast Surg 1:87-88, 1948.
33. Gingold BS, Arvanitis M. Y-V anoplasty for treatment of anal stricture. Surg Gynecol Obstet 162:241-242, 1986.
34. Angelchik PD, Harms BA, Starling JR. Repair of anal stricture and mucosal ectropion with Y-V or pedicle flap anoplasty. Am J Surg 166:55-59, 1993.
35. Ramanujan PS, Venkatesh KS, Cohen M. Y-V anoplasty for severe anal stenosis. Contemp Surg 3:62-68, 1988.
36. Rosen L. V-Y advancement for anal ectropion. Dis Colon Rectum 29:596-598, 1986.
37. Christensen MA, Pitsch RM, Cali RL, Blatchford GJ, Thorson AG. "House" advancement pedicle flap for anal stenosis. Dis Colon Rectum 35:201-203, 1992.
38. Caplin DA, Kodner IJ. Repair of anal stricture and mucosal ectropion by simple flap procedures. Dis Colon Rectum 29:92, 1986.

CHAPTER 15

Surgery for Pilonidal Disease and Hidradenitis Suppurativa

DOUGLAS A. KHOURY

Pilonidal disease and hidradenitis suppurativa provide common challenges for the surgeon. Because of the proximity of these diseases to the anus rather than their cause, patients often are referred to colorectal surgeons. High recurrence rates and significant morbidity highlight the difficulty in treating what appear to be simple cutaneous infections. A thorough understanding of these diseases and their treatment options is important to successful outcome with minimal morbidity.

PILONIDAL DISEASE

Pilonidal disease was first reported by Anderson[1] in 1847 as a complication of surgical therapy. He had drained a midline fistulous opening, believed to be caused by tuberculosis, near the coccyx in a young adult male patient. The wound failed to heal after 3 weeks, and careful examination at that time revealed a 2-inch long hair within the wound. Removal of the hair resulted in prompt wound healing. Thirty-three years later, the term *pilonidal sinus* (L. *pilus*, hair; *nidus*, nest) was coined for this disease, which was believed to be unique to the gluteal cleft region.[2]

Over the next 60 years, treatment was predicated on the widespread premise that pilonidal disease was a congenital malformation.[3,4] Most surgeons believed pilonidal sinuses were distal remnants of the medullary canal; others thought pilonidal disease was caused by faulty infoldings of the natal cleft epithelium. The purpose of surgical therapy seemed obvious: complete removal of the congenitally malformed tissues.[5] Experience soon demonstrated that pilonidal sinus excision resulted in a significant number of unhealed wounds and recurrence of disease. Acquired theories of pilonidal disease development were subsequently reconsidered and refined and are now regarded by most as more plausible.[6] Treatment has also advanced beyond simple excision to include elimination of the conditions that favor pilonidal disease development. To successfully treat the complications of pilonidal disease surgery, one must first appreciate the mechanism of pilonidal disease development.

Pathophysiology

Midline pits, also known as skin dimples, are usually found at the base of the gluteal cleft in patients with pilonidal disease. Bascom[7] examined these pits microscopically and deduced that they were distorted hair follicles. He suggested that normal gluteal cleft hair follicles enlarge in the following manner. Keratin accumulates concentrically around the intrafollicular portion of the hair shaft. This generates outward pressure on the follicular wall, thereby increasing its diameter. The follicle enlarges to become a cavity, after which a vacuum effect is created from normal gluteal cleft motion[8]: when a person is in a sitting position, air and loose debris (e.g., keratin) are expelled out of the dilated follicle as the gluteal tissues are pushed against the sacrum. When the person stands, the gluteal tissues fall away from the sacrum, creating a vacuum within the enlarged follicle.

As the dilated follicle diameter increases, so does its wall tension, according to Laplace's law (Tension = Pressure × Diameter × p), which makes it more prone to rupture. The most likely point of rupture is the bottom of the follicle.[9,10] The retained hair is pushed down through the bottom of the follicle because of the orientation of scales on the hair surface.[11,12] The scales lie with their free ends toward the hair tip, which causes the hair root to move deeper into the dilated follicle but not in the reverse direction. Hair and keratin extrude into the underlying subcutaneous fat, provoking an inflammatory response followed by microabscess formation. The associated edema occludes the follicle's skin orifice, causing pus to accumulate within the ruptured follicle and underlying fat.

When the edema subsides, the follicle's skin orifice becomes patent, allowing pus and follicular debris to drain spontaneously. Epithelium grows down into the follicular remnant and underlying abscess cavity to become a chronic pilonidal sinus. The previously mentioned vacuum effect promotes enlargement of the pilonidal sinus cavity and lateral extensions into the adjacent subcutaneous fat.

This acquired theory appears applicable to the majority of patients with pilonidal disease: hirsute men between the ages of 16 and 40 years.[13] However, a significant number of men and women with pilonidal disease have little if any natal cleft hair. In these persons, three gluteal cleft factors have been identified that foster pilonidal sinus formation: catch basin effect, gluteal cleft friction, and intergluteal cleft depth.

Loose hairs from the back and head accumulate within the gluteal cleft.[14,15] Normal motion of the buttocks creates friction that aligns the loose hairs into a drill-shaped configuration.[8,10] Continued buttocks motion drives these hairs into the base of the gluteal cleft, resulting in skin puncture. Loose hair and other gluteal cleft debris pass through the skin puncture site into the subcutaneous fat, provoking the same inflammatory response described earlier. Persons with deeper gluteal clefts are believed to accumulate more loose hair and generate more intergluteal friction than those with smaller clefts, which suggests they are at greater risk for pilonidal disease.

Complications

Most surgeons treat pilonidal abscesses with simple incision and drainage.[15-19] Although this effectively treats the abscess, in as many as 42% of patients the wounds do not heal and require additional surgical treatment.[20] In those in whom the wounds do heal, chronic pilonidal sinuses that require additional treatment develop in 15% to 40%.[15,20] Lundhus and Gottrup[21] recently reported their attempts to definitively treat pilonidal abscesses with excision and primary closure coupled with perioperative antibiotic therapy. In 70% of their patients the wounds healed primarily; however, a recurrence rate of 30% prompted the investigators to conclude that this was not a better treatment option.

Chronic pilonidal disease. Although conservative management is an effective alternative,[19] most surgeons recommend surgery in patients with chronic pilonidal disease because it is believed to be curative. Several surgical procedures have been described, but without consensus as to which is best.[7,14,22-36] The controversy is fueled by a wide range of healing times, variable recurrence rates, and a significant number of unhealed wounds (Table 15-1). Regardless of which operation is performed, most wounds heal and patients return to their normal lifestyles with no recurrence of pilonidal disease. However, in a significant number, as many as 12% in some series, the wounds fail to heal and these patients are unable to resume normal daily activities. In addition, in 15% to 50% of patients in whom surgical wounds heal, recurrent disease develops, usually within 3 years. These treatment failures can ultimately result in significant personal and financial hardship.

Unhealed presacral wound. The initial approach to any nonhealing wound is to rule out infection. Presacral wounds purposely left open to heal by secondary intention rarely become infected because they are completely drained. Conversely, any presacral wound closed primarily is at greater risk for infection. With careful physical examination of the wound and the surrounding soft tissues, infection is readily identified. The presence of fluctuance, excessive tenderness, drainage, and erythema in these wounds indicates infection and requires immediate opening and debridement of nonviable tissue. Supplemental antibiotic therapy is indicated only if there is evidence of systemic infection.[37] With standard local wound care, these wounds will heal the same as those left to heal by secondary intention after simple pilonidal sinus excision.[15]

Failure to remove all diseased tissue is another significant cause of the unhealed presacral wound. Meticulous examination of the wound with the patient in the prone jackknife position is the best way to examine for residual

Table 15-1 Elective surgical treatment options for pilonidal disease

Technique	Author (year)	No. of patients	Hospital time (days)	Average healing time (days)	Recurrence rate (%)	Unhealed wounds (%)
Pilonidal cystostomy	Weinstein et al.[22] (1977)	126	3	<60	20.9	ND
Excision with healing by secondary intention	Goodall[23] (1961)	36	18	ND	20.7	ND
	Eftaiha and Abcarian[24] (1977)	175	2	42	0.6	0
	Kronborg et al.[25] (1985)	32	ND	64	14.8	9.4
	Sondenna et al.[26] (1992)	60	Outpatient	86	2	3
	Kooistra[27] (1942)	24	10.7	84	21	ND
	Khawaja et al.[28] (1992)	23	Outpatient	41	0	0
Excision with partial closure	McLaren[29] (1984)	22	20	20	0	0
Excision with semiprimary closure	Abramson[30] (1978)	234	Outpatient	26	5.8	ND
Excision with primary closure	Kooistra[27] (1942)	53	10.4	27	28.3	ND
	Goodall[23] (1961)	126	18.3	ND	38.2	ND
	Kronborg et al.[25] (1985)	33	ND	14	33.3	12.1
	Khawaja et al.[28] (1992)	23	Outpatient	14	0	0
	Sondenna et al.[26] (1992)	60	Outpatient	23	7	0
Marsupialization	Buie and Curtiss[31] (1952)	618	3	20	0	ND
Follicle excision and lateral drainage	Bascom[7] (1980)	50	Outpatient	21	8	ND
	Bascom[32] (1983)	161	Outpatient	21	5.6	ND
Dufourmentel technique	Manterola et al.[33] (1991)	25	4	14	0	ND
Advancement flap	Karydakis[34] (1973)	1687	8.2	ND	0.5	ND
Z-plasty	Mansoory and Dickson[14] (1982)	120	2	8	1.6	ND
	Toubanakis[35] (1986)	110	ND	ND	0	ND
Phenol injection	Maurice and Greenwood[36] (1964)	21	2	31	19	ND

ND = not described.

pilonidal disease. Patients with deep gluteal clefts, large amounts of subcutaneous fat, and multiple lateral sinus tracts are at greatest risk for unhealed wounds. If found, all residual diseased tissue should be excised intraoperatively with the patient under regional or general anesthesia. The remainder of the wound should be debrided of all nonviable tissue and allowed to heal by secondary intention.

Although less common, failure to make the correct diagnosis is another possible explanation for unhealed presacral wounds. Complex fistulas in ano or hidradenitis suppurativa can be mistaken for pilonidal disease. Careful physical and microscopic examination of previously resected tissue will best determine whether the correct disease has been identified. If one ascertains that pilonidal disease is not the primary diagnosis, treatment options need to be redirected to the true primary disease.

Suboptimal postoperative wound care is the most easily corrected cause of unhealed presacral wounds. Wounds closed primarily require little more than twice daily cleansing with soap and water, whereas those intended to heal by secondary intention require diligent dressing changes. The wounds must be kept meticulously clean, free of nonviable tissue, and devoid of foreign material.[38] Intraoperative debridement may be required initially, after which saline solution wet-to-dry dressings are essential. Dressing changes three times daily will prevent wound desiccation, remove accumulated exudates, and debride necrotic tissue. It is imperative that the gauze closest to the wound be in contact with all wound surfaces to ensure optimal debridement with each dressing change. Sitz baths are also recommended before placing each new dressing; however, more important, the wound should be gently wiped with moistened gauze to remove all residual debris. Use of Water Pik lavage has been reported with enthusiasm both for its success and ease of patient use.[39]

Each week, any hair at and around the wound edges should be removed. Because hairs in this region grow medial and cephalad, their tips can extend into midline presacral wounds. Just one hair within the wound can prevent healing because there is no natural mechanism to push it out.[40] Shaving is quicker, but plucking the hairs individually usually produces longer-lasting results.

Despite eliminating infection, excising residual pilonidal disease, and optimizing local wound care, in some patients the wounds still fail to heal. In these patients the most likely reason for incomplete healing can be linked to the factors that led initially to development of pilonidal disease. The catch basin effect of the gluteal cleft promotes foreign body contamination of presacral wounds, and normal buttocks motion generates wound surface friction and movement that prevents epithelialization.[41] These two effects are believed to be enhanced in patients with deep gluteal clefts. Several surgeons have subsequently recognized the importance of making the gluteal cleft less steep.[14,35,41-43]

Rosenberg[41] reported his success with reverse bandaging of the buttocks; however, this method has not been widely used. Two additional surgical options are cleft closure[44] and creation of a rotational buttock flap.[45] Both are designed to close the unhealed presacral wound and eliminate the associated portion of the gluteal cleft.

With Bascom's method,[44] cleft closure is accomplished with the patient in the prone jackknife position under spinal or general anesthesia. The buttocks are pushed together and their outer line of contact is marked (Fig. 15-1, *A*). After spreading the buttocks with tape and preparing the operative field, the skin and subcutaneous tissues are infiltrated with a bupivacaine-epinephrine solution to control bleeding and postoperative pain.

Operative incisions to create an island of skin are placed on the side with the most skin damage (Fig. 15-1, *B*). The skin within the operative incisions is excised with care to preserve as much underlying fat as possible. The apex of the excised skin lies superior and lateral to the top of the gluteal cleft; its lateral border coincides with the ipsilateral line of buttocks contact. An oblique incision extends from the apex across the midline to a point immediately cephalad and lateral to the most superior extent of the unhealed wound. The incision continues inferiorly to a point immediately caudad and lateral to the most inferior extent of the unhealed wound. From there it crosses the midline at a right angle and becomes comma-shaped (pointing toward the anus), which creates the inferior apex of the operative wound. A full-thickness fat-free skin flap is created from the remaining midline wound edge and elevated laterally to the previously marked line of buttocks contact. Loose granulation tissue and debris are wiped from the sides and base of the unhealed wound with gauze.

A

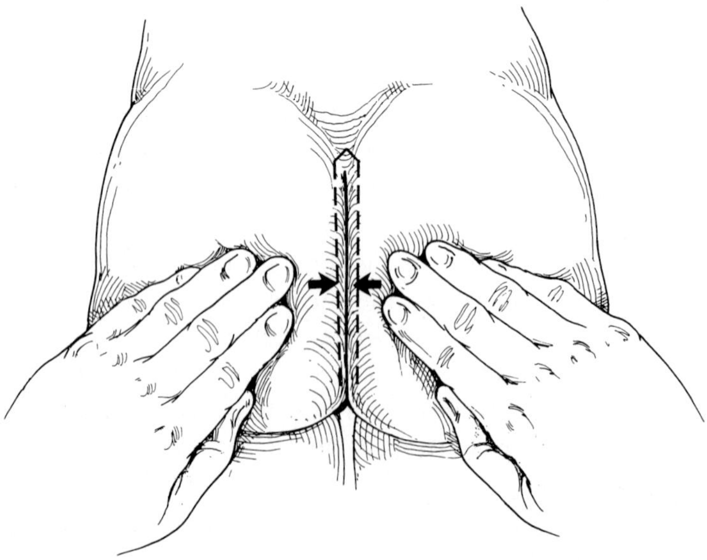

Fig. 15-1 **A,** Cleft closure technique. The buttocks are marked at their natural line of contact.

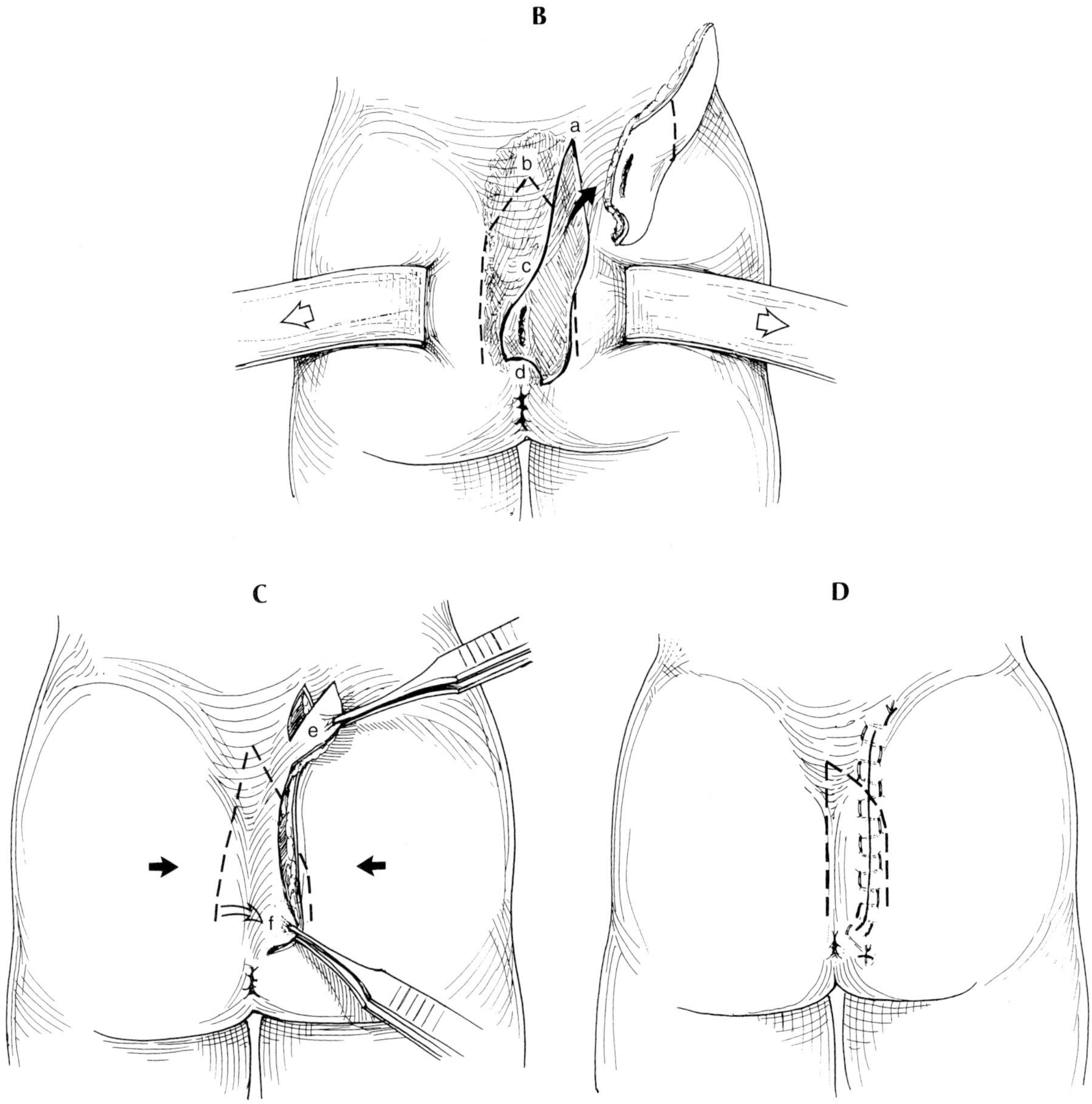

Fig. 15-1, cont'd **B**, The buttocks are spread apart with tape, and a local anesthetic with epinephrine is injected to reduce intraoperative bleeding and early postoperative pain. An island of skin that includes the unhealed wound's superficial edges is created by placing operative incisions on the side with the most skin damage. Its apex *(a)* lies superior and lateral to the top of the gluteal cleft *(b)*. The incision crosses the midline at an acute angle superior to the unhealed wound *(c)* and at a right angle inferior to the wound *(d)*. **C**, Release of the retraction tapes allows the subcutaneous wound edges to come together. Excess skin *(e)* in the upper half of the flap is excised. The flap's inferior portion *(f)* is rotated toward the anus to avert a dog-eared appearance. **D**, After obliterating wound dead space with interrupted absorbable sutures in the subcutaneous tissues, the skin edges are approximated with 3-0 polypropylene running horizontal mattress sutures. (Modified from Bascom J. Pilonidal sinus. In Fazio VW, ed. Current Therapy in Colon and Rectal Surgery. Toronto: BC Decker, 1990, pp 32-39. With permission.)

After irrigating the wound and obtaining meticulous hemostasis, the retracting tapes are removed. With the buttocks pushed together, the elevated skin flap is brought across the midline to cover the exposed subcutaneous fat. The flap's inferior edge is rotated toward the anus to prevent a dog-eared appearance. Overlapping skin is excised with special care to create a tension-free anastomosis (Fig. 15-1, *C*).

A soft, closed-suction drain is placed at the base of the wound and brought out through a separate stab wound incision. Interrupted 4-0 polydioxanone sutures are placed in the subcutaneous tissue to approximate the fatty edges and obliterate dead space. The skin is closed with 3-0 polypropylene running horizontal mattress sutures in the subcuticular layer (Fig. 15-1, *D*). Steri-Strips are applied, followed by a light dressing. Bascom[43,44] recommends preoperative intravenous cefazolin and metronidazole followed by 4 days of the same antibiotics orally. He removes the drain on postoperative day 4, and the subcuticular polypropylene suture 3 days later. Patients are seen weekly until their wounds heal.

Complications were infrequent in Bascom's series of 40 patients[44] treated with cleft closure. Infection was treated with opening of the lower 2 cm of the wound and antibiotics. Focal skin flap necrosis did delay healing but did not affect the end result.

Although it has been described as a closure technique for use after primary excision of new or recurrent pilonidal diseases, the method of Fishbein and Handelson,[45] creation of a rotational buttock flap, is useful for treating unhealed sacral wounds. It not only covers the sacral defect with a significant amount of soft tissue but also flattens the gluteal cleft. The flap consists of skin, subcutaneous fat, and the adjacent fascial covering of the gluteus maximus muscle. The technique is shown in Fig. 15-2. This technique may be a better option than

A

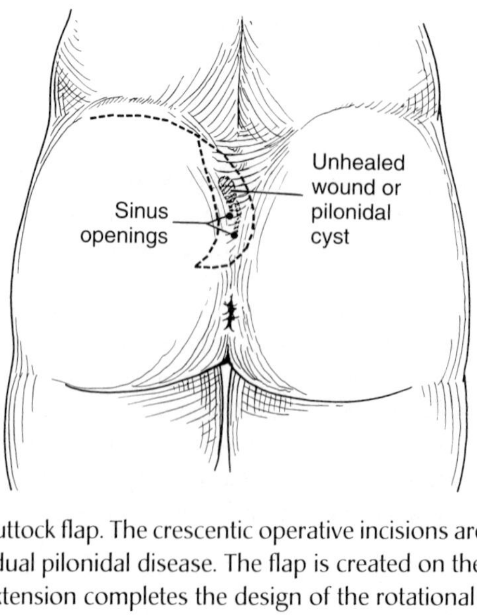

Fig. 15-2 **A,** Rotational buttock flap. The crescentic operative incisions are planned to include the unhealed wound and any residual pilonidal disease. The flap is created on the side with the least disease. Superiorly, the curvilinear extension completes the design of the rotational flap.

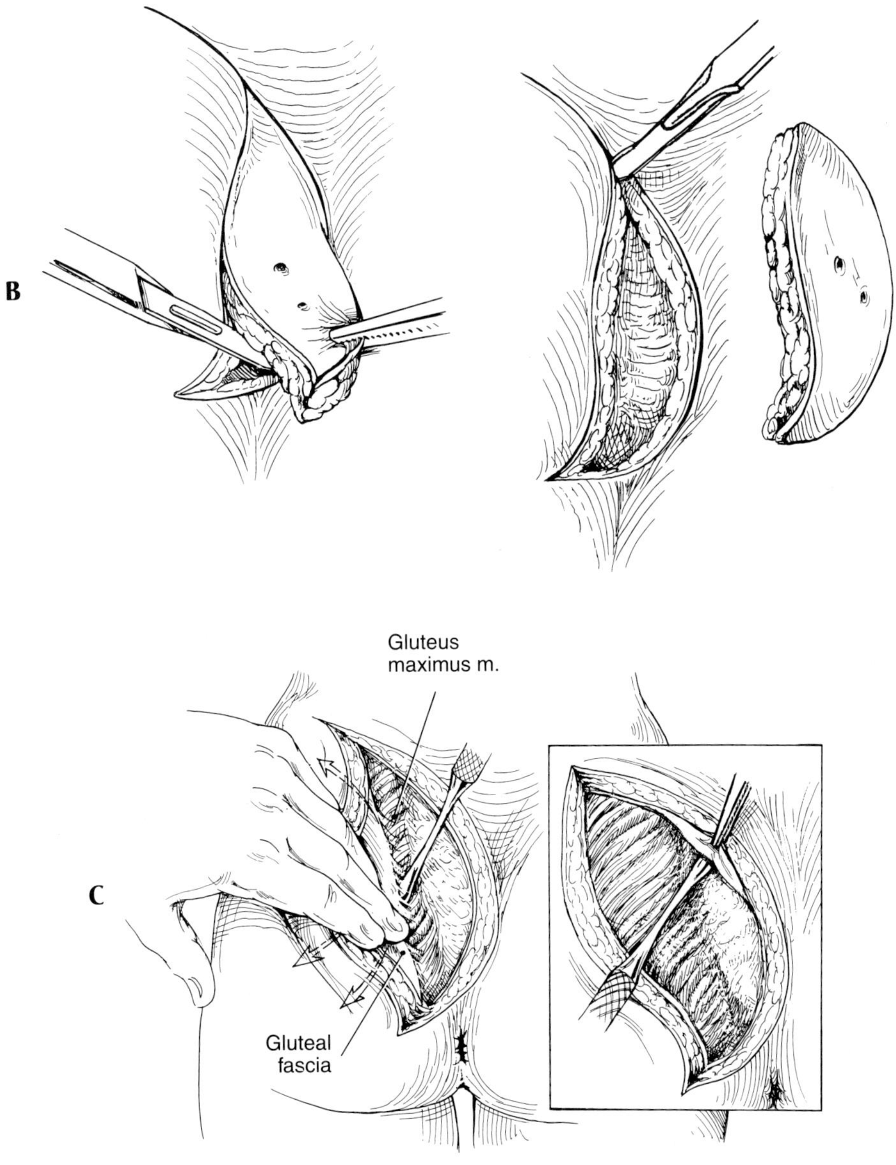

Fig. 15-2, cont'd **B**, The island of skin and underlying subcutaneous tissues are excised, exposing the musculofascial origins of the paired gluteus maximus muscles and the sacrococcygeal ligament. It is essential that the walls of the resultant defect remain perpendicular to the base of the wound. **C**, The curvilinear extension is extended down through the gluteus maximus muscle fascia. The subfascial plane is entered and opened to create the flap, which is composed of skin, subcutaneous tissues, and underlying gluteal fascia. The flap is elevated a distance that corresponds to the length of the new midline defect.

Continued.

D

E

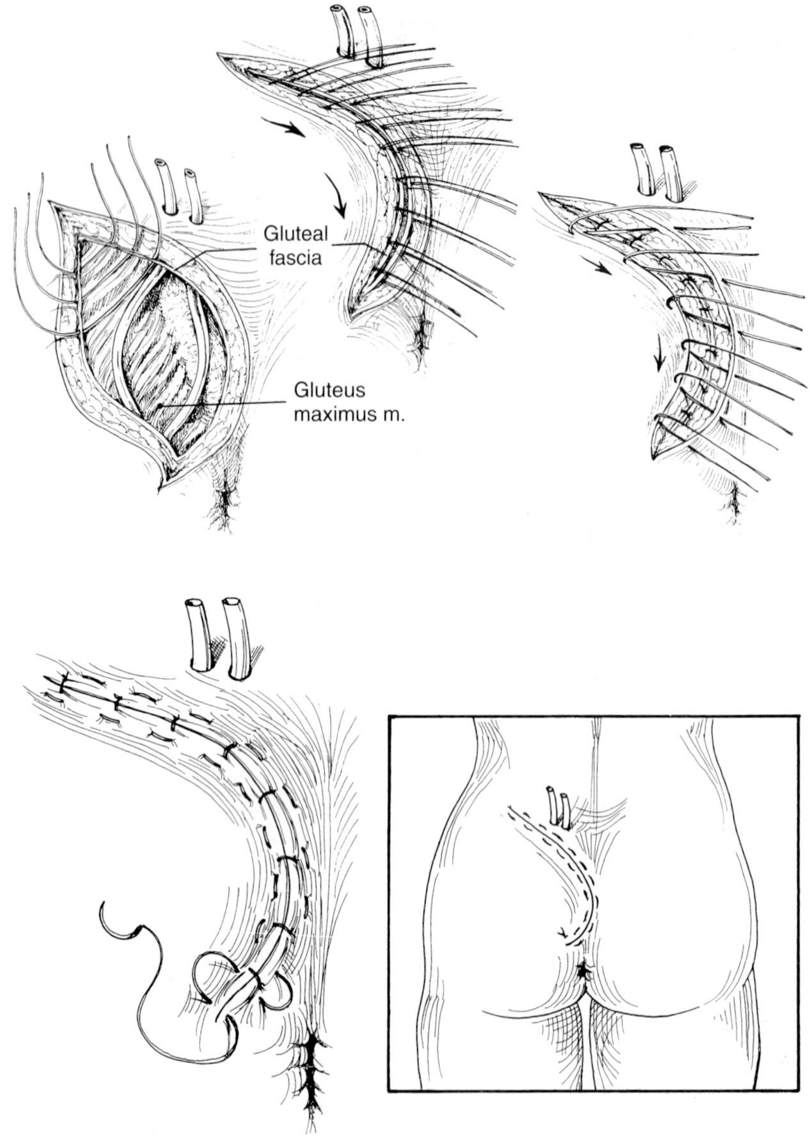

Fig. 15-2, cont'd **D**, After mobilization of an appropriately sized flap, one or two closed-suction drains are placed superiorly opposite the free edge of the flap. The flap is drawn medially and rotated caudally until its free margin meets the midline defect's fixed edge. Interrupted absorbable sutures are used to approximate the fascia and the subcutaneous tissues. The dermal edges are approximated with smaller, inverted absorbable sutures. **E,** The skin is closed with monofilament nylon vertical mattress sutures. The closed-suction drains are removed after 4 days, provided drainage is minimal. (Modified from Fishbein RH, Handelson JC. A method for primary reconstruction following radical excision of sacrococcygeal pilonidal disease. Ann Surg 190:231-235, 1979. With permission.)

Bascom's cleft closure in patients with larger wounds and limited laxity of the gluteal skin and subcutaneous tissues.

Patients with large sacral wounds (transverse diameter greater than 10 cm) may be better served with a gluteus maximus myocutaneous flap.[46] Like the rotational flap, this flap obliterates the gluteal cleft and covers large sacral defects with a significant amount of soft tissue. In addition, it has its own blood supply and can provide a better sacral cushion, which may be required for patients with deep and wide soft tissue defects.

The patient is placed in the prone jackknife position under spinal or general anesthesia. All scar tissue and granulation tissue is debrided to expose normal fat and a clean base. A buttock rotational flap is created in a fashion similar to that for the cleft closure technique but includes the superior portion of the gluteus maximus muscle. It is important to use only half of this muscle, based either on the superior or inferior gluteal vessels, to prevent impaired hip joint extension (Fig. 15-3). Identification of the gluteus medius and piriformis muscles signifies that an adequate amount of gluteus maximus has been transected. The flap is rotated into place over a closed-suction drain, and the wound is closed in layers.

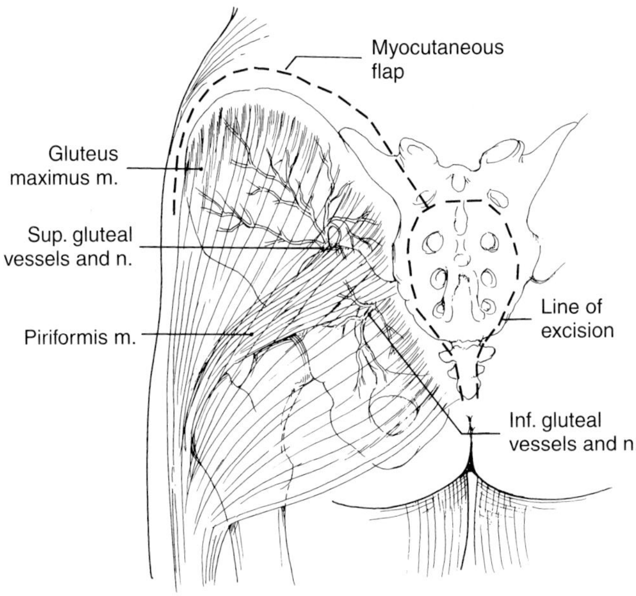

Fig. 15-3 Gluteus maximus myocutaneous flap. The flap free edge is marked out *(dashed line)*, along with the defect. Its blood supply is from the superior gluteal vessels, which exit about 5 cm lateral to the midline sacrum, above the sciatic nerve, and superior to the piriformis muscle. (From Perez-Gurri JA, Temple WJ, Ketcham AS. Gluteus maximus myocutaneous flap for the treatment of recalcitrant pilonidal disease. Dis Colon Rectum 27:262-264, 1984. With permission.)

The patient is instructed not to lie or sit on the flap for 1 week, and the drain is removed when drainage is minimal.

Recurrent pilonidal disease. Recurrent pilonidal disease can be defined as pilonidal disease found after complete wound healing following definitive surgical treatment of pilonidal disease. Recurrent disease can be either residual pilonidal disease or true recurrent pilonidal disease. Residual pilonidal disease can be the result of inadequate intraoperative exposure, failure to recognize lateral sinus tracts, and/or insufficient cyst excision.[15,47] True recurrent pilonidal disease is probably more common; however, there is no means by which to distinguish the two. One would presume that residual disease in patients with healed surgical wounds would become manifest earlier than true recurrent disease. Distinguishing between the two forms of disease does not affect treatment options but can be a useful self-assessment tool for surgical technique.

Although many published reports outline primary surgical treatment of pilonidal disease, considerably fewer data are available that specifically address the treatment of recurrent pilonidal disease. Treatment recommendations are often based on data derived from the initial definitive surgical procedures.[15] As with unhealed sacral wounds, treatment options for recurrent disease should be aimed at eliminating the conditions that promote pilonidal disease formation: catch basin effect, gluteal cleft friction, and intergluteal cleft depth.

Small areas of recurrent disease in the presence of a shallow gluteal cleft and disease initially treated with a primary closure technique is best excised, with healing by means of secondary intention. Scar tissue from prior surgical procedures can impair mobilization of clean wound edges and preclude primary closure. Excision with split-thickness skin grafting has also been reported as treatment for recurrent pilonidal disease. In their series of 58 patients, Guyuron et al.[47] reported a recurrence rate of 1.7%, a graft failure rate of 3.4%, and a mean hospital stay of 9.8 days (range 7 to 22 days). Excision with healing by secondary intention can be done on an outpatient basis, averts the morbidity of a skin donor wound, and has the lowest risk for postoperative wound infection.[24] Complete removal of all diseased tissue followed by meticulous postoperative wound care is essential.

In patients with more significant recurrent disease or those with deep gluteal clefts, the focus of treatment should be elimination of the conditions that promoted the recurrence. Adequate excision of extensive recurrent pilonidal disease often results in a large wound that is best treated with a rotational flap. Patients with good buttock soft tissue laxity and wounds smaller than 10 cm in diameter are good candidates for a rotational buttock flap. In those with minimal soft tissue laxity and wounds greater than 10 cm in diameter, gluteus maximus myocutaneous flaps should be considered. Preoperative selection of the appropriate wound closure method is essential to optimize the chances for cure and minimize the risks for an unhealed wound.

HIDRADENITIS SUPPURATIVA

First described by Velpeau[48] in 1832, hidradenitis suppurativa is a chronically progressive inflammatory disease of the apocrine sweat glands.[49] Found primarily in the axilla and groin, apocrine glands can also be found in the perineum, scrotum, and labial and perianal regions.[50,51] Woollard[52] coined the term *anal organ* to describe the concentrated mass of apocrine glands located in the circumanal skin. Perianal hidradenitis suppurativa affects men and women of all races but is most commonly seen in men, especially among black men.[50,53] It typically begins during adolescence and peaks in the third or fourth decade of life.[51,54]

Pathophysiology

Like its eccrine sweat gland counterpart, an apocrine gland consists of a coiled secretory portion and a less tortuous duct.[55] Whereas the eccrine gland duct extends to the skin surface, the apocrine gland duct empties into a hair follicle. In lower mammals the apocrine gland is significant in animal recognition, protection, and mating; in humans, however, the gland is believed to be a vestigial structure.[50] Secretions are scentless, but they do contain substances readily degraded by bacteria into distinctly odoriferous breakdown products.

Although the exact cause is unknown, most authors agree that hidradenitis suppurativa begins with obstruction of the apocrine gland duct with keratinous material.[50] Inspissated secretions coupled with secondary bacterial infections lead to gland rupture and extension of the inflammatory process into the dermis. Perianal hidradenitis suppurativa, unlike that found in the axilla, generally involves enteric aerobic and anaerobic bacteria in addition to *Staphylococcus* species.[50,51,56] Early episodes often respond to simple incision and drainage with or without antibiotic therapy.[51] The inflammation resolves, and scarring is initially minimal.

Recurrent disease extends deeper into the dermis to involve neighboring glands and ducts and the adjacent subcutaneous fat.[49,50] Cellulitis and abscess formation ensue, which require antibiotic therapy along with more extensive incision and drainage procedures. Despite successful treatment of the acute infectious processes, perianal sinuses and fistulas surrounded by subcutaneous scars and fibrosis frequently develop.[54,56] In more severe cases, the scarring can extend throughout the perineum to involve the buttocks, scrotum, labia, and sacral region.[51]

Nonsurgical Treatment

Nonsurgical treatment of perianal hidradenitis suppurativa includes skin cleansing agents, sitz baths, topical and systemic antibiotic therapy, hormonal agonists and antagonists, isotretinoin, and immunomodulating agents.[50,51,56-59] These treatment options are helpful in early or minimal disease but rarely produce successful long-term results. Recurrence is generally the rule with extensive involvement.[59,60]

Surgical Treatment

Primary surgical treatment of perianal hidradenitis suppurativa consists of incision and drainage, unroofing of sinuses and fistulas, and local excision of diseased skin and subcutaneous tissues.[51,56,59] Incision and drainage of abscesses is effective for early limited disease.[61] Combined with antibiotic therapy, it alleviates pain and helps resolve localized cellulitis. Most patients have recurrent episodes, which are usually more severe.[59] Repeated episodes lead to sinus tract formation, which requires unroofing and curettage of residual tract surfaces.[49] Meticulous wound care is essential for successful healing.

Local excision is generally more successful in the perianal region than in the inguinal, perineal, or axillary areas.[49,57,59,60] Harrison et al.[60] offer two explanations for improved results with perianal disease. Perianal excisions tend to be more radical than those done elsewhere in the body, and perianal apocrine glands are more concentrated in the immediate circumanal skin compared with more diffuse distributions in the axillary and inguinal regions. Recurrence rates are reduced if entire sinus tracts and diseased glands are excised before hidradenitis becomes widespread.[61]

Complications

Despite early medical and surgical intervention, recurrent or progressive perianal hidradenitis suppurativa can develop.[50] Confirmation of the diagnosis is essential before additional surgical therapy can be considered.[49] Thorough inspection and palpation of the axillae, groin, and entire perineum should be performed to evaluate for generalized apocrine gland disease. Meticulous examination of the presacral region, anal verge, and anorectum will help determine whether disorders other than hidradenitis, such as pilonidal disease, anal fistulas, or perirectal suppurative disease, are present. Anal canal or rectal involvement is rarely seen with perianal hidradenitis and suggests other underlying disease.[53] In regions of induration, erythema, or tenderness, biopsy specimens should be examined to rule out Crohns' disease, tuberculosis, actinomycosis, lymphogranuloma venereum, cystic acne, and squamous cell carcinoma.[51,61]

It is important to keep in mind that patients with long-standing hidradenitis (i.e., 20 years or more) are at risk for squamous cell carcinoma.[51,62] Delayed diagnosis is common, not so much from late patient presentation but from missed diagnosis. Squamous cell carcinoma arising from perianal hidradenitis begins in and spreads along deep subcutaneous sinuses.[62] This makes superficial biopsy specimens of suspect nonhealing wounds inadequate and unreliable; analysis of multiple deep biopsy samples is required to accurately identify the true underlying disease.[62]

Recurrent Hidradenitis

Recurrent perianal hidradenitis suppurativa is best treated with wide local excision of all diseased skin and subcutaneous tissue.[49-51,54,60,61,63] All indurated and palpably involved tissue must be extirpated. Minimally involved areas need only be excised down to normal appearing subcutaneous fat, whereas extensively diseased regions often require excision down to and sometimes through the fascial level.[54,61] Some authors advocate removal of adjacent apocrine glandular tissue to reduce the risk for future recurrence.[49,50,54] Removal of normal skin and subcutaneous tissue is of no benefit, but ensuring that the resultant wound is lined with disease-free tissue will optimize chances for cure.

Before definitive surgical therapy, acute cellulitis is treated with broad-spectrum antibiotics, and undrained abscesses with incision and drainage.[44,61] Preoperative mechanical bowel preparation along with postoperative antimotility agents will help reduce fecal contamination of the wound.[61] The operation is performed with the patient in the prone jackknife or lateral decubitus position under regional or general anesthesia. After excision, subsequent wound management includes primary closure, grafting, marsupialization, or healing by secondary intention.[51,54] Wound configuration, presence of underlying infection, overall patient health, and patient body habitus will dictate which methods are appropriate.

Narrow wounds whose edges can be approximated without tension or associated dead space can be considered for primary closure; however, the risk for infection is not negligible.[51,54,64] Wound contamination, as well as the highest recurrence rates (greater than 50%), make this technique less than desirable.[57,60] Inadvertent compromise of the excision margin to achieve primary wound closure is believed to be the most likely explanation for recurrence after primary closure.[60]

Larger wounds, which are generally the rule after excision of recurrent or long-standing disease, are not amenable to primary closure because of their size. Grafting with split-thickness skin grafts or plastic soft tissue flap technique (Z-plasty, rotation, or pedicle grafts) has been used with variable success.[51,56] The presence of purulence at the time of grafting poses the greatest risk of graft failure.[49,61] Recurrence rates after grafting are variable, ranging from 0% to 50%.[49,56,61,65] This wide variability may once again reflect a compromise in the excised margin to achieve a smaller grafting surface.

Wound marsupialization has been advocated by some but is generally not possible after wide local excision.[49-51] Unlike pilonidal disease, hidradenitis suppurativa does not lead to development of a large central sinus; rather, multiple burrowing sinus tracts develop adjacent to distorted apocrine glands. Marsupialization of multiple sinuses separated by islands of soft tissue with diseased glands enhances the risk for recurrence.

Healing by secondary intention has become the most popular wound management method.[49,51,53,54,61,63] After removal of all diseased tissue and achievement of meticulous hemostasis, the wound is packed with dilute povidone-iodine–moistened gauze and an occlusive dressing is applied. All packing is removed after 24 hours, and local wound care is begun. The wound is cleansed with sitz baths or a hand-held shower head three times a day, after which saline wet-to-dry gauze dressings are applied. Oral analgesics are usually adequate.[54,61,65] The patient is discharged when he or she is able to care for the wound and is seen in follow-up 1 week later. Thornton and Abcarian[54] reported highly favorable results in their retrospective review of 104 patients with recurrent hidradenitis treated with wide local excision with healing by secondary intention. The average hospital stay was 7.2 days, and 80% of patients were discharged by postoperative day 10. Mean healing time ranged from 3½ weeks for small wounds (2 × 2 cm) to 7 weeks for larger ones (>5 cm in any dimension.). Only 4 patients (3.8%) required repeat surgery because of recurrent disease. All wounds healed without grafting, wound contractures were minimal, and the perineums remained pliable and nontender when healing was complete. Others have reported similar healing rates, with recurrence ranging from 0% to 21%.[53,65,66]

In most patients who undergo wide excision with healing by secondary intention, the wounds heal uneventfully; patients return to work 2 to 3 weeks after discharge and at 12 months report considerable improvement over their preoperative state.[65]

Fecal diversion. Because perianal hidradenitis infrequently extends proximal to the subcutaneous external sphincter, fecal incontinence is rarely a problem provided the anal sphincter mechanism has not been altered by other preceding or coexistent diseases.[51,53,54] Excision of recurrent disease should not include any sphincter muscle.[53,61] In theory, inflammation may extend into the subcutaneous external sphincter, which may necessitate some muscle excision; however, this should not affect continence.

Creation of a diverting colostomy should only be considered in patients unable to ambulate postoperatively for perianal wound care, with chronic diarrhea that cannot be controlled medically, and with fecal incontinence secondary to anal sphincter dysfunction.[53,54,56]

REFERENCES

1. Anderson AW. Hair extracted from an ulcer. Boston Med Surg J 36:74, 1847.
2. Hodges RM. Pilonidal sinus. Boston Med Surg J 103:485-486, 1880.
3. Gage M. Pilonidal sinus: An explanation of its embryologic development. Arch Surg 31: 175-189, 1935.
4. Hanley PH. The dilemma of pilonidal disease. Dis Colon Rectum 20:278, 1977.
5. Goligher J. Pilonidal sinus. In Goligher J. Surgery of the Anus, Rectum, and Colon, 5th ed. London: Baillière Tindall, 1984, pp 221-236.
6. Patey DH, Scarff RW. Pathology of postanal pilonidal sinus: Its bearing on treatment. Lancet 25:484-486, 1946.
7. Bascom J. Pilonidal disease: Origin from follicles of hairs and results of follicle removal as treatment. Surgery 87:567-572, 1980.
8. Brearly R. Pilonidal sinus: A new theory of origin. Br J Surg 43:62-68, 1955.

9. Weale FE. A comparison of Barber's and postanal pilonidal sinuses. Br J Surg 51:513-516, 1964.
10. Patey DH, Scarff RW. The hair of the pilonidal sinus. Lancet 1:772-773, 1955.
11. Page BH. The entry of hair into a pilonidal sinus. Br J Surg 56:32, 1969.
12. Patey DH. A reappraisal of the acquired theory of sacrococcygeal pilonidal sinus and an assessment of its influence on surgical practice. Br J Surg 56:463-466, 1969.
13. Culp CE. Pilonidal disease and its treatment. Surg Clin North Am 47:1007-1014, 1967.
14. Mansoory A, Dickson D. Z-plasty for treatment of disease of the pilonidal sinus. Surg Gynecol Obstet 155:409-411, 1982.
15. Allen-Mersh TG. Pilonidal sinus: Finding the right track for treatment. Br J Surg 77:123-132, 1990.
16. Hanley PH. Acute pilonidal abscess. Surg Gynecol Obstet 150:9-11, 1980.
17. Nivatvongs S. Pilonidal disease. In Gordon PH, Nivatvongs S. Principles and Practice of Surgery for the Colon, Rectum, and Anus. St. Louis: Quality Medical Publishing, 1992, pp 267-279.
18. Hanley PH. The dilemma of pilonidal disease: Discussion. Dis Colon Rectum 20:292-298, 1977.
19. Armstrong JH, Barcia PJ. Pilonidal sinus disease: The conservative approach. Arch Surg 129:914-918, 1994.
20. Jensen SL, Harling H. Prognosis after simple incision and drainage for a first-episode acute pilonidal abscess. Br J Surg 75:60-61, 1988.
21. Lundhus E, Gottrup F. Outcome at three to five years of primary closure of perianal and pilonidal abscess. Eur J Surg 159:555-558, 1993.
22. Weinstein MA, Rubin RJ, Salvati EP. The dilemma of pilonidal disease: Pilonidal cystostomy, reappraisal of an old technique. Dis Colon Rectum 20:287-289, 1977.
23. Goodall P. The aetiology and treatment of pilonidal sinus: A review of 163 Patients. Br J Surg 49:212-218, 1961.
24. Eftaiha M, Abcarian H. The dilemma of pilonidal disease: Surgical treatment. Dis Colon Rectum 20:279-286, 1977.
25. Kronborg O, Christensen K, Zimmermann-Nielson C. Chronic pilonidal disease: A randomized trial with a complete 3-year follow-up. Br J Surg 72:303-304, 1985.
26. Sondenna K, Andersen E, Soreide JA. Morbidity and short term results in a randomised trial of open compared with closed treatment of chronic pilonidal sinus. Eur J Surg 158: 351-355, 1992.
27. Kooistra HP. Pilonidal sinuses: Review of the literature and report of 350 cases. Am J Surg 55:3-17, 1942.
28. Khawaja HT, Bryan S, Weaver PC. Treatment of natal cleft sinus: A prospective clinical and economic evaluation. Br Med J 304:1282-1283, 1992.
29. McLaren CA. Partial closure and other techniques in pilonidal surgery: An assessment of 157 cases. Br J Surg 71:561-562, 1984.
30. Abramson DJ. Out-patient management of pilonidal sinuses: Excision and semiprimary closure technic. Milit Med 143:753-757, 1978.
31. Buie LA, Curtiss RK. Pilonidal disease. Surg Clin North Am 32:1247-1259, 1952.
32. Bascom J. Pilonidal disease: Long-term results of follicle removal. Dis Colon Rectum 26: 800-807, 1983.
33. Manterola C, Barroso M, Araya JC, Fonseca L. Pilonidal disease: 25 cases treated by the Dufourmentel technique. Dis Colon Rectum 34:649-652, 1991.
34. Karydakis GE. New approach to the problem of pilonidal sinus. Lancet 2:1414-1415, 1973.
35. Toubanakis G. Treatment of pilonidal sinus disease with the Z-plasty procedure (modified). Am Surg 52:611-612, 1986.

36. Maurice BA, Greenwood RK. A conservative treatment of pilonidal sinus. Br J Surg 51: 510-512, 1964.
37. Moosa AR, Mayer AD, Lavelle-Jones M. Surgical complications. In Sabistion DC, ed. Textbook of Surgery: The Biological Basis of Modern Surgical Practice. Philadelphia: WB Saunders, 1991, pp 299-316.
38. Ehrlichman RJ, Seckel BR, Bryan DJ, Moschella CJ. Common complications of wound healing, prevention and management. Surg Clin North Am 71:1323-1351, 1991.
39. Hoexter B. Use of Water Pik lavage in pilonidal wound care. Dis Colon Rectum 19:470-471, 1976.
40. Lord PH. Anorectal problems: Etiology of pilonidal sinus. Dis Colon Rectum 18:661-664, 1975.
41. Rosenberg I. The dilemma of pilonidal disease: Reverse bandaging for care of the reluctant wound. Dis Colon Rectum 20:290-291, 1977.
42. Azab ASG, Kamal MS, Saad RA, Abou al Atta KA, Ali NA. Radical cure of pilonidal sinus by a transposition rhomboid flap. Br J Surg 71:154-155, 1984.
43. Bascom J. Pilonidal sinus. In Fazio VW, ed. Current Therapy in Colon and Rectal Surgery. Toronto: BC Decker, 1990, pp 32-39.
44. Bascom JU. Repeat pilonidal operations. Am J Surg 154:118-122, 1987.
45. Fishbein RH, Handelson JC. A method for primary reconstruction following radical excision of sacrococcygeal pilonidal disease. Ann Surg 190:231-235, 1979.
46. Perez-Gurri JA, Temple WJ, Ketcham AS. Gluteus maximus myocutaneous flap for the treatment of recalcitrant pilonidal disease. Dis Colon Rectum 27:262-264, 1984.
47. Guyuron B, Dinner MI, Dowden RV. Excision and grafting in treatment of recurrent pilonidal sinus disease. Surg Gynecol Obstet 156:201-204, 1983.
48. Velpeau AA. In Dictionnaire de Médecine, un Répertoire Général des Sciences Médicales sous le Rapport Théorique et Pratique, 2nd ed, vol 2. Bechet Jeune, 1839, p 91.
49. Rubin RJ, Chinn BT. Perianal hidradenitis suppurativa. Surg Clin North Am 74:1317-1325, 1994.
50. Paletta CP, Jurkiewicz MJ. Hidradenitis suppurativa. Clin Plast Surg 14:383-390, 1987.
51. Corman ML. Suppurative hidradenitis or hidradenitis suppurativa. In Corman ML, ed. Colon and Rectal Surgery, 3rd ed. Philadelphia: JB Lippincott, 1993, pp 392-397.
52. Woollard HH. The cutaneous glands of man. J Anat 64:415-421, 1930.
53. Wiltz O, Schoetz DJ, Murray JJ, Roberts PL, Coller JA, Veidenheimer MC. Perianal hidradenitis suppurativa: The Lahey Clinic experience. Dis Colon Rectum 33:731-734, 1990.
54. Thornton JP, Abcarian H. Surgical treatment of perianal and perineal hidradenitis suppurativa. Dis Colon Rectum 21:573-577, 1978.
55. Ham AW, Cormack DH. Histology, 8th ed. Philadelphia: JB Lippincott, 1979, pp 621-623.
56. O'Connell PR. Hidradenitis suppurativa. In Wexner SD, Vernava AM, eds. Clinical Decision Making in Colorectal Surgery. New York: Igaku-Shoin Medical Publishers, 1995, pp 169-172.
57. Banerjee AK. Surgical treatment of hidradenitis. Br J Surg 79:863-866, 1992.
58. Brown CF, Gallup DS, Brown VM. Hidradenitis suppurativa of the anogenital region: Response to Isotretinoin. Am J Obstet Gynecol 158:12-15, 1988.
59. Jemec GBE. Effect of localized surgical excisions in hidradenitis suppurativa. J Am Acad Dermatol 18:1103-1107, 1988.
60. Harrison BJJ, Mudge M, Hughes LE. Recurrence after surgical treatment of hidradenitis suppurativa. Br Med J 294:487-489, 1987.

61. Williams ST, Billingham RP. In Fazio VW, ed. Current Therapy in Colon and Rectal Surgery. Toronto: BC Decker, 1990, pp 39-41.
62. Shukla VK, Hughes LE. A case of squamous cell carcinoma complicating hidradenitis suppurativa. Eur J Surg Oncol 21:106-109, 1995.
63. Karulf RE. In Beck DE, Wexner SD, eds. Fundamentals of Anorectal Surgery. New York: McGraw-Hill, 1992, pp 189-190.
64. Broadwater JR, Bryant RL, Petrino RA. Advanced hidradenitis suppurativa: Review of surgical treatment in 23 patients. Am J Surg 144:668-670, 1982.
65. Silverberg B, Smoot CE, Landa SJF, Parsons RW. Hidradenitis suppurativa: Patient satisfaction with wound healing by secondary intention. Plast Reconstr Surg 79:555-559, 1987.
66. Culp CE. Chronic hidradenitis suppurativa of the anal canal: A surgical skin disease. Dis Colon Rectum 26:669-676, 1983.

CHAPTER 16

Surgery for Fecal Incontinence

ALAN E. TIMMCKE
DANIEL A. NG

Fecal incontinence, the inability to limit the passage of flatus or stool to a socially acceptable time and place, is a common and incapacitating condition. A recent study of the prevalence of fecal incontinence in Wisconsin households found that 2.2% of the general population, including all age groups, reported some fecal incontinence.[1] Many patients experience fecal incontinence, but few discuss it with their physician, believing that there is nothing that can be done, that no effective treatment is available. Although fecal incontinence may be common, there is wide variance in its severity and underlying cause. Although no uniform classification system exists, most studies use the following: complete incontinence (incontinence of gas, liquid, and solid stool), partial incontinence (incontinence of gas and liquid stool), and minor incontinence (e.g., fecal seepage and soiling or incontinence of gas).

Recent advances in anorectal physiologic evaluation have resulted in better understanding of the factors that contribute to fecal incontinence. Physiologic tests that for the most part are no more uncomfortable for the patient than a digital rectal examination aid the surgeon in differentiating the causes of incontinence (i.e., idiopathic, neurogenic, or myopathic factors or sphincter lacerations or other sphincter trauma). To minimize poor results and complications, management of fecal incontinence should be guided by findings at a complete history and physical examination and additional colorectal physiologic tests. Such findings enable determination of which patients might benefit most from surgical intervention and permit formulation of an alternative treatment plan for those patients who will likely not benefit from surgery. Quantification of anal pressures with manometry may be valuable to document the degree of incontinence and provide baseline values before sphincter repair. Determination of anal sensation and rectal capacity can also be helpful. Electromyography (EMG) and pudendal nerve terminal motor latency studies can reveal neuropathies that may significantly influence the results of specific surgical interventions. Finally, endorectal ultrasound can assist in localizing sphincter defects and determining the amount of undamaged muscle remaining. Videodefecography can occasionally be useful in documenting the presence of perineal descent, rectoceles, rectal intussusception, and other associated disease that may negatively affect the results of surgical procedures to correct incontinence. Limitations of these studies are discussed in Chapter 26. In this chapter, we concentrate on complications associated with the surgical management of incontinence.

NONSURGICAL TREATMENT

Nonsurgical therapy is a reasonable initial step in the management of most anal incontinence. A well-balanced high-fiber diet, drugs that decrease intestinal motility, perineal strengthening exercises, and biofeedback conditioning may benefit patients without demonstrated sphincter muscle defects. If there is no improvement with simple measures, surgery is advised in appropriately selected patients. Surgical treatments for fecal incontinence are often associated with complications, not the least of which is no improvement in continence. When considering surgery to correct incontinence, we must be sure the remedy is not worse than the disease.

SURGICAL TREATMENT

The five main surgical options for the correction of sphincter dysfunction are encirclement procedures, sphincteroplasty or sphincter reconstruction, Parks' postanal repair, muscle transfer reconstructions such as of gracilis or gluteus muscle, and insertion of a prosthetic anal sphincter. If these fail, fecal diversion with a colostomy is a final surgical option. Preoperative preparation of all patients undergoing surgery for anal incontinence includes a mechanical bowel cleansing, preoperative and perioperative antibiotic therapy, and placement of an indwelling urinary catheter.

Encirclement

An encirclement, or Thiersch, procedure involves encircling the anal sphincters with a wire, suture, strip of fascia, or more recently with a Dacron mesh–impregnated Silastic band. Originally described for treatment of rectal prolapse, the encirclement procedures effectively replace the anal sphincters in impeding fecal spillage. The original Thiersch procedure, which involved encircling the anal canal with silver wire, was fraught with problems that included breakage or erosion of the wire, subsequent perineal sepsis, and fecal impaction. Of the materials currently available, the Dacron mesh–impregnated Silastic sling (Fig. 16-1) offers the advantages of an elastic ring, which more easily allows a bolus of fecal material to pass. Marlex, Mersilene, and Teflon are also available but have been reported to cause patients considerable discomfort. Labow et al.[2] reported

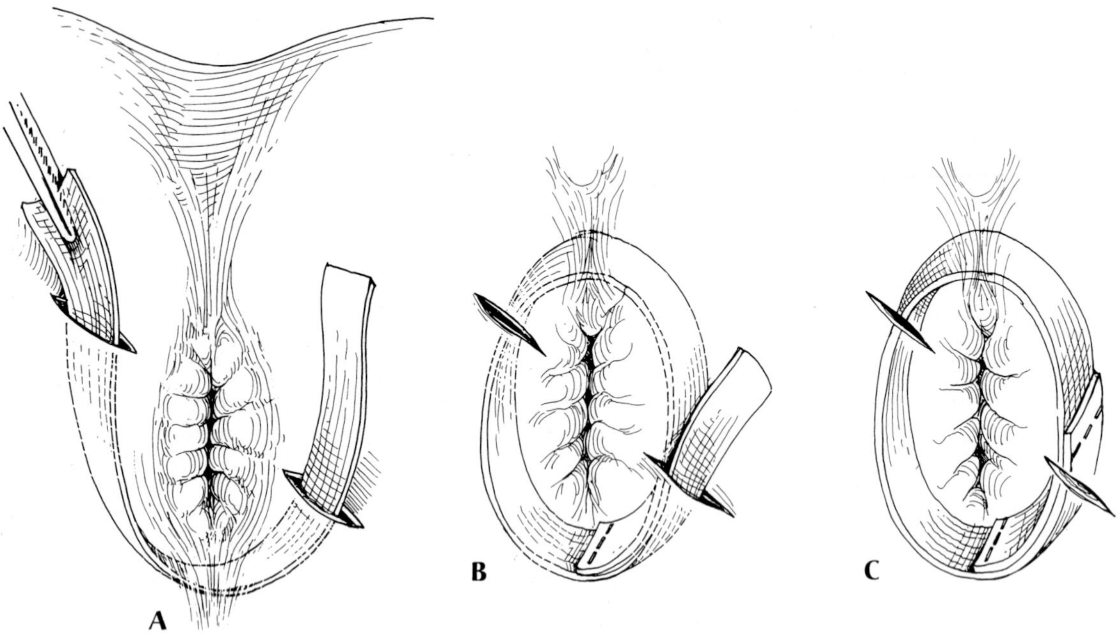

Fig. 16-1 Encirclement procedure. **A,** Insertion of Dacron mesh–impregnated Silastic. **B** and **C,** Deep encirclement of the external sphincter with overlap secured with either sutures or staples.

nine patients in whom use of the Silastic sling produced good to excellent continence and no complications. On the other hand, in 11 patients in whom the Silastic sling was used, Horn et al.[3] reported that six have good to excellent continence, three had urinary retention, and in 4 patients infection developed that necessitated removal of the sling. In two of these 4 patients, however, the Silastic sling was successfully reimplanted after resolution of the infection.

Direct Sphincter Repair

Patients who have had a traumatic disruption of the internal and external sphincters are ideal candidates for direct repair of the sphincters. The technique of overlapping repair was originally described by Parks and McPartlin[4] in 1971 and modified by Slade et al.[5] This repair involves mobilization of both ends of the disrupted sphincter and overlapping the cut edges of muscle (Fig. 16-2). Generally 50% of the circumference of the sphincter must be intact and able to actively contract to allow success of this technique. Other keys to successful repair include establishment of the presence of an intact neurovascular bundle (pudendal nerve) with pudendal nerve terminal motor latency studies, delay of repair of obstetric injury for at least 3 months in patients with failure of primary

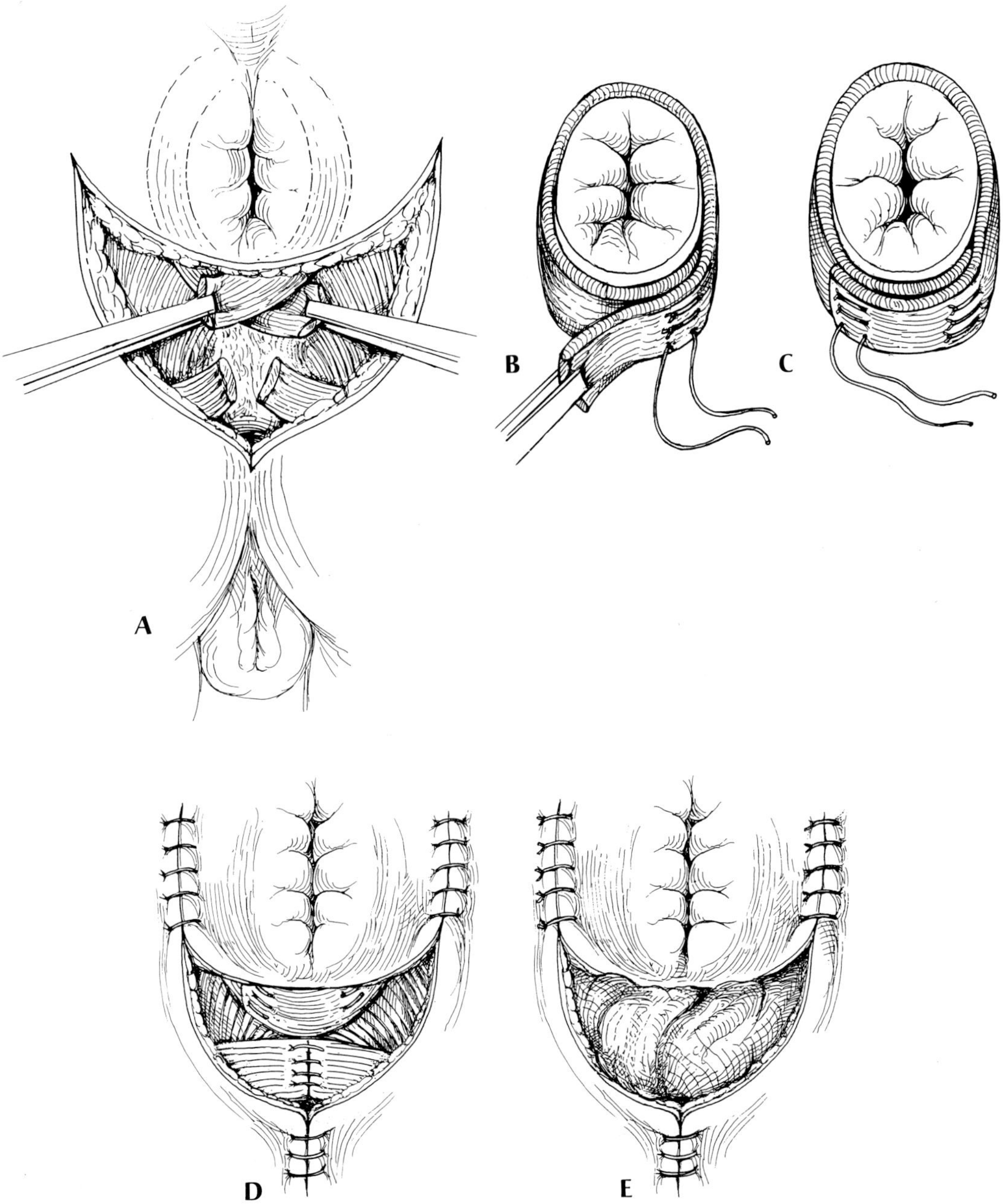

Fig. 16-2 Overlapping sphincter repair. **A,** Overlapping of the dissected ends of the external sphincter. **B** and **C,** The technique of overlapping the dissected sphincter muscles using horizontal mattress sutures placed through the scarred ends of the external sphincter muscle. **D,** Repair of the transverse perineal muscles. **E,** Partial closure of the wound with wet-to-dry gauze dressing inserted.

repair, preservation of scar tissue at the ends of the sphincter muscle to ensure that sutures do not cut through, and eradication of infection before repair. In some cases such as multiple previous attempts at repair, massive perineal trauma or impalement injury, perineal wound disruption, and perineal sepsis a diverting colostomy may be needed to allow adequate healing.

A review of the literature supporting direct sphincter repair reveals good to excellent continence rates. Most authors report continence of solid stool in 80% to 90% of patients and continence of solid and liquid stool in 50% to 80%.[4-13] Comparison of existing reports is difficult because of their nonrandomized, retrospective nature, difference in criteria for grading degree of incontinence, selection bias in determining which patients will undergo repair, mixed population of patients (i.e., various ages, sex, and causes of incontinence), and the variety of surgical procedures performed.

Fang et al.[8] reported 79 patients who underwent overlapping sphincter repair. Of the 76 patients available for follow-up, complete continence of solid and liquid stool and flatus resulted in 58%, and only occasional liquid stool incontinence remained in 31%, yielding an 89% continence rate for solid and liquid stool. Five patients (6%) were continent of solid stool only. Of the 79 patients, 16% had complications that included urinary retention (6%), abscess (2%), fecal impaction (2%), hemorrhage (2%), and hematoma (1%). One patient died of a myocardial infarction in the immediate postoperative period. All incisions were left open and allowed to heal secondarily, which contributed to the lower infection rate in this series. Their report included a mixed population of patients, with obstetric injuries in 54% of the patients. This large percentage of obstetric injuries may explain the lower rates of complete continence in contrast to other series in which operative injuries predominate.

Similarly, in the series of Fleshman et al.,[9] 48 of 55 patients with obstetric trauma underwent overlapping sphincteroplasty. Fifty percent of their population achieved complete continence, and 24% achieved partial continence. The authors report a 15% morbidity rate, primarily wound infection. Although use of a perineal drain was associated with a lower infection rate, this was not found to be statistically significant. In a later series,[10] the same group reported an improved complete continence rate of 75%.

Browning and Motson[6] reported a 78% rate of complete continence in a series of 97 patients. Of no surprise, 60% of their patient population had a history of previous anal operations, and 27% had nonobstetric, noniatrogenic, traumatic disruption; only 13% of their patients had obstetric trauma. Conversely, they reported a 28% morbidity rate, secondary to dehiscence (4%), fistulas (9%), strictures (16%), delayed healing (9%), and perineal sinus formation (6%). The sinus rate diminished after changing from wire to polyglycolic acid sutures.

Complication rates for overlapping sphincter repair vary from 10% to 30%. Wound infection and perineal sepsis account for a large proportion (13% to 20%) of complications. Wound infection is usually managed with intravenous antibiotic agents and establishment of adequate drainage. Other less common complications include wound dehiscence (9% in one series after wound infection), urinary retention, bleeding, and sinus formation.

Although overlapping direct repair of the anal sphincter is the preferred method of treatment by most authors, recent reports indicate that in some selected cases, repair without overlap (i.e., by apposition of the muscle ends) may be feasible with an acceptable success rate. Arnaud et al.[14] reported 31 of 40 patients (78%) treated with end-to-end repair with good (continence of solid stool and only occasional leakage of liquid stool) to excellent results. Seven patients from this series did require diversion because of nonobstetric trauma. Three of five patients with wound infection had dehiscence. All these patients had posterolateral defects. Christiansen and Pedersen[7] reported using direct sphincter repair without overlap in seven patients with complex defects. All had improvement in continence, which was complete in four of the seven. It is unclear whether diverting colostomy was used in these patients.

The effect of denervation injury on the success of sphincter repair was demonstrated in the study by Jacobs et al.[15] Of 37 patients with obstetric trauma, 30 had an obvious muscle defect. Overlap repair yielded an 83% rate of complete continence. The 17% failure rate was largely attributed to denervation injury (high fiber density was noted at single-fiber EMG). In contrast, of the seven patients with no apparent defect, all had increased fiber density suggestive of neuropathy. Five of the seven were seen immediately postpartum and received conservative treatment with dietary measures. In four of these patients, continence improved within 1 year. Thus pudendal nerve conduction studies may prove valuable in the evaluation and management of fecal incontinence in obstetric patients (Table 16-1).

Table 16-1 Results of overlapping sphincteroplasty

Author	No. of patients	Grade of continence* (%)		
		1	2	3
Browning and Motson[6] (1984)	83	78	13	9
Fang et al.[8] (1984)	76	58	38	4
Hawley[44] (1985)	100	52	30	18
Morgan et al.[45] (1987)	45	82	9	9
Ctercteko et al.[46] (1988)	44	54	32	14
Abcarian et al.[47] (1989)	43	100	—	—
Yoshioka and Keighley[13] (1989)	27	26	48	26
Jacobs et al.[15] (1990)	30	83	17	—
Fleshman et al.[9] (1991)	55	51	43	5
Fleshman et al.[10] (1991)	28	75	21	4

Adapted from Gordon PH, Nivatvongs S. Principals and Practice of Surgery for the Colon, Rectum, and Anus. St. Louis: Quality Medical Publishing, 1992.

*1, Continent for solid and liquid stool; 2, continent for solid but not always for liquid stool; 3, little or no continence.

Postanal Repair and Plication

Postanal repair, as championed by Parks,[16] was originally designed to restore the anorectal angle and lengthen the anal canal. Patients with neuropathic or idiopathic fecal incontinence were thought to be ideal candidates for this repair because it mechanically increased the barrier to the passage of stool. However, it has been demonstrated by several authors that despite decreasing the anorectal angle, continence in some patients does not improve. Moreover, in some patients continence improves even if the angle is not decreased by the operation. Lengthening of the sphincter is thought to be the primary benefit of the Parks method of postanal repair. This method involves plicating the puborectalis muscle through a posterior, intersphincteric approach, effectively lengthening and narrowing the anal passage (Fig. 16-3). Clinical results of this procedure have varied widely. Few groups have been able to reproduce the excellent results of Parks et al.[16,17] (86% rate of fecal continence).

Henry and Simson[18] reported a 58% rate of fecal continence in a series of 242 patients undergoing postanal repair. The patient population was mixed and included some with fecal incontinence, rectocele, prolapse, and solitary rectal ulcer syndrome. Nineteen percent of the patients in the series had complications, primarily wound sepsis (15%), wound dehiscence, and fistula. Womack et al.[19] reported an 88% rate of solid and liquid continence in 16 patients. Yoshioka et al.[20-22] reported on a series of 124 patients from 1976 to 1987. Although 85% of the patients reported "improvement," with a decrease in the frequency of bowel movements, 60% of patients still reported urgency. Seventy-six percent demonstrated fecal leakage, and more than half of the patients still used pads to prevent soiling. Fifteen percent of the patients in their series experienced complications, including wound infection (6%), ischemic necrosis of the skin (8%), fistulas, and hematomas. One patient died of a massive pulmonary embolus.

Most authors reported limited success with the Parks method of postanal repair. This may reflect the population of patients selected. Most patients have "idiopathic incontinence," and may have concomitant conditions (e.g., perineal descent, rectocele, solitary rectal ulcer syndrome) that may contribute to the poor results with this operation. Scheuer et al.,[23] in their series of 39 patients, found postanal repair to be "effective" in 70%. However, only 43% were made continent for solid and liquid stool. He clearly demonstrated that correction of the anorectal angle is not critical to the success of the procedure. Laurberg et al.,[24] in their series of 18 patients, reported continence for solid and liquid stool and flatus, with occasional soiling in 32% of the patients studied. Forty-three percent of patients demonstrated some liquid stool incontinence (Table 16-2).

Snooks et al.[25] showed that patients in whom continence was not improved with postanal repair had low resting anal canal pressures, prolonged pudendal nerve terminal motor latency, and increased fiber density, indicating reinner-

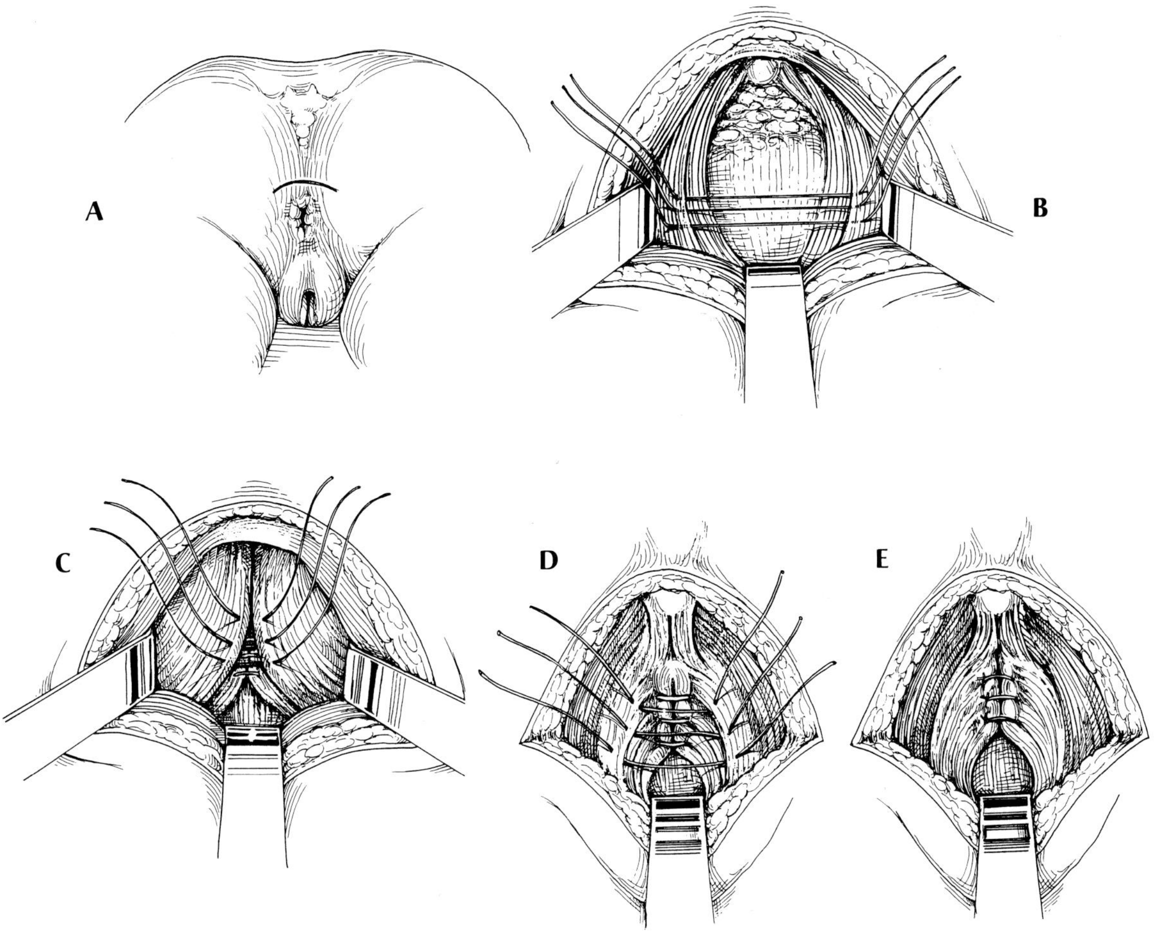

Fig. 16-3 Parks' postanal repair. **A,** Location of the curvilinear incision posterior to the anal sphincter. **B,** Deep dissection and plication of the levator muscles. **C-E,** Additional plication of the levator muscles in layers, progressing superficially.

Table 16-2 Results of Parks' postanal repair

Author	No. of patients	Grade of continence* (%)		
		1	2	3
Browning and Motson[6] (1984)	83	78	13	9
Henry and Simson[18] (1985)	204	58	12	30
Habr-Gama et al.[48] (1986)	42	52	41	7
Keighley[49] (1987)	114	32	62	6
Miller et al.[50] (1988)	17	59	—	41
Womack et al.[19] (1988)	16	88	—	12
Scheuer et al.[23] (1989)	39	15	54	31
Laurberg et al.[24] (1990)	28	32	43	25

Adapted from Gordon PH, Nivatvongs S. Principals and Practice of Surgery for the Colon, Rectum, and Anus. St. Louis: Quality Medical Publishing, 1992.

*1, Continent for solid stool—successful; 2, sporadic episodes of fecal incontinence—significant improvement; 3, incontinent for stool—failure.

vation of the external sphincter muscle, compared with a control group. Rainey et al.[26] reported that patients with only mild degrees of fecal incontinence did poorly with postanal repair. It has been suggested that progressive neurologic damage to the muscles of the pelvic floor occurs after postanal repair and may be responsible for poor functional results.[24,25]

Complications of postanal repair include wound infection, hematoma, skin ischemia and necrosis, and fistula formation. Keighley[27] noted that since altering the type of incision and flap technique, as well as replacing the use of epinephrine solution with closed-suction drainage, the prevalence of hematoma and skin flap ischemia has diminished. These authors do not advocate routine colostomy. Patients should be informed that immediate continence after postanal repair should not be anticipated. Postoperative pelvic exercises, training, and rehabilitation are important to the success of the operation.

As a result of the poor results of postanal repair and the high frequency of rectocele in many of these patients with idiopathic incontinence, several authors have explored use of an anterior plication approach. Miller et al.[28] reported results in 30 patients who underwent anterior levatorplasty with anal sphincter plication. Fourteen patients had anterior defects, and 16 patients had no identifiable defects. With this combined approach, 62% to 70% of patients were continent for solid and liquid stool. This success is thought partly due to improved sensory function within the anal canal. Pinho et al.[29] have advocated total pelvic floor repair, which involves combined postanal repair, anterior levatorplasty, and direct sphincter repair. In a series of 22 patients with neuropathic fecal incontinence, a 96% continence rate for liquid and solid stool was achieved. Follow-up of this series is short. However, this operation may prove to be a viable option in this population of patients.

Muscle Transposition

Various muscles have been used to augment the failing anal sphincter. The transposed gracilis muscle is the most widely used pedicle graft; others include the gluteus maximus, tensor fascia lata, sartorius, and adductor longus muscles. When the external anal canal has been severely damaged (loss of at least half the musculature), if there has been extensive loss of tissue secondary to cancer, trauma, infection, or if previous attempts at repair have failed, surgical reconstruction with a gracilis flap is a reasonable option. The gracilis transposition supplants the function of the anal sphincters by creating a barrier to the passage of stool.

Originally introduced by Pickrell et al.[30] for use in young children with congenital anomalies, Corman[31-35] has pioneered the use of this technique to treat adult fecal incontinence. The procedure involves mobilization of the gracilis muscle at its insertion and wrapping this graft around the anal sphincter through subcutaneous tunnels. The muscle is reattached to the contralateral ischial tuberosity and thus functions as an artificial sphincter (Fig. 16-4).

Corman[32] reported good to excellent results in nine of 13 patients. He defined an excellent result as complete continence without the use of pads, suppositories, or enemas and a good result as complete continence with occasional or frequent use of enemas and suppositories but no need for a pad. Corman reported one incidence of perineal sepsis, three of fecal impaction requiring operative disimpaction, and the need for repeat surgery after infection. Patients with diarrhea, neurologic disorders, and advanced age are poor candidates for this procedure. Other authors have had similar success rates and complications. Leguit et al.[36] reported 10 patients with incontinence from a variety of causes. Seven of the 10 patients were continent for solid and liquid stool. The authors noted that several of their patients sustained scarring of the muscle, resulting in a fibrotic, noncontractile, albeit functional sphincter substitute. This, in effect, converts the gracilis flap to a "living Thiersch" band. In a recent series of patients reported by Faucheron et al.,[37] 22 patients underwent graciloplasty. Twelve patients achieved continence of solid and liquid stool. However, morbidity was considerable and included perineal sepsis that necessitated repeat surgery in one patient and was managed with antibiotic agents and drainage in three other patients. Impaction developed in six patients, dyspareunia in one, and one patient had a parastomal hernia. Poorer results were attributed to sepsis, and

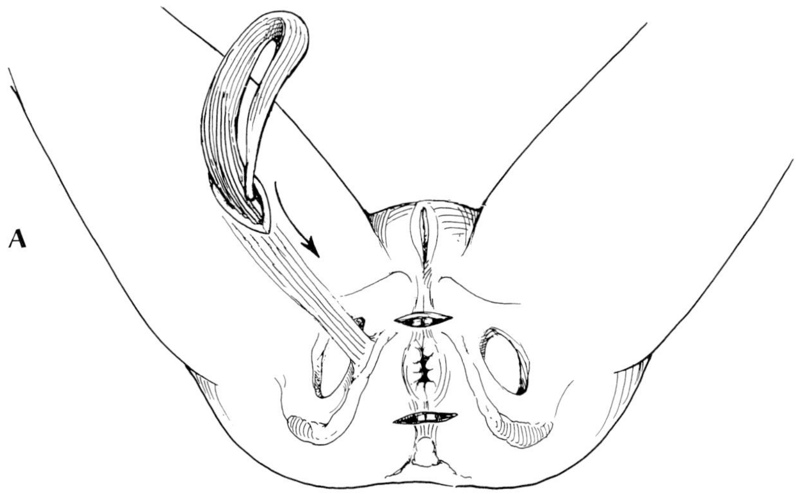

Fig. 16-4 Gracilis muscle transposition. **A,** Dissection of the gracilis muscle of the right medial thigh, carefully preserving its proximal neurovascular supply.

Continued.

B

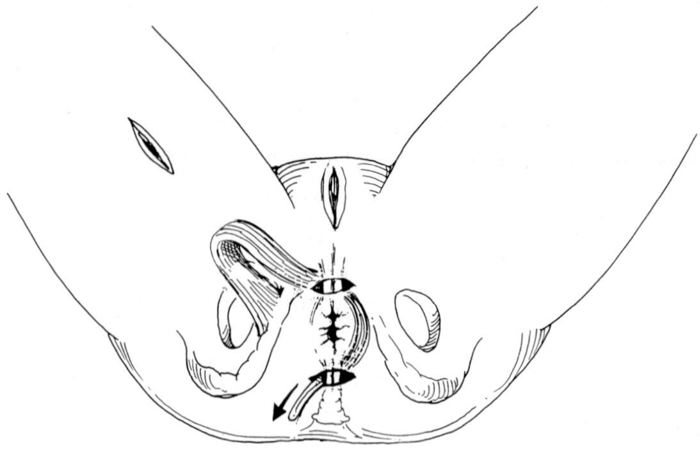

C

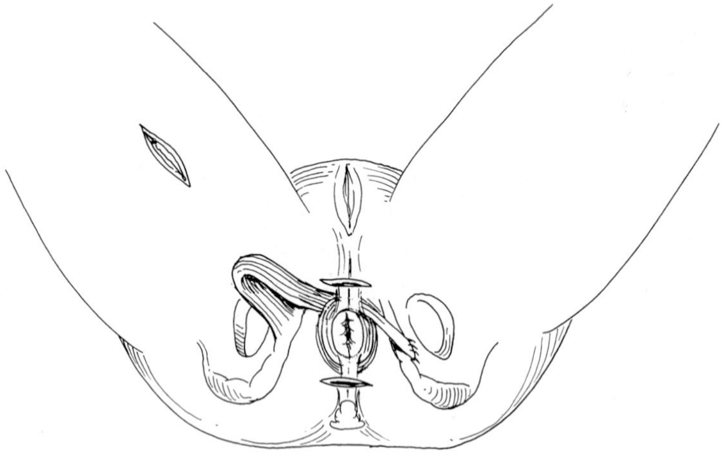

Fig. 16-4, cont'd **B,** Incisions used to deeply encircle the external sphincter. **C,** Attachment of the gracilis tendon to the contralateral ischial tuberosity.

multiple previous operations with resulting fibrosis. Yoshioka and Keighley[38] in a series of six patients, reported poor results in all six, which they attributed to advanced age (Table 16-3).

Devesa et al.[39] recently reported use of gluteus maximus transposition in the management of fecal incontinence in a series of 10 patients. Initially, this operation was plagued by perianal wound sepsis and subsequent need for repeat surgery. After modification of the technique, they have noted fewer complications. They found that muscle under tension predisposes the muscle to become fibrotic, resulting in a sling somewhat like a Thiersch encirclement. Table 16-3 illustrates the success authors have had with gracilis muscle transposition.

In an effort to improve on the technique of gracilis transposition, some authors have added electrostimulation of the muscle for two purposes: to at-

Table 16-3 Results of gracilis muscle transposition

Author	No. of patients	Grade of continence* (%)		
		1	2	3
Corman[35] (1985)	14	50	28	21
Leguit et al.[36] (1985)	10	70	20	10
Yoshioka and Keighley[38] (1988)	6	—	—	100
Williams et al.[40] (1991)	18	50	17	33
Faucheron et al.[37] (1994)	22	50	18	36

*1, continent for solid and liquid stool; 2, continent for solid stool only and may use pads, enemas, or suppositories; 3, incontinent for formed stool, obstruction, or colostomy.

tempt to convert the fast-twitch muscle fibers in the gracilis muscle to slow-twitch, less fatiguable muscle fibers, and, on converting these fibers, to attain the tonic contractile nature of the sphincter musculature. Williams et al.[40] reported on 32 patients who underwent dynamic (electrically stimulated) graciloplasty. Twelve of 20 patients with idiopathic incontinence had resultant continence of stool with only occasional loss of liquid stool. Seven of 12 patients who underwent reconstruction of the anal canal with graciloplasty after abdominal perineal resection because of cancer achieved acceptable continence. Initial results were marginal with this technique. However, with modification of the technique, including use of an implantable stimulator (for fewer infectious complications), stimulation of the main nerve to the gracilis versus the more peripheral branches (to exercise the whole muscle), and delayed gracilis transposition (to ensure adequate blood supply), complication rates have decreased. Complications included severe perineal sepsis (28%), muscle necrosis (13%), electrode migration (13%), difficult evacuation (13%), and transient neuralgia (6%).

Patients are instructed to use the magnet to activate the stimulator. Deactivating the stimulator causes relaxation of the muscle and resultant defecation. Baeten et al.,[41] in a series of 10 patients, reported excellent results with respect to continence with the dynamic graciloplasty. Complications were similar to those of the series by Williams et al.[40] Fistula from an eroding gracilis flap, wound infection that necessitated removal of the stimulator, and atrophic gracilis muscle pedicle were all noted. Other potential problems with the presence of hardware include malfunction of the stimulator and potential infectious complications secondary to foreign body. Best results are obtained in patients with intact anal sensation. Williams et al.[42] also reported a series of patients who received electrically stimulated gracilis neoanal sphincters in conjunction with reconstruction after abdominal perineal resection because of cancer. Their patients did not fare so well because of the lack of sensation of a fecal bolus. These patients required extensive postoperative training to effectively benefit from this technique.

IMPLANTABLE DEVICES

Christiansen and Sparso[43] reported an implantable device similar to that used in patients with urinary incontinence that can be used to manage fecal incontinence. The device consists of a cuff that encircles the anal canal, a pressure regulator, and a pump that is implanted in the scrotum or labia. Continence is achieved by pumping the device. For defecation to occur, the cuff is deflated. This device provides an alternative to a permanent stoma in patients with idiopathic fecal incontinence or failed attempts at direct repair. In their series of 12 patients, Christiansen and Sparso reported excellent results (occasional leakage of flatus) in five and good results (continent to solid and usually to liquid stool) in three. However, two patients required removal of the device because of infection, and four others required eight revisions because of mechanical failure (ruptured cuff). Correct placement of the cuff is also essential to prevent migration and sliding of the device. After modification of the technique to stabilize the device, the authors have reported fewer complications.

REFERENCES

1. Nelson R, Norton N, Cautley E. Prevalence of fecal incontinence in Wisconsin households. Presented at the American Society of Colon and Rectal Surgeons, 93rd Annual Convention, Orlando, Fla.: May 10, 1994.
2. Labow S, Rubin RJ, Hoexter B, Salvati E. Perineal repair of rectal procidentia with an elastic fabric sling. Dis Colon Rectum 23:467-469, 1980.
3. Horn HR, Schoetz DJ Jr, Coller JA, Veidenheimer MC. Sphincter repair with a silastic sling for anal incontinence and rectal procidentia. Dis Colon Rectum 28:868-872, 1985.
4. Parks AG, McPartlin JF. Late repair of injuries of the anal sphincter. Proc R Soc Med 64: 1187-1189, 1971.
5. Slade MS, Goldberg SM, Schottler JL, Balcos EG, Christenson CE. Sphincteroplasty for acquired anal incontinence. Dis Colon Rectum 20:33-35, 1977.
6. Browning GGP, Motson RW. Anal sphincter injury: Management and results of Parks sphincter repair. Ann Surg 199:351-357, 1984.
7. Christiansen J, Pedersen IK. Traumatic anal incontinence: Results of surgical repair. Dis Colon Rectum 30:189-191, 1987.
8. Fang DT, Nivatvongs S, Vermeulen FD, Herman FN, Goldberg SM, Rothenberger DA. Overlapping sphincteroplasty for acquired anal incontinence. Dis Colon Rectum 27:720-722, 1984.
9. Fleshman JW, Peters WR, Shemesh EI, Fry RD, Kodner IJ. Anal sphincter reconstruction: Anterior overlapping muscle repair. Dis Colon Rectum 34:739-743, 1991.
10. Fleshman JW, Dreznik Z, Fry RD, Kodner IJ. Anal sphincter repair for obstetric injury: Manometric evaluation of functional results. Dis Colon Rectum 34:1061-1067, 1991.
11. Pezim ME, Spencer RJ, Stanhope CR, Beart RW Jr, Ready RL, Illstrup DM. Sphincter repair for fecal incontinence after obstetrical or iatrogenic injury. Dis Colon Rectum 30: 521-525, 1987.
12. Wexner SD, Marchetti F, Jagelman DG. The role of sphincteroplasty for fecal incontinence re-evaluated: A prospective physiologic and functional review. Dis Colon Rectum 34:22-30, 1991.

13. Yoshioka K, Keighley MRB. Sphincter repair for fecal incontinence. Dis Colon Rectum 32:39-42, 1989.
14. Arnaud A, Sarles JC, Sielezneff I, Orsoni P, Joly A. Sphincter repair without overlapping for fecal incontinence. Dis Colon Rectum 34:744-747, 1991.
15. Jacobs PPM, Scheuer M, Kuijpers JH, Vingerhoets MH. Obstetric fecal incontinence: Role of pelvic floor denervation and results of delayed sphincter repair. Dis Colon Rectum 33: 494-497, 1990.
16. Parks AG. Postanal pelvic floor repair (and the treatment of anorectal incontinence). In Rob C, Smith E, eds. Operative Surgery, 3rd ed. Colon, Rectum and Anus. London: Butterworth, 1977, pp 249-253.
17. Browning GGP, Parks AG. Postanal repair for neuropathic faecal incontinence: Correlation of clinical results and anal canal pressures. Br J Surg 70:101-104, 1983.
18. Henry MM, Simson JNL. Results of postanal repair: A retrospective study. Br J Surg 72(Suppl):S17-S19, 1985.
19. Womack NR, Morrison JFB, Williams NS. Prospective study of the effects of postanal repair in neurogenic faecal incontinence. Br J Surg 75:48-52, 1988.
20. Yoshioka K, Hyland G, Keighley MRB. Clinical and physiological evaluation of postanal repair [abstract]. Gut 28:1362, 1987.
21. Yoshioka K, Hyland G, Keighley MRB. Physiological changes after postanal repair and parameters predicting outcome. Br J Surg 75:1220-1224, 1988.
22. Yoshioka K, Keighley MRB. Critical assessment of the quality of continence after postanal repair for faecal incontinence. Br J Surg 76:1054-1057, 1989.
23. Scheuer M, Kuijpers HC, Jacobs PP. Postanal repair restores anatomy rather than function. Dis Colon Rectum 32:960-963, 1989.
24. Laurberg S, Swash M, Henry MM. Effect of postanal repair on progress of neurogenic damage to the pelvic floor. Br J Surg 77:519-522, 1990.
25. Snooks SJ, Swash M, Henry M. Electrophysiologic and manometric assessment of failed postanal repair for anorectal incontinence. Dis Colon Rectum 27:733-736, 1984.
26. Rainey JB, Donaldson DR, Thomson JPS. Postanal repair: Which patients derive most benefit. J R Coll Surg Edinb 35:101-105, 1990.
27. Keighley MRB. Fecal incontinence. In Keighley M, Williams N, eds. Surgery of the Anus, Rectum and Colon. Philadelphia: WB Saunders, 1993, p 567.
28. Miller R, Orrom WJ, Cornes H, Duthie G, Bartolo DCC. Anterior sphincter plication and levatorplasty in the treatment of faecal incontinence. Br J Surg 76:1058-1060, 1989.
29. Pinho M, Ortiz J, Oya M, Panagamuwa B, Asperer, J, Keighley MRB. Total pelvic floor repair for the treatment of neuropathic fecal incontinence. Am J Surg 163:340-343, 1992.
30. Pickrell KL, Broadbent TR, Masters FW, Metzger JT. Construction of a rectal sphincter and restoration of anal continence by transplanting the gracilis muscle. Ann Surg 135:853-862, 1952.
31. Corman ML. Management of faecal incontinence by gracilis muscle transposition. Dis Colon Rectum 22:290-292, 1979.
32. Corman ML. Follow up evaluation of gracilis muscle transposition for fecal incontinence. Dis Colon Rectum 23:552-555, 1980.
33. Corman JL. The management of anal incontinence. Surg Clin North Am 63:177-192, 1983.
34. Corman ML. Colon and Rectal Surgery. Philadelphia: JB Lippincott, 1984, pp 129-134.
35. Corman ML. Gracilis muscle transposition for anal incontinence: Late results. Br J Surg 72(Suppl):S21, 1985.

36. Leguit R Jr, van Baal JG, Brummelkamp WH. Gracilis muscle transposition in the treatment of fecal incontinence: Long term follow up and evaluation of anal pressure recordings. Dis Colon Rectum 28:1-4, 1985.
37. Faucheron J, Hannoun L, Thome C, Parc R. Is fecal continence improved by nonstimulated gracilis muscle transposition? Dis Colon Rectum 37:979-983, 1994.
38. Yoshioka K, Keighley MRB. Clinical and manometric assessment of gracilis muscle transplant for fecal incontinence. Dis Colon Rectum 31:767-769, 1988.
39. Devesa JM, Vicente E, Enriquez JM, Nuno J, Bucheli P, de Blas G, Villaneuva MG. Total fecal incontinence—A new method of gluteus maximus transportation: Preliminary results and report of previous experience with similar procedures. Dis Colon Rectum 35:339-349, 1992.
40. Williams NS, Patel J, George BD, Hallan RI, Watkins ES. Development of an electrically stimulated neoanal sphincter. Lancet 338:1166-1169, 1991.
41. Baeten CG, Konsten J, Spaans F, Visser R, Habets AM, Bourgeois IM, Wagenmakers AJ, Soeters PB. Dynamic graciloplasty for treatment of faecal incontinence. Lancet 338:1163-1165, 1991.
42. Williams NS, Hallan RI, Koeze TH, Watkins ES. Restoration of gastrointestinal continuity and continence after abdomino-perineal excision of the rectum arising in an electrically stimulated neoanal sphincter. Dis Colon Rectum 33:561-565, 1990.
43. Christiansen J, Sparso B. Treatment of anal incontinence by an implantable prosthetic anal sphincter. Ann Surg 214:383-386, 1992.
44. Hawley PR. Anal sphincter reconstruction. Langenbecks Arch Chir 366:269-272, 1985.
45. Morgan S, Bernard D, Tasse D, Wassef R. Results of Parks' sphincteroplasty for post traumatic anal incontinence. Can J Surg 30:229(R212), 1987.
46. Ctercteko GC, Fazio VW, Jagelman DG, Lavery IC, Weakley FL, Melia M. Anal sphincter repair: A report of 60 cases and review of the literature. Aust N Z J Surg 58:703-710, 1988.
47. Abcarian H, Orsay CP, Pearl R, Nelson RL, Briley SC. Traumatic cloaca. Dis Colon Rectum 32:783-787, 1989.
48. Habr-Gama A, Alves PR, da Silva e Sousa AH. Treatment of fecal incontinence by postanal repair. Coloproctology 8:244-246, 1986.
49. Keighley MRB. Postanal repair. How I do it. Int J Colorect Dis 2:236-239, 1987.
50. Miller R, Bartolo DCC, Locke-Edmunds JC, Mortensen NJ. Prospective study of conservative and operative treatment for fecal incontinence. Br J Surg 75:48-52, 1988.

CHAPTER 17

Surgery for Rectal Prolapse

PETER W. MARCELLO
PATRICIA L. ROBERTS

Although rectal prolapse was recognized as early as 1500 BC, the optimal surgical procedure for rectal prolapse is still debated. With more than 50 surgical procedures to choose from, the surgeon must select the procedure most likely to have a low complication rate, low failure rate, and reasonable chance of ensuring a good functional result for the particular patient. Factors that must be considered include the age and sex of the patient, medical status, bowel function, continence, history of previous repairs, and expertise of the surgeon. To that end, we will discuss the complications of the most common abdominal and perineal procedures.

ABDOMINAL PROCEDURES

A variety of abdominal procedures have been described for the treatment of rectal prolapse, including rectosacral fixation (using sutures, mesh, or sponge), anterior resection, combined resection and fixation, and recently the addition of laparoscopically assisted procedures. Each of these is performed in an attempt to correct some of the anatomic defects that may predispose to the development of rectal prolapse. These defects include redundancy of the sigmoid colon, laxity in the normal posterior fixation of the rectum, a deep pouch of Douglas, and diastasis of the pelvic floor musculature.

In the patient at good risk for surgery, abdominal procedures are preferred to perineal procedures for several reasons. The most compelling of these is a reported lower frequency of recurrence with abdominal procedures compared with perineal procedures. In appropriately selected patients, an abdominal procedure can be performed with relatively low morbidity and mortality and with improved functional results.

Mortality

Perioperative mortality after abdominal procedures has remained consistently low (0% to 3%; Tables 17-1 to 17-3). In earlier studies, mortality rates as high

Table 17-1 Fixation procedures

Author	Year	No. of patients	Mortality	Recurrence	Type of recurrence	Incontinence		Constipation	
						Preoperative	Postoperative	Preoperative	Postoperative
Mesh rectopexy									
Gordon and Hoexter[1]	1978	1111	NS	26 (2.3)*	C	NS		NS	
Eisenstat et al.[2]	1979	30	0	0		NS		NS	
Romero-Torres[3]	1979	24	1 (4.2)	0		NS	0	NS	
Failes et al.[4]	1979	53	0	3 (5.7)	C	NS	7 (13)	NS	
				6 (11)	M				
Hilsabeck[5]	1981	14	0	1 (7.1)	M	NS	4 (29)	NS	
Keighley et al.[6]	1983	100	0	4 (4.0)	M	67 (67)	24 (24)	NS	
Loygue et al.[7]	1984	257	2 (0.7)	13 (5.6)	C	107 (42)	90 (35)	NS	
Holmstrom et al.[8]	1986	108	3 (2.8)	4 (3.7)	C	37 (40)	9 (10)	25 (27)	40 (43)
McMahan and Ripstein[9]	1987	23	0	0		0	0	0	0
Roberts et al.[10]	1988	135	1 (0.7)	13 (9.6)	C	58 (43)	27 (22)	51 (38)	38 (31)
				4 (3.0)	M				
Sayfan et al.[11]	1990	16	0	0		12 (75)	9 (56)	3 (19)	7 (44)
Speakman et al.[12]	1991	26	0	4 (15)	C	21 (81)	20 (77)	9 (35)	17 (65)
				2 (7.7)	M				
Luukkonen et al.[13]	1992	15	1 (6.7)	0		9 (60)	2 (13)	5 (33)	2 (13)
Duthie and Bartolo[14]	1992	20	0	0		15 (75)	5 (25)	NS	
Tjandra et al.[15]	1993	142	1 (0.7)	13 (9.1)	C	48 (37)	25 (19)	47 (36)	42 (33)
Winde et al.[16]	1993	47	0	5 (14)	M	22 (63)	10 (29)	22 (47)	6 (17)
Scaglia et al.[17]	1994	16	0	0		8 (50)	4 (25)	6 (37)	6 (37)

Ivalon sponge rectopexy									
Morgan et al.[18]	1972	150	4 (2.7)*	3 (3.2)	C	83 (81)	40 (39)	67 (65)	28 (27)
				8 (8.6)	M				
Penfold and Hawley[19]	1972	101	0	3 (3.2)	C	48 (61)	32 (41)	NS	23 (29)
				31 (33)	M				
Stewart[20]	1972	41	0	3 (7.5)	C	16 (48)	2 (6.1)	NS	—
				10 (25)	M				
Atkinson and Taylor[21]	1984	40	0	4 (10)	C	14 (35)	4 (10)	NS	—
				12 (30)	M				
Mann and Hoffman[22]	1988	59†	0	4 (6.8)	M	21 (36)	11 (19)	17 (29)	28 (47)
McCue and Thomson[23]	1991	53	0	2 (3.8)	C	37 (70)	23 (43)	12 (23)	8 (15)
				10 (19)	M				
Duthie and Bartolo[14]	1992	9	0	0		5 (56)	3 (33)	NS	—
Novell et al.[25]	1994	31	0	1 (3.2)	C	10 (32)	9 (29)	NS	15 (48)
Scaglia et al.[26]	1994	16	0	0		4 (25)	1 (6.2)	7 (44)	13 (81)
Suture rectopexy									
Kirkman[27]	1975	30	3 (10.0)	1 (3.7)	C	NS	—	NS	—
Carter[28]	1983	32	0	1 (3.1)	C	NS	—	NS	—
Blatchford et al.[29]	1989	43	0	1 (2.4)	C	27 (64)	11 (26)	20 (48)	30 (71)
				4 (9.6)	M				
McKee et al.[30]	1992	8	0	0		5 (63)	1 (13)	5 (63)	7 (88)
Duthie and Bartolo[14]	1992	10	0	0		8 (80)	1 (10)	NS	—
Novell et al.[25]	1994	32	0	1 (3.1)	C	10 (31)	5 (16)	NS	10 (31)

C = complete prolapse; M = mucosal prolapse; NS = not stated.

*Numbers in parentheses represent percent of patients and may be derived from fewer than the total number of patients.

†Patients also had suturepexy.

Table 17-2 Resection and combination procedures

Author	Year	No. of patients	Mortality	Recurrence	Indication	Incontinence		Constipation	
						Preoperative	Postoperative	Preoperative	Postoperative
Rectosigmoid resection									
Wolff and Dietzen[31]	1991	150	1 (0.7)*	11 (8.9)	C	66 (54)	47 (38)	NS	—
Cirocco and Brown[32]	1993	41	0	3 (7.3)	C	21 (51)	11 (27)	17 (41)	14 (34)
Resection and suture rectopexy									
Watts et al.[33]	1985	138	0	2 (1.9)	C	15 (25)	9 (15)	? (63)	? (44)
Sayfan et al.[34]	1990	13	0	0		9 (69)	3 (23)	5 (38)	1 (7.7)
Luukkonen et al.[35]	1992	15	0	0		11 (73)	1 (6.7)	7 (47)	0
McKee et al.[30]	1992	9	0	0		3 (33)	3 (33)	4 (44)	2 (22)
Madoff et al.[36]	1992	47	0	3 (6.3)	C	21 (45)	19 (40)	20 (43)	10 (21)
				4 (8.5)	M				
Duthie and Bartolo[14]	1992	29	0	0		6 (21)	24 (83)	NS	—
Tjandra et al.[37]	1993	18	0	0		5 (28)	3 (17)	12 (67)	2 (11)
Deen et al.[38]	1994	10	0	2 (20)	M	10 (100)	1 (10)	NS	0

C = complete prolapse; M = mucosal prolapse; NS = not stated.

*Numbers in parentheses represent percent of patients and may be derived from fewer than the total number of patients.

Table 17-3 Laparoscopic procedures

Author	Year	No. of patients	Mortality	Recurrence
Mesh rectopexy				
Berman[39]	1992	1	0	0
Kusminsky et al.[40]	1992	1	0	0
Munro et al.[41]	1993	1	0	0
Cuesta et al.[42]	1993	4	0	0
Kwok et al.[43]	1994	1	0	0
Cushieri et al.[44]	1994	5	0	0
Eu et al.[45]	1995	10	0	0
Rectosigmoid resection				
Ballantyne[46]	1992	1	0	0
Senagore et al.[47]	1993	6	0	0
Baker et al.[48]	1995	8	0	0

as 10% were reported.[27] The majority of deaths were related to myocardial infarction, pulmonary emboli, and rarely septic complications. With improvements in perioperative monitoring, anesthetic technique, and the selection of a perineal procedure for the debilitated patient at highest risk, perioperative mortality has become uncommon in recent years. Appropriate preoperative screening of cardiopulmonary status is necessary in this heterogeneous group of patients that often includes patients in their eighth, ninth, and occasionally tenth decade of life.

Presacral Hemorrhage

Presacral hemorrhage, a potentially life-threatening complication, can occur after any procedure in which the posterior rectum is mobilized. This is an inherent step in all abdominal procedures performed to treat rectal prolapse. The prevalence of presacral hemorrhage is 0% to 8%[37,49,50] and appears to occur more frequently after rectopexy than after resectional procedures. This is probably related to puncture of the anterior presacral plexus or basivertebral veins while the rectopexy sutures are placed.

The exact cause of presacral bleeding has been carefully evaluated by Qinyao et al.[51] (Fig. 17-1). Significant hemorrhage can occur if the basivertebral veins are transected at the level of the lower sacral foramina. These veins communicate with the internal vertebral venous system, a large valveless venous pool that in turn communicates with the inferior vena cava. The rapid blood loss associated with injury to the basivertebral veins is related to high hydrostatic pressure in the

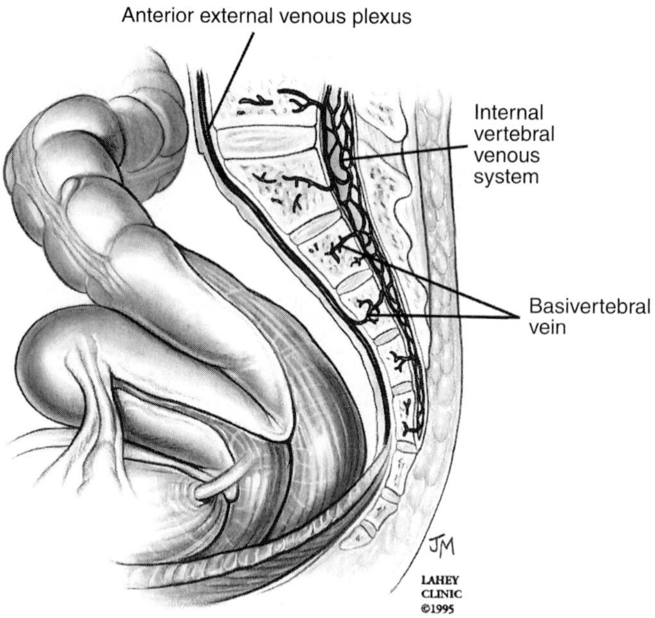

Fig. 17-1 Presacral hemorrhage may result from any procedure that requires rectal mobilization. Bleeding from the anterior external venous plexus may be controlled with cautery or suture ligation, whereas bleeding from large basivertebral veins is generally best controlled with use of thumbtacks.

depth of the pelvis and is accentuated by the lithotomy position, which increases venous pooling within the pelvis.

If hemorrhage is the result of injury to the presacral plexus of veins, bleeding may be controlled with sutures or electrocautery. When the injury involves disruption of the basivertebral veins at the sacral foramina, the use of suture ligation, electrocoagulation, or thrombogenic agents is often unsuccessful, because these large veins, when transected, retract into the sacral foramina. Abdominal packing and bone wax have been used in this situation. Numerous reports over the past years, however, have advocated the use of thumbtacks to successfully occlude the foramina and arrest the bleeding.[51-53] Newly designed titanium tacks are now available for this specific use.[54] A modified technique of indirect coagulation using a muscle fragment has also been successful in 11 cases of presacral hemorrhage.[55] Meticulous attention during rectal mobilization can often avoid this life-threatening complication.

Recurrence

Recurrence of rectal prolapse has been noted with every abdominal procedure described, which emphasizes our incomplete understanding of the cause of rectal prolapse. After abdominal surgery, rectal prolapse recurs in as many as

10% of patients. However, the rate of recurrence reported in the literature varies considerably, even among authors using similar procedures (see Tables 17-1 to 17-3). This is related to numerous factors, including the length and completeness of follow-up study, the experience of the surgeon, the type of procedure performed, and extent of recurrence. Recurrent prolapse may occur as long as 16 years after surgery.[31] Tjandra et al.[37] reported that nearly one third of recurrent rectal prolapse after a successful Ripstein procedure occurred after 3 years. Many of the smaller reports lack an adequate duration of follow-up, which falsely lowers the true rate of recurrence they report.

Recurrent rectal prolapse may be complete, involving the full thickness of the bowel wall, or mucosal. Mucosal recurrence is more common than complete recurrence (see Tables 17-1 and 17-2). When reporting the rate of recurrence, some authors have combined both mucosal and complete recurrence, whereas others have noted each individually or have excluded mucosal recurrence. This has only added to the discrepancies among the rates of recurrence recorded in the literature. Recurrent mucosal prolapse occurs in 0% to 15% of patients, although rates as high as 33% have been reported.[19,21] In general, mucosal prolapse is self-limiting and can be treated by banding or injection if symptoms persist.

Complete recurrence of rectal prolapse occurring within 1 year of the original procedure is likely the result of a specific technical failure. Limited mobilization of the rectum, inadequate fixation of the rectum to the sacrum, or incomplete resection of a redundant rectosigmoid colon have been associated with early recurrence. Early recurrence has also been noted after vigorous physical activity or in patients with continued postoperative constipation who exhibit persistent straining, resulting in disruption of the rectopexy from the hollow of the sacrum. Disruption of a rectal sling occurred in one of our patients after childbirth.[50] Management of early recurrent prolapse depends on the type of procedure performed and the cause of recurrence and is discussed later for each procedure. When one procedure has failed, however, another procedure should generally be performed. In patients at good risk, a different abdominal procedure may be performed. If the patient is not a good candidate for abdominal surgery, a perineal approach is preferred.

Incontinence

Over the past decade, the relative efficacy of any procedure for repair of complete rectal prolapse has been judged not only by the recurrence rate and morbidity but also by its functional results. Patients with rectal prolapse often have disturbances in their bowel habits, either progressive incontinence or persistent constipation. The ideal surgical procedure for rectal prolapse should not only correct the prolapse but also improve these bowel disturbances. The frequency of preoperative incontinence reported in the literature varies widely, from 25% to 100% (Tables 17-1, 17-2, 17-4, and 17-5), although most larger studies have

Table 17-4 Perineal rectosigmoidectomy

Author	Year	No. of patients	Mortality	Recurrence	Indication	Incontinence	
						Preoperative	Postoperative
Hughes[56]	1949	108	0	65 (60)*	C	NS	—
Porter[57]	1962	110	1 (0.9)	55 (50)	C	52 (66)	60 (76)
				9 (8)	M		
Altemeier et al.[58]	1971	106	0	3 (2.8)	C	NS	—
Friedman et al.[59]	1983	27	0	12 (54)	C	11 (41)	NS
Gopal et al.[60]	1984	18	1 (5.5)	1 (5.5)	C	NS	—
Watts et al.[33]	1985	33	0	0		2 (12)	5 (28)
Prasad et al.[61]	1986	25	0	0		25 (100)	0
Williams et al.[62]	1992	114	0	11 (10)	C	67 (64)	34 (33)
Johansen et al.[63]	1993	20	1 (5)	2 (11)	M	14 (70)	8 (42)
Ramanujam et al.[64]	1994	72	0	4 (5.5)	C	54 (75)	24 (33)
				4 (5.5)	M		
Deen et al.[38]	1994	10	0	1 (10)	C	10 (100)	6 (60)
				2 (20)	M		

C = complete prolapse; M = mucosal prolapse; NS = not stated.

*Numbers in parentheses represent percent of patients and may be derived from fewer than the total number of patients.

Table 17-5 Delorme procedure

Author	Year	No. of patients	Mortality	Recurrence	Indication	Incontinence	
						Preoperative	Postoperative
Swinton and Palmer[65]	1960	19	0	6 (30)*	C	NS	—
Nay and Blair[66]	1972	30	0	3 (10)	C	NS	8 (27)
Uhlig and Sullivan[67]	1979	44	0	3 (6.8)	C	NS	19 (43)
Christiansen and Kirkegaard[68]	1981	12	0	2 (17)	C	6 (50)	3 (25)
Gundersen et al.[69]	1985	18	0	1 (5.5)	C	NS	1 (5.5)
Monson et al.[70]	1986	27	0	2 (7.4)	C	18 (67)	3 (11)
Houry et al.[71]	1987	18	0	3 (17)	C	9 (50)	4 (22)
Abulafi et al.[72]	1990	22	0	1 (4.5)	C	8 (36)	3 (14)
Senapati et al.[73]	1994	32	0	4 (12)	C	28 (88)	15 (47)
				3 (9)	M		
Oliver et al.[74]	1994	40	1 (2.5)	8 (22)	C	17 (45)	15 (39)
Lechaux et al.[75]	1995	85	1 (1.2)	11 (14)	C	65 (82)	36 (45)

C = complete prolapse; M = mucosal prolapse; NS = not stated.
*Numbers in parentheses represent percent of patients and may be derived from fewer than the total number of patients.

reported that at least half of patients will have some degree of incontinence. Abnormalities in both the internal and external sphincter complexes have been identified in patients with rectal prolapse and incontinence. Manometric evaluations have noted significantly lower anal pressure at rest, indicating damage to the internal anal sphincter.[76,77] Duthie et al.[78] confirmed this and noted a low frequency of response of the internal anal sphincter as demonstrated by ambulatory EMG. The anorectal inhibitory reflex is also inhibited by the persistent rectal prolapse, and sensation along the anal canal is reduced. Anal pressure during maximal contraction is abnormally low, signifying injury to the external sphincter and rectal sling.[78,79] Radiologic assessment of these patients has identified an obtuse anorectal angle and abnormally elongated perineal descent, which may also contribute to incontinence.

After correction of the rectal prolapse with an abdominal procedure, approximately 75% of patients regain continence or at least have improved continence. The improvement is associated with return of function of the internal and external sphincter exhibited by increased resting and squeeze pressures and return of the anorectal inhibitory reflex. Sensation along the anal canal and awareness of rectal filling have also improved after surgery.[78,80]

The onset of new incontinence after successful correction of rectal prolapse has been reported in 5% to 13% of patients and appears to occur more frequently after rectosigmoid resection than after rectopexy alone.[23,31,36] After anterior resection in 123 patients, Wolff and Dietzen[31] identified 16 patients (13%) with postoperative incontinence; five patients eventually needed colostomies. Madoff et al.[36] noted the development of incontinence after resection and rectopexy in six of 47 patients (13%); in three patients, permanent diversion was required. The occurrence of postoperative incontinence did not correlate with length of bowel resected. The development of postoperative incontinence may be related to decreased compliance of the bowel after resection or, by correction of associated constipation with resection, previously unrecognized incontinence may become apparent. In patients with persistent postoperative incontinence, Parks postanal repair or anterior sphincteroplasty has been performed with relative short-term success.[18,81,82]

Constipation

Preoperative constipation is noted in 25% to 50% of patients with rectal prolapse. The cause is unclear, although a delay in colonic transit has been demonstrated with marker studies.[30,35] Postoperative constipation, whether persistent or of new onset, has been a continued problem with all procedures performed to correct rectal prolapse. Although some authors have noted improvement in symptoms of constipation after surgery, others have noted worsening symptoms of constipation or the development of constipation in patients who did not have this problem before surgery. The development of constipation after correction of rectal prolapse is more common after abdominal rectopexy than rectosigmoid resection or resection plus rectopexy (see Tables 17-1 and 17-2). In a prospective randomized trial, McKee et al.[30] compared suture rectopexy with sigmoidectomy and suture rectopexy and found that postoperative constipation occurred in 88% and 22% of patients, respectively. In a similar study in which posterior mesh rectopexy was compared with sigmoidectomy and suture rectopexy, preoperative constipation improved in 100% and 60% of patients, respectively. However, the onset of new constipation occurred in one third of patients who underwent rectopexy alone.[35]

Although constipation or delayed transit may be a predisposing factor to the development of rectal prolapse because of persistent straining, the cause of postoperative constipation is unknown, but several mechanisms have been proposed. After posterior rectopexy, redundant sigmoid colon may fold over the fixed rectal attachments and create a relative outlet obstruction. This finding, however, has not been confirmed with radiographic defecography.[83,84] A delay in colonic transit above the rectopexy has also been identified in some patients with constipation.[84] Autonomic denervation of the rectosigmoid colon after mobilization and division of the lateral ligament has been proposed as an etiologic factor.[26,34,85] In a prospective randomized trial by Speakman et al.,[85] results in 12 patients who underwent posterior mesh rectopexy without lateral ligament division were compared with those in 14 patients who underwent posterior polyvinyl alcohol sponge (Ivalon; Downs Surgical, Sheffield, England) rectopexy with division of the lateral ligaments. In the group without lateral ligament division, three of six patients with constipation before surgery showed improvement, but constipation developed in four patients who had not had preoperative constipation. In the 14 patients with division of the lateral ligaments, one of three patients had improvement in constipation after surgery, whereas constipation developed in eight patients. Other studies have reported similar results with division of the lateral ligaments. However, in a prospective nonrandomized evaluation of various rectopexy techniques in which the lateral ligaments were divided in all 68 patients, no patient reported a new complaint of constipation.[14] It seems likely that the cause of constipation after successful repair of prolapse is multifactorial. However, in the patient with severe preoperative constipation or colonic inertia, sigmoid resection with rectopexy appears to offer superior functional results compared with rectopexy alone.

Mesh Rectopexy

Fixation of the rectum to the sacrum was originally described by Orr,[86] who used two strips of fascia to suspend the rectum. The technique was modified by Loygue et al.,[87] who used nylon strips and fully mobilized the bowel. These authors noted recurrence of rectal prolapse in 13 of 233 patients (5.6%), of which half were followed up for 5 years or more (see Table 17-1). Among the complications were intervertebral disk space infections in three patients, which responded to conservative management. The passage of sutures through the presacral fascia and bone likely caused the infections. Although not usually reported, intervertebral infection can occur after any of the rectopexy procedures.

Mesh rectopexy, as described by Ripstein,[71] is one of the most commonly performed abdominal procedures for repair of complete rectal prolapse in North America. In this procedure the rectum is affixed to the hollow of the sacrum with Teflon or Marlex (C.R. Bard, Billerica, Mass.) mesh, or, more recently, a Gore-Tex (W.L. Gore & Associates, Elkton, Md.) patch. Early experience with the procedure produced a low rate of recurrence (see Table 17-1). Significant morbidity has been noted with this procedure, however, occurring in as many as 52% of patients.[50] Postoperative complications reported include presacral hemorrhage (0% to 8%); pelvic sepsis (0% to 5%) including pelvic abscess, infected mesh, and fistula formation; small bowel obstruction (0% to 2%); wound infection (0% to 10%); and urinary tract infection (0% to 10%). In an attempt to prevent pelvic infection related to permanent mesh rectopexy, some authors have used polyglycolic acid absorbable mesh, with similar results.[89]

Late complications associated with the Ripstein procedure are fecal impaction and stricture at the level of the mesh. A survey of members of the ASCRS by Gordon and Hoexter[49] in 1978 recorded complications in 1111 procedures performed by 129 surgeons. Of these, 183 complications (16.5%) were directly related to the rectal sling and included fecal impaction in 74 cases (6.7%) and stricture in 20 (1.8%). At that time, the procedure was performed by attaching the mesh circumferentially around the mobilized rectum. If the mesh was wrapped too tightly, a stricture would form, which resulted in outlet obstruction (Fig. 17-2). This was also thought to predispose to postoperative constipation. Delayed stricture formation secondary to fibrosis around the mesh has been noted. Surgical correction of an early stricture has been performed by removal of the mesh, division of the mesh anteriorly, or anterior resection if a dense fibrotic reaction has occurred.[49,50,90] In a modification of the procedure, McMahan and Ripstein[91] recommended that the mesh be secured posteriorly to the sacral hollow and then attached three quarters of the circumference around the rectum, leaving the anterior rectum free to expand. This is the technique we currently use (Fig. 17-3). Since modification of the technique, the rates of reported fecal impaction and stricture formation have decreased.

Rectal prolapse may occur after the Ripstein procedure because the sling has become detached from the sacrum, was placed too high in the pelvis, or was loosely fixed to the bowel or sacrum. Although a new sling has been successfully placed after recurrent prolapse, resection of the rectosigmoid colon with or without rectopexy is recommended in the patient at good risk. In patients who are not candidates for an abdominal procedure, perineal rectosigmoidectomy can be performed.

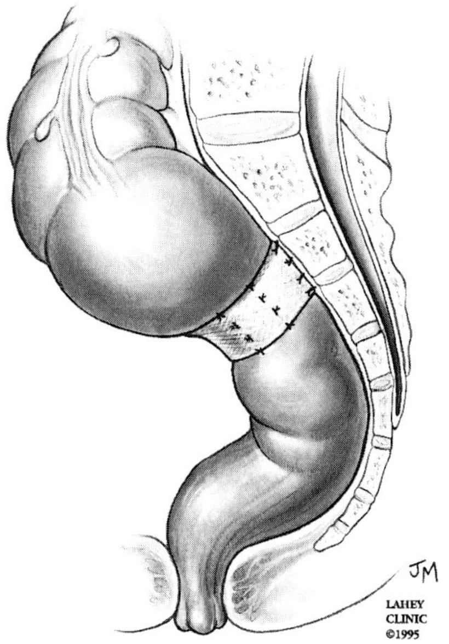

Fig. 17-2 During the performance of the Ripstein procedure, placement of the sling so that it is too tight and compromises the rectal lumen results in progressive obstructive symptoms and rectal stricture.

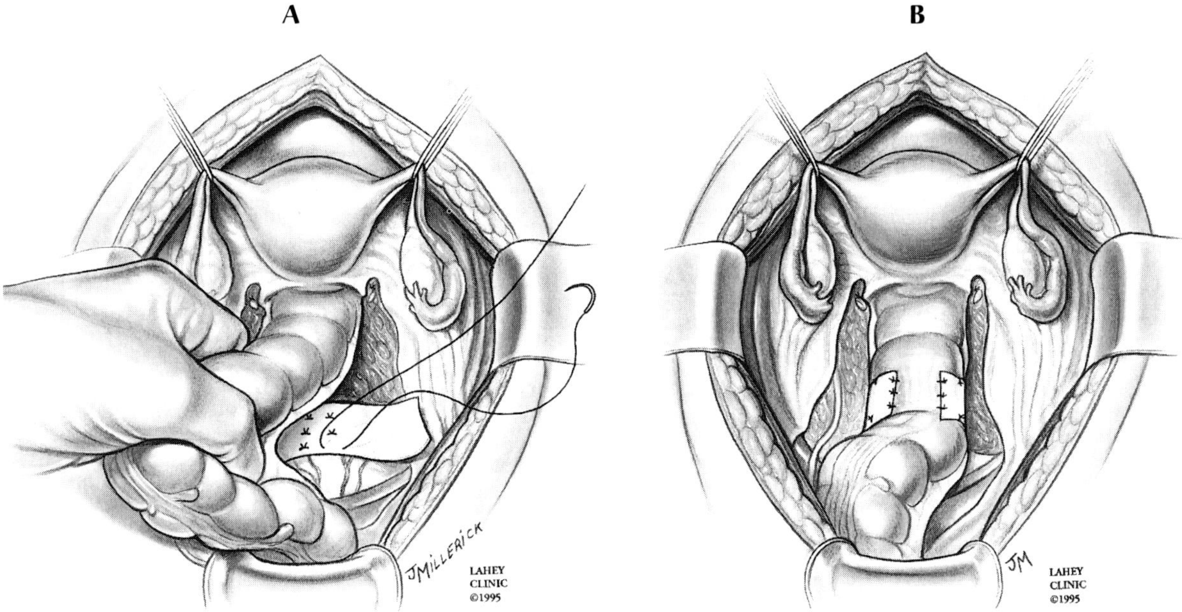

Fig. 17-3 **A,** To avoid the potential complication of a rectal stricture from the Ripstein procedure, the sling is secured to the periosteum of the sacrum. **B,** The sling is then secured to either side of the rectum, leaving the anterior wall of the rectum free to distend and preventing formation of a stricture.

Polyvinyl Alcohol Sponge Rectopexy

Polyvinyl alcohol sponge posterior rectopexy was popularized in 1959 by Wells.[75] The procedure is similar to the modified Ripstein procedure, with full mobilization of the rectum and fixation of a foreign body to the hollow of the sacrum that in turn is attached posteriorly to the rectum. The polyvinyl alcohol sponge was chosen because it creates a fibrous reaction that fosters fixation of the rectum to the sacrum. Complications of the Wells procedure are similar to those of the Ripstein procedure. Pelvic sepsis has been reported in 0% to 2.7% of patients.[1-9] This often requires removal of the sponge and repair of the prolapse with anterior resection. However, in four patients with pelvic sepsis related to an infected sponge reported by Morgan et al.,[18] the sponge had partially or completely eroded through the rectal wall. The sponge was therefore removed transanally. Follow-up study of these four patients revealed no recurrent prolapse and normal bowel function.

Fecal impaction has also been noted in as many as 3.8% of patients, and stricture formation in 1.7%.[22,23] These are related to the dense fibrotic reaction created by the polyvinyl alcohol sponge, and the involved bowel is resected if surgery is required.

The rate of complete recurrent prolapse after polyvinyl alcohol sponge rectopexy is similar to that of the Ripstein procedure (see Table 17-1). The cause of early recurrence is the same technical failure as with mesh rectopexy. Likewise, the management of complete recurrence should be the same: resection and rectopexy in the patient at good risk for surgery and perineal rectosigmoidectomy in the patient at poor risk.

Suture Rectopexy

Fixation of the mobilized rectum to the sacrum with sutures alone has been advocated by some[25,27-29] because it reduces the amount of prosthetic material at risk for subsequent infection and offers results equal to those with the mesh and polyvinyl alcohol sponge rectopexy procedures. In a randomized prospective trial that compared polyvinyl alcohol sponge rectopexy (31 patients) with suture rectopexy (32 patients), Novell et al.[25] noted recurrent prolapse in two patients (one in each group) (median follow-up, 47 months). Morbidity was higher in the sponge group (6 patients, 19%) than in the suture group (3 patients, 9%). The higher morbidity was not related to the sponge, however, and the authors concluded that the outcome of both procedures was equivalent. Functional results are also similar to those of mesh procedures. Constipation after suture rectopexy has been noted in 50% to 88% of patients (see Table 17-1).

If recurrent prolapse occurs after suture rectopexy, a mesh rectopexy, resection and rectopexy, or perineal rectosigmoidectomy can be performed.

Rectosigmoid Colon Resection

Muir[93] described anterior resection for the treatment of complete rectal prolapse in 1955. The procedure removes the redundant loosely fixed bowel and allows adhesions to form between the rectum and sacrum. Wolff and Dietzen[14] reported the largest series (150 patients) of anterior resection performed to correct rectal prolapse. The rate of recurrence was 8.9% among 123 patients who were followed up from 3 months to 20 years (mean, 10 years). Fifty-two complications occurred in 42 patients (28%), of which 25 complications (23 patients, 15%) were related to bowel mobilization, resection, or anastomosis. Five anastomotic leaks (3.3%) were noted, as well as four pelvic collections, five wound infections, and two anastomotic strictures. In a previous report of 113 anterior resections from the same institution, Schlinkert et al.[94] reported a significantly higher prevalence of complications associated with anastomosis below the peritoneal reflection (52%) than above it (19%). Opponents of anterior resection for the treatment of rectal prolapse criticize its high overall morbidity and anastomotic complications. However, in the larger reports of mesh or sponge rectopexy, the morbidity, mortality, and prevalence of anastomotic or prosthetic complications are comparable.

Recurrent rectal prolapse after anterior resection can be treated with abdominal rectopexy in the fit patient. Repeat resection has been performed but is likely to be technically challenging. In the patient at poor risk, an encirclement procedure can be used.

Sigmoid Colon Resection and Rectopexy

Sigmoidectomy combined with posterior suture rectopexy permits both resection of redundant bowel and fixation of the rectum to the sacrum. The complications associated with this procedure should be comparable to those with anterior resection. However, in review of the literature, the frequency of anastomotic complications appears to be less with resection and rectopexy than with resection alone.[7,16,19] In a series 138 patients, Watts et al.[33] noted only four anastomotic complications (2.9%), two of which required surgery. Similarly few anastomotic complications have been noted by other authors.[13,17,18,21] This may be related to the smaller sample size of the other reports.

Proponents of resection and rectopexy advocate its improved functional results compared with those achieved with mesh or polyvinyl alcohol sponge rectopexy (see Tables 17-1 and 17-2). Postoperative constipation has rarely deteriorated and often is improved after a combined procedure. Incontinence is also improved in the majority of patients after resection and proctopexy. However, in a small subset of patients after resection with or without rectopexy, disabling postoperative incontinence will develop and may require permanent diversion.

The rate of recurrent rectal prolapse after resection and rectopexy is comparable to that with mesh or polyvinyl alcohol sponge rectopexy (0% to 6%; see Table 17-2). This appears to be lower than that with resection alone. The addition of suture rectopexy may allow more complete fixation of the bowel to the sacral hollow, thereby reducing the likelihood of recurrence. If prolapse should recur after sigmoid resection and rectopexy, anterior resection or mesh rectopexy can be performed. Perineal resection after sigmoid resection should be performed cautiously because of the possibly tenuous blood supply of the intervening bowel. A perineal encirclement procedure is recommended as a last resort in the patient at poor risk.

Laparoscopically Assisted Procedures

Over the past 3 years, isolated reports of laparoscopically assisted procedures for the treatment of rectal prolapse have been reported (see Table 17-3). The two most commonly performed procedures are laparoscopic mesh rectopexy and rectosigmoid resection. These procedures enable the surgeon to perform an abdominal operation in some patients at poor risk who may not be able to tolerate a laparotomy. Additional advantages include a relatively short hospital stay and early resumption of bowel activity. However, no randomized prospective trial comparing laparoscopic procedures with conventional abdominal procedures for the treatment of rectal prolapse has been reported.

Complications associated with laparoscopic procedures include gas embolism, cardiopulmonary compromise related to the pneumoperitoneum, and trocar-related injuries. Bleeding, hernia formation, and inadvertent injury to abdominal structures can occur after any trocar placement. These complications are discussed in much greater depth in Chapter 10.

With a relatively short follow-up, no study has noted a recurrence of rectal prolapse after a laparoscopically assisted procedure. Continued follow-up of these patients will be necessary to ensure that the recurrence rate after laparoscopic procedures remains the same as with open procedures.

PERINEAL PROCEDURES

Perineal procedures for rectal prolapse have generally been reserved for use in elderly patients and patients with medical conditions that preclude performance of a laparotomy. Although the surgical risk is generally less with perineal procedures, the trade-off is an increase in potential recurrence of the prolapse, which may be reasonable in an elderly patient.

The most common perineal procedures performed include perineal rectosigmoidectomy and Delorme's procedure. Anal encirclement procedures, uncommonly performed, have been reserved for patients at extremely poor risk; however, such patients probably can tolerate perineal rectosigmoidectomy and anal encirclement procedures.

Perineal Rectosigmoidectomy

Originally described by Mikulicz[95] in 1889, perineal rectosigmoidectomy is probably the most popular perineal procedure performed to correct rectal prolapse. The procedure (frequently referred to as an Altemeier procedure) is performed by prolapsing the rectum and incising circumferentially within 1 to 2 cm of the dentate line through the full thickness of the bowel. The prolapsed segment is unfolded and the mesentery ligated and divided. The anastomosis may be either sutured or stapled (Fig. 17-4).

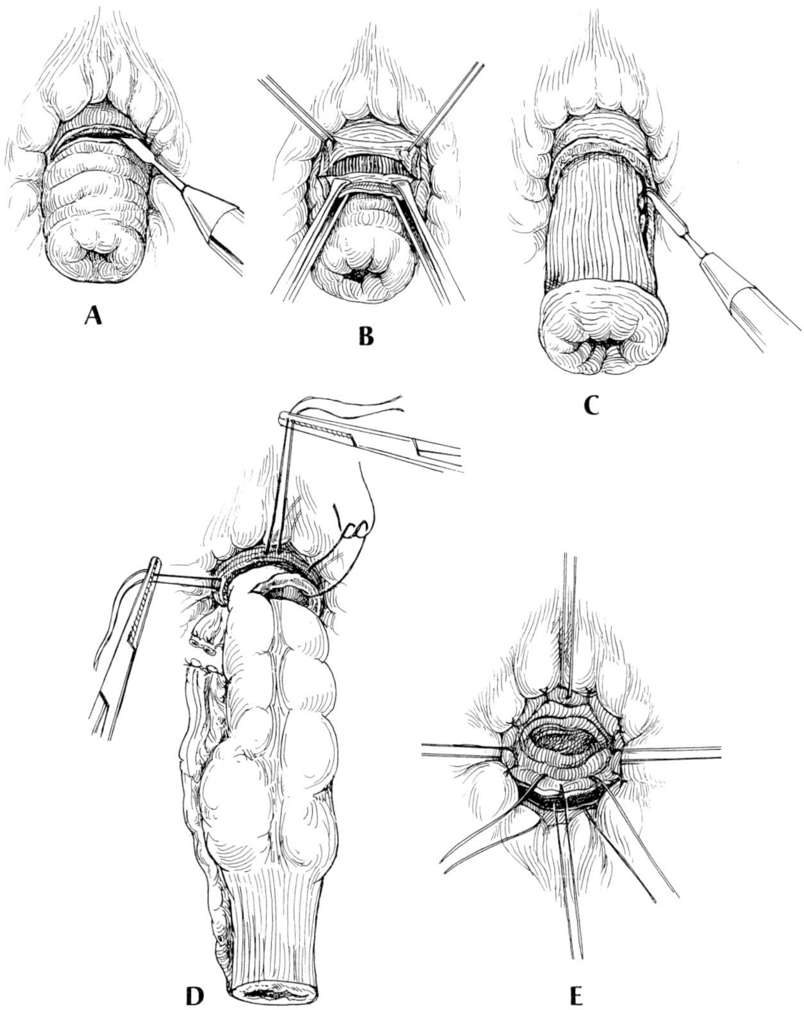

Fig. 17-4 Perineal rectosigmoidectomy. **A**, A circumferential incision is made in the anal canal just above the dentate line. **B** and **C**, The prolapsed rectum is separated and everted. The peritoneal reflection is incised sharply, allowing the redundant bowel to be fully mobilized. **D** and **E**, Once the mesentery is divided, the bowel is opened and full-thickness interrupted sutures are placed between the divided bowel and the residual cuff.

Recurrence rates of 0% to 60% have been reported, although in more recent series the recurrence rate is generally about 10% (see Table 17-4). It should be noted that the follow-up in these series was relatively short, reflecting the older age of patients undergoing the procedure. Higher recurrence rates may be the result of not continuing the dissection high enough and not entering the anterior peritoneal reflection. If prolapse recurs, repeated perineal rectosigmoidectomy can be performed.

Constipation is rarely a problem after perineal rectosigmoidectomy; rather, many patients will have transient incontinence because of resection of the rectal reservoir. The addition of posterior levatoroplasty, as advocated by Prasad et al.[61] may decrease the risk for postoperative incontinence.

Anastomotic dehiscence is rare and results from tension on the anastomosis or from poor blood supply. Therefore care must be taken to avoid undue tension on the anastomosis. Similarly, care must be taken to not ligate the mesentery too far above the redundant bowel.

Other complications, such as anastomotic stricture, are relatively uncommon. Minor narrowing at the anastomosis can usually be treated by dilation and bulking agents.

Delorme's Operation

Edmund Delorme, a French military surgeon, originally reported his operation for treatment of rectal prolapse in 1900.[96] The operation has had a resurgence in interest recently, because preservation of the rectal reservoir may improve continence. In the Delorme operation, the mucosa of the rectum is stripped circumferentially, the denuded rectal wall is plicated, and the mucosal edges are anastomosed (Fig. 17-5).

Recurrence rates of 0% to 30% have been reported (see Table 17-5). More proximal extension of the dissection may decrease the frequency of recurrence.[97] In general, if the mucosal tube is twice the length of the prolapse, the rate of recurrence is reduced.

As with perineal rectosigmoidectomy, constipation is rarely a problem, and fecal incontinence may be improved in 50% to 75% of patients.

Significant bleeding from the denuded rectum occurs in 1.5% of patients as a result of the extensive dissection and may be lessened with the use of electrocautery or a dilute saline-epinephrine solution.[65-75] Anastomotic complications, such as separation and stenosis, may be averted with the use of accurately placed plicating sutures and by prevention of tension on the anastomosis.

Anal Encirclement Procedures

With the increasing popularity and advantages of perineal rectosigmoidectomy and Delorme's operation, interest in anal encirclement procedures is largely historic only. The potential value of the anal encirclement procedures is that

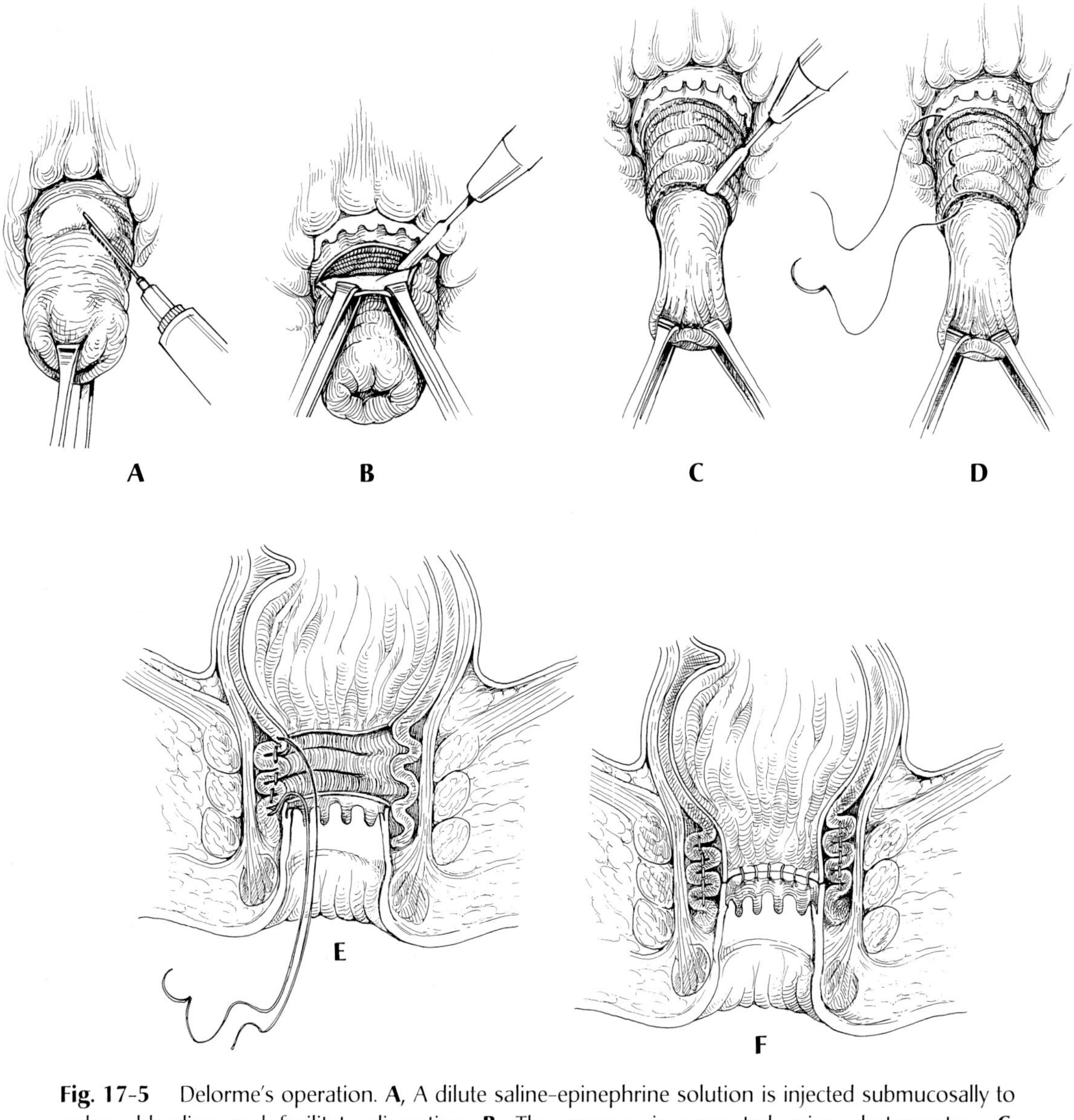

Fig. 17-5 Delorme's operation. **A**, A dilute saline-epinephrine solution is injected submucosally to reduce bleeding and facilitate dissection. **B**, The mucosa is separated using electrocautery. **C**, Circumferential stripping is continued as far cephalad as is possible. **D**, Before excision of the redundant mucosa, plicating sutures are placed in the circular muscle of the rectum. **E** and **F**, Plication is performed, the redundant mucosa amputated, and the mucosal anastomosis completed with absorbable suture.

Table 17-6 Encirclement procedures

Author	Year	No. of patients	Indication	Breakage	Erosion infection	Fecal impaction	No. removed
Metal							
Gabriel[98]	1953	25	I, P	7	11	0	4
Burke and Jackman[99]	1959	29	P	5	3	4	5
White[100]	1961	7	NS	0	1	0	1
Porter[57]	1962	100	P	16	12	4	4
Total (%)		161		28 (17)	27 (17)	8 (5)	14 (9)
Elastic							
Schwartz and Marin[101]	1962	11	P	2	0	0	3
Haskell and Rovner[102]	1963	12	P	0	4	0	3
Plumley[103]	1966	16	P	0	0	0	0
Baker[104]	1970	62	P	3	14	4	7
Lomas and Cooperman[105]	1972	25	I, P	0	6	0	1
Hopkinson and Hardman[106]	1973	16	P	0	3	3	0
Notaras[107]	1973	18	P	0	0	0	0
Jackman et al.[108]	1980	52	P	4	5	NS	1
Labow et al.[109]	1980	9	P	0	0	0	0
Horn et al.[110]	1985	16	I, P	0	4	0	4
Hunt et al.[111]	1985	41	P	3	15	5	4
Poole et al.[112]	1985	15	P	2	5	0	6
Larach and Vazquez[113]	1986	15	I, P	1	1	0	2
Khanduja et al.[114]	1988	16	I, P	3	2	0	0
Khalili and Fleshner[115]	1995	43	P	3	8	0	NS
Total (%)		367		21 (6)	67 (18)	12 (4)	31 (10)

I = incontinence; NS = not stated; P = prolapse.

they may be performed with use of local anesthesia and entail relatively minimal surgical trauma. Although Theirsch initially used silver wire to encircle the anus, other materials such as polypropylene or polyethylene mesh, Silastic tubing, monofilament nylon suture, Dacron-impregnated Silastic, and transposed gracilis muscle have all been used to encircle the anus. These procedures are performed by making two small incisions around the anus (either anterior and posterior or left and right lateral), tunneling the selected material around the anus, and securing it over a dilator or the surgeon's index finger.

The rate of complications associated with encirclement procedures is high (Table 17-6). Despite relatively short follow-up, breakage or erosion of the encircling material occurred in more than 25% of patients; in addition, fecal impaction and infection of the sling developed in a number of patients. Infection generally requires removal of the foreign material.

Mucosal prolapse occurs frequently, because the rectal prolapse has not been corrected; encirclement merely prevents it from passing beyond the anal verge. Recurrent full-thickness prolapse is common, and approximately 25% of patients require repeat surgery because of recurrence or other complications such as erosion or breakage of the sling.[116]

CONCLUSION

The ideal procedure for correction of complete rectal prolapse should result in low morbidity and rate of recurrence and improve the bowel disturbances often associated with rectal prolapse. As of yet, no such procedure has been described. Any procedure, whether abdominal or perineal, is associated with recurrence of rectal prolapse and some morbidity. The goal of the surgeon is to select the appropriate operation for each patient. Selection criteria should include the patient's age and fitness for surgery and degree of procedure-associated incontinence or constipation.

REFERENCES

1. Gordon PH, Hoexter B. Complications of the Ripstein procedure. Dis Colon Rectum 21: 277-280, 1978.
2. Eisenstat TE, Rubin RJ, Salvati EP. Surgical treatment of complete rectal prolapse. Dis Colon Rectum 22:522-523, 1979.
3. Romero-Torres R. Sacrofixation with Marlex mesh in massive prolapse of the rectum. Surg Gynecol Obstet 149:709-711, 1979.
4. Failes D, Killingback M, Stuart M, DeLuca C. Rectal prolapse. Aust N Z J Surg 49:72-75, 1979.
5. Hilsabeck JR. Transabdominal posterior proctopexy using an inverted T of synthetic material. Arch Surg 116:41-44, 1981.
6. Keighley MRB, Fielding JWL, Alexander-Williams J. Results of Marlex mesh abdominal rectopexy for rectal prolapse in 100 consecutive patients. Br J Surg 70:229-232, 1983.

7. Loygue J, Nordlinger B, Cunci O, Malafosse M, Huguet C, Parc R. Rectopexy to the promontory for the treatment of rectal prolapse: report of 257 cases. Dis Colon Rectum 27:356-359, 1984.
8. Holmstrom B, Broden G, Dolk A. Results of the Ripstein operation in the treatment of rectal prolapse and internal rectal procidentia. Dis Colon Rectum 29:845-848, 1986.
9. McMahan JD, Ripstein CB. Rectal prolapse: An update on the rectal sling procedure. Am Surg 53:37-40, 1987.
10. Roberts PL, Schoetz DJ Jr, Coller JA, Veidenheimer MC. Ripstein procedure. Lahey Clinic experience: 1963-1985. Arch Surg 123:554-557, 1988.
11. Sayfan J, Pinho M, Alexander-Williams J, Keighley MRB. Suture posterior abdominal rectopexy with sigmoidectomy compared with Marlex rectopexy for rectal prolapse. Br J Surg 77:143-145, 1990.
12. Speakman CTM, Madden MV, Nicholls RJ, Kamm MA. Lateral ligament division during rectopexy causes constipation but prevents recurrence: Results of a prospective randomized study. Br J Surg 78:1431-1433, 1991.
13. Luukkonen P, Mikkonen U, Jarvinen H. Abdominal rectopexy with sigmoidectomy vs. rectopexy alone for rectal prolapse: A prospective, randomized trial. Int J Colorect Dis 7: 219-222, 1992.
14. Duthie GS, Bartolo DCC. Abdominal rectopexy for rectal prolapse: A comparison of techniques. Br J Surg 79:107-113, 1992.
15. Tjandra JJ, Fazio VW, Church JM, Milsom JW, Oakley JR, Lavery IC. Ripstein procedure is an effective treatment for rectal prolapse without constipation. Dis Colon Rectum 36:501-507, 1993.
16. Winde G, Reers B, Nottberg H, Berns T, Meyer J, Bunte H. Clinical and functional results of abdominal rectopexy with absorbable mesh-graft for the treatment of complete rectal prolapse. Eur J Surg 159:301-305, 1993.
17. Scaglia M, Fasth S, Hallgren T, Nordgren S, Oresland T, Hulten L. Abdominal rectopexy for rectal prolapse: Influence of surgical technique on functional outcome. Dis Colon Rectum 37:805-813, 1994.
18. Morgan CN, Porter NH, Klugman DJ. Ivalon (polyvinyl alcohol) sponge in the repair of complete rectal prolapse. Br J Surg 59:841-846, 1972.
19. Penfold JC, Hawley PR. Experience of Ivalon-sponge implant for complete rectal prolapse at St. Mark's Hospital, 1960-70. Br J Surg 59:846-848, 1972.
20. Stewart R. Long-term results of Ivalon wrap operation for complete rectal prolapse. Proc R Soc Med 65:777-778, 1972.
21. Atkinson KG, Taylor DC. Wells procedure for complete rectal prolapse: A ten-year experience. Dis Colon Rectum 27:96-98, 1984.
22. Mann CV, Hoffman C. Complete rectal prolapse: The anatomical and functional results of treatment by extended abdominal rectopexy. Br J Surg 75:34-37, 1988.
23. McCue JL, Thomson JPS. Clinical and functional results of abdominal rectopexy for complete rectal prolapse. Br J Surg 78:921-923, 1991.
24. Reference deleted in galleys.
25. Novell JR, Osborne MJ, Winslet MC, Lewis AAM. Prospective randomized trial of Ivalon sponge versus sutured rectopexy for full-thickness rectal prolapse. Br J Surg 81:904-906, 1994.
26. Scaglia M, Fasth S, Hallgren T, Nordgren S, Oresland T, Hulten L. Abdominal rectopexy for rectal prolapse: Influence of surgical technique on functional outcome. Dis Colon Rectum 37:805-813, 1994.
27. Kirkman NF. Procidentia of the rectum: Results of abdominal rectopexy in the elderly. Dis Colon Rectum 18:470-472, 1975.

28. Carter AE. Rectosacral suture fixation for complete rectal prolapse in the elderly, the frail and the demented. Br J Surg 70:522-523, 1983.
29. Blatchford GJ, Perry RE, Thorson AG, Christensen MA. Rectopexy without resection for rectal prolapse. Am J Surg 158:574-576, 1989.
30. McKee RF, Lauder JC, Poon FW, Aitchison MA, Finlay IG. A prospective randomized study of abdominal rectopexy with and without sigmoidectomy in rectal prolapse. Surg Gynecol Obstet 174:145-148, 1992.
31. Wolff BG, Dietzen CD. Abdominal resectional procedures for rectal prolapse. Semin Colon Rectal Surg 2:184-186, 1991.
32. Cirocco WC, Brown AC. Anterior resection for the treatment of rectal prolapse: A 20-year experience. Am Surg 59:265-269, 1993.
33. Watts JD, Rothenberger DA, Buls JG, Goldberg SM, Nivatvongs S. The management of procidentia: 30 years' experience. Dis Colon Rectum 28:96-102, 1985.
34. Sayfan J, Pinho M, Alexander-Williams J, Keighley MRB. Suture posterior abdominal rectopexy with sigmoidectomy compared with Marlex rectopexy for rectal prolapse. Br J Surg 77:143-145, 1990.
35. Luukkonen P, Mikkonen U, Jarvinen H. Abdominal rectopexy with sigmoidectomy vs. rectopexy alone for rectal prolapse: A prospective, randomized trial. Int J Colorect Dis 7:219-222, 1992.
36. Madoff RD, Williams JG, Wong WD, Rothenberger DA, Goldberg SM. Long-term functional results of colon resection and rectopexy for overt rectal prolapse. Am J Gastroenterol 87:101-104, 1992.
37. Tjandra JJ, Fazio VW, Church JM, Milsom JW, Oakley JR, Lavery IC. Ripstein procedure is an effective treatment for rectal prolapse without constipation. Dis Colon Rectum 36:501-507, 1993.
38. Deen KI, Grant E, Billingham C, Keighley MRB. Abdominal resection rectopexy with pelvic floor repair versus perineal rectosigmoidectomy and pelvic floor repair for full-thickness rectal prolapse. Br J Surg 81:302-304, 1994.
39. Berman IR. Sutureless laparoscopic rectopexy for procidentia: Technique and implications. Dis Colon Rectum 35:689-693, 1992.
40. Kusminsky RE, Tiley EH, Boland JP. Laparoscopic Ripstein procedure. Surg Laparosc Endosc 2:346-347, 1992.
41. Munro W, Avramovic J, Roney W. Laparoscopic rectopexy. J Laparoendosc Surg 3:55-58, 1993.
42. Cuesta MA, Borgstein PJ, deJong D, Meijer S. Laparoscopic rectopexy. Surg Laparosc Endosc 3:456-458, 1993.
43. Kwok SP, Carey DP, Lau WY, Li AKC. Laparoscopic rectopexy. Dis Colon Rectum 37:947-948, 1994.
44. Cushieri A, Shimi SM, Vander Velpen G, Banting S, Wood RAB. Laparoscopic prosthesis fixation rectopexy for complete rectal prolapse. Br J Surg 81:138-139, 1994.
45. Eu KW, Milsom JW, Hull T, Fazio VW. Laparoscopic suture rectopexy for rectal prolapse without constipation. [abst]. Dis Colon Rectum 38:P24, 1995.
46. Ballantyne GH. Laparoscopically assisted anterior resection for rectal prolapse. Surg Laparosc Endosc 2:230-236, 1992.
47. Senagore AJ, Luchtefeld MA, MacKeigan JM. Rectopexy. J Laparoendosc Surg 3:339-343, 1993.
48. Baker R, Senagore AJ, Luchtefeld MA. Laparoscopic-assisted vs. open resection: Rectopexy offers excellent results. Dis Colon Rectum 38:199-201, 1995.
49. Gordon PH, Hoexter B. Complications of the Ripstein procedure. Dis Colon Rectum 21:277-280, 1978.

50. Roberts PL, Schoetz DJ Jr, Coller JA, Veidenheimer MC. Ripstein procedure. Lahey Clinic experience: 1963-1985. Arch Surg 123:554-557, 1988.
51. Qinyao W, Weijin S, Youren Z, Wenqing Z, Zhengrui H. New concepts in severe presacral hemorrhage during proctectomy. Arch Surg 120:1013-1020, 1985.
52. Nivatvongs S, Fang DT. The use of thumbtacks to stop massive presacral hemorrhage. Dis Colon Rectum 29:589-590, 1986.
53. Timmons MC, Kohler MF, Addison WA. Thumbtack use for control of presacral bleeding, with description of an instrument for thumbtack application. Obstet Gynecol 78:313-315, 1991.
54. Stolfi VM, Milsom JW, Lavery IC, Oakley JR, Church JM, Fazio VW. Newly designed occluder pin for presacral hemorrhage. Dis Colon Rectum 35:166-169, 1992.
55. Xu J, Lin J. Control of presacral hemorrhage with electrocautery through a muscle fragment pressed on the bleeding vein. J Am Coll Surg 179:351-352, 1994.
56. Hughes ESR. Discussion on rectal prolapse. Proc R Soc Med 42:1007-1011, 1949.
57. Porter N. Collective results of operations for rectal prolapse. Proc R Soc Med 55:1087 1092, 1962.
58. Altemeier WA, Culbertson WR, Schowengerdt C, Hunt J. Nineteen years' experience with one-stage perineal repair of rectal prolapse. Ann Surg 173:993-1006, 1971.
59. Friedman R, Muggia-Sulam M, Freund HR. Experience with the one-stage perineal repair of rectal prolapse. Dis Colon Rectum 26:789-791, 1983.
60. Gopal KA, Amshel AL, Shonberg IL, Eftaiha M. Rectal procidentia in elderly and debilitated patients. Experience with the Altemeier procedure. Dis Colon Rectum 27:376-381, 1984.
61. Prasad ML, Pearl ML, Abcarian H, Orsay CP, Nelson RL. Perineal proctectomy, posterior rectopexy and postanal levator repair for the treatment of rectal prolapse. Dis Colon Rectum 29:547-552, 1986.
62. Williams JG, Rothenberger DA, Madoff RD, Goldberg SM. Treatment of rectal prolapse in the elderly by perineal rectosigmoidectomy. Dis Colon Rectum 35:830-834, 1992.
63. Johansen OB, Wexner SD, Daniel N, Nogueras JJ, Jagelman DG. Perineal rectosigmoidectomy in the elderly. Dis Colon Rectum 36:767-772, 1993.
64. Ramanujam PS, Venkatesh KS, Fietz MJ. Perineal excision of rectal procidentia in elderly high-risk patients. Dis Colon Rectum 37:1027-1030, 1994.
65. Swinton NW, Palmer TE. The management of rectal prolapse and procidentia. Am J Surg 99:144-151, 1960.
66. Nay HR, Blair CR. Perineal surgical repair of rectal prolapse. Am J Surg 123:577-579, 1972.
67. Uhlig BE, Sullivan ES. The modified Delorme operation: Its place in the surgical treatment for massive rectal prolapse. Dis Colon Rectum 22:513-521, 1979.
68. Christiansen J, Kirkegaard P. Delorme's operation for complete rectal prolapse. Br J Surg 68:537-538, 1981.
69. Gundersen AL, Cogvill TH, Landercasper J. Reappraisal of Delorme's operation for rectal prolapse. Dis Colon Rectum 28:721-724, 1985.
70. Monson JRT, Jones NAG, Vowden P, Brennan TG. Delorme's operation: The first choice in complete rectal prolapse. Ann R Coll Surg Engl 68:143-146, 1986.
71. Houry S, Lechaux JP, Huguier M, Molkhou JM. Treatment of rectal prolapse by Delorme's operation. Int J Colorect Dis 2:149-152, 1987.
72. Abulafi AM, Fiddian RV, Sherman IW, Rothwell-Jackson RL. Delorme's operation for rectal prolapse. Ann R Coll Surg Engl 72:382-385, 1990.
73. Senapati A, Nicholls RJ, Thomson JPS, Phillips RKS. Results of Delorme's procedure for rectal prolapse. Dis Colon Rectum 37:456-460, 1994.
74. Oliver GC, Vachon D, Eisenstat TE, Rubin RJ, Salvati EP. Delorme's procedure for complete rectal prolapse in severely debilitated patients: An analysis of 41 cases. Dis Colon Rectum 37:461-467, 1994.

75. Lechaux JP, Lechaux D, Perez M. Results of Delorme's procedure for rectal prolapse: Advantages of a modified technique. Dis Colon Rectum 38:301-307, 1995.
76. Keighley MRB, Makuria T, Alexander-Williams J, Arabi Y. Clinical and manometric evaluation of rectal prolapse and incontinence. Br J Surg 67:54-56, 1980.
77. Hiltunen KM, Matikainen M. Improvement of continence after rectopexy for rectal prolapse. Int J Colorect Dis 7:8-10, 1992.
78. Duthie GS, Farouk R, Bartolo DCC. The functional results of surgery for rectal prolapse. Semin Colon Rectal Surg 2:205-211, 1991.
79. Farouk R, Duthie GS, Bartolo DCC, MacGregor AB. Restoration of continence following rectopexy for rectal prolapse and recovery of the internal anal sphincter electromyogram. Br J Surg 79:439-440, 1992.
80. Spencer RJ. Manometric studies in rectal prolapse. Dis Colon Rectum 27:523-525, 1984.
81. Failes D, Killingback M, Stuart M, DeLuca C. Rectal prolapse. Aust N Z J Surg 49:72-75, 1979.
82. Keighley MRB, Fielding JWL, Alexander-Williams J. Results of Marlex mesh abdominal rectopexy for rectal prolapse in 100 consecutive patients. Br J Surg 70:229-232, 1983.
83. Ahlback S, Broden B, Broden G, Ewerth S, Holmstrom B. Rectal anatomy following Ripstein's operation for prolapse studied by cineradiography. Dis Colon Rectum 22:333-335, 1979.
84. Siproudhis L, Ropert A, Gosselin A, Bertagne JF, Heresbach D, Raoul J, Gosselin M. Constipation after rectopexy for rectal prolapse. Where is the obstruction? Dig Dis Sci 38:1801-1808, 1993.
85. Speakman CTM, Madden MV, Nicholls RJ, Kamm MA. Lateral ligament division during rectopexy causes constipation but prevents recurrence: Results of a prospective randomized study. Br J Surg 78:1431-1433, 1991.
86. Orr TG. A suspension operation for prolapse of the rectum. Ann Surg 126:833-842, 1947.
87. Loygue J, Nordlinger B, Cunci O, Malafosse M, Huguet C, Parc R. Rectopexy to the promontory for the treatment of rectal prolapse: Report of 257 cases. Dis Colon Rectum 27:356-359, 1984.
88. Ripstein CB. Surgical care of massive rectal prolapse. Dis Colon Rectum 8:34-38, 1965.
89. Winde G, Reers B, Nottberg H, Berns T, Meyer J, Bunte H. Clinical and functional results of abdominal rectopexy with absorbable mesh–graft for the treatment of complete rectal prolapse. Eur J Surg 159:301-305, 1993.
90. Lescher TJ, Corman ML, Coller JA, Veidenheimer MC. Management of late complications of Teflon sling repair for rectal prolapse. Dis Colon Rectum 22:445-447, 1979.
91. McMahan JD, Ripstein CB. Rectal prolapse: An update on the rectal sling procedure. Am Surg 53:37-40, 1987.
92. Wells C. New operation for rectal prolapse. Proc R Soc Med 52:602-603, 1959.
93. Muir EG. Rectal prolapse: Presidential address. Proc R Soc Med 48:33-44, 1955.
94. Schlinkert RT, Beart RW, Wolff BG, Pemberton JH. Anterior resection for complete rectal prolapse. Dis Colon Rectum 28:409-412, 1985.
95. Mikulicz J. Zur operativen behandlung des prolapsus Recti et Coli invaginati. Arch Klin Chir 38:74, 1889.
96. Delorme E. On the treatment of total prolapse of the rectum by excision of the rectal mucous membranes or rectocolic. Dis Colon Rectum 28:544-553, 1985.
97. Williams JG. Perineal approaches to repair of rectal prolapse. Semin Colon Rectal Surg 2:198-204, 1991.
98. Gabriel WB. Theirsch's operation for anal incontinence and minor degrees of rectal prolapse. Am J Surg 86:583-590, 1953.
99. Burke RM, Jackman RJ. A modified Theirsch operation in the treatment of complete rectal prolapse. Dis Colon Rectum 2:555-561, 1959.

100. White MEE. Operation for rectal prolapse using stainless steel ring. Lancet 1:858-859, 1961.
101. Schwartz A, Marin R. Use of polyethylene in the Theirsch operation. Dis Colon Rectum 5:302-305, 1962.
102. Haskell B, Rovner H. A modified Theirsch operation for complete rectal prolapse using a Teflon prosthesis. Dis Colon Rectum 6:192-195, 1963.
103. Plumley P. A modification to Theirsch's operation for rectal prolapse. Br J Surg 53:624-625, 1966.
104. Baker WNM. Results of using a monofilament nylon in Theirsch's operation for rectal prolapse. Br J Surg 57:37-39, 1970.
105. Lomas MI, Cooperman H. Correction of rectal procidentia by use of polypropylene mesh (Marlex). Dis Colon Rectum 15:416-419, 1972.
106. Hopkinson BR, Hardman J. Silicone rubber perianal suture for rectal prolapse. Proc R Soc Med 66:1095-1098, 1973.
107. Notaras MJ. The use of Mersilene mesh in rectal prolapse repair. Proc R Soc Med 66:684 686, 1973.
108. Jackman FR, Francis JN, Hopkinson BR. Silicone rubber band treatment of rectal prolapse. Ann R Coll Surg Engl 62:386-387, 1980.
109. Labow S, Rubin RJ, Hoexter B, Salvati EP. Perineal repair of rectal procidentia with an elastic fabric sling. Dis Colon Rectum 23:467-468, 1980.
110. Horn HR, Schoetz DJ Jr, Coller JA, Veidenheimer MC. Sphincter repair with a Silastic sling for anal incontinence and rectal procidentia. Dis Colon Rectum 28:868-872, 1985.
111. Hunt TM, Fraser IA, Maybury NK. Treatment of rectal prolapse by sphincter support using Silastic rods. Br J Surg 72:491-492, 1985.
112. Poole GV Jr, Pennell TC, Myers RD, Hightower F. Modified Theirsch operation for rectal prolapse. Am Surg 51:226-229, 1985.
113. Larach SW, Vazquez B. Modified Theirsch procedure with Silastic mesh implant: A simple solution for fecal incontinence and severe prolapse. South Med J 79:307-309, 1986.
114. Khanduja KS, Hardy TG, Aquilar PS, Plasencia G, Hartmann RF, Bowers F, Stewart WRC. A new silicone prosthesis in the modified Theirsch operation. Dis Colon Rectum 31:380-383, 1988.
115. Khalili T, Fleshner PR. Anal encirclement procedures for rectal prolapse: The final chapter [abst]. Dis Colon Rectum 38:P10-11, 1995.
116. Heine JA, Wong WD. Rectal prolapse. In Mazier WP, Levien DH, Luchtefeld MA, Senagore AJ, eds. Surgery of the Colon, Rectum and Anus. Philadelphia: WB Saunders, 1995, pp 515-537.
117. Eisentat TE, Rubin RJ, Salvati EP. Surgical treatment of complete rectal prolapse. Dis Colon Rectum 22:522-523, 1979.
118. Romero-Torres R. Sacrofixation with Marlex mesh in massive prolapse of the rectum. Surg Gynecol Obstet 149:709-711, 1979.
119. Hilsabeck JR. Transabdominal posterior proctopexy using an inverted T of synthetic material. Arch Surg 116:41-44, 1981.
120. Holmstrom B, Broden G, Dolk A. Results of the Ripstein operation in the treatment of rectal prolapse and internal rectal procidentia. Dis Colon Rectum 29:845-848, 1986.

CHAPTER 18

Small Bowel Resection and Strictureplasty

JAMES M. CHURCH

Small bowel is most commonly resected as part of a right colectomy, or ileocolic resection, for cancer or Crohn's disease. Isolated small bowel resection is less common and is mainly performed in the treatment of five conditions: small bowel obstruction due to adhesions, complications of Crohn's enteritis, complications of radiation enteritis, small bowel involvement with tumors, and vascular disorders such as ischemia, infarction, or hemorrhage (Table 18-1). (The proportions of each of these diagnoses will of course vary according to the practice patterns of individual surgeons and hospitals.) Complications of small bowel surgery are an important cause of morbidity. Some are technical, independent of the underlying diagnosis, some are disease related, and some are the result of unwise decision making during surgery. In addition to procedural complications of small bowel resection, there may be metabolic sequelae.

In this chapter we will discuss complications of isolated small bowel resection. Ileocolic resection is not specifically addressed, although most of the principles apply equally to it. Measures for the prevention and management of complications are outlined, and a section of the chapter is devoted to strictureplasty.

TECHNICAL COMPLICATIONS

Sound technique is important in preventing complications in all areas of surgery and is no less important in procedures carried out on the small bowel. The consequences of technical complications, which can usually be easily prevented, may prove to be disastrous for the patient. The technique of small bowel resection includes mobilization, resection, and anastomosis. The complications of each component will be considered separately in this chapter. As can be seen in the box on p. 264 and Fig. 18-1, most serious complications are related to the anastomosis.

Table 18-1 Author's personal experience with small bowel resection, 1989 to 1993

Indication	No. of patients (N = 54)	Complication (n = 11)	Treatment
Crohn's disease	21	Enterocutaneous fistula (n = 3)	Repair (n = 2)
		1 Prolonged ileus (n = 1)	TPN (n = 1)
		Short bowel syndrome (n = 1)	
Resection with ileostomy closure	6	None	
Familial polyposis (desmoid tumor)	6	Abscess (n = 1)	Diversion/TPN
(Kock pouch excision, n = 3)		Short bowel syndrome (n = 1)	
Radiation enteritis	4	None	
Colon cancer metastasis	3	None	
Vascular malformations	3	None	
Infarction or ischemia	3	Enterocutaneous fistula (n = 1)	TPN, octreotide acetate
		Short bowel syndrome (n = 2)	
Enterocutaneous fistula	3	Short bowel syndrome (n = 1)	
Lymphoma	2	None	
Ileitis (unspecified)	1	None	
Adhesion or obstruction	2	None	

TECHNICAL COMPLICATIONS OF SMALL BOWEL RESECTION

- Leaking anastomosis
- Ischemic anastomosis
- Stenotic anastomosis
- Dysfunctional anastomosis
- Bleeding anastomosis
- Mesenteric hemorrhage
- Hernia through mesenteric defect
- Missed enterotomy

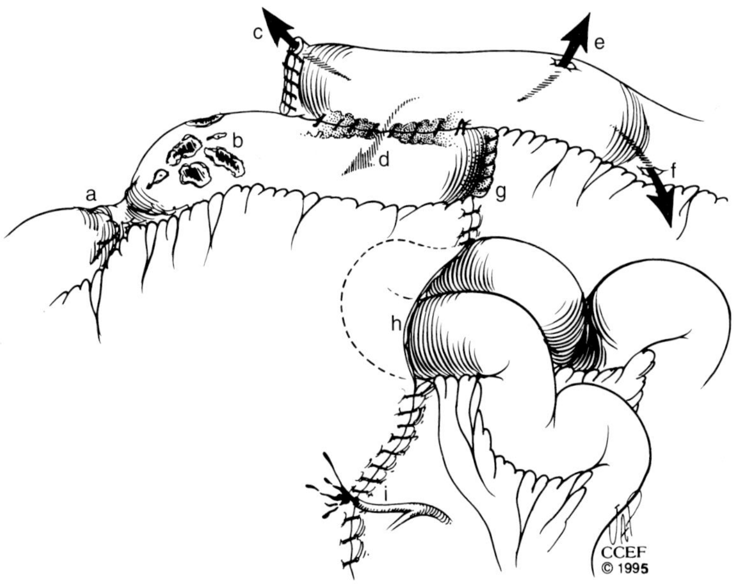

Fig. 18-1 Common complications of small bowel resection: *a,* downstream obstruction predisposing to anastomotic leak; *b,* serosal tears; *c,* defect at oversewn end (a common site of a leak); *d,* strictured anastomosis; *e,* inadvertent enterotomy; *f,* damage from occluding tape; *g,* ischemic bowel end; *h,* hernia through mesentery; *i,* hemorrhage from mesenteric vessel.

Mobilization

Mobilization of small bowel is easy in the case of a patient who has not undergone previous abdominal surgery, because the only adhesions will be disease related or congenital (usually some minor tethering of the terminal ileum to the brim of the pelvis). In patients who have undergone previous abdominal surgery, the severity and density of adhesions range from obliterative peritonitis to no adhesions at all. Most patients have some adhesions, and correct technique in dissecting them is important to prevent inadvertent enterotomy or serosal tears.

In mobilizing the small bowel, several complications can occur. An enterotomy or hole in the bowel can occur when the bowel is cut or torn. A tear usually occurs because excess force is applied during retraction of the bowel. The small bowel is at particular risk when the abdomen is opened through an old incision or when dense adhesions bind it in an area that is relatively inaccessible (such as deep in the pelvis). When possible, the abdomen is opened through an area not previously operated on. If this is not possible, the fascia is carefully and gradually incised through the least indurated part of the wound. Hemostasis is maintained, and the abdominal wall is elevated with clamps or retractors. A sharp scalpel, scissors, or electrocautery is used to divide the adhesions. It is better to leave some fascia on the bowel rather than risk bowel injury.

Mobilization of the small bowel is most difficult when it must be performed 10 to 30 days after a previous laparotomy. The development of intra-abdominal adhesions is most vigorous during this time, and there is a possibility of surgeons doing more harm than good. Therefore most surgeons attempt to avoid repeat laparotomy for at least 30 days.

It is important to assess the fragility of the bowel and density of the adhesions to determine how easily the bowel will tear and how gently it must be handled. Chronically obstructed or inflamed bowel is more fragile than normal bowel. Filmy adhesions may be squeezed or gently pulled apart; denser adhesions are approached frontally and divided with sharp dissection with blunt-tipped scissors (e.g., Harrington) or electrocautery. Small snips are made to develop a feel for where the bowel edge is. Adhesions are isolated by gentle squeezing. If division of an adhesion proves too difficult, attention should be directed elsewhere. If dissection at the front of the adhesions is difficult, the posterior area of the adhesion should be examined. The dissection should also be kept close to the small bowel wall to minimize the chances of damaging adjacent organs. The surgeon must be particularly careful when dissecting small bowel that is adherent to the pelvis as a result of previous pelvic surgery. In repeat pelvic surgery, ureteric stents should be considered. These stents enhance recognition of ureteric damage when it occurs.

In case of enterotomy, fecal spill must be minimized. Bare spots or enterotomies should be marked with sutures or repaired when they occur. To repair an enterotomy, enough small bowel is mobilized to allow the enterotomy to be closed without tension. The ragged edges are trimmed to remove all fascia, tumor, or devitalized tissue. The hole is repaired transversely with interrupted seromuscular absorbable sutures (e.g., 3-0 polyglycolic acid). Proper placement of the sutures avoids gaps in the suture line. After mobilization and before construction of an anastomosis, the at-risk bowel is tested to ensure that all repairs are watertight and all enterotomies are identified.

Partial loss of serosa and muscle (tear) occurs more frequently than enterotomy. In evaluation of a serosal tear, it is important to note the depth of the defect. If adequate muscle is left intact, no repair is necessary. If the mucosa protrudes through the defect in the muscle and serosa, the injury should be repaired. Injuries of intermediate depth should also be repaired if possible. If the repair narrows or distorts the bowel or if the area of the defect is too wide to cover, the segment of bowel should be resected. All repairs should be tested.

The bowel mesentery can also be damaged or cut during mobilization, especially when two adjacent bowel loops are adherent. Careful retraction helps avoid inadvertent incision or tearing of mesenteric vessels. This is especially important with the fragile tissue in elderly patients or those receiving long-term steroid therapy. The surgeon must also be especially careful when the "hard part" is over, because there is a tendency to relax, which increases the chances of a complication.

Small, easily identifiable mesenteric hemorrhages can be controlled with electrocautery. Spurting arteries are underrun with precisely placed sutures. The bowel adjacent to mesenteric damage is evaluated to assess its viability. Any hole in the mesentery capable of accommodating a loop of bowel is repaired. Division of the mesentery can lead to troublesome hemorrhage if arteries are not clamped and sutured. Attempts to stop the bleeding can compromise the blood supply of the adjacent bowel.

When adhesions are particularly dense, other organs can be damaged during mobilization of the small bowel. Those at particular risk include the ureter, ovaries, fallopian tubes, and large bowel. If the adhesions are too difficult to dissect and frequent enterotomies are produced, it may be prudent to terminate the operation. The new enterotomies should be repaired, and the most distal loop of bowel available can be used to create a stoma. The fold of Treves (the antimesenteric or dorsal fatty attachment of the terminal ileum) is useful to identify the terminal ileum in an extremely adhesed abdomen. If the created stoma is high in the jejunum, the patient may require home total parenteral nutrition (TPN) for a time. Although not a preferred option, this method of management allows the patient to survive with minimal loss of bowel (Fig. 18-2).

Small bowel adhesions can lead to bowel obstruction. Failure to identify and correct bowel obstruction downstream from an anastomosis can result in an anastomotic leak. To avoid missed adhesions the small bowel is "run" to ensure that it is normal and there are no potentially obstructing kinks. Nonobstructing

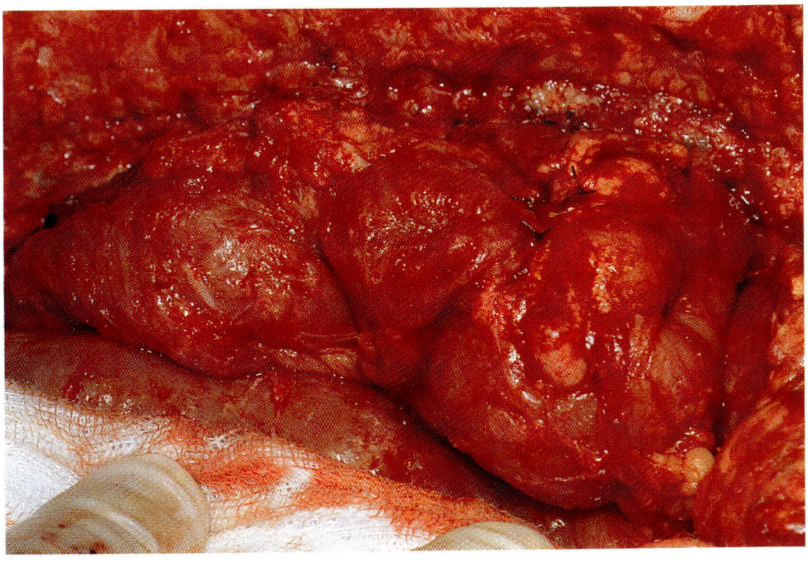

Fig. 18-2 Obliterative, dense adhesions of small bowel to the midline incision in a patient with familial polyposis and desmoid tumors who underwent repeat surgery 14 days after small bowel resection. Adhesiolysis was abandoned, and a jejunostomy was made.

A

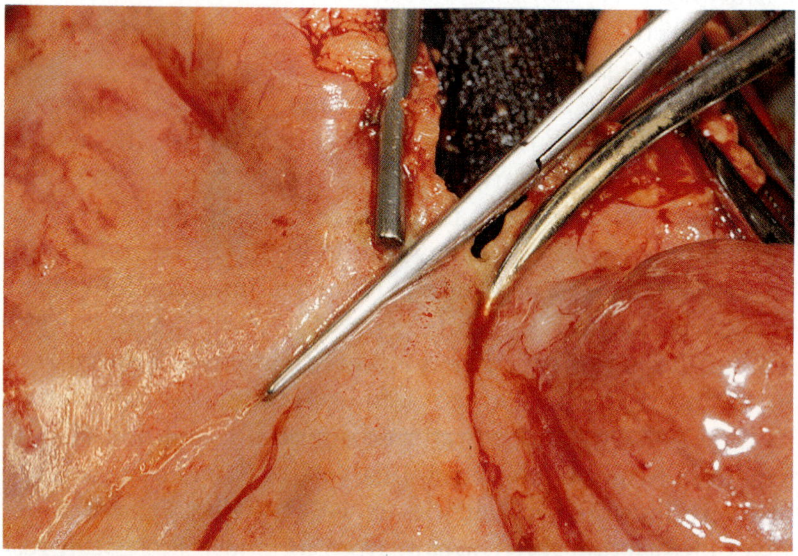

B

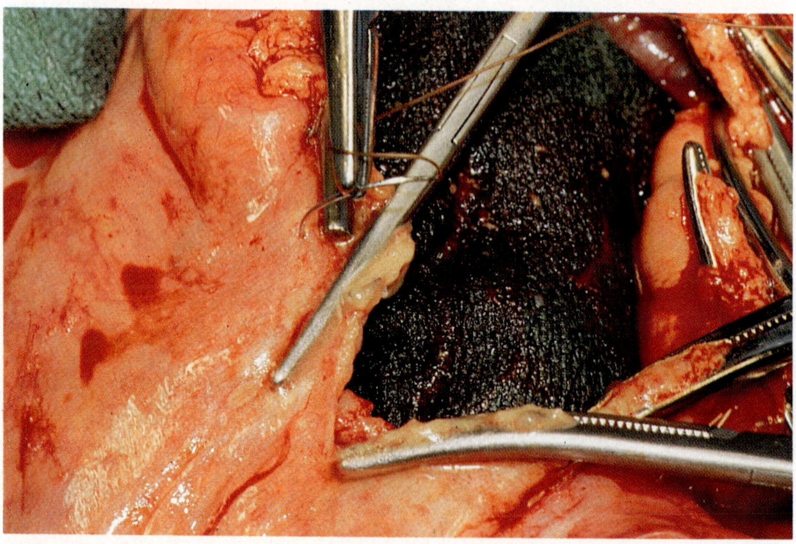

Fig. 18-3 Technique for dividing thick mesentery. **A,** The mesentery is divided with overlapping toothed clamps on the patient side. **B,** Each clamp is suture-ligated, with care taken to ensure that suture ligatures overlap tissue contained in each.

adhesions in normal bowel can be left alone. As stated previously, the small bowel downstream of an anastomosis or repair is mobilized to identify and deal with any potentially obstructing band.

Resection

After the length of bowel to be resected is mobilized, the resection can proceed. This involves division of the mesentery and bowel.

Failure to control the mesenteric vessels leads to mesenteric hemorrhage. This leads to unnecessary loss of blood, makes the operation untidy, and wastes time. Delayed mesenteric hemorrhage can be life threatening. An expanding mesenteric hematoma occurs when an artery slips out of a tie and bleeds into the mesentery below the line of resection. This is more likely when thick mesenteries are ligated with simple ties but can be prevented with suture ligation of the thickened mesentery in small "bites" an adequate distance proximal to the occluding clamp. An expanding mesenteric hematoma can be managed by incising the mesenteric peritoneum and religating the mesentery with sutures below the hematoma.

Thick or fatty mesentery should be divided in small steps and controlled with suture ligatures (Fig. 18-3). Transilluminating the mesentery helps to identify windows and vessels. The peritoneum needs to be incised carefully over the mesentery. The vessels can be isolated with blunt dissection. The mesenteric resection line should be designed as a wedge but should not approach the base of the mesentery unless necessary or malignancy is suspected. Extra care must be taken when loops of bowel have been previously isolated for ileal conduits or ileal reservoirs. These loops may be devascularized with careless mesenteric resection.

The superior mesenteric vein can be ligated inadvertently during blind attempts to suture-ligate bleeding from the base of the small bowel mesentery. This complication carries a high morbidity and mortality (Fig. 18-4) and can be prevented by not suturing near the base of the mesentery. If the vein is damaged, the injury should be isolated and repaired with precisely placed vascular sutures.

If mesenteric division undermines the bowel ends they can become ischemic, which predisposes to anastomotic failure. Fresh bleeding from the bowel edges confirms adequate vascularity. If there is any doubt, excision of additional bowel should be performed. If large segments of mesentery are contained in each clamp and ligature, the mesentery will be appreciably shortened. This "concertina-like" mesentery may cause distortion of the anastomosis and tension at the bowel ends.

Some surgeons use tape to occlude the lumen on either side of the resection. The tape is passed through the mesentery, just underneath the bowel wall. It is possible to damage the bowel wall when inserting the tape, causing a stricture or perforation. If the tape is not removed, bowel obstruction is inevitable. It is

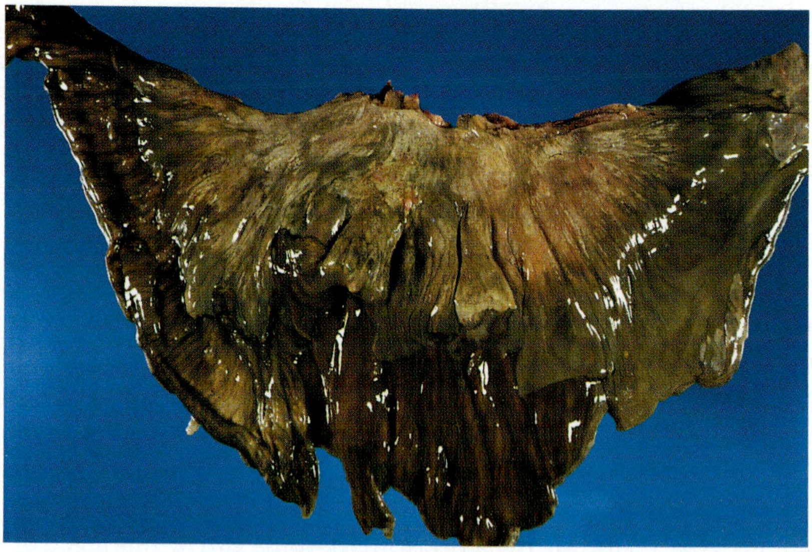

Fig. 18-4 Complete necrosis of the small bowel resulting from thrombosis of the superior mesenteric vein. The patient survived with a duodenocolic anastomosis but requires permanent home parenteral nutrition.

therefore a good idea to place a clamp on the tape to prevent it from being forgotten. When the tape is removed, it should be checked for yellow-green-brown discoloration. Staining of this type may come from stool, which suggests bowel perforation.

Anastomosis

Anastomosis is the part of the small bowel resection procedure associated with the highest risk for complications. Some of the many ways to join two ends of small bowel together are shown in Figs. 18-5 and 18-6. The simplest and least costly method is to suture the two bowel ends together with absorbable sutures. Staplers have the advantage of speed, but their use means relatively distorted side-to-side or end-to-side anastomoses (see Fig. 18-5), multiple (sometimes overlapping) staple lines, and added expense. Aside from technical matters, the health of the patient and of the bowel ends are the important factors in determining the risk for complications.

Leakage of stool through an anastomotic suture or staple line is one of the worst complications of small bowel resection. If the leak is not contained, peritonitis and sepsis will develop. If the leak is contained, an abscess or delayed fistula may develop. Anastomotic leaks may be immediate or delayed, related to technique or disease, and be detected at clinical or radiologic examination.

Immediate leakage suggests a technical cause such as a gap in the suture line from misplacement of sutures or misfire of the stapler, or an enterotomy or tear

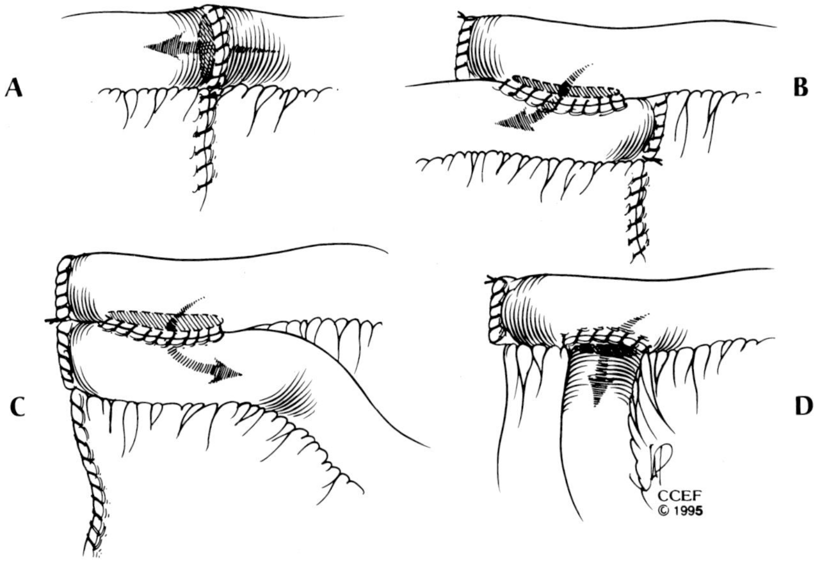

Fig. 18-5 Methods of anastomosing bowel after resection. **A,** End-to-end (usually hand sutured). **B,** Side-to-side, isoperistaltic (stapled). **C,** Side-to-side, antiperistaltic (stapled). **D,** End-to-side; used when bowel ends are of differing diameter (stapled).

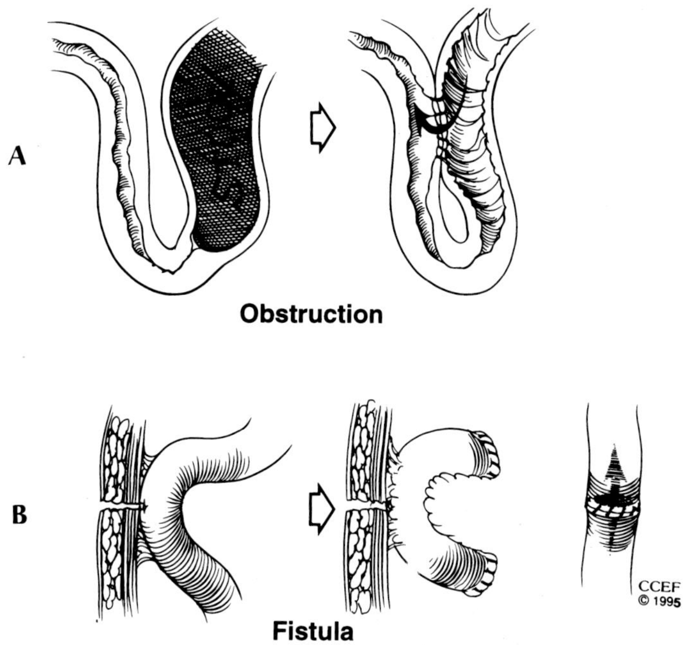

Fig. 18-6 Methods of anastomosing small bowel in a bypass procedure. **A,** Side-to-side when bypassing an obstruction. **B,** End-to-end in an exclusion bypass of a fistula.

near the suture line. Delayed leakage is probably related to disease such as ischemia or distal obstruction. This becomes apparent when the diseased bowel sloughs or when resolution of postoperative ileus places stress on the suture line.

Small leaks may be contained and manifest with muted or absent clinical signs. In low anterior resections of the rectum, there is a well-documented incidence of "subclinical" leakage[1] and this probably occurs with small bowel anastomoses as well. It is much easier to detect small leaks from a colorectal anastomosis with barium contrast studies than to detect leaks from a small bowel anastomosis with small bowel contrast studies, so their true incidence in the small bowel in unknown. Large leaks from a small bowel anastomosis usually cause peritonitis or large abscesses (Fig. 18-7), although this is not always the case. An anastomosis also may leak when an inflammatory mass drains into the bowel through the anastomosis. This can occur after resection of a perforated bowel with an associated abscess. An inflammatory "nest" of granulation tissue is sometimes left behind (Fig. 18-8). This can produce a recurrent abscess that may drain into a nearby anastomosis, producing an apparent leak.

Before constructing an anastomosis, it is wise to consider whether to perform the anastomosis in the first place or whether the anastomosis should be protected by diversion of stool. Factors that enter into this consideration are discussed in detail later.

To minimize the chances of an anastomotic leak, it is important to ensure that the bowel ends are intact, viable, and without active disease. Extra care is needed if there is a discrepancy in the bowel diameters. Obstructed, thickened or inflamed bowel should be sutured with an inverting technique. Doubtful areas are reinforced. I reinforce stapled-over ends of the bowel with a continuous 3-0 polyglycolic acid suture. The anastomosis is tested whenever possible by instilling saline solution and air under pressure to identify any small inadvertent or unrecognized enterotomies. Omentum is also placed around the anastomosis if feasible. Other important considerations are to exclude downstream obstruction and to avoid placing the anastomosis near an abscess cavity or inflammatory "nest." If there is a "nest," the anastomosis should be separated from the inflammation with omentum or a Silastic dam. One should strongly consider not performing an anastomosis at all.

Management of an anastomotic leak depends on its presentation. The early, obvious leak is characterized by the appearance of stool through the wound or in drains during the first postoperative week or the development of peritonitis. Any of these findings is an indication for laparotomy, during which the perforation is treated on its merits. Depending on the status of the patient and the bowel, the leak is repaired, resected, exteriorized, or defunctioned. If repair or resection is performed, it is wise to create a proximal diverting stoma.[2]

A B

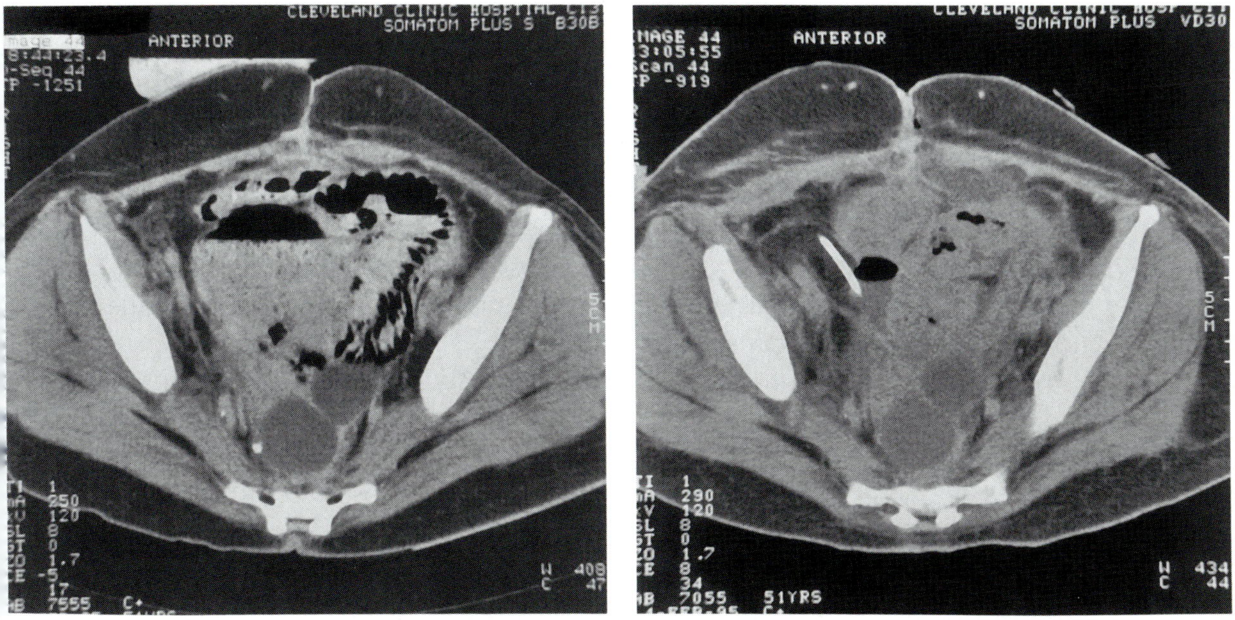

Fig. 18-7 **A,** CT scan of the abdomen shows a large abscess that formed 2 weeks after small bowel resection. **B,** The abscess has been drained percutaneously with CT guidance. The patient required a proximal diverting jejunostomy and home parenteral nutrition.

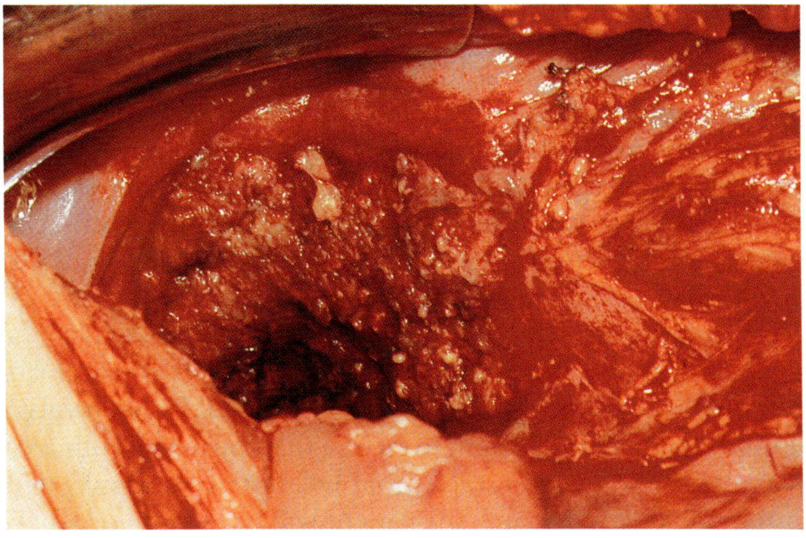

Fig. 18-8 An inflammatory "nest" left in the pelvis after resection of a loop of inflamed small bowel in a patient with Crohn's disease. An anastomosis was made but was separated from the nest with a Silastic dam.

Less obvious leaks are mainifested by postoperative fever and abdominal pain but no peritonitis. An abdominal CT scan may show a phlegmon or abscess (see Fig. 18-7, *A*). An abscess may be percutaneously drained[2,3] (see Fig. 18-7, *B*). If drainage and antibiotic therapy fail to resolve the fever and pain, proximal diversion of stool is necessary.

Most late leaks are manifested as an enterocutaneous fistula and are also managed according to their symptoms. They are given an opportunity to close spontaneously, as long as there are no factors present that will make this unlikely (e.g., distal obstruction, associated abscess, diseased bowel). Intravenous nutrition and octreotide[4] can be used to accelerate healing and reduce fistula output. Persistent fistulas must be resected.

Well-vascularized small bowel bleeds vigorously when cut. When bowel ends are anastomosed, the vessels may not be completely occluded by the staples or the sutures and hemorrhage can occur. If possible, the anastomosis is checked from the lumenal side and any spurting vessels are suture ligated. Bleeding from small vessels at the bowel ends may be controlled with cautery, whereas large hemorrhages are managed with suture ligation. Bleeding is less common if variable gap staplers are closed to the minimal thickness.

Anastomotic hemorrhage identified after completing the operation is uncommon and can be managed in a number of ways. If the anastomosis is very close to the colon or duodenum, endoscopic treatment may be possible. Coagulation with electrocautery or heater probe can be effective if the site of bleeding is accessible. Interventional radiologic techniques such as arteriography with intraarterial vasopressin injection may be used if the anastomosis is not endoscopically accessible. If these techniques fail and the bleeding does not stop by itself, a repeat laparotomy may be required. Fortunately, this is an uncommon event.

Most anastomoses narrow initially as a result of postsurgical edema. If localized perianastomotic inflammation is present because of a small leak, this can prolong or accentuate the effects of the edema. Two-layer sutured anastomoses can also narrow the bowel, especially if the "bites" are generous. Short inflammatory stenoses may cause no symptoms or temporary symptoms of bowel obstruction. Structural stenoses from a narrow anastomosis or fibrosis from ischemia may be more persistent problems.

To prevent anastomotic stenosis, the surgical technique should be adapted to the diameter of the bowel ends. When the diameter is small, a single-layer inverting suture line with deep, narrow "bites" is used. Wide bowel ends allow more latitude. Again, it is important to ensure that the bowel ends are well vascularized and to use the largest stapler that will fit into the bowel ends.

If anastomotic stenosis occurs, the patient will have symptoms of bowel obstruction. Postoperative bowel obstruction is managed conservatively as long as there is no evidence of compromised bowel (e.g., leukocytosis, peritonitis, severe abdominal pain, extreme dilatation of bowel loops). If the symptoms do not resolve within 7 to 10 days, intravenous nutrition may be needed (earlier in patients who were undernourished in the preoperative period). If possible, most surgeons prefer to wait until the immediate postlaparotomy period (10 to 30 days) is over before planning a repeat laparotomy. A contrast material–enhanced study of the small bowel is helpful to distinguish ileus from a mechanical obstruction and may localize the site of obstruction. A fibrotic stenosis may be dilated endoscopically if it can be reached (e.g., an ileocolonic anastomosis). An inflamed small bowel anastomosis is almost impossible to dilate, and the procedure is extremely risky; resection is preferred.

The small bowel is well vascularized, but ischemic anastomoses can occur if the mesenteric excision is badly planned or there is a generalized vascular problem. In patients who have undergone a previous small bowel resection (or especially isolation, such as a continent urinary reconstruction), the mesentery may be distorted, and devascularization of bowel ends or isolated bowel loops is possible. A relatively easy way to produce anastomotic ischemia is to traumatize the mesenteric vessels either during mobilization or repair of the mesenteric defect after anastomosis. When the bleeding mesenteric vessels are ligated, the blood supply to the anastomosis may be critically reduced.

It is sometimes difficult to distinguish bruised bowel ends from ischemic bowel ends: both look blue. The amount of bleeding from the bowel ends is an important factor.[1] Minor ischemia can resolve without sequelae, but sometimes anastomotic stenosis or leakage can follow.

To minimize anastomotic ischemia, the mesenteric resection is carefully planned so that the lines of bowel resection are not undercut. The surgeon must be extremely cautious if previous mesenteric resections have been performed. The bowel ends must be well vascularized,[1] and if there is any doubt, additional bowel should be resected. It is important to handle the mesentery carefully to prevent tears and to take care when repairing the mesenteric defect not to puncture the marginal artery.

Chronic anastomotic ischemia is manifest clinically as a stenosis or fistula, which will need to be resected and redone. For emergent acute ischemia, an end ileostomy and mucous fistula is a good option that enables early detection of recurrent ischemia and minimizes its consequences. If there is doubt about the viability of the bowel after an anastomosis, a "second look" laparotomy within 24 hours can resolve the issue. Intraoperative fluorescein infusion or the use of Doppler ultrasound can be helpful in assessing intestinal viability.

When linear stapling instruments are used to perform side-to-side small bowel anastomoses, the efferent loop of the proximal bowel and the afferent loop of the distal bowel are essentially defunctioned. This is not a problem so long as the length of the defunctioned bowel is short. Long, blind bowel ends can lead to stasis with the potential for bacterial overgrowth and blind loop syndrome, manifested by diarrhea, abdominal cramps, and a variety of nutritional deficiencies.

If this is suspected, it can be managed with empiric treatment with metronidazole. A more scientific approach uses a hydrogen breath test to confirm the diagnosis, but treatment is the same.

SHORT BOWEL SYNDROME

Short bowel syndrome is a metabolic complication of small bowel resection resulting from the effect of the resection on the ability of the bowel to absorb and digest fluids, electrolytes, minerals, vitamins, trace elements, and nutrients. A brief discussion of a complex subject follows.

Pathogenesis

Short bowel syndrome occurs after resection or bypass of a large amount of small bowel. The clinical circumstances in which this occurs include volvulus or internal herniation of a large segment of bowel, a mesenteric embolus or thrombosis, resection of mesenteric desmoid tumors, repeated bowel resection to treat Crohn's disease or malignancy, bypass to treat malignant obstruction, or temporary high jejunostomy in patients with sepsis. The main symptom of short bowel syndrome is diarrhea. The main sequelae are malabsorption and malnutrition. Complications of short bowel syndrome include calcium oxalate renal calculi, gastric hyperacidity with peptic ulceration, and a variety of syndromes of nutritional deficiency (e.g, zinc deficiency, vitamin B_{12} deficiency, folate deficiency).

Three factors determine whether short bowel syndrome will develop after small bowel resection: the amount of small bowel left, the presence or absence of a colon, and the rapidity with which the bowel is lost. Gradual loss by means of multiple resections over several year's allows adaptation and increases tolerance; sudden loss predisposes to short bowel syndrome because adaptation cannot occur. In my experience, a patient with 18 inches of jejunum between the duodenum and transverse colon has been able to maintain nutrition orally. This is the absolute minimum length of small bowel, however, and after such resection many patients will need parenteral nutrition to supplement oral intake. The presence of a colon is beneficial in three ways: it enables sufficient oral nutrition with as little as 20 inches of small bowel left (as opposed to the 40 inches needed when there is no colon),[5,6] provides for some absorption of calories,[7] and reduces the degree of salt and magnesium depletion.[5]

Treatment

Treatment of short bowel syndrome includes control of diarrhea by avoidance of dietary fat (and sometimes lactose) and the use of antidiarrheal agents (e.g., codeine elixir, tincture of opium, and subcutaneous injection of octreotide).[8] Nutritional supplementation by oral or parenteral routes is needed but should be reevaluated as bowel adaptation occurs. Calcium oxalate urinary stones can be prevented by maintaining high oral fluid intake, avoiding foods rich in oxalate, and taking calcium citrate. Hydrogen ion blocking drugs can control the gastric hyperacidity, which usually is a problem only in the immediate postoperative period. Gallstones may develop in patients receiving parenteral nutrition for prolonged periods, but prophylactic cholecystectomy is not a good idea.

Surgery to lengthen or widen bowel is not popular,[9] and small intestinal transplantation is still experimental. Sometimes a colostomy is necessary if diarrhea is intolerable. The colostomy should be made like an ileostomy, with a spout.

TERMINAL ILEAL RESECTION

Specific nutritional problems follow resection of the terminal ileum. Resection of the terminal ileum can lead to diarrhea because ileal absorption of bile salts is reduced and bile salts spill into the colon. This can be treated with cholestyramine resin. Gradual development of vitamin B_{12} deficiency is likely because absorption stops and stores are depleted. If more than 100 cm of terminal ileum has been resected, the bile salt pool becomes inadequate as losses exceed the liver's capacity to synthesize replacements. Fat absorption is impaired, and steatorrhea results. A low-fat diet is necessary, with consultation with a nutritionist or dietitian.

DISEASE-SPECIFIC CONSIDERATIONS

One way to avoid the anastomotic complications of small bowel resection is to not make an anastomosis. The decision to unite bowel ends is based on consideration of factors known to increase the risk for complications: poor nutritional status, associated sepsis, blood loss, chronic uremia, and diseased bowel.[10,11] Sometimes the decision can be made only when all factors are considered intraoperatively.

Crohn's Disease

Patients undergoing small bowel resection because of Crohn's disease are subject to several factors that put them at risk for complications.[12] These include the "three *S*s"—sepsis, starvation,[13] and steroids[14]—as well as chronic anemia and a thick mesentery.

Sepsis. Crohn's disease is characterized by a tendency for bowel perforation. This can lead to a variety of clinical findings, including free perforation, intra-abdominal abscess, psoas abscess, phlegmon, and fistula. Patients may be toxic or have acute or localized sepsis. In patients with sepsis, surgical principles demand that the source of the sepsis be removed. Immediate anastomosis after such resection may be risky because of the catabolic state of the patient, the often-fragile bowel, and the drastic consequences of further sepsis from an anastomotic leak. The safest procedure is ileostomy. If the bowel is relatively normal and all the sepsis can be removed with the specimen, protect an anastomosis with proximal diversion.

Starvation. Severe starvation (loss of >15% of ideal body weight) is associated with an increased risk for complications after abdominal surgery.[13] Pure starvation can be repleted with preoperative nutritional support, and some evidence suggests that this may decrease surgical risk.[13,15] In patients with Crohn's disease, however, starvation is often associated with sepsis, and nutritional support is ineffective.[16] Septic, malnourished patients with Crohn's disease should not be left with an unprotected anastomosis.

Steroids. There is evidence that chronic steroid use weakens tissues and impairs wound healing.[14] In practice, however, it is difficult to determine the dosage of steroid that is too much and the course of therapy that is too long. Evaluate the other factors operative in the patient and, in particular, assess the strength of tissues throughout the abdominal cavity. If in doubt, it is safest to divert.

Anemia. Anemia is one factor found to be associated with anastomotic complications[10] and needs to be taken into account when intraoperative decisions are made.

Mesenteric thickening. Patients with Crohn's disease often have a mesentery thickened by enlarged nodes or the effects of chronic sepsis. Mesenteric vessels cannot be seen with transillumination, and the practice of "punching" through the mesentery is likely to create problems. A technique for resecting thickened mesentery is shown in Fig. 18-3. Kocher (toothed) clamps are applied in 2 cm, slightly overlapping "bites" across the mesentery, with untoothed Kelly clamps on the specimen side. After the specimen is removed, the tissue in the toothed clamps is suture ligated. The tie for one clamp overlaps the tissue in the next. The mesenteric resection is tidy, and the vessels are well controlled. The line of resection is inspected, and any oozing areas are underrun.

Obstructed Small Bowel

Several factors potentially operative in patients with small bowel obstruction influence the risk for complications after small bowel resection.[17] These vary according to the duration and cause of the obstruction.

State of the patient. Patients with chronic small bowel obstruction may be significantly undernourished. If severe undernutrition (recent weight loss of

>15% of well weight)[13] is present with no significant sepsis, preoperative nutritional support is indicated. Significant improvement in the severely malnourished patient's impaired physiology cannot be expected before a minimum of 4 days.[13] Acute bowel obstruction can cause dangerous dehydration that must be corrected before surgery.

Adhesions. The severity of obstructive adhesions varies from a single band to obliteration of the entire peritoneal cavity. Adhesions are at their worst between 10 and 30 days after surgery (see Fig. 18-2). Attempts at laparotomy during this time may cause damage to bowel involved by the adhesions, leading to postoperative sepsis. Avoid this situation by postponing a laparotomy that could cause more problems than the surgery was intended to solve.

Even if adhesiolysis is possible, it is often a long, tedious procedure that is associated with increased risk for prolonged postoperative ileus, pulmonary complications, and DVT.

Remember to inspect mobilized bowel for damage and to ensure there are no potentially obstructing adhesions below an anastomosis or repair.

State of the bowel. Obstructed bowel is dilated, thickened, and edematous. Unobstructed bowel is collapsed and of normal thickness. Stapling these different types of bowel together is not recommended because of the thick, edematous obstructed end. Anastomosis of two bowel ends of different diameters requires precise suturing with interrupted sutures and a "halving" technique. A Cheatle slit may be needed to even the diameters of the ends.

Ischemia or Infarction

Resection of ischemic or infarcted small bowel can pose difficult problems that carry risks for significant postoperative complications. Surgeons have an urge to conserve bowel that is sometimes at odds with the need to provide two well-vascularized bowel ends for anastomosis.

State of the patient. Patients with chronic intestinal ischemia are often undernourished. Acute ischemia sometimes occurs in association with chronic ischemia, with the undernourished, possibly septic patient at high risk for postoperative complications. Comorbidity may have predisposed to the infarction or ischemia (e.g., cardiac arrhythmia, recent myocardial infarction, cancer), and that bears on surgical risk.

State of the bowel. Quality of life after extensive enterectomy can be acceptable with the current methods available to treat short bowel syndrome. The top priority is therefore to get the patient through the surgery without serious complication or the need for a second major operation. All dead bowel must be removed. If bowel ends are obviously viable, anastomosis is a satisfactory option, but also consider diversion or just bringing bowel ends out as a stoma and mucous fistula. The latter is the least risky. Techniques and tips for assessing the viability of bowel ends and preventing anastomotic ischemia have been discussed.

Radiation

Radiation enteritis is fairly common in patients who undergo radiation therapy for pelvic malignancies. Cancers of the anus, cervix, prostate gland, and rectum are likely to be treated with irradiation. When surgery is necessary to treat complications of radiation enteritis (e.g., fistula, obstruction), the combined effects of the prior pelvic surgery and irradiation produce technical difficulties with a high risk for complications.

State of the patient. Radiation enteritis, especially when it or its complications are severe enough that surgery is necessary, is associated with significant weight loss in a high proportion of patients. There may also be sepsis, and thus the patient is at high risk for complications of any major surgery.

State of the bowel. In the radiation-affected small bowel, chronic obliterative vasculitis causes stiffening and scarring of all layers of its wall. The bowel is fragile, often involved in dense adhesions, and does not hold sutures or staples reliably. Do not anastomose or suture radiation-damaged bowel. Either resect damaged bowel (it is not working properly, anyway) or bypass it. The anastomosis must be in normal bowel. Remember the safe option of proximal diversion or temporary end stoma in difficult situations.

Tumor

Patients with small bowel involved with tumor are least at risk for complications of resection because the bowel itself is usually normal. Treatment strategies depend largely on the state of the tumor. In cases of chronic obstruction, the same considerations as for obstructed small bowel apply.

If the cancer, arising either in another organ (usual) or in the small bowel itself (rare), is localized and potentially curable, one should perform a wide mesenteric excision and suture-ligate thick mesentery as described for Crohn's disease. Adhesions should not be squeezed or divided between the small bowel and the tumor but resected en bloc. If the tumor is incurable and surgery is palliative, the surgeon should perform the minimum procedure necessary (usually a bypass) to alleviate the symptoms. The steps outlined for prevention of complications should be followed carefully, because a complication in a palliative procedure is particularly tragic: one set of symptoms is replaced by another. If palliative resection or bypass is contemplated, one must ensure that *all* potential points of obstruction are treated.

COMPLICATIONS OF STRICTUREPLASTY

Strictureplasty is a relatively recent addition to the surgical options for treatment of stenosing Crohn's disease of the small bowel. In its simplest terms, it involves widening of a stricture with techniques designed for pyloroplasty (e.g., Heineke-Mickulicz and Finney operations). In the Heineke-Mickulicz strictureplasty, used for short strictures, a longitudinal incision is centered on the middle of the stricture and closed transversely. The Finney procedure, used for long strictures, is a side-to-side anastomosis with its apex at the middle of the stricture. Incising and suturing rather than removing small bowel affected by Crohn's disease seems to contravene surgical principles. This is not associated with unduly high complication rates,[18] and strictureplasty has become widely used and valued as a means of conserving bowel in patients at risk of losing too much bowel.

Table 18-2 is a compilation of results from the large series reported by Fazio et al.[18] from the Cleveland Clinic and other series summarized in their paper. The incidence of septic complications is low considering the poor nutritional state of many of the patients, the preoperative steroids many were taking, and the multiple suture lines and anastomoses involved in many of the procedures (Fig. 18-9). Recurrence of stricture is uncommon, and sites of previous stricture-plasties often show complete resolution of Crohn's disease at a later laparotomy. The rate of recurrence of Crohn's disease, hardly a complication in these high-risk patients, who usually have jejunoileitis, is reasonable considering the relatively short follow-up in most series.

Table 18-2 Complications of strictureplasty*

Complication	Number	Percent
Mortality	0	0
Perioperative hemorrhage (>3 units of blood)	7	3
Fistula or abscess	17	7
Prolonged ileus	8	3
Repeat surgery because of sepsis	8	3
Recurrence of symptoms	69	30
Recurrence of stricture	18	8

Data from Fazio VW, Tjandra JJ, Lavery IC, et al. Dis Colon Rectum 36:355-361, 1993.
*Data for 231 patients from nine studies, with follow-up of 6 to 84 months.

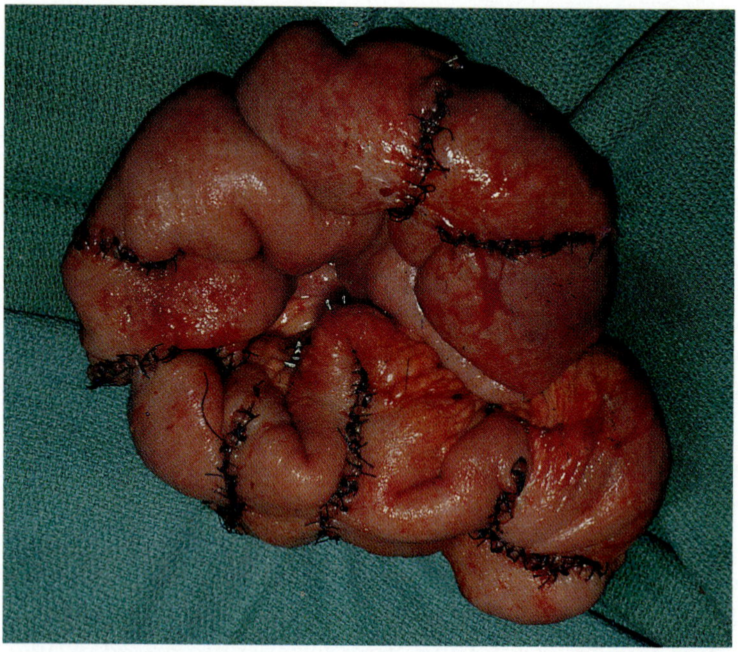

Fig. 18-9 Multiple strictureplasties in a patient with Crohn's jejunoileitis. The patient was symptom free at 2-year follow-up.

The same measures to prevent complications of small bowel resection in general and Crohn's disease in particular apply to strictureplasty. In addition, the following points deserve emphasis:

1. Select strictures carefully. Short, tight, fibrotic strictures are ideal for strictureplasty. Beware of inflammatory strictures. Resect strictures associated with a fistula, abscess or phlegmon. Strictures that are close together can be treated as one with strictureplasty or resection.
2. Perform an adequate strictureplasty. Extend the longitudinal incision on the antimesenteric margin for a full 2 cm into normal bowel on either side of the stricture. Close the defect transversely with interrupted absorbable sutures. Make the "bites" narrow but deep into the muscle, excluding mucosa.
3. Ensure adequate mucosal hemostasis without charring the whole length of the incision. Postoperative hemorrhage can be significant and difficult to treat.
4. Ensure no downstream strictures are left untreated. Crohn's disease characteristically includes "skip" lesions, that is, patches of disease separated by normal bowel. Feel for the mesenteric marginal thickening that betrays mucosal disease and check for a stricture. Pass a Foley catheter

with its 5 ml balloon inflated through the bowel to ensure no occult strictures survive to precipitate anastomotic leakage.

5. Look for cancer. Chronic small bowel Crohn's disease has been associated with carcinoma. Biopsy suspect strictures.
6. Use long Finney-type operations with caution. These produce large diverticula that may give rise to stasis (blind loop) syndrome, especially if a recurrent stricture narrows their inflow and outflow.

CONCLUSION

Small bowel resection can be a difficult procedure in patients with severe intra-abdominal disease. Many factors that involve the patient and his or her abdomen and bowel influence the risk for complications of resection. Good surgical technique and sound judgment are important to minimize complications and their sequelae.

REFERENCES

1. Novell Jr, Lewis AA. Preoperative observation of marginal artery bleeding: A predictor of anastomotic leakage. Br J Surg 77:137-138, 1990.
2. Church JM. Surgical management of anastomotic leaks and intra-abdominal sepsis. Prob Gen Surg 9:634-640, 1992.
3. Gerzof SG, Johnson WC, Robbins AH, Nasbeth DC. Expanded criteria for percutaneous abscess drainage. Arch Surg 120:227-232, 1985.
4. Nubiola P, Badia JM, Martinez-Rodenas F, Gil MJ, Segura M, Sancho J, Sitges-Serra A. Treatment of 27 postoperative enterocutaneous fistulas with the long half-life somatostatin analog SMS 201-995. Ann Surg 210:56-60, 1989.
5. Nightingale JM, Lennard-Jones JE. The short bowel syndrome: What's new and old? Dig Dis 11:12-31, 1993.
6. Nightingale JM, Lennard-Jones JE, Gertner DJ, Wood SR, Bartram CI. Colonic preservation reduces need for parenteral therapy, increases incidence of renal stones, but does not change high prevalence of gall stones in patients with a short bowel. Gut 33:1493-1497, 1992.
7. Nordgaard I, Hansen BS, Mortensen PB. Colon as a digestive organ in patients with short bowel. Lancet 343:373-376, 1994.
8. O'Keefe SJ, Peterson ME, Fleming CR. Octreotide as an adjunct to home parenteral nutrition in the management of permanent end-jejunostomy syndrome. J Parenter Enter Nutr 18:26-34, 1994.
9. Thompson JS. Surgical considerations in the short bowel syndrome. Surg Gynecol Obstet 176:89-101, 1993.
10. Schrock TR, Deveny CW, Dunphy JE. Factors contributing to leakage of colonic anastomosis. Ann Surg 177:513-517, 1972.
11. Jex RK, van Heerden JA, Wolff BG, Ready RL, Ilstrup DM. Gastrointestinal anastomosis. Factors affecting early complications. Ann Surg 206:138-141, 1987.
12. Post S, Betzler M, von Ditfurth B, Schurman G, Kuppers P, Herfarth C. Risks of intestinal anastomoses in Crohn's disease. Ann Surg 213:37-42, 1991.

13. Hill GL. Body composition research: Implications for the practice of clinical nutrition. J Parenter Enter Nutr 16:197-218, 1992.
14. Aszodi A, Ponsky JL. Effects of corticosteroid on the healing bowel anastomosis Am Surg 10:546-548, 1984.
15. Haydock DA, Hill GL. Improved wound healing response in surgical patients receiving intravenous nutrition. Br J Surg 74:320-323, 1987.
16. Church JM, Hill GL. The ability of intravenous nutrition to restore body protein in patients with severe inflammatory bowel disease. Dis Colon Rectum 33:2, 1990.
17. Jonsson K, Jiborn H, Zederfeldt B. Healing of anastomoses after obstruction of small intestine. Surg Gynecol Obstet 167:324-330, 1988.
18. Fazio VW, Tjandra JJ, Lavery IC, Church JM, Milsom JW, Oakley JR. Long-term follow-up of strictureplasty in Crohn's disease. Dis Colon Rectum 36:355-361, 1993.

CHAPTER 19

Diverticulosis

JOHN J. MURRAY

The prevalence of acquired diverticular disease of the colon increases with advancing age. Radiologic studies and autopsy series have identified diverticulosis in 5% to 10% of patients older than 45 years and 65% of those 70 years of age or older.[1] Only 10% to 25% of patients with diverticulosis experience inflammatory complications.[2] In the majority of patients, acute diverticulitis can be managed successfully without surgery through diet modification and broad-spectrum antibiotic therapy. Approximately 30% of patients with symptomatic diverticular disease eventually require surgery to treat complications of the disorder.[1-4] The potential morbidity associated with surgical treatment of diverticular disease is influenced by the indication for surgery and the type of operative procedure undertaken. Whether surgery is undertaken on an elective or emergency basis also influences the risk of complications.[5]

SURGICAL INDICATIONS

Urgent laparotomy is required in patients with pneumoperitoneum and diffuse peritonitis indicative of free perforation of a diverticulum. Perforated diverticulitis is among the most lethal intra-abdominal catastrophies when associated with feculent peritonitis. This complication is uncommon because acute diverticulitis is usually accompanied by a progressive pericolonic adhesive reaction that serves to contain the inflammatory process. Patients with localized disease that does not respond to antibiotic treatment and bowel rest will also require surgery. These patients typically exhibit lower abdominal tenderness and frequently have an associated soft tissue mass that reflects the presence of a nonresolving phlegmon or abscess. A review of indications for surgery in patients with complicated diverticulosis treated at Massachusetts General Hospital identified these septic complications as the precipitant for surgery in 58% of patients.[3] A similar study of patients requiring surgery for diverticular disease at the Lahey Clinic identified sepsis, perforation, or a persistent abdominal mass as the indication for surgery in 75% of cases.[6]

Acute diverticulitis may be complicated by partial obstruction of the intestinal tract as a result of extrinsic compression of the colon or entrapment of a segment of small intestine by an expanding pericolic phlegmon or abscess. Relief of the obstruction rarely serves as the sole indication for surgery in the acute setting. The symptoms of obstruction usually subside with appropriate medical therapy or obstruction is relieved during definitive surgery to treat the nonresponding septic process. Repeated episodes of acute diverticulitis may produce distortion and fibrous scarring of the bowel wall. This may result in a symptomatic stricture of the large intestine, which is the indication for surgery in 10% to 20% of patients who require less urgent surgery because of complicated diverticular disease.[3,6] Although the availability of flexible endoscopes has facilitated examination of strictures to exclude the presence of carcinoma, the inability to exclude malignancy remains an indication for surgery in a small number of patients.

Internal or external fistulas that involve the abdominal wall, perineum, bladder, small intestine, or vagina result from erosion of a pericolic or pelvic abscess into an adjacent structure. These fistulas represent the chronic stage of complicated diverticulitis. Their symptomatic expression can be alleviated only with surgery.

SURGICAL OPTIONS

Surgical management of complicated diverticular disease has been controversial. The relative merit and safety of resecting the diseased segment of large intestine at the initial operation and the appropriate time for restoration of intestinal tract continuity have been the central issues of debate. Lack of consensus has produced a variety of treatment options (Fig. 19-1).

Critical analysis of the results achieved with these therapeutic alternatives has been complicated by the unpredictable course of symptomatic diverticular disease and the variable severity of its clinical presentation. Attempts to develop a clinical staging system to facilitate standardization of therapy for complicated diverticulitis have met with limited success.[7,8]

The traditional three-stage approach to the surgical management of complicated diverticular disease evolved before broad-spectrum antibiotics were available and also preceded the development of supportive measures currently available for the care of critically ill patients. In 1942, Smithwick[9] reported a mortality rate of 6% with diverting colostomy and drainage of the pericolic phlegmon in patients with acute diverticulitis. This report established the three-stage approach as the standard of care for patients with complicated diverticular disease. Although a three-stage approach may be successful for managing diverticulitis complicated by abscess, fistula, or obstruction, it has been associated with a mortality rate of 20% to 50% when used to treat perforated diverticulitis and peritonitis.[10-13] The significant mortality accompanying drainage and fecal diversion in patients with perforated diverticulitis results from persistent intra-abdominal sepsis. Preservation of the perforated segment of sigmoid colon,

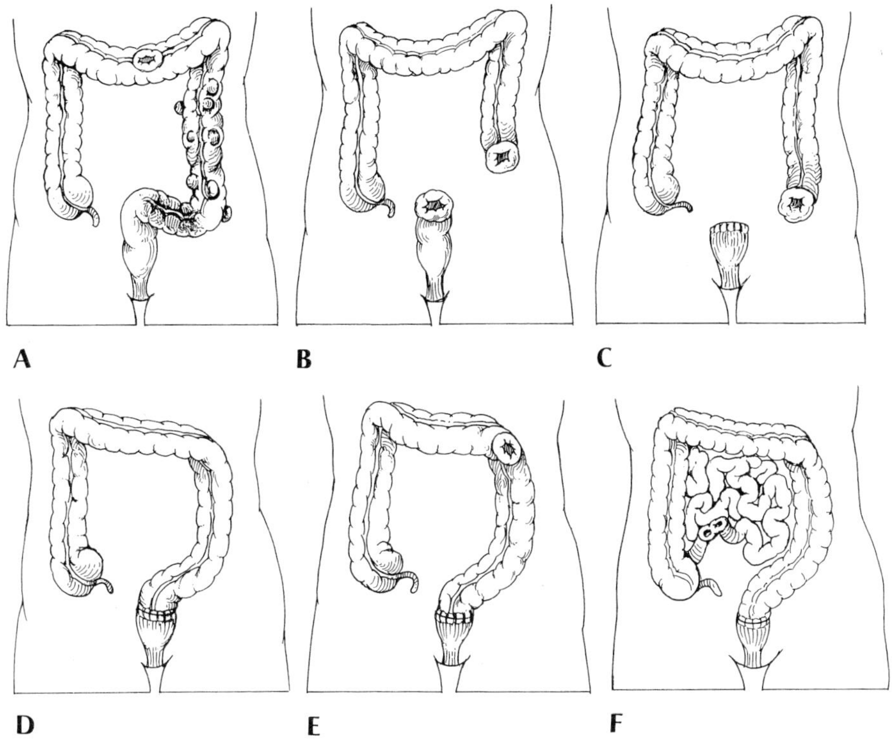

Fig. 19-1 Treatment options for complicated diverticulitis. **A**, Proximal loop colostomy and drainage of a paracolic phlegmon. **B**, Sigmoid colectomy with a colostomy and a mucous fistula. **C**, Hartmann resection. **D**, Sigmoid colectomy with a primary anastomosis. **E** and **F**, Sigmoid colectomy with a primary anastomosis and diverting loop colostomy or loop ileostomy.

often filled with a column of fecal material, provides a source for continued contamination of the peritoneal cavity. A poor response to fecal diversion can also result from inadequate drainage of a pericolic abscess or less frequently from progression of disease in the excluded segment of large intestine. Treatment of complicated diverticulitis with fecal diversion and drainage has been accompanied by development of a colocutaneous fistula in 10% to 20% of cases.[14,15] These fistulas may represent persistent discharge from a drain tract established at the initial operation or may reflect spontaneous eruption of a new or inadequately drained paracolic or intra-abdominal abscess. These fistulas typically drain through an established surgical wound. Fistulas to the bladder or vaginal stump have also been reported to occur under similar circumstances. Contrary to the proposed rationale for preliminary drainage and fecal diversion, resection of the sigmoid colon at a subsequent operation can be technically challenging because of the dense fibrotic reaction that accompanies long-standing inflammation. Unlike the acute setting, where gentle, blunt dissection through edematous tissue planes can be successful, delayed resection usually requires sharp dissection through dense scar tissue that may place the ureters and great vessels at substantial risk for injury.

Critical analysis of the efficacy of multistaged surgical procedures for the treatment of complicated diverticular disease must consider the cumulative mortality and morbidity and the prolonged cumulative disability that may complicate multiple surgical procedures. Failure to complete all phases of a three-staged approach to treatment of diverticular disease occurs in 16% to 54% of patients[3,16,17] and reflects postoperative complications and the influence of comorbid conditions.

Concern about the cumulative morbidity and prolonged disability associated with the traditional three-stage approach to the surgical management of diverticular disease has promoted enthusiasm for the practice of resection of the involved segment of large intestine at the initial operation. In general, this is accomplished by one of several options that include Hartmann resection, resection with colostomy and mucous fistula, or resection with primary anastomosis and diverting loop colostomy. Depending on the circumstances encountered, intestinal tract continuity can be restored in 6 weeks to 6 months. The extent of mesocolic induration determines the length of intestine that should be resected. For disease confined to the sigmoid colon, resection should proceed distally to include the rectosigmoid junction. It is unusual for there to be sufficient length in the distal segment of intestine to permit exteriorization on the abdominal wall as a mucous fistula. In most instances, a mucous fistula can be created only if residual disease or active inflammation is left intact. This may serve as a potential source for septic complications.

Fistulas that involve the bladder, small intestine, or the vaginal cuff may be divided, debrided, and closed primarily after resection of the involved segment of large intestine. Colocutaneous fistulas are simply divided and the cutaneous tract drained. Small pericolic abscesses can often be excised with the specimen, especially when the abscess is encompassed by the sigmoid mesentery. Larger abscesses require drainage in conjunction with sigmoid colectomy. Large, well-localized pelvic or pericolic abscesses identified on preoperative CT scans can usually be drained percutaneously.[18] This is followed by definitive resection in 4 to 6 weeks. A staged approach to the management of diverticular abscesses facilitates subsequent single-stage resection and primary colorectal anastomosis in 75% of cases.[19]

As many as 20% of patients who undergo emergency sigmoid colectomy or anterior resection because of a presumptive diagnosis of perforated diverticulitis are found to have carcinoma of the colon.[13] Distinguishing a perforated carcinoma from diverticulitis may be difficult when a large phlegmon is found in the left lower quadrant of the abdomen. Removing the involved segment of intestine at the initial operation averts the potential consequences of delaying treatment of undiagnosed carcinoma.

Although comparison of results obtained with two-stage and three-stage procedures for treatment of complicated diverticular disease is flawed by the retrospective design of most studies, colon resection at the initial operation appears to provide consistently better results, especially when diverticulitis is complicated by perforation and peritonitis.[10,20,21] Resection of the involved segment of intestine at the initial operation improves survival and reduces the risk of postoperative complications.[12,14,22] A review of the Lahey Clinic experience with two-stage procedures used to treat complicated diverticulitis reveals that duration of hospitalization is decreased by 25% and duration of postoperative disability by 50% compared with results in patients undergoing a traditional three-stage approach.[6]

Given the advantages associated with primary resection of the diseased intestinal segment, a traditional three-stage approach to the management of diverticulitis has become primarily a procedure of historic interest. The Hartmann resection is the most widely used approach to emergency treatment of complicated diverticulitis. Compared with primary anastomosis and diverting colostomy, Hartmann resection provides a more satisfactory stoma and obviates potential complications associated with anastomotic dehiscence. Leakage from the rectal stump has been reported in as many as 5% of patients after Hartmann resection for carcinoma or diverticulitis.[23] Dehiscence of the Hartmann stump may occur if blood supply to the apex of the stump is compromised or if the closure is under tension from distention of the stump by gas or fecal material. Gentle dilation of the anal sphincter and evacuation of the rectal stump may reduce the risk for dehiscence and minimize the consequences if a leak develops. Leakage from the rectal stump usually results in a pelvic abscess. In many cases the abscess will drain spontaneously through the anus.

Patients with signs of pelvic sepsis after Hartmann resection should be examined with CT. Instillation of contrast material into the rectum before examination may confirm extravasation from the apex of the rectal stump. If a pelvic abscess is identified after dehiscence of the Hartmann stump, it can often be successfully managed with percutaneous drainage of the abscess and catheter drainage of the rectal stump. Evacuation of residual fecal material from the rectal stump may facilitate resolution of pelvic sepsis. Surgical intervention will be required if the abscess is not accessible to percutaneous drainage or signs of progressive peritonitis are present. If surgery is necessary, closure of the rectal stump at a more distal site with a linear stapling instrument can be attempted. When there is insufficient length in the Hartmann pouch to permit secure closure without extensive or hazardous dissection, placement of closed suction drains adjacent to the Hartmann pouch in combination with catheter drainage of the rectum should facilitate resolution of the septic process.[24]

Reanastomosis after Hartmann resection can be a challenging procedure. Identification and mobilization of the rectal stump is difficult if the stump was contained within the walls of a pelvic abscess cavity. Extensive pelvic dissection to facilitate anastomosis may result in injury to the ureters, iliac vessels, or the autonomic nerves that control bladder and sexual function. The availability of the circular stapling instrument and the development of the double-staple technique for performing a distal colorectal anastomosis have simplified Hartmann reanastomosis and limited the extent of requisite pelvic dissection. Failure to mobilize the rectum adequately, however, may lead to inadvertent inclusion of the bladder or the vagina in the stapling instrument and result in rectovesical or rectovaginal fistulas. In contrast to the experience with sigmoid colectomy and primary anastomosis, restoration of intestinal tract continuity after Hartmann resection usually requires mobilization of the splenic flexure of the colon to create a tension-free anastomosis.[5]

Primary anastomosis with diverting loop colostomy at the time of sigmoid colectomy to treat acute diverticulitis averts some of the disadvantages associated with Hartmann resection. An uninvolved margin of proximal rectum above the level of the peritoneal reflection that is suitable for anastomosis to the descending colon is invariably present during surgery for acute diverticulitis. In this situation, anastomosis rarely requires mobilization of the splenic flexure. Subsequent closure of the loop colostomy is generally simpler than Hartmann reanastomosis. Fecal diversion does not prevent anastomotic dehiscence, however, but merely minimizes the consequences. Dehiscence can result in serious septic complications if there is extensive fecal loading of the colon between the colostomy and the colorectal anastomosis. Most anastomotic leaks identified on follow-up lower GI barium studies will close spontaneously, but colostomy closure must await successful healing.

Colon resection with primary anastomosis is an additional option for the surgical management of acute diverticulitis. Compared with other alternatives, resection with primary anastomosis is associated with the shortest period of hospitalization and the briefest duration of postoperative disability.[6,17] This procedure has been used to manage all stages of complicated diverticulitis. The reported prevalence of anastomotic dehiscence ranges from 0% to 33%, and associated mortality of 0% to 20%.[20,25,26] In general, however, these results involve small numbers of patients and may reflect a bias in patient selection for those with less complicated stages of diverticulitis.[25] Candidates for primary intestinal anastomosis include those with acute diverticulitis complicated by localized peritonitis, intestinal obstruction, or a pericolic abscess that can be drained and largely excised at sigmoid colectomy. The usual criteria for safe construction of an intestinal anastomosis must be observed. The intestine must be approximated without tension, and the anastomosis should utilize segments that are well perfused, pliable, and uninflamed.

The decision to create a primary anastomosis is influenced frequently by the amount of fecal material in the proximal colon. Inadequate mechanical cleansing of the colon before surgery is associated with an increased risk of anastomotic dehiscence.[27] The technique for intraoperative antegrade lavage of the proximal colon (as described in Chapter 2) facilitates primary anastomosis in patients undergoing nonelective resection of the sigmoid colon to treat complications of diverticular disease. Although the experience reported in the literature with this technique in patients with complicated diverticulitis is limited, an increased incidence of anastomotic complications has not been identified.[28] This option should be considered when the primary contraindication to single-stage resection is lack of preoperative mechanical bowel preparation. Primary anastomosis should not be performed in patients with diffuse peritonitis or the pulmonary and hemodynamic complications of intra-abdominal sepsis. These patients are best served with expeditious surgery to remove the focus of contamination, thereby minimizing the chances for further intra-abdominal complications. Hartmann resection would seem to be the most appropriate choice in this clinical setting.

Despite improved results with more aggressive surgical intervention for diverticulitis and its complications, surgery is associated with substantial morbidity and mortality. Sepsis with attendant multiorgan system failure remains the leading cause of death.[3] Postoperative morbidity is influenced by the indication for surgery, the type of operation performed, and the presence of comorbid conditions. Respiratory failure, wound sepsis, intra-abdominal abscess, and the consequences of anastomotic dehiscence are the postoperative complications seen most frequently. When colectomy is performed under urgent or complicated circumstances, morbidity increases threefold.[5]

RECURRENCE

Recurrent diverticulitis is uncommon in patients who undergo sigmoid colectomy to treat symptomatic diverticular disease. Benn et al.[29] at the Mayo Clinic identified recurrent diverticulitis in 10.4% of 501 patients followed for a minimum of 5 years after sigmoid colectomy. Only 3% of patients required further surgery for treatment of recurrent diverticulitis. Although all patients underwent resection of the proximal sigmoid colon, anastomosis was performed to the distal sigmoid colon in 321 patients and to the rectum in 180 patients. The distal level of anastomosis did not influence the need for further surgery because of diverticular disease, but diverticulitis recurred in 12.5% of patients with anastomosis to the distal sigmoid colon compared with only 6.7% of patients undergoing complete sigmoid colectomy. This suggests that the risk of recurrent diverticulitis is increased in patients with residual diverticular disease distal to the colon anastomosis after segmental colectomy. The potential for recurrent diverticulitis does not appear to be influenced by involvement of the proximal colon with diverticular disease. Approximately 15% of patients who undergo sigmoid colectomy will demonstrate progression of diverticular disease in the proximal colon on follow-up lower GI barium examination.[30] Pancolonic diverticular disease carries a similar prognosis after sigmoid resection to that of disease confined to the sigmoid colon.

Patients who develop anastomotic complications after sigmoid colectomy for diverticular disease and patients with recurrent diverticulitis after sigmoid colectomy should be examined carefully for the presence of Crohn's colitis masquerading as diverticular disease. The second peak in the bimodal age distribution for Crohn's disease consists largely of patients with distal colitis.[31] These patients may have symptoms that suggest diverticulitis. The two diseases may coexist in the same patient. It has been proposed that diverticulitis may result from infection of an aphthous ulcer in the mucosa of a colonic diverticulum.[32] Distinguishing Crohn's colitis from diverticulitis can be of crucial importance when surgery is indicated. Procedures designed to treat sigmoid diverticulitis may be associated with a high incidence of anastomotic dehiscence and death from septic complications when performed in patients with Crohn's colitis. A review from the Lahey Clinic identified four deaths (24%) from septic complications among 17 patients undergoing segmental resection with end colostomy or primary anastomosis to treat an inflammatory process involving the sigmoid colon that displayed features of Crohn's colitis and diverticular disease.[33] In contrast, there were no operative deaths among eight patients in whom the surgical procedure included proctectomy. When the original operative procedure was designed to treat inflammatory bowel disease rather than diverticulitis, no patients had symptoms of recurrent Crohn's disease at follow-up ranging from 2 to 5 years. In contrast, 61% of patients undergoing segmental sigmoid colectomy had symptoms of recurrent colitis. Features that should raise suspicion of Crohn's disease rather than diverticulitis include the presence of anal disease, abnormal sigmoidoscopic findings, a history of rectal bleeding, or unexpected technical difficulty when attempting sigmoid colectomy. A soft, uninflamed, pliable segment of intraperitoneal rectum is almost invariably encountered during surgery in patients with acute diverticulitis or its complications. When Crohn's disease involves the distal colon, however, the inflammatory process frequently extends to involve both the intraperitoneal and extraperitoneal segments of the rectum and mesorectum.

Complications associated with diverticulosis can be grouped into two broad categories: those that reflect progression of the disease process and those that accompany surgical treatment of the disease. Strategies to reduce the morbidity associated with symptomatic diverticular disease should encourage surgical intervention before serious complications of the disease have developed. In our experience, operative morbidity increases threefold when colectomy is performed under urgent or complicated circumstances.[34] Elective resection of the sigmoid colon in patients at risk for complications of diverticular disease offers the best chance to reduce the morbidity and disability that may accompany the disorder.

Based on experience in treating complicated diverticular disease, the Lahey Clinic has developed criteria for elective sigmoid colectomy in patients with diverticulosis[34]:

1. Two or more admissions for treatment of acute diverticulitis
2. One hospital admission for treatment of diverticulitis complicated by:
   a. Radiographic or clinical evidence of perforation
   b. Urinary tract symptoms
   c. Clinical or radiographic evidence of persistent obstruction
   d. Patient age <50 years
3. Inability to rule out carcinoma as a diagnosis

We believe that these criteria identify patients at increased risk for complications of diverticular disease and therefore justify prophylactic sigmoid colectomy.

REFERENCES

1. Almy TP, Howell DA. Diverticular disease of the colon. N Engl J Med 302:324-331, 1980.
2. Parks TG. Natural history of diverticular disease of the colon. Clin Gastroenterol 4:53-69, 1975.
3. Rodkey GV, Welch CE. Changing patterns in the surgical treatment of diverticular disease. Ann Surg 200:466-478, 1984.
4. Parks TG, Connell AM. The outcome in 455 patients admitted for the treatment of diverticular disease of the colon. Br J Surg 57:775-778, 1970.
5. Veidenheimer MC. Clinical presentation and surgical treatment of complicated diverticular disease. In Allan RN, Keighley MR, Alexander-Williams J, Hawkins C, eds. Inflammatory Bowel Disease. London: Churchill Livingstone, 1983, pp 519-528.
6. Hackford AW, Schoetz DJ, Coller JA, Veidenheimer MC. Surgical management of complicated diverticulosis: The Lahey Clinic experience, 1967 to 1982. Dis Colon Rectum 28: 317-321, 1985.
7. Hinchey EJ, Schaal PG, Richards GK. Treatment of perforated diverticular disease of the colon. Adv Surg 12:85-109, 1978.
8. Killingback M. Management of perforative diverticulitis. Surg Clin North Am 63:97-115, 1983.
9. Smithwick RH. Experiences with surgical management of diverticulitis of the sigmoid. Ann Surg 115:969-985, 1942.
10. Grief JM, Fried G, McSherry CK. Surgical treatment of perforated diverticulitis of the sigmoid colon. Dis Colon Rectum 23:483-487, 1980.
11. Alexander-Williams J. Management of the acute complications of diverticular disease: The dangers of colostomy. Dis Colon Rectum 19:289-292, 1976.
12. Nagorney DM, Adson MA, Pemberton JH. Sigmoid diverticulitis with perforation and generalized peritonitis. Dis Colon Rectum 28:71-75, 1985.
13. Krukowski ZH, Koruth NM, Matheson NA. Evolving practice in acute diverticulitis. Br J Surg 72:684-686, 1985.
14. Finlay IG, Carter DC. A comparison of emergency resection and staged management in perforated diverticular disease. Dis Colon Rectum 30:929-933, 1987.
15. Saran S, Boulos PB. Evaluation of current surgical management of acute inflammatory diverticular disease. Ann R Coll Surg Engl 73:278-282, 1991.

16. Classen JN, Bonardi R, O'Mara CS, Wharton Finney DC, Sterioff S. Surgical treatment of acute diverticulitis by staged procedures. Ann Surg 184:582-585, 1976.
17. Auguste LJ, Wise L. Surgical management of perforated diverticulitis. Am J Surg 141: 122-127, 1981.
18. Hachigian MP, Honickman S, Eisenstat TE, Rubin RJ, Salvati EP. Computed tomography in the initial management of acute left-sided diverticulitis. Dis Colon Rectum 35:1123-1130, 1992.
19. Stabile BE, Puccio E, Van Sonnenberg E, Neff CC. Preoperative percutaneous drainage of diverticular abscesses. Am J Surg 159:99-105, 1990.
20. Rodkey GV, Welch CE. Colonic diverticular disease with surgical treatment: A study of 338 cases. Surg Clin North Am 54:655-674, 1974.
21. Kronborg O. Treatment of perforated sigmoid diverticulitis: A prospective randomized trial. Br J Surg 80:505-507, 1993.
22. Krukowski ZH, Matheson NA. Emergency surgery for diverticular disease complicated by generalized and fecal peritonitis: A review. Br J Surg 71:921-927, 1984.
23. Lubbers EJ, de Boer HH. Inherent complications of Hartmann's operation. Surg Gynecol Obstet 155:717-721, 1982.
24. Schein M, Kopelman D, Nitecki S, Hashmonai M. Management of the leaking rectal stump after Hartmann's procedure. Am J Surg 165:285-286, 1993.
25. Eng K, Ranson JH, Localio SA. Resection of the perforated segment. Am J Surg 133:67-72, 1977.
26. Eisenstat TE, Rubin RJ, Salvati EP. Surgical management of diverticulitis: The role of the Hartmann procedure. Dis Colon Rectum 26:429-432, 1983.
27. Irvin TT, Goligher JC. Aetiology of disruption of intestinal anastomoses. Br J Surg 60: 461-464, 1973.
28. Murray JJ, Schoetz DJ, Coller JA, Roberts PL, Veidenheimer MC. Intraoperative colonic lavage and primary anastomosis in nonelective colon resection. Dis Colon Rectum 34: 527-531, 1991.
29. Benn PL, Wolff BG, Ilstrup DM. Level of anastomosis and recurrent colonic diverticulitis. Am J Surg 151:269-271, 1986.
30. Wolff BG, Ready RL, MacCarty RL, Dozois RR, Beart RW. Influence of sigmoid resection on progression of diverticular disease of the colon. Dis Colon Rectum 27:645-647, 1984.
31. Roberts PL, Schoetz DJ, Pricolo R, Veidenheimer MC. Clinical course of Crohn's disease in older patients. Dis Colon Rectum 33:458-462, 1990.
32. Meyers MA, Alonso DR, Morson BC, Bartram C. Pathogenesis of diverticulitis complicating granulomatous colitis. Gastroenterology 74:24-31, 1978.
33. Berman IR, Corman ML, Coller JA, Veidenheimer MC. Late onset Crohn's disease in patients with colonic diverticulitis. Dis Colon Rectum 22:524-529, 1979.
34. Hackford AW, Veidenheimer MC. Diverticular disease of the colon: Current concepts and management. Surg Clin North AM 65:357-363, 1985.

CHAPTER 20

Resection for Colorectal Cancer

BRUCE A. ORKIN

Resection of the colon and rectum because of carcinoma remains among the most common procedures performed by general and colorectal surgeons. Although these major procedures are generally well tolerated, many complications can ensue. The careful and experienced surgeon knows how to avoid many of the problems associated with this type of surgery but still will have difficulties from time to time. In this chapter I will discuss some of the preoperative, intraoperative, and postoperative problems and prognostic factors and review the treatment of recurrent carcinoma. Complications of intra-abdominal and wound infections, hand-sewn and stapled anastomoses, bleeding, stomas, the urinary system, and small bowel obstruction are discussed elsewhere in this text.

PREOPERATIVE EVALUATION

Patients with colorectal cancer should be examined and prepared for surgery as described in Chapters 1 and 2. In addition, whenever possible, the entire colon should be examined before surgical resection of a colorectal malignancy because of the frequency of synchronous lesions. About 5% (2% to 7%) of patients have a second carcinoma, and about half (25% to 75%) have other adenomatous polyps.[1-7] Most of these polyps may be treated at colonoscopy, but occasionally a large lesion will require resection. Clearly, it is best to know this before surgery so that the appropriate procedure may be planned and the patient informed. In addition, a missed lesion that requires later intervention or that is allowed to remain and grow may become a major complication itself. Preoperative colonoscopy is the best method of examining the colon, because most small lesions will be seen, and diagnostic and therapeutic maneuvers may be carried out.[6,8] Lower GI barium studies and sigmoidoscopy together are acceptable, particularly when colonoscopy is technically difficult in a particular individual. In some cases, preoperative clearance of the colon is not possible, usually because of partial or complete luminal obstruction. Alternative approaches include preoperative laser recannulation of an obstructing rectosigmoid carcinoma, careful intraoperative palpation and colonoscopy after 3 to 6 months, or intraoperative colonoscopy.

INTRAOPERATIVE MANAGEMENT

During surgery to treat colorectal cancer, the patient is at risk for many complications. This section will cover the potential for splenic injury and the risks associated with a coloanal anastomosis.

Splenic Injury

Splenic injury is an all too common intraoperative complication of colectomy.[9] Injuries may occur when the tumor lies in this area and a segmental splenic flexure, transverse colon, or descending colon resection is being performed or when the splenic flexure of the colon is being mobilized to increase distal length to allow a tension-free sigmoid or rectal anastomosis. Splenic injury may occur during traction on the splenic flexure of the colon or on the omentum. This traction is transmitted to the spleen through the various attachments in this area, resulting in tears of the splenic capsule, parenchyma, or hilum. Injuries are most common along the lower and medial poles of the spleen, where most of the pericolonic, peritoneal, and omental attachments lie. A significant splenic injury may be immediately apparent with copious bleeding or may be occult and not noticed until later when a large hematoma is discovered.

When resecting a tumor adjacent to the splenic flexure, the omentum is generally resected with the specimen. Splenic injury may be avoided by initially entering the lesser sac and ligating the omental vessels from medial to lateral. The omentum and colon are then carefully freed from the lower pole of the spleen with sharp dissection. With the patient in the synchronous position with the legs in stirrups, the surgeon stands between the legs, with the first assistant on the patient's right and the second assistant on the left. Good visualization and left upper quadrant retraction along with an adequate incision and minimal traction are important. Splenectomy may be indicated if there is any suspicion of invasion by the tumor. When mobilizing the splenic flexure to create a distal anastomosis, one may approach the splenic attachments from both the medial and lateral directions. After initial careful mobilization of the omentum off of the splenic flexure of the colon and the spleen, the bowel is freed.

Most superficial tears of the capsule may be controlled with a combination of packing and later examination, electrocautery, and various hemostatic agents placed beneath the packing as necessary. If this fails to stop the hemorrhage, more aggressive local means may be used, such as grasping and clipping individual bleeding vessels in the parenchyma, figure-of-eight sutures, or pledget-controlled full-thickness sutures. Deeper lacerations or injuries of the hilum may require mobilization of the spleen and segmental ligation of the feeding hilar arteries.

Partial splenectomy may be necessary for deep, devascularizing injuries. Total splenectomy is rarely necessary and carries the risk of postsplenectomy sepsis from organisms such as *Pneumococcus, Haemophilus influenzae, Meningococcus, Streptococcus,* and *Staphylococcus.*[10] Treatment with pneumococcal vaccine (Pneumovax) to reduce the rate of pneumococcal infection and prophylaxis with penicillin is recommended. There is a suggestion that patients with Dukes stage C colorectal carcinoma have a decreased survival rate after splenectomy.[11]

Coloanal Anastomosis

Very low colorectal anastomoses and coloanal anastomoses are being performed with greater frequency in patients with middle and lower rectal carcinomas. The goal is to maintain the normal route of evacuation while still obtaining good surgical results. A large volume of literature confirms that there is no difference in survival or recurrence rate between a correctly performed abdominoperineal resection with colostomy and rectal resection with anastomosis. Coloanal anastomosis may be chosen when the neoplasm is in the lower rectum and the entire rectum and a portion of the internal sphincter must be removed to obtain an adequate distal margin. These anastomoses may be created at various levels and with a variety of techniques. The level of anastomosis may be at the anorectal junction, in the transitional zone mucosa, at the dentate line, or even below. The plane of dissection may progress down along the rectal wall into the intersphincteric space, with removal of part of the internal sphincter, or a mucosectomy may be performed transanally beginning at the dentate line. The anastomosis may be constructed with sutures or with staples. Many surgeons are now using a double-stapled technique, transecting the upper anal canal with a 30 mm linear stapler and then placing the intraluminal circular stapler transanally. In most patients in whom a coloanal anastomosis is created, a diverting ostomy is created as well. This is closed after 2 to 3 months and after performance of lower GI gastrograffin studies to detect anastomotic leaks. More recently, some surgeons omit the diversion, especially when the anastomosis is created with a stapler, and find no higher complication rates.

Anastomotic leakage is the most feared problem when a surgeon performs a coloanal anastomosis. Even when the anastomosis is sutured under direct vision and is protected by a diverting colostomy, the leakage rate is 2% to 11%.[12-14] Many more leaks may be demonstrated radiographically before closure of the ostomy. When these leaks are small, they usually do not require further intervention, and most will close over time. The healing of long narrow anastomotic sinuses can be hastened by dividing the bowel wall septum between the sinus and the bowel lumen. This converts a narrow-necked sinus to an open cavity or diverticulum. The technique described by Whitlow et al. is suitable for colorectal or ileoanal anastomosis. A proctoscope or anoscope is used to visualize the opening on the sinus.[15] The septum is divided with laparoscopic cautery scissors passed through the scope, residual granulation tissue is removed with a curet, and suction cautery is used to control any residual bleeding. The authors reported excellent healing in a selected group of patients, most of whom had undergone proximal intestinal diversion before surgical manipulation of the sinus.

Occasionally, formal revision of the anastomosis may be necessary. Symptomatic anastomotic leaks usually are associated with pelvic sepsis, which may be treated with percutaneous or transanastomotic drainage. These will often heal, but caution must be exerted to prevent further problems when the colostomy is closed.

Anastomotic stenosis is fairly common after coloanal anastomosis and may occur in as many as 42% of patients.[13,15] Many of these stenoses can be managed with simple digital dilation; in some cases, however, marked narrowing develops with a more rigid and constricting fibrosis. Even with dilation under anesthesia, these stenoses may recur rapidly. Treatment options for these stenoses include frequent self-dilation at home with a digit or graduated dilators, transabdominal revision of the anastomosis, transanal excision of the stenotic ring and reconstitution of the anastomosis, and transanal release of the stricture. All of these options are associated with morbidity and the significant possibility that the sphincters will be further damaged. Conversion to a permanent colostomy is the ultimate treatment option and is occasionally necessary because of stenosis, leakage, or incontinence.

Function after coloanal anastomosis is generally good, given the nature of the procedure. It is important to carefully counsel patients before surgery so that their expectations are reasonable. Because there is some compromise in sphincter function and the rectal reservoir is entirely lost, they will initially have frequent, loose stools. They often have urgency and may experience soiling, especially at night. Function usually improves over time and with dietary and medical management. Biofeedback to improve sphincter function has been helpful in selected patients. About 85% of patients have good control, although often with minor nocturnal soiling; 3% will be totally incontinent. Bowel movements average three to four per day after 6 months, and most patients are happy with the outcome compared with their function with a diverting ostomy.[13,14,16,17] Physiologic testing has demonstrated that there is a modest drop in resting pressures after all types of coloanal anastomosis. Squeeze pressure changes are more variable and seem to be related to the surgical technique. This drop in pressure is more marked when the anal canal is everted but does improve over time. Neorectal capacity and compliance are initially poor, as would be expected from a segment of sigmoid or descending colon. Over time, however, the neorectum becomes dilated and is able to accommodate larger volumes with less pressure. This allows the patient to defer evacuation more easily, improves continence, and decreases the frequency of bowel movements. Failure rates range from 3% to 11%, and most failures are the result of sepsis or poor function. Recurrence rates are similar to those after low anterior resection or abdominoperineal resection.

Addition of a colonic J pouch to increase early neorectal capacity and compliance and improve functional results has been suggested by several authors.[19-22] Several nonrandomized retrospective and prospective studies have been published, but these often do not clearly demonstrate the advantage of a colonic pouch over a straight anastomosis. In two recent randomized studies that do seem to support a functional advantage of a pouch, less urgency, fewer bowel movements per day, and less soiling at night were noted.[23,24] When creating a colonic J pouch, the splenic flexure should always be mobilized. The pouch is best made from the descending colon rather than the sigmoid colon. High ligation of the inferior mesenteric artery rarely compromises perfusion of the remaining colon, but this should be checked. Stenosis of the pouch–anal anastomosis is also common but usually responds to simple digital dilation. Anastomotic leakage is no more common when a colonic pouch is created, although all patients reported had temporary diversion. Some patients may have incomplete emptying. In general, a colonic J pouch may be added to the coloanal procedure with the expectation that there will be some early functional benefit. Nevertheless, this has not become general practice because it is technically more difficult, adds to the operative time, and a longer segment of bowel must be mobilized.

PROGNOSTIC FACTORS AND RECURRENCE

Estimating the prognosis in patients with colorectal carcinoma has been attempted for more than a century. Countless studies have evaluated all types of factors, and recent journals contain many articles about this issue. Prognosis with and without a particular therapy is the major determinant of that therapy's usefulness, and this information guides the clinician's decisions about treatment recommendations. Patients also like to have an idea of what to expect so they may plan their lives. Prognosis is usually described in terms of 5-year survival and local or distant recurrence. This is directly related to the spread of these tumors, by either direct invasion or lymphatic or hematogeneous dissemination. Classic work in this area was performed by Ernest Miles, a British surgeon, and Cuthbert Dukes, a pathologist at St. Mark's Hospital in London.

Miles' work early in the twentieth century demonstrated the importance of lymphatic spread of rectal carcinoma.[25,26] He described three routes of lymphatic drainage: upward along the superior hemorrhoidal vessels to the inferior mesenteric and periaortic nodes, laterally through the perirectal tissues into the iliac system along the pelvic side walls, and inferiorly through the perianal tissues to the inguinal nodes. Miles believed that a curative operation for cancers of the rectum and sigmoid colon had to include all three areas. These three lymphatic drainage areas were clearly important in the advanced lesions that Miles saw; however, it has since been shown that lymphatic spread from earlier lesions is almost exclusively upward along the inferior mesenteric distribution. In the

1930s and subsequently, Dukes performed a comprehensive, retrospective analysis of possible prognostic factors in patients who were operated on because of rectal carcinoma.[27,28] He found that penetration of the rectal wall and spread to the regional lymph nodes were the most significant factors. Almost every analysis of prognostic factors in patients with colon and rectal carcinoma since that time has confirmed this. Thus the Dukes staging system and all of its modifications, as well as the TNM classification system, rely heavily on these two features (see Table 25-1).

Clearly, curative treatment of carcinoma cannot be achieved unless the tumor is completely removed, and obtaining adequate surgical margins is a major axiom of extirpative therapy. Margins may be expressed in terms of proximal and distal bowel wall clearance or as radial and mesenteric clearance.

Proximal and Distal Margins

Proximal and distal bowel margins are generally not a problem in resection of carcinomas of the intra-abdominal colon. Five centimeters is the general rule for these margins, although a much larger segment of colon and mesentery is usually removed with the goal of wide lymphatic clearance. The distal margin of resection is a significant issue when treating rectal carcinoma, however, because of the limits imposed by the tumor's proximity to the pelvic floor and anal sphincter complex. The "5 centimeter rule" may be suspended in such cases because it has little real scientific basis. The currently accepted safe distal margin is 2 cm, although a margin between 1 and 2 cm in the unstretched, fresh specimen is probably adequate. These recommendations are based on a series of studies that concluded that intramural spread beyond 1.5 cm from the raised edge of the lesion is uncommon.[29-33] Indeed, spread to more than 5 mm from the palpable edge of the tumor is almost always associated with extensive lymphatic metastasis, poorly differentiated or mucinous histologic findings, and advanced disease.[30,34-37] Margins greater than 2 cm do not influence survival or local recurrence rates; however, margins less than 1 cm are associated with increased local recurrence rates.[31,38,39]

Radial Margins

Radial or lateral clearance of colonic tumors becomes an issue when the lesion is adherent to or invades an adjacent structure. Neoplasms of the abdominal colon occasionally invade whatever tissues they are against. For example, a cecal or right colonic lesion may invade the abdominal wall, duodenum, bladder, ureter or kidney, uterus, or other loops of bowel; carcinomas of the transverse colon and flexures may invade the liver, gallbladder, stomach, duodenum, pancreas, or spleen. In as many as 70% of lesions that are adherent to an adjacent structure, carcinomatous invasion is demonstrated at pathologic examination. Therefore excision of all involved tissues with a margin of normal tissue is a major goal of surgery. Simply releasing an adherent lesion is associated with a high recurrence rate. When the lesion and all adherent tissues are removed en bloc with clear margins, the prognosis is almost the same as for nonadherent lesions of similar stage.[40,41] Further radial spread tends to occur into the mesenteric tissues along the lymphatic channels, and this is addressed by wide mesenteric resection.

Radial clearance is more difficult when resecting rectal carcinomas for two reasons. First, the rectum is located within the confines of the pelvis, and the bones, vessels, and soft tissue structures limit the amount of lateral tissue typically removed. Invasion into adjacent structures is much more common than with colonic primary tumors. Posterolateral structures such as the sacrum, lateral pelvic side walls and vessels, and ureters may be invaded. Anteriorly, in male patients the bladder, seminal vesicles, and prostate gland may be invaded, whereas in female patients the uterus and vagina are not infrequently involved. The same tenets hold true for rectal carcinoma as for colonic tumors: en bloc resection with a clear margin is the best and perhaps only method of attaining cure. This may involve posterior exenteration in women or total pelvic exenteration in men.[41-45] En bloc resection of the sacrum up to the level of S2-3 may be performed but is associated with significant morbidity. Again, the prognosis after wide resection with clear margins is similar by stage to that in other patients.[40,41,46] The second difficulty with lateral rectal clearance occurs because the low rectal mesenteric tissues are not organized into a confined mesentery as they are in the colon. These tissues spread into the retrorectal and lateral pelvic spaces, making wide mesenteric clearance essential to a curative operation.

Lymphatic Spread

Adenocarcinoma spreads preferentially along lymphatic channels but is exceedingly uncommon when the tumor is limited to the lamina propria. However, once the lesion has invaded the submucosa, which contains intramural lymphatic channels, the rate of lymph node disease rises to 10%. The rate of lymph node involvement is 30% to 40% when the muscularis propria has been breeched.[47,48] The lymphatic channels parallel the vascular supply. As the tumor spreads, shed cells get caught up in the lymph nodes along these channels and multiply. Spread to the regional lymph nodes has repeatedly been shown to be a major prognostic factor; thus examination of the regional lymph nodes is a critical component of all staging systems. Because the routes of spread follow the major vessels that supply each segment of bowel, tumors of the cecum, right colon, and right half of the transverse colon will spread to the lymph nodes along the ileocolic, right colic, and right branch of the middle colic arteries. Splenic flexure, left colon, and sigmoid cancers will spread along the left branch of the middle colic artery, the left colic artery, and the sigmoid branches and to the inferior mesenteric artery, respectively. As noted by Miles, lymphatic spread from the rectum may progress upward along the superior hemorrhoidal vessels to the inferior mesenteric and periaortic nodes, laterally through the perirectal tissues into the iliac system along the pelvic side wall, and inferiorly through the perianal tissues to the inguinal nodes. Spread from the mid and upper rectum and sigmoid colon is almost exclusively proximally along the inferior mesenteric vessels.[27,49] Lateral and distal spread may occur with tumors of the lower third of the rectum but is uncommon in the absence of extensive proximal lymphatic obstruction.[28,29,32,35,50-52] There has been a major shift from abdominoperineal resection to low anterior resection for the treatment of rectal carcinoma.[53-56] It has been clearly established that these two procedures produce equivalent oncologic outcomes if a distal margin of 2 cm is achieved with wide lateral and proximal lymphatic clearance.[34,57-61]

The proximal limit of mesenteric resection has been debated. For lesions of the abdominal colon, the dissection is limited by the need to maintain blood supply to the remaining intestine. Sigmoid and rectal lesions may be resected with high ligation of the inferior mesenteric vessels. The inferior mesenteric artery may be ligated above or below the takeoff of the left colic artery. If ligated below, the left colic artery is preserved and the left colon retains its normal vascular supply, reducing the risk of colonic ischemia. This does leave the lymphatic tissue between this level and the takeoff of the inferior mesenteric artery in situ. Transection of the inferior mesenteric artery just as it comes off the aorta allows a more complete lymphatic clearance but sacrifices the left colic artery. In general, adequate perfusion is maintained through the marginal artery of Drummond from the superior mesenteric vasculature.[62,63] This also frees up the descending colon significantly, which is helpful when performing a very low anastomosis. It appears that removing these highest lymph nodes provides important prognostic information but does little to improve outcome.[64-69] If these nodes are involved with tumor, the disease is invariably systemic and will not be cured with surgery alone.

Complete mesorectal excision appears to be of benefit in lowering local recurrence rates. Typical series report local recurrence rates of 12% to 20%, and one group has reported a rate of 3% to 4% when the entire mesorectum was meticulously removed to the anorectal ring distally and circumferentially.[70-73] This removes all lateral mesenteric lymphatic tissue. More radical lateral and high lymphatic dissections that begin at level of the duodenum and remove the periaortic and parailiac tissues have been advocated by some.[74] However, these procedures are associated with unacceptably high complication rates, with frequent ureteric injuries and urinary dysfunction (39% versus 9%) and impotence (76% versus 38%), and early reports of improved survival have not been duplicated in other centers.[73,75-78]

"No Touch" Technique

Intraoperative dissemination of tumor cells may occur during manipulation of the tumor[79-81] but may be reduced with lymphovascular and luminal isolation of the tumor before mobilization. The "no touch" technique, as popularized by

Turnbull, attempts to do this.[82,83] This operative technique is easily learned, easily performed, and adds no morbidity to the procedure. Although Turnbull's data suggest that this method confers a survival benefit, results from a recent randomized trial from The Netherlands approached but failed to reach significance.[84] When comparing no-touch and conventional operation groups, the rates of liver metastases (14% versus 22%), 5-year survival (60% versus 56%), and total deaths (40% versus 44%), deaths from recurrent disease (25% versus 31%), or deaths from vascular invasion (31% versus 52%) were not statistically different.

DNA Ploidy

Flow cytometric analysis of tumor cells yields information about DNA structure from which mitotic activity may be inferred. Normal cells at rest are diploid, with two sets of chromosomes. Dividing cells have different complements, dependent on their state of reproduction. Malignant cells divide at a faster than normal rate and may harbor abnormal chromosomal numbers. Thus, aneuploid or tetraploid peaks may be more prominent in these malignancies. Fifty percent to 70% of colorectal tumors demonstrate a significant increase in the nondiploid peaks on flow cytometry histograms. S phase analysis estimates the percentage of cells that are actively dividing. Normal colorectal mucosal cells have an S phase fraction of 4% to 10%, whereas in malignant cells the fraction may be as high as 20%. The presence of increased nondiploid peaks and increases in S phase fraction are correlated with poor prognosis and in some studies are independent predictors of tumor behavior.[85-89] In practice, these determinations are most useful in decisions as to whether a patient with cancer without lymphatic spread should receive adjuvant therapy.

Obstruction and Perforation

Near or complete bowel obstruction presents a particular surgical challenge. The preoperative management of this problem is discussed in Chapter 2. Several studies have shown obstruction to be a significant prognostic factor; however, patients generally have more advanced lesions that are full thickness and often produce lymphatic or distant metastases.[90-92] Patients may have perforation of the colon, either at the site of the cancer from tumor necrosis or in the cecum from distal obstruction. A tumor perforation may be walled off and contained, may fistulize into an adjacent structure, or may communicate freely with the peritoneal cavity. Free perforation carries the risk of tumor dissemination within the abdominal cavity and subsequent carcinomatosis. Perforation may also occur during surgical resection because of close margins or necrotic tissues. As early as 1913, Mayo[93] stated his belief that recurrence of rectal carcinoma could be the result of spillage of tumor cells in the operative field after traumatic manipulation. Perforation that occurs during the operation is clearly associated with increased recurrence rates.[94-96]

Differentiation

Colorectal carcinomas may be classified as well, moderately, or poorly differentiated, dependent on criteria observed by the pathologist during microscopic examination. Tumors that are well differentiated and have cells that look like adenomatous tissue tend to behave more benignly than lesions with poorly differentiated and anaplastic cells.[97,98] Although these features do differentiate these tumors, the majority are classified as moderately differentiated. Other pathologic features associated with poor prognosis include mucinous and signet cell histologic findings and vascular and neural invasion.[99-102]

Local Recurrence

Local recurrence is relatively uncommon in patients who have undergone resection of carcinoma of the abdominal colon unless the lesion had perforated or invaded adjacent structures.[103-105] Local recurrence after resection of a rectal lesion remains a significant problem and is more common as the level of the tumor in the rectum decreases.[36] Distal intramural invasion is hardly ever more than 5 mm from the palpable edge of the tumor, so increasing the margin beyond 2 cm has no effect on local recurrence.[36,59,70,106] Thus there is no difference in local recurrence rates between low anterior resection with sphincter preservation and abdominoperineal resection as long as a good margin is obtained.[36] Lateral margins are critical because they are limited by the bony confines of the pelvis. Excision of all mesorectal tissue flush with the pelvic side walls and the presacral fascia and down to the anorectal ring has been shown to reduce local recurrence. Adjuvant radiation therapy further reduces local recurrence rates, and this effect may be potentiated by simultaneous chemotherapy (see Chapter 24).

True anastomotic recurrence after resection of the abdominal colon is rare because of the wide margins of resection obtained. Occasionally a lesion will recur and the treatment of choice is repeat resection. A larger tumor or widespread disease is often discovered during exploratory surgery, and resection may not be possible. Even if the cure cannot be achieved, palliative resection and anastomosis is often reasonable to prevent or delay malignant obstruction. If resection is not possible, bypass is a good option. If obstruction is imminent, a proximal ostomy is another alternative. Anastomotic recurrence at a colorectal anastomosis is a more common finding and may be related to an inadequate distal margin or tumor seeding at the time of the original operation.[66,107-109]

Occasionally these lesions may be resected for either cure or palliation. Although it may appear to be a limited problem, there may also be unrecognized extensive disease or invasion into the pelvic structures. Abdominoperineal resection with an end colostomy usually is the best procedure in these patients. Occasionally another low anterior resection may be possible if the original anastomosis was in the upper rectum, and good distal and lateral margins may be obtained. Cure is effected with resection in fewer than 50% of these patients, and after resection the 5-year survival is less than 50%.[107-113] Pelvic recurrence is the most common form of local recurrence. These recurrent lesions may invade any of the pelvic structures and are often unresectable when found.[112-115] Some authors have suggested that regular follow-up endorectal ultrasound in patients after low anterior resection of rectal carcinomas will enable identification of local recurrence earlier and will increase resectability rates. If resection is possible, an extensive procedure is likely necessary. Pelvic exenteration or sacral resection may be offered to selected patients without distant disease if they are willing to accept the significant morbidity associated with these procedures. In highly selected patients who undergo these procedures, the 5-year survival rate is 8% to 34%.[116-118] Otherwise, palliation with proximal bypass, laser recannulation for obstructing lesions, or radiation therapy may be helpful. Rarely, an isolated recurrence will develop in the perineal closure wound after an abdominoperineal resection. After searching for other sites of recurrence, wide local excision may be performed.[119,120] Radiation may be added if not already performed. Most local recurrent lesions are detected at advanced stages and and are not amenable to curative treatment.

REFERENCES

1. Heald RJ, Bussey HJR. Clinical experiences at St. Mark's Hospital with multiple synchronous cancers of the colon and rectum. Dis Colon Rectum 18:6-10, 1975.
2. Lasser A. Synchronous primary adenocarcinomas of the colon and rectum. Dis Colon Rectum 21:20-22, 1978.
3. Welch JP. Multiple colorectal tumors: An appraisal of natural history and therapeutic options. Am J Surg 142:274-280, 1981.
4. Reilly JC, Russin LC, Theuerkauf FJ Jr. Colonoscopy: Its role in cancer of the colon and rectum. Dis Colon Rectum 25:532-538, 1982.
5. Langevin JM, Nivatvongs S. The true incidence of synchronous cancer of the large bowel: A prospective study. Am J Surg 147:330-333, 1984.
6. Thorson AG, Christensen MA, Davis SJ. The role of colonoscopy in the assessment of patients with colorectal cancer. Dis Colon Rectum 29:306-311, 1986.
7. Carlsson G, Petrelli NJ, Herrera L, Nava H, Mittelman A. Endoscopic surveillance of patients following a curative resection for colorectal cancer. J Surg Oncol 38:80-82, 1988.
8. Wolff WI, Shinya H, Geffen A, Ozoktay S, DeBeer R. Comparison of colonoscopy and the contrast enema in five hundred patients with colorectal disease. Am J Surg 129:181-186, 1975.
9. Langevin JM, Rothenberger DA, Goldberg SM. Accidental splenic injury during surgical treatment of the colon and rectum. Surg Gynecol Obstet 159:139-144, 1984.
10. Leonard AS, Giebink GS, Baesl TJ, Krivit W. The overwhelming postsplenectomy sepsis problem. World J Surg 4:423-432, 1980.
11. Davis EJ, Ilstrup DM, Pemberton JH. Influence of splenectomy on survival rate of patients with colorectal cancer. Am J Surg 155;173-179, 1988.
12. Parks AG, Percy JP. Resection and sutured colo-anal anastomosis for rectal carcinoma. Br J Surg 69:301-304, 1982.

13. Drake DB, Pemberton JH, Beart RW Jr, Dozois RR, Wolff BG. Coloanal anastomosis in the management of benign and malignant rectal disease. Ann Surg 206:600-605, 1987.
14. Hautefeuille P, Valleur P, Perniceni T, et al. Functional and oncological results after coloanal anastomosis for low rectal cancer. Ann Surg 207:61-64, 1988.
15. Whitlow CB, Beck DE, Opelka GF, Gathright JB. Operative management of anastomotic sinus (in press).
16. Bernard D, Morgan S, Tasse D, Wassef R. Preliminary results of coloanal anastomosis. Dis Colon Rectum 32:580-584, 1989.
17. Vernava AM III, Robbins PL, Brabbee GW. Restorative resection: Coloanal anastomosis for benign and malignant disease. Dis Colon Rectum 32:690-693, 1989.
18. Pappalardo G, Toccaceli S, Dionisio P, Castrini G, Ravo B. Preoperative and postoperative evaluation by manometric study of the anal sphincter after coloanal anastomosis for carcinoma. Dis Colon Rectum 31:119-122, 1988.
19. Lazorthes F, Fages P, Chiotasso P, Lemozy J, Bloom E. Resection of the rectum with construction of a colonic reservoir and coloanal anastomosis for carcinomas of the rectum. Br J Surg 73:136-138, 1986.
20. Parc R, Tiret E, Frileux P, Moszkowski E, Jygue J. Resection and coloanal anastomosis with colonic reservoir for rectal carcinoma. Br J Surg 73:139-141, 1986.
21. Nicholls RJ, Lubowski DZ, Donaldson Dr. Comparison of colonic reservoir and straight coloanal reconstruction after rectal excision. Br J Surg 75:318-320, 1988.
22. Leo E, Belli F, Baldini MT, et al. Total rectal resection and coloanal anastomosis with colonic reservoir for low rectal cancer. Int J Colorect Dis 9:82-86, 1994.
23. Hallbook O, Krog M, Pahlman L, Wexner SD, Sjodahl R. Colonic pouch versus straight reconstruction in low anterior resection for cancer—A randomized trial [abstract]. Presented at the World Congress of Gastroenterology Meeting. Los Angeles: Oct 2-7, 1994.
24. Seow-Choen F, Goh HS. Colonic pouch is superior to straight low colorectal anastomosis [abst]. Presented at the American Society of Colon and Rectal Surgeons 92nd Annual Convention. Chicago: May 2-7, 1993.
25. Miles WE. A method of performing abdominoperineal excision for carcinoma of the rectum and of the terminal portion of the pelvic colon. Lancet 2:1812, 1908.
26. Miles WE. Cancer of the Rectum. London: Harrison, 1926.
27. Dukes CE. The spread of cancer of the rectum. Br J Surg 17:643, 1930.
28. Dukes CE. The surgical pathology of rectal cancer. Proc R Soc Med (Lond) 37:131, 1943.
29. Black WA, Waugh JM. The intramural extension of carcinoma of the descending colon, sigmoid and rectosigmoid: A pathologic study. Surg Gynecol Obstet 87:457-464, 1948.
30. Grinnell RS. Distal intramural spread of carcinoma of the rectum and rectosigmoid. Surg Gynecol Obstet 99:421, 1954.
31. Madsen PM, Christiansen J. Distal intramural spread of rectal carcinomas. Dis Colon Rectum 29:279-282, 1986.
32. Pollett WG, Nicholls RJ. The relationship between the extent of distal clearance and survival and local recurrence rates after curative anterior resection for carcinoma of the rectum. Ann Surg 198:159-163, 1983.
33. Williams NS, Dixon MF, Johnston D. Reappraisal of the 5 centimetre rule of distal excision for carcinoma of the rectum: A study of distal intramural spread and of patients' survival. Br J Surg 70:150-154, 1983.
34. Quer EA, Dahlin DC, Mayo CW. Retrograde intramural spread of carcinoma of the rectum and rectosigmoid: A microscopic study. Surg Gynecol Obstet 96:24-30, 1953.
35. Grinnell RS. Lymphatic metastasis and spread in carcinoma of the colon and rectum. Ann Surg 163:272-280, 1966.

36. McDermott FT, Hughes ES, Pihl E, Johnson WR, Price AB. Local recurrence after potentially curative resection for rectal cancer in a series of 1008 patients. Br J Surg 72:34-37, 1985.
37. Lazorthes F, Voigt JJ, Roques J, Chiotasso P, Chevreau P. Distal intramural spread of carcinoma of the rectum correlated with lymph nodal involvement. Surg Gynecol Obstet 170:45-48, 1990.
38. Wilson SM, Beahrs OH. The curative treatment of carcinoma of the sigmoid, rectosigmoid, and rectum. Ann Surg 183:556-565, 1976.
39. Wolmark N, Fisher B. An analysis of survival and treatment failure following abdominoperineal and sphincter-saving resection in Dukes' B and C rectal carcinoma. A report of the NSABP clinical trials. National Surgical Adjuvant Breast and Bowel Project. Ann Surg 204:480-489, 1986.
40. Durdey P, Williams NS. The effect of malignant and inflammatory fixation of rectal carcinoma on prognosis after rectal excision. Br J Surg 71:787-790, 1984.
41. Orkin BA, Dozois RR, Beart RW Jr, Patterson DE, Gunderson LL, Ilstrup DM. Extended resection for locally advanced primary adenocarcinoma of the rectum. Dis Colon Rectum 32:286-292, 1989.
42. Ledesma EJ, Bruno S, Mittelman A. Total pelvic exenteration in colorectal disease: A 20-year experience. Ann Surg 194:701-703, 1981.
43. Wanebo HJ, Gaker DL, Whitehill R, Morgan RF, Constable WC. Pelvic recurrence of rectal cancer. Options for curative resection. Ann Surg 205:482-495, 1987.
44. Kraybill WG, Lopez MJ, Bricker EM. Total pelvic exenteration as a therapeutic option in advanced malignant disease of the pelvis. Surg Gynecol Obstet 166:259-263, 1988.
45. Williams LF, Jr, Huddleston CB, Sawyers JL, Potts JR III, Sharp KW, McDougal SW. Is total pelvic exenteration reasonable primary treatment for rectal carcinoma? Ann Surg 207:670-678, 1988.
46. Fedorov VD, Shelygin YA. Treatment of patients with rectal cancer. Dis Colon Rectum 32:138-145, 1989.
47. Nivatvongs S, Rojanasakul A, Reiman HM, Dozois RR, Wolff BG, Pemberton JH, Beart RW, Jacques LF. The risk of lymph node metastasis in colorectal polyps with invasive adenocarcinoma. Dis Colon Rectum 34:323-328, 1991.
48. Wolmark N, Cruz I, Redmond CE, Fisher B, Fisher E, and contributing NSABP investigators. Tumor size and regional lymph node metastasis in colorectal cancer: A preliminary analysis from the NSABP Clinical trials. Cancer 51:1315-1322, 1983.
49. Villemin F, Huard P, Montagne M. Anatomical study of the lymphatics of the rectum and the anus for application in the surgical treatment of cancer. Rev Chir 63:39, 1925.
50. Batholdson L, Hultborn A, Hulten L, Roos B, Rosencrantz M, Ahnen C. Lymph drainage from the upper and middle third of the rectum as demonstrated by Au. Acta Radiol Ther 16:352-360, 1977.
51. Goligher JC, Dukes GE, Bussey HJ. Local recurrences after sphincter-saving excisions for carcinoma of the rectum and rectosigmoid. Br J Surg 39:199-211, 1951.
52. Hojo K, Koyama Y, Moriya Y. Lymphatic spread and its prognostic value in patients with rectal cancer. Am J Surg 144:350-354, 1982.
53. Dixon CF. Surgical removal of lesions occurring in the sigmoid and rectosigmoid. Am J Surg 46:12-17, 1939.
54. Lockhart-Mummery HE, Ritchie JK, Hawley PR. The results of surgical treatment for carcinoma of the rectum of St. Mark's Hospital from 1948-1972. Br J Surg 63:673-677, 1976.
55. Smart CR. Rectal cancer patterns of care. Bull Am Coll Surg 65:414-415, 1980.

56. McDermott FT, Hughes ES, Pihl EA, Johnson WR, Polglase AL, Milne BA, Katrivessis H. Changing survival prospects in rectal carcinoma. A series of 1,306 patients managed by one surgeon. Dis Colon Rectum 29:798-803, 1986.
57. Frigell A, Ottander M, Stenbeck H, Pahlman L. Quality of life of patients treated with abdominoperineal resection or anterior resection for rectal carcinoma. Ann Chir Gynaecol 79:26-30, 1990.
58. Slanetz CA, Herter FP, Grinnell RS. Anterior resection versus abdominoperineal resection for cancer of the rectum and rectosigmoid. Am J Surg 123:110, 1972.
59. Heimann TM, Szporn A, Bolnick K, Aufses AH Jr. Local recurrence following surgical treatment of rectal cancer. Comparison of anterior and abdominoperineal resection. Dis Colon Rectum 29:862-864, 1986.
60. Neville R, Fielding LP, Amendola C. Local tumor recurrence after curative resection for rectal cancer. A ten-hospital review. Dis Colon Rectum 30:12-17, 1987.
61. Athlin L, Bengtsson NO, Stenling R. Local recurrence and survival after radical resection of rectal carcinoma. Acta Chir Scand 154:225-229, 1988.
62. Goligher JC. The adequacy of the marginal blood supply to the left colon after high ligation of the inferior mesenteric artery during excision of the rectum. Br J Surg 41:351, 1954.
63. Griffiths JD. Surgical anatomy of the blood supply of the distal colon. Ann R Coll Surg Engl 19:241, 1956.
64. Morgan CN, Griffiths JD. High ligation of the inferior mesenteric artery during operations for carcinoma of the distal colon and rectum. Surg Gynecol Obstet 108:641, 1959.
65. Grinnell RS. Results in the treatment of carcinoma of the colon and rectum. Surg Gynecol Obstet 19:241, 1953.
66. Anet GW, Castro AF, Smith RS. Clinical study of ligation of the inferior mesenteric artery in left colon resection. Surg Gynecol Obstet 94:223-228, 1952.
67. Grinnell RS. Results of ligation of inferior mesenteric artery at the aorta in resections of carcinoma of the descending and sigmoid colon and rectum. Surg Gynecol Obstet 120:1031-1039, 1965.
68. Pezim ME, Nicholls RJ. Survival after high or low ligation of the inferior mesenteric artery during curative surgery for rectal cancer. Ann Surg 200:729-733, 1984.
69. Surtees P, Ritchie JK, Phillips RKS. High versus low ligation of the inferior mesenteric artery in rectal cancer. Br J Surg 77:618-621, 1990.
70. Karanjia ND, Schache DJ, North WRS, Heald RJ. 'Close shave' in anterior resection. Br J Surg 77:510-512, 1990.
71. Heald RJ, Husband EM, Ryall RD. The mesorectum in rectal cancer surgery—The clue to pelvic recurrence? Br J Surg 69:613-616, 1982.
72. Heald RJ, Ryall RD. Recurrence and survival after total mesorectal excision for rectal cancer. Lancet 1:1476, 1986.
73. McAnena OJ, Heald RJ, Lockhart-Mummery HE. Operative and functional results of total mesorectal excision with ultra-low anterior resection in the management of carcinoma of the lower one-third of the rectum. Surg Gynecol Obstet 170:517-521, 1990.
74. Koyama Y, Moriya Y, Hojo K. Effects of extended systematic lymphadenectomy for adenocarcinoma of the rectum—Significant improvement of survival rate and decrease of local recurrence. Jpn J Clin Oncol 14:623-632, 1984.
75. Stearns MW, Deddish MR. Five year results of abdominal lymph node dissection for carcinoma of the rectum. Dis Colon Rectum 2:169-172, 1959.
76. Enker WE, Pilipshen SJ, Heilweil ML, Stearns MW Jr, Janov AJ, Hertz RE, Sternberg SS. En block pelvic lymphadenectomy and sphincter preservation in the surgical management of rectal cancer. Ann Surg 203:426-433, 1986.

77. Kodaira S, Teramoto T. Extended radical operation of cancer of the rectum. Gan No Rinsho 32:1328-1332, 1986.
78. Michelassi F, Block GE. Morbidity and mortality of wide pelvic lymphadenectomy for rectal adenocarcinoma. Dis Colon Rectum 35:1143-1147, 1992.
79. Cole WH, Packard D, Southwick HW. Carcinoma of the colon with special reference to the prevention of recurrence. JAMA 155:1549, 1954.
80. Fisher ER, Turnbull RB. The cytologic demonstration and significance of tumor cells in the mesenteric venous bleed in patients with colorectal carcinomas. Surg Gynecol Obstet 100:102, 1955.
81. Griffiths JD, McKenna JA, Rowbotham HD, Tsolkidis P, Salsbury AJ. Carcinoma of the colon and rectum: Circulating malignant cells and five year survival. Cancer 31:226, 1973.
82. Barnes JP. Physiologic resection of the right colon. Surg Gynecol Obstet 94:722, 1952.
83. Turnbull RB, Kyle K, Watson FR, Spratt J. Cancer of the colon: The influence of the no-touch isolation technique on survival rates. Ann Surg 166:420-427, 1967.
84. Wiggers T, Jeekel J, Arends JW, Brinkhorst AD, Kluck HM, Luyk CI, Munting JDK, Dovel J, Rutten A, Volvovics A, Greep J. No-touch isolation technique in colon cancer: A controlled prospective trial. Br J Surg 75:409-415. 1988.
85. Tribukait B, Hammarberg C, Rubio C. Ploidy and proliferation patterns in colo-rectal adenocarcinomas related to Dukes' classification and to histopathological differentiation. A flow-cytometric DNA study. Acta Pathol Microbiol Immunol Scand [A] 91:89-95, 1983.
86. Forsslund G, Cedermark B, Ohman U, Erhardt K, Zetterberg A, Auer G. The significance of DNA distribution pattern in rectal carcinoma. Dis Colon Rectum 27:579-584, 1984.
87. Banner BF, Tomas-de la Vega JE, Roseman DL, Coon JS. Should flow cytometric DNA analyses precede definitive surgery for colon carcinoma? Ann Surg 202:740-744, 1986.
88. Scott NA, Rainwater LM, Wieand HS, Wieland LH, Pemberton JH, Beart RW, Lieber MM. The relative prognostic value of flow cytometric DNA analysis and conventional clinicopathologic criteria in patients with operable rectal carcinoma. Dis Colon Rectum 30:513-520, 1987.
89. Hood DL, Petras RE, Edinger M, Fazio V, Tubbs RR. Deoxyribonucleic acid ploidy and cell cycle analysis of colorectal carcinoma by flow cytometry. A prospective study of 137 cases using fresh whole cell suspensions. Am J Clin Pathol 93:615-620, 1990.
90. Wolmark N, Wieand HS, Rockette HE, Fisher B, Glass A, Lawrence W, Lerner H, Cruz A, Volk H, Shibata H, Evans J, Prager D, and contributing NSABP investigators. The prognostic significance of tumor location and bowel obstruction in Dukes B and C colorectal cancer: Findings from the NSABP clinical trials. Ann Surg 198:743-752, 1983.
91. Pescatori M, Maria G, Beltrani B, Mattana C. Site, emergency, and duration of symptoms in the prognosis of colorectal cancer. Dis Colon Rectum 25:33-40, 1982.
92. Steinberg SM, Barkin JS, Kaplan RS, Stablein DM. Prognostic indicators of colon tumors: The Gastrointestinal Tumor Study Group experience. Cancer 57:1866-1870, 1986.
93. Mayo WJ. Grafting and traumatic dissemination of carcinoma in the course of operations for malignant disease. JAMA 60:512-513, 1913.
94. Ranbarger KR, Johnston WD, Chang JC. Prognostic significance of surgical perforation of the rectum during abdominoperineal resection for rectal carcinoma. Am J Surg 143:186-188, 1982.
95. Slanetz CA Jr. The effect of inadvertent intraoperative perforation on survival and recurrence in colorectal cancer. Dis Colon Rectum 27:792-797, 1984.
96. Zirngibl H, Husemann B, Hermanek P. Intraoperative spillage of tumor cells in surgery for rectal cancer. Dis Colon Rectum 33:610-614, 1990.

97. Dukes CE, Bussey HJ. The spread of rectal cancer and its effects on prognosis. Br J Cancer 12:309-320, 1958.
98. Spratt JS Jr, Spjut HJ. Prevalence and prognosis of individual clinical and pathological variables associated with colorectal carcinoma. Cancer 10:1976-1985, 1967.
99. Bentzen SM, Balslev I, Pedersen M, Teglbjaerg PS, Hanberg-Soerensen F, Bone J, Jacobsen NO, Overgaard J, Sell A, Bertelsen K, Hagee, Fenger C, Kronburg O, Hansen L, Hoestrup H, Noergaard-Pedersen B. A regression analysis of prognostic factors after resection of Dukes' B and C carcinoma of the rectum and rectosigmoid. Does postoperative radiotherapy change the prognosis? Br J Cancer 58:195-201, 1988.
100. Horn A, Dahl O, Morild I. The role of venous and neural invasion on survival in rectal adenocarcinoma. Dis Colon Rectum 33:598-601, 1990.
101. Minsky BD, Mies C, Recht A, Tich TA, Chaffey JT. Resectable adenocarcinoma of the rectosigmoid and rectum: The influence of blood vessel invasion. Cancer 61:1417-1428, 1988.
102. Talbot IC, Ritchie S. Leighton MH, Hughes AO, Bussey HJ, Morson BC. Invasion of veins by carcinoma of rectum: Method of detection, histological features and significance. Histopathology 5:141-163. 1981.
103. Russell AH, Tong D, Dawson LE, Wisbeck W. Adenocarcinoma of the proximal colon: Sites of initial dissemination and patterns of recurrence following surgery alone. Cancer 53:360-366, 1984.
104. Gunderson LL, Sosin H. Areas of failure found at reoperation (second or symptomatic look) following "curative surgery" for adenocarcinoma of the rectum: Clinicopathologic correlation and implications for adjuvant therapy. Cancer 34:1278-1292, 1974.
105. Welch JP, Donaldson GA. The clinical correlation of an autopsy study of recurrent colorectal cancer. Ann Surg 189:496-502, 1979.
106. Rubbini M, Vettorello GF, Guerrera C, Mari C, DeAnna D, Mascoli F, Pozza E, Gasbarro V, Donini I. A prospective study of local recurrence after resection and low stapled anastomosis in 183 patients with rectal cancer. Dis Colon Rectum 33:117-121, 1990.
107. Andersen B, Clemmesen T, Sprechler M, Baden H. Anastomotic recurrences and five-year survival rate after low anterior resection for cure in 128 patients with rectal cancer. Scand J Gastroenterol 6:449-451, 1971.
108. Pihl E, Hughes ES, McDermott FT, Price AB. Recurrence of carcinoma of the colon and rectum at the anastomotic suture line. Surg Gynecol Obstet 153:495-496, 1981.
109. Pacini P, Cionini L, Pirtoli L, Clatto S, Tucci E, Sebaste L. Symptomatic recurrences of carcinoma of the rectum and sigmoid. Dis Colon Rectum 29:865-868, 1986.
110. Sannella NA. Abdominoperineal resection following anterior resection. Cancer 38:378-381, 1976.
111. Segall MM, Goldberg SM, Nivatvongs S, Balcos EG, Nemer FD, Schottler JL, Christenson CE, Rothenberger DA. Abdominoperineal resection for recurrent cancer following anterior resection. Dis Colon Rectum 24:80-84, 1981.
112. Pilipshen AJ, Heilweil M, Quan SH, Sternberg SS, Enker WE. Patterns of pelvic recurrence following definitive resections of rectal cancer. Cancer 53:1354-1362, 1984.
113. Vassilopoulos PP, Yoon JM, Ledesma EJ. Mittelman A. Treatment of recurrence of adenocarcinoma of the colon and rectum at the anastomotic site. Surg Gynecol Obstet 152:777-780, 1981.
114. Stearns MW Jr. Diagnosis and management of recurrent pelvic malignancy following combined abdominoperineal resection. Dis Colon Rectum 23:359-361, 1980.
115. Cohen AM, Minsky BD. Aggressive surgical management of locally advanced primary and recurrent rectal cancer. Current status and future directions. Dis Colon Rectum 33:432-438, 1990.

116. Vassilopoulos PP, Ledesma EJ, Yoon JM, Jung O, Mittelman A. Surgical treatment of metastatic colorectal adenocarcinoma. Dis Colon Rectum 24:265-271, 1981.
117. Benotti PN, Bothe A, Eyere RC, Cady B, McDermott MV, Steele G. Management of recurrent pelvic tumors. Arch Surg 122:457-460, 1987.
118. Sardi A, Bolton JS, Hicks TC, Skenderis BS II. Total pelvic exenteration with and without sacral resection in patients with recurrent colorectal cancer. South Med J 87:363-369, 1994.
119. Polk HC Jr, Spratt JS Jr. The results of treatment of perineal recurrence of cancer of the rectum. Cancer 43:952-955, 1979.
120. Wilking N, Herrera L, Petrelli NJ, Mittelman A. Pelvic and perineal recurrences after abdominoperineal resection for adenocarcinoma of the rectum. Am J Surg 150:561-563, 1985.

CHAPTER 21

Abdominoperineal Resection

JOHN M. MacKEIGAN
PETER A. CATALDO

Rectal resection to treat malignant disease or complicated benign disease is often performed under less than ideal conditions and in an older patient population with significant comorbid conditions. Abdominoperineal resection (APR) is an extensive operation performed in a confined space. This, coupled with anatomic variation, tumor extension, surrounding fibrosis, and inflammatory reaction, leads to a higher frequency of complications.

With the recent ability to perform low anastomoses and coloanal procedures, abdominoperineal resection is reserved mainly for rectal carcinoma involving the pelvic floor or upper anal canal. Anal cancers that do not respond to chemotherapy and radiation are appropriate for such therapy. Patients with unfavorable lesions at high risk of local recurrence and those at significant risk of anal incontinence and in whom anastomosis is inappropriate also should undergo abdominoperineal resection.

Small arteries and veins, many under high pressure, are at high risk of injury in an otherwise well-conducted operation. Collection of blood and serum in a confined space leads to infection and contributes to unhealed perineal wounds. Previous surgery coupled with a large primary tumor or radiation may obliterate normal tissue planes and relationships. A narrow pelvis in an obese patient may present a challenge even to a skilled operator. Complications that occur intraoperatively include hemorrhage and ureteral injury. Postoperative urinary retention, perineal hemorrhage or abscess, delayed wound healing, and colostomy-related problems are the most common complications of even a well-conducted APR.

PATIENT PREPARATION AND POSITIONING

APR necessitates denuding large areas and opening spaces. Appropriate monitoring for anticipated shifts in fluid balance and stress of surgery is essential. A Foley catheter is inserted in the operating room. The surgeon's direct role in premarking the stoma site is important.

Extra assistance for holding and changing position of retractors facilitates the operation. Whether the procedure is performed by one or two teams depends on the surgeon's training and the tumor characteristics. We prefer a one-team approach. Most of the pelvic dissection to the level of the levator muscles is performed from above; this minimizes the extent of the perineal portion and allows easier access to the perineum.

Proper positioning of the legs, which allows a well-executed operation, reduces the potential for neurologic injury, and may help to minimize DVT.[1] We customarily use low-dose heparin therapy preoperatively and sequential compression devices on the legs despite the paucity of evidence to support this approach.

Since we do the operation with one team, the patient's legs are placed in the stirrups only after the abdominal component is completed. The patient's buttocks are brought to the break in the table, and adequate padding is ensured. When possible, Allen stirrups (Fig. 21-1) or similar devices should be used to allow the legs to be held without compression and easily positioned. The feet in stirrups must be well padded and wrapped with an elastic or gauze bandage once positioned.

The legs should be positioned symmetrically with regard to flexion, abduction, and rotation (Fig. 21-2). The hips are mildly flexed and mildly abducted with minimal external rotation. Extension and adduction of the knees is avoided, and the fibular head is well padded and not subject to compression. The leg is balanced in the stirrup with the weight resting on the foot, with care that the calf does not rest on the upper edge of the stirrup. (The commonly used Lloyd Davies stirrup has no foot piece, and the calf rests directly on the pad.) If the ankle and knee are in line with the opposite shoulder and without much external rotation,

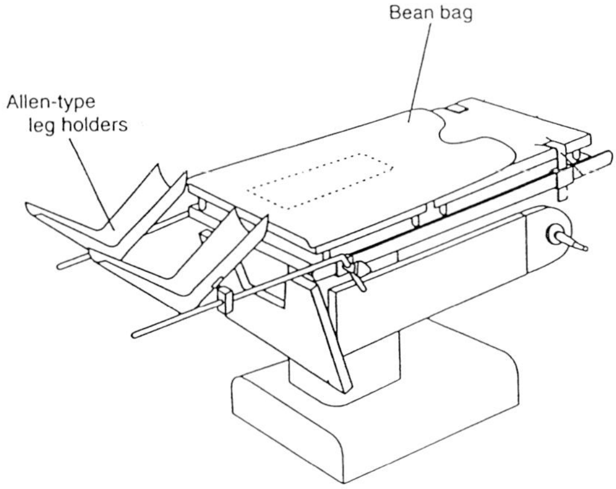

Fig. 21-1 Allen stirrups.

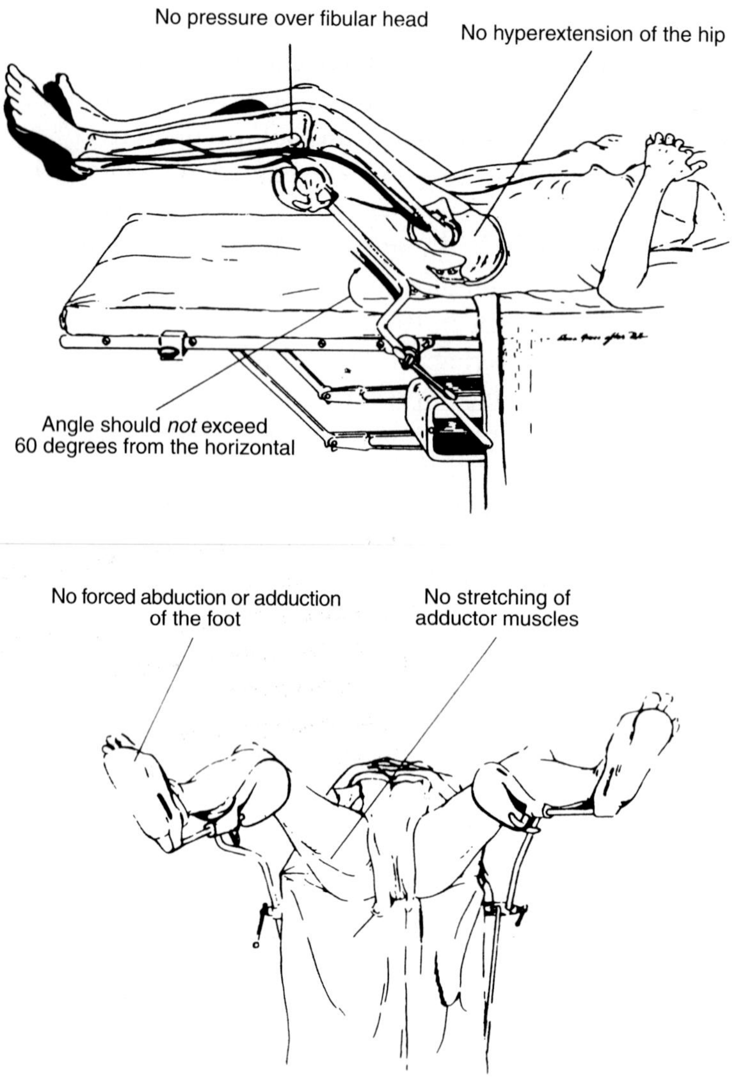

Fig. 21-2 Leg positioning for abdominoperineal resection. (From Herrera-Ornelas L, et al. Common perineal nerve palsy associated with pelvic surgery for cancer. Dis Colon Rectum 29:395, 1986.)

a fairly neutral position is attained. If it is customary to use two teams, then this position, with only mild hip flexion, will allow access by assistants.

If the patient's arms are tucked at the side, support and padding of the hand, wrist, and elbow should be ensured. Before surgery we check pulses and constantly remind staff members not to lean anything on the legs during surgery.

OPERATIVE TECHNIQUE

The operation is conducted through a midline incision extended to the right of the umbilicus. The stoma site is premarked. The left colic vessel is generally left in place unless obvious nodal disease dictates high transection of the origin of the inferior mesenteric artery. This helps minimize vascular compromise of the stoma. The descending colon is mobilized as necessary to ensure a tension-free stoma, which may require that the inferior mesenteric artery be divided at its origin.

Once the primary vessels are ligated, resectability determined, and the ureters identified, retrorectal dissection is begun. It is not necessary to denude the aorta or bifurcation. It may be possible to retain the hypogastric nerve trunks. Dissection is facilitated with suspension of the uterus to the lower aspect of the incision and self-retaining retractors. An able assistant using a deep ribbon retractor or a St. Mark's or Herrington retractor facilitates dissection, because repositioning is frequent. Staying in the avascular plane posteriorly and laterally minimizes bleeding. Despite all reasonable efforts, some patients have attenuated retrorectal fascia and high-pressure presacral vessels may be easily disrupted.

By combining anterior dissection to the midportion of the posterior vaginal wall (or beyond the prostate gland) and posterior dissection down to the tip of the coccyx on the levator floor, the lateral stalks are easily isolated. Usually no ligation of vessels to this point is necessary. Even the lateral stalks may be divided on the pelvic side wall with minimal bleeding. If the bleeding does not stop immediately, direct clipping or ligation is usually possible. When dissection is carried outside the pelvic fascial covering, significant bleeding from the internal iliac branch on the side wall of the pelvis may occur. Once the pelvic dissection is completed, the colon is transected, the colostomy created, and the abdomen closed.

The perineal dissection is then begun with proper patient preparation and draping. The rectum will have been previously irrigated and the anus closed. The legs are placed in the stirrups and the hips flexed. This shortens the length of the perineal dissection and thereby the time of hip flexion. Exaggerated hip flexion should be avoided if possible.

A wide elliptical incision from perineal body to coccyx is made down to the levator muscles. Some surgeons prefer cautery to minimize bleeding. The most prominent bleeding originates from the inferior hemorrhoidal vessels that pass through the ischioanal space. Usually the bleeding stops directly with minimal pressure. The anococcygeal attachment is divided in a plane toward the umbilicus, entering the pelvis above the levator muscles. With a finger above the levators, the muscle is incised toward the side walls. The anterior dissection is then carried to the transverse perineal musculature. With the proximal portion of the specimen delivered, the dissection is carried out from either side, and with minimal traction to prevent urethral injury in male patients. The posterior wall of the vagina is included in most anterior malignant lesions. The pelvis is irrigated and inspected for bleeding, particularly from the posterior aspect of the vagina, prostate gland, and bladder, along with the lateral stalks. A closed suction drain is inserted through a separate skin wound but delivered between the divided levator, if a drain has not been used from above. It is generally removed after 24 to 48 hours. The perineal wound is closed with two or three layers of running, absorbable suture. If there has been significant bleeding or fecal contamination or the perineal dissection is extremely wide, the wound is packed. The most common complications of perineal dissection are disruption of the rectum, urethral injury in male patients, and peripheral neuropathy of the legs secondary to positioning.

METHODS OF CLOSURE

The perineal wound can be packed open, partially closed, or completely closed. The peritoneal defect above the pelvic space can also be sutured closed or left open. Adjunctive procedures such as drainage of the pelvic space, with or without continuous irrigation, and omental plugging may also be considered.

Rates of primary healing after perineal wounds are closed range from 4% to 92%.[2-9] Open packing relegates all wounds to secondary healing, is inconvenient, and often is painful, but may result in a lower rate of chronic perineal sinus formation.[5] Closure of the pelvic peritoneum has been advocated to prevent perineal evisceration and postoperative small bowel obstruction. However, it may prevent obliteration of the pelvic cavity, leading to formation of a persistent perineal sinus.[10] Loops of small bowel may also become incarcerated in small defects in the peritoneal closure, resulting in postoperative bowel obstruction.

Two studies compared various methods of peritoneal and perineal closure. Irvin and Goligher[5] prospectively randomized 106 patients undergoing proctectomy to one of three methods of perineal closure: open packing of the perineal wound, with peritoneal closure; primary closure of the perineal wound and pelvic peritoneum, with suction drainage of the pelvis; and primary closure of the perineum, with suction drainage of the pelvis and without closure of the pelvic peritoneum. The overall complication rate was high: repeated surgery was necessary in 21% of patients in the open packing group, most often because of hemorrhage, and in 25% and 19% of the two closed groups, most commonly for drainage of abscesses. Primary healing occurred in 45% of the patients with primary closure of both the perineum and peritoneum and in 43% of patients with open peritoneums and closed perineums.[5]

Campos et al.[11] prospectively evaluated 102 patients undergoing proctectomies because of inflammatory bowel disease or cancer. Perineal wounds were treated with open packing, perineal closure with open peritoneum and continuous irrigation, or primary peritoneal and perineal closure. The best results were obtained in the group with open peritoneum, closed perineum, and continuous irrigation; 85% of these patients achieved primary healing of their perineal wounds.

Continuous irrigation was also advocated by Lieberman and Feldman.[12] In 27 patients undergoing proctectomy because of inflammatory bowel disease, 85% achieved primary healing of perineal wounds. In all cases intersphincteric dissections were performed with careful approximation of the levator muscles and closure of the perineal wound. The peritoneum was left open and the pelvic space was drained with large sump catheters. For 48 hours after surgery, the pelvic space was irrigated with saline solution, 125 ml/hr, through a third catheter, thus preventing accumulation of pelvic fluid. Again, primary healing was achieved in 85% of patients, with only a 3% incidence of perineal sinus formation. The authors credit continuous irrigation with maintaining a well-drained pelvic space, thereby preventing formation of a fibrotic pelvic cavity with secondary perineal sinus formation.[12]

In an effort to fill the pelvic space after rectal resection, Page et al.[13] advocate an omental plug. They describe mobilization of the omentum on the left gastroepiploic arterial pedicle, with subsequent placement in the pelvis. Advantages include increased local blood flow and lymphatic drainage, and obliteration of the pelvic space. The omental plug also has the advantage of keeping the small bowel out of the pelvis, thereby decreasing the chance of radiation enteritis in patients who require postoperative radiation therapy. The authors report primary healing in 26 of 34 patients (77%). This technique is relatively simple. It seems to improve perineal healing and prevent radiation enteritis and therefore is appealing.

PERINEAL WOUND COMPLICATIONS

When comparing abdominoperineal resection with other abdominal and pelvic procedures, the most striking difference is the perineal dissection and ensuing perineal wound. Treatment of this wound has long been the center of debate and controversy. Miles,[2] in his original description in 1908, recommended open packing, and his technique is still used by some surgeons. Over the following 75 years, many techniques to treat the perineal wound have been developed, including partial closure, primary closure, and closure with continuous irrigation or omental plugging.

For purposes of discussion, perineal wound complications of abdominoperineal resection can be divided into four categories: hemorrhage, abscess, perineal sinus, and perineal hernia.

Hemorrhage

Perineal hemorrhage is nearly always associated with open packing of the perineal wound. Its frequency varies from 0% to 4%.[3,14-16] Petrelli et al.[15] reported a postoperative death secondary to exsanguinating hemorrhage after packing removal on postoperative day 12. Open perineal packing is sometimes used as a procedure of last resort to treat uncontrolled pelvic (usually presacral) hemorrhage. Early postoperative perineal bleeding is related to persistent technical hemostatic problems. It is found at the first packing change because the pelvic packing temporarily tamponades bleeding vessels but does not definitively treat the underlying cause. Perineal bleeding may also be found after packing has been changed several times. This hemorrhaging is caused by erosion into the previously controlled pelvic vessels. Repacking of the wound results in temporary hemostasis. Bed rest is prescribed, and appropriate resuscitation is performed. Packing is removed after 48 to 72 hours of observation if the patient remains hemodynamically stable and there are no signs of ongoing bleeding. Generally this results in control of the bleeding vessels, but occasionally it fails and repeat surgery is required to control hemorrhage.

Abscess

Perineal abscess, unlike hemorrhage, is nearly always associated with primary closure of the pelvic wound. Rothenberger and Wong[3] reported an 11% incidence of abscess after primary closure in 143 patients undergoing abdominoperineal resection. In a series of 158 patients who underwent abdominoperineal resection with primary closure at the Mayo Clinic, postoperative perineal abscesses developed in 25 (15.8%),[16] compared with 25 (11%) of 230 patients at the Lahey Clinic.[4] Fecal contamination during rectal excision is highly predictive of postoperative perineal infection and failure of primary healing of the perineal wound. Irvin and Goligher[5] reported a 100% rate of perineal infection and no primarily healed wounds in 9 of 100 patients who underwent APR complicated by fecal contamination. Baudot et al.[17] noted similar findings in eight cases of APR with fecal soiling.

As with most subcutaneous abscesses, opening of the wound followed by local care is the preferred treatment. Thus a primarily closed perineum must now close by secondary intention. However, persistent perineal sinus may be more likely to result in wounds opened postoperatively than in those left open at the time of surgery.[17] Alternatively, presacral and perineal abscesses, particularly those associated with well-healed or healing incisions, can be treated with percutaneous drainage, averting the need for an open perineal wound.[18]

Nonhealing Wound and Perineal Sinus

Perineal sinus is defined as a perineal wound that remains unhealed for a minimum of 6 months. Characteristics include a fixed fibrotic pelvic cavity; a long, narrow track lined with a thick unyielding peel; and a small external opening.[19]

Silen and Glotzer,[10] on the basis of their extensive experience, compared the pelvic space after APR with the fixed pleural space after pneumonectomy. The pelvic space is bound posteriorly and laterally by the rigid bony pelvis, anteriorly by the relatively unyielding genitourinary structures, inferiorly by the slightly mobile perineal floor (if surgically closed), and superiorly by the peritoneal contents. Of all these borders, certainly the peritoneal structures are the most mobile. Silen and Glotzer contended that the pelvic space after abdominoperineal resection is filled not with granulation tissue but with a combination of upward migration of the perineal soft tissues and descent of the peritoneal contents. They argue that any forces (either iatrogenic, such as closure of the peritoneum or prolonged packing of the pelvis, or secondary to complications, such as pelvic abscess or hematoma) that produce a fixed fibrotic cavity are likely to result in a nonhealing perineal wound.

They recommended that the peritoneal contents be allowed to descend into the pelvis, the space be kept irrigated and well drained to prevent fluid accumulation, and any packing used in the perineal wound be removed early to prevent development of fibrotic wound edges. Despite the excellent description of perineal healing by Silen and Glotzer and the development of multiple techniques for perineal closure, nonhealing perineal wounds remain a common problem. Bacon and Nuguid[20] noted a 40% incidence of persistent perineal sinus in 1042 patients after rectal resection. In 230 patients who underwent APR at the Lahey Clinic, 32 (14%) had unhealed perineal wounds at 6 months compared with 38 of 158 (24%) at the Mayo Clinic.

Risk factors

Inflammatory bowel disease versus carcinoma. Rectal resection is most commonly performed to treat low rectal cancer or inflammatory bowel disease. Often the extent of soft tissue resection is much greater in the treatment of rectal cancer, with complete removal of the levator musculature and posterior vaginectomy advocated by some versus the intersphincteric proctectomy (sparing the external anal sphincter and the levator ani) often used in surgical treatment of inflammatory bowel disease. On this basis, an increase in perineal wound complications might be expected after APRs to treat cancer—yet just the opposite is true. Irvin and Goligher[5] reported a 9% incidence of unhealed perineal wounds in the treatment of cancer, compared with a 33% incidence in proctectomies performed because of inflammatory bowel disease. Baudot et al.[17] found persistent perineal sinus in 14% of rectal resections for malignancy compared with 34% in association with inflammatory bowel disease.

The reasons for poor healing in patients with inflammatory bowel disease remain unknown.[7,8] Steroid therapy does not appear to increase the incidence of unhealed wounds.[21] Tolstedt et al.[22] believe pararectal inflammation in inflammatory bowel disease, particularly Crohn's disease, leads to a fibrotic pelvic cavity that cannot collapse and that removal of the proximal colon leaves less bowel to fill the pelvis after surgery.

Radiation therapy. Radiation therapy is often used in the treatment of rectal and anal neoplasia both preoperatively and postoperatively. Local radiation impairs wound healing in animal models. Page et al.[13] reported primary healing in 4 of 5 patients (80%) undergoing APR without radiation therapy but in only 6 of 11 patients (55%) when APR was performed after radiation therapy.

Fecal contamination. Fecal contamination during proctectomy significantly decreases primary healing and may increase the risk of chronic perineal sinus formation.[5,17] This complication is presumably related to the development of pelvic infection with secondary development of a fixed abscess cavity that makes obliteration of the pelvic space more difficult. Fecal contamination may also lead to a higher incidence of perineal wound recurrence.

Treatment. Nonhealing perineal wounds develop in 8% to 69% of patients undergoing APR.[2-6,16] Because of the scope of the problem, many techniques have been developed to ensure complete healing. Early efforts included operative debridement with wide drainage, including coccygectomy and even partial sacral resection.[10] These measures were designed to eliminate the rigid fibrotic space that always accompanies a nonhealing perineal wound. Often these measures resulted in eventual healing but required extensive wound care for many months. Despite this treatment, some wounds failed to heal.

Alternative methods to improve healing and decrease wound care have been developed. Skin grafting alone often fails, because the pressure demands of the perineal area combined with the low oxygenation in these wounds prevent primary graft healing. Myocutaneous flaps have become the procedure of choice for closure of persistent perineal sinuses. Mathes et al.[23] described the advantages of myocutaneous flaps in the chronic, nonhealing, often infected wound to include increasing oxygen tension in ischemic tissues, improved leukocyte migration and function, and obliteration of dead space. They found these wounds colonized and/or infected with *S. faecalis, E. coli,* and *Staphylococcus epidermitis.* Treatment included operative debridement followed in a single stage, or in a second stage 3 to 4 days later, by closure with unilateral or occasionally bilateral gracilis myocutaneous flaps. Results were impressive, with 100% healing of five perineal sinuses that had been present on average for 2.2 years.[23]

In 1994, Ryan[24] reported his experience with gracilis myocutaneous flaps for closure of 15 nonhealing perineal sinuses after proctectomy performed because of inflammatory bowel disease. Preoperative workup included bone scans to rule out osteomyelitis and contrast material–enhanced studies to evaluate the possibility of enteric fistulas. His operative treatment consisted of debridement, including coccygectomy, with reconstruction in a single stage or at a second stage. Eighty percent of wounds could be closed with a single gracilis flap; 20% required bilateral flaps. Complete primary healing was achieved in only three patients; eventually healing occurred in 80%, and all but one demonstrated significant improvement.[24] As an alternative to gracilis flaps, Baird et al.[25] described the use of inferior gluteal flaps. In 13 patients with persistent perineal sinuses after rectal resection and in three patients with large perineal defects 16 inferior gluteal flaps (15 unilateral and one bilateral) were used to close the perineal defect. Primarily healing was achieved in 50%, and in 15 of 16 patients, healing was complete within 2 months.

Operative debridement and myocutaneous flap reconstruction creates an environment conducive to healing of these chronic wounds by obliteration of the fibrotic cavity, elimination of infection, improvement in local oxygenation, and coverage of dead space with viable tissue. It is not surprising, therefore, that these procedures result in maximum healing and are now popular for the treatment of the unhealed perineal wound.

Perineal Hernia and Evisceration

Perineal hernia after abdominoperineal resection is defined as bulging of peritoneal contents through an intact perineal wound, and perineal evisceration describes extrusion of small or large bowel through an open perineal wound. Evisceration occurs immediately after surgery and necessitates repeat surgery with reduction of intestines and repeat packing. Perineal hernias occur in about 1% of patients after APR.[26] The rate increases to 3% after pelvic exenteration.[27] Initial symptoms include perineal bulging, often associated with fullness or pain on sitting. Occasionally, patients complain of voiding problems if herniated bowel compresses the bladder.[28] Rarely, skin breakdown occurs, resulting in exposed bowel in the perineum. Perineal hernias, like peristomal and incisional hernias, do not always require repair. Indications for surgery are similar for all three postoperative hernias: patient discomfort refractory to conservative therapy, bowel obstruction, incarceration, and impending skin loss. Cosmesis alone should rarely merit surgical repair.

Several case reports delineate various techniques for repair. There are, however, no large series that compare different techniques. Brotschi et al.[28] reported repair of a perineal hernia after abdominoperineal resection and reviewed the literature. Further review revealed primary repairs without prosthetic material through both the abdominal and pelvic approaches, tensor fascia lata grafts placed transperitoneally, and prosthetic patches placed both peritoneally and transabdominally. Primary repair seemed to fail more often. Bell et al.[29] reported successful repair of a perineal hernia after pelvic exenteration with the use of a gracilis myocutaneous flap. Sarr et al.[30] used a combined abdominoperineal repair with a Marlex patch without recurrence of hernia. Although no clear consensus can be gleaned from the literature, the following principles should be followed: operate only because of symptoms refractory to nonsurgical therapy, fully examine patients before surgery, and adhere to sound principles proved successful in all hernia surgery (i.e., obtain good exposure, identify the defect well, anchor the repair to strong tissue, and use prosthetic material liberally to prevent tension).[31]

• • •

It is clearly better to prevent perineal wound complications if possible. Attention to technical details during both rectal resection and perineal closure will avert most complications. The following areas are important: (1) meticulous hemostasis, (2) prevention of fecal contamination, (3) effective drainage of the pelvic space to prevent development of a fibrotic pelvic cavity, (4) handling of the peritoneum so that abdominal contents can descend to close the pelvic space, and (5) careful closure of the perineal wound (closing the levator musculature if possible and eliminating perineal dead space with approximation of infralevator soft tissues). Attention to these details should result in higher rates of primary perineal wound healing.

INTRAOPERATIVE INJURY

Ureters

The ureters lie in the retroperitoneum on the psoas muscle and cross anterior to the iliac bifurcation before coursing into the pelvis. Once in the pelvis, the ureters fall to the pelvic side wall anterolateral to the rectum and descend anteromedially to enter the bladder. They are particularly vulnerable during five maneuvers performed in the course of rectal sigmoid resection: medial mobilization of the sigmoid colon, ligation of the inferior mesenteric artery, rectal mobilization adjacent to the sacral promontory, division of the lateral stalks, and reperitonealization of the pelvis.[32]

Ureteral injury is most common after gynecologic pelvic surgery, accounting for 61 of 87 injuries in one series.[33] However, colorectal surgical procedures are second only to gynecologic procedures in causing ureteral injury. In this series, 12 ureteral injuries followed colorectal operations: 11 after abdominoperineal resection and 1 after stoma creation. The prevalence ranges from 0.3% to 6%.[34,35] In 1605 resections performed because of rectal cancer, Graham and Goligher[36] reported 15 ureteral injuries, for a rate of 0.9%. In 105 abdominoperineal resections, Baumrucker and Shaw[34] found a 6% incidence of ureteral injury. Injuries have been described as ligation, transection, stenosis secondary to suture, crush injury, partial laceration, and devascularization.[32]

Only approximately 20% to 30% of injuries are recognized at surgery,[37] and the incidence of injury requiring nephrectomy increases 700% if injuries are not identified at surgery.[38] For this reason, some surgeons have advocated prophylactic preoperative ureteral catheterization.

Ureteral catheterization is performed immediately before colorectal resection. Cystoscopy enables identification of both ureteral orifices within the bladder. Stents are then passed retrograde into the proximal ureters. In some cases, lighted filaments are passed within the stents to illuminate the ureters during surgery. This has been particularly helpful in laparoscopic rectosigmoid resections.

Bothwell et al.[39] retrospectively reviewed 561 cases of rectosigmoid resection. In 92 cases (16%), an attempt at ureteral catheterization was made before surgery. Bilateral placement was possible in 87%, and at least unilateral cannulation was accomplished in 98% of cases. In two of 469 procedures (0.71%) performed without catheterization, intraoperative injury to the ureter occurred. The injury was discovered intraoperatively in one procedure, and postoperatively in the second. Two of 92 patients (2.2%) who underwent preoperative catheter placement also sustained ureteral injuries. In one case, the injury occurred intraoperatively and was discovered and repaired; in the second case, catheters could not be placed at cystoscopy. On the third postoperative day, an intravenous pyelogram revealed extravasation of contrast medium at the ureterovesical junction, presumably as a result of perforation during attempted catheter placement.

Leff et al.[40] evaluated 198 cases of distal rectosigmoid resection with preoperative placement of ureteral stents. Unilateral stent placement was possible in 99% and bilateral stent placement in 91%. Four ureteral injuries occurred intraoperatively. Three were recognized and repaired; in the fourth case, the right ureter was devascularized during reestablishment of intestinal continuity after a Hartmann procedure. This was not identified intraoperatively and resulted in a ureterocutaneous fistula. One case of reflux anuria on stent removal, caused by ureteral edema, responded to postoperative replacement of the ureteral stents.

There is no evidence that preoperative catheterization of the ureters prevents ureteral injury. Retrospective reviews can be misleading, however, because often catheterization is reserved for the most difficult cases. Consensus indicates, however, that ureteral catheters do increase intraoperative recognition of injury, thereby leading to prompt repair and decreased morbidity.[38]

Bladder and Urethra

Bladder injuries occur in 0% to 5% of distal colorectal resections[41-43] and are generally recognized either intraoperatively or at removal of the Foley catheter. Most injuries respond to prolonged catheter drainage of the bladder, but occasionally, surgical repair is required. The urethra is at risk only during the most distal rectal resections (i.e., ultra-low anterior and abdominoperineal resections). Injury is found in 0.7% to 6.7% of these cases.[44,45] Intraoperative recognition is often possible because of an indwelling bladder catheter. Direct repair with absorbable sutures is recommended. Unrecognized injuries usually are manifested as urethroperineal fistulas or urethral stenosis.

The general surgeon or colorectal surgeon and urologist must cooperate in the treatment of most genitourinary complications of abdominoperineal resection.[46]

Pelvic and Presacral Hemorrhage

In the course of mobilization of the rectum and sigmoid colon, a number of potential sites are at risk for significant bleeding. Rarely, a middle sacral artery over the sacral promontory or a large left common iliac vein may be injured during initiation of the pelvic dissection. Patients with portal hypertension with large and numerous retroperitoneal vessels are at particular risk of bleeding.

The pelvic side walls in the lower third of the pelvis may cause significant bleeding. This occurs when the pelvic fascia is pulled medially by surrounding perirectal fibrosis from the tumor reaction or radiation therapy. Dissection is then initiated outside the fascia, and the internal iliac vessels are injured. This necessitates direct control and occasionally prolonged pelvic packing. When performed in the correct plane, most of the dissection is avascular down to the lateral stalks immediately above the levator muscles. Even when divided without clipping or clamping, they seldom bleed vigorously.

Presacral hemorrhage is sometimes unavoidable and is often a difficult complication to manage. A thin and variable presacral fascia overlies the high-pressure anterior venous plexus. Risk of injury is minimized if presacral dissection is sharp. Despite this, some patients have very thin or almost nonexistent presacral fascia. Others have significant adhesions or fibrotic reaction retrorectally that leads to disruption of the fascia and vessels in the course of the dissection. Most bleeding can be controlled with packing, suture ligation, clips, or cautery.[48,49]

In 1985, Wang et al.[49] reported a study of the sacral venous complexes. They noted a large connection between the basivertebral vein connecting the internal vertebral venous system to the presacral system. This seems to occur in 15% of patients and is located between S3 and S5. When such bleeding occurs, the site can be controlled with fingertip pressure over the depression in the sacrum or immediately over the foramen (Fig. 21-3). When thus controlled, a sterile thumbtack, preferably titanium, is placed directly into the site (Fig. 21-4). Commercial devices have been developed,[50] but a long clamp and finger insertion of the tack will usually stop the bleeding.[51] Such a maneuver may be lifesaving in instances where other methods have failed and may prevent the need for significant transfusion if applied early.

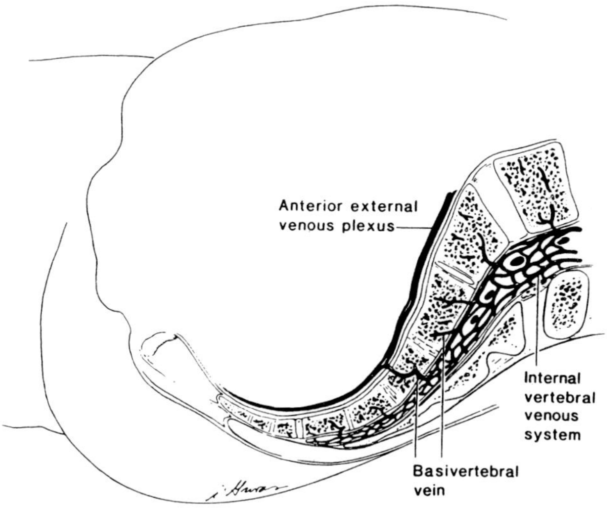

Fig. 21-3 Venous system of the sacrum (sagittal view). (From Nivatvongs S, Fang DT. The use of thumbtacks to stop massive presacral hemorrhage. Dis Colon Rectum 29:590, 1986.)

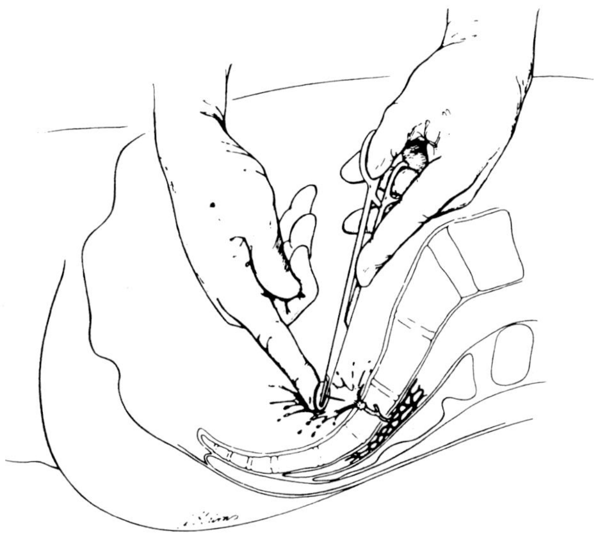

Fig. 21-4 Thumbtack occlusion of a bleeding basivertebral vein. (From Nivatvongs S, Fang DT. The use of thumbtacks to stop massive presacral hemorrhage. Dis Colon Rectum 29:590, 1986.)

Peripheral Neuropathy and Compartment Syndromes

Peripheral neuropathies in pelvic surgery may not be avoidable but may be minimized by observation of some basic principles.[52-57] The most common mechanism of injury is compression leading to local ischemia.[58-60] Damage may occur with the stretch force from hyperextension of the hip or knee.[58,61-64] Patients with diabetes, alcoholism, nutritional deprivation, peripheral vascular disease, recent weight loss, or primary neuropathies are at greatest risk. Hypoxemia and hypothermia are contributing factors. Intraoperatively, moving of the patient or the stirrup itself, leaning on the legs, poorly placed retractors, hypertension, and an operative time of more than 6½ hours have been associated with neuropathies.[53,65,66]

Positioning Injuries

The sciatic, tibial, sural, common peroneal, femoral, obturator, genitofemoral, and lateral cutaneous nerves to the thigh are all at potential risk for injury during APR.[67-71] Information about each of these nerves and mechanisms of injury is given in Chapter 3. Careful positioning in relatively neutral position, good padding, and avoidance of prolonged surgery minimizes the development of pelvic neuropathies. Adherence to the same principles also assists in minimizing development of DVT.

GENITOURINARY COMPLICATIONS

Genitourinary complications of APR include operative trauma to the urinary tract (i.e., ureter, bladder, and urethra), voiding dysfunction after surgery, and postoperative sexual dysfunction. Some genitourinary complications are unavoidable, particularly in resections for carcinoma. However, a sound grasp of pelvic anatomy and strict attention to surgical detail will minimize many unnecessary complications and result in improved quality of life after surgery.

Anatomy

Ureters. The ureters drain in the renal pelves into the bladder and can be divided into abdominal and pelvic components. The abdominal ureter lies in the retroperitoneum on the psoas muscle and crosses over the bifurcation of the iliac arteries as it enters the pelvis. An additional landmark helpful in identification of the left ureter is the intersigmoid fossa, found at the base of the sigmoid mesocolon. On medial mobilization to the sigmoid, the left ureter is found in the deep recess of this fossa. Once in the pelvis, the ureters fall to the pelvic side walls laterally and terminate on entering the posterior aspect of the bladder anterior to the distal rectum.

Pelvic neuroanatomy. Innervation of the distal genitourinary tract is divided into sympathetic, parasympathetic, and somatic components. Each is important in both sexual function and micturition. The sympathetic innervation arises from T1-2 to L3 via the thoracolumbar trunk. The superior hypogastric plexus, which contains sympathetic fibers, lies anterior to the aorta at the takeoff of the inferior mesenteric artery and descends in front of the left common iliac artery. In the area of the sacral promontory, the plexus splits into the left and right hypogastric nerves, which course along the pelvic side walls lateral to the rectum but medial to the ureters and iliac vessels. The superior hypogastric plexus and hypogastric nerves contain both preganglionic and postganglionic sympathetic nerve fibers and visceral afferent fibers. Parasympathetic innervation, known as nervi erigentes, arises from S2-4. These fibers join the hypogastric nerves to form the inferior hypogastric plexus or pelvic plexus. These plexuses now contain sympathetic, parasympathetic, and visceral afferent fibers and descend laterally and anteriorly to innervate the base of the bladder and proximal urethra. In male patients, innervation includes the prostate gland and seminal vesicles (Figs. 21-5 and 21-6).

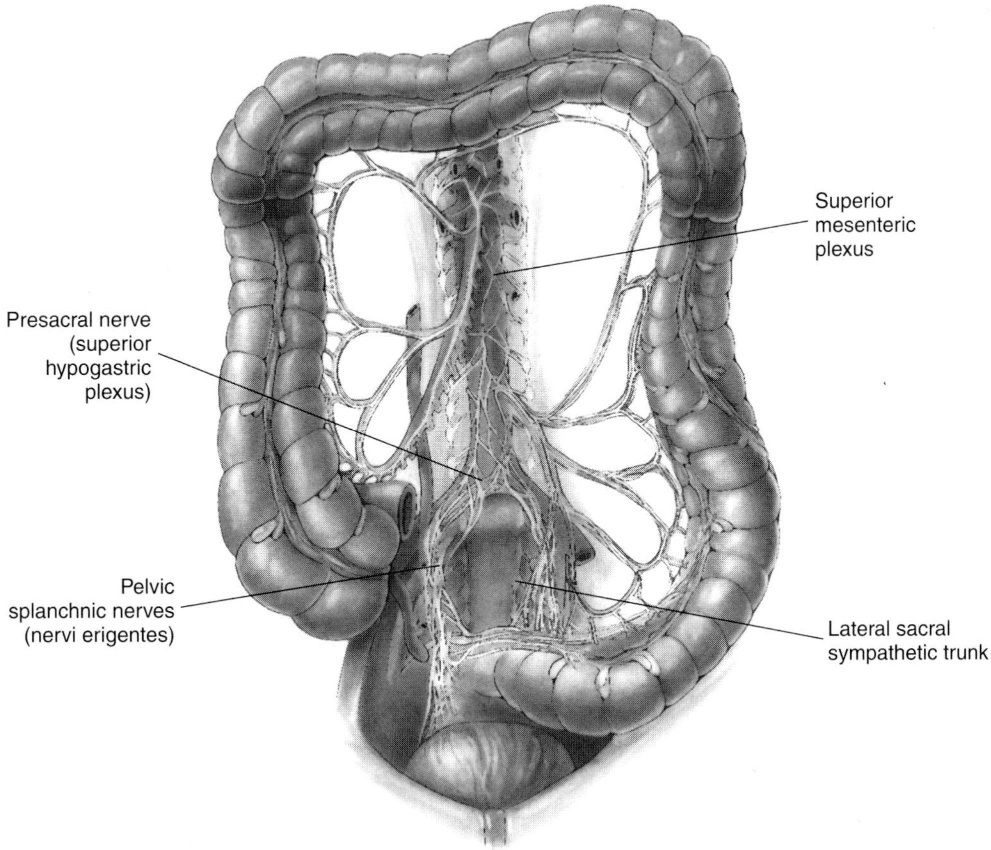

Fig. 21-5 Nerve supply to the rectum (frontal view). (From Gordon PH, Nivatvongs S. Principles and Practice of Surgery for the Colon, Rectum, and Anus. St. Louis: Quality Medical Publishing, 1992.)

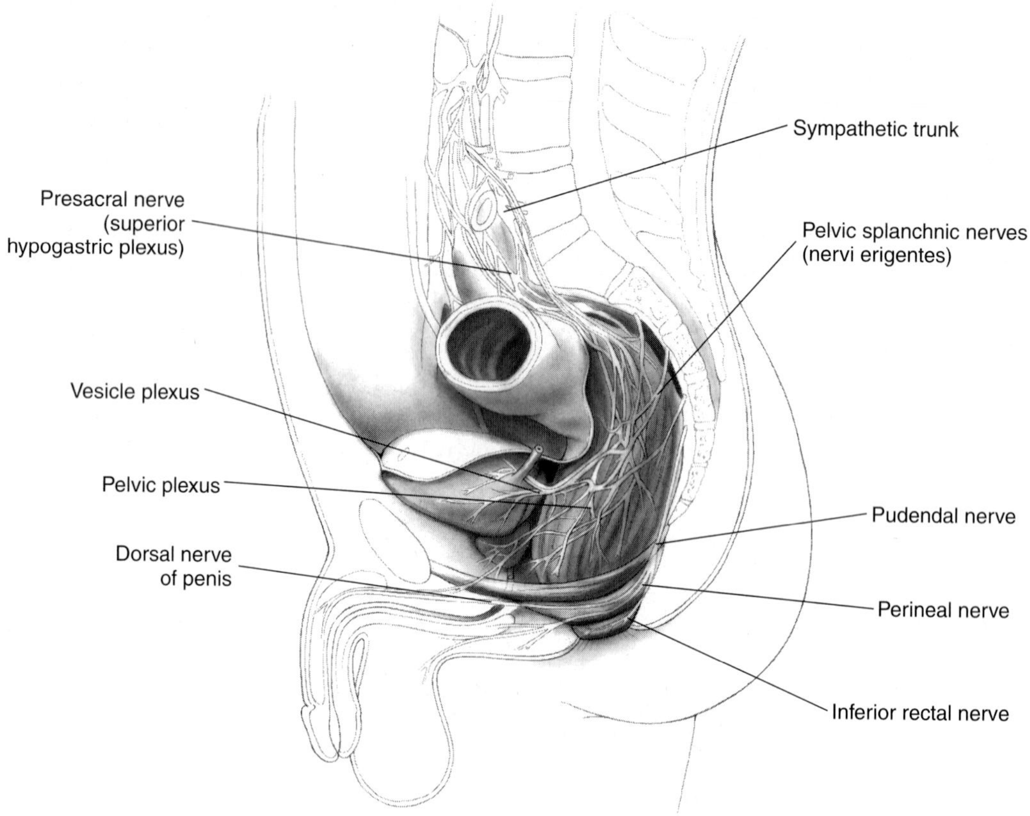

Fig. 21-6 Nerve supply to the rectum (lateral view). (From Gordon PH, Nivatvongs S. Principles and Practice of Surgery for the Colon, Rectum, and Anus. St. Louis: Quality Medical Publishing, 1992.)

Somatic innervation is provided by the pudendal nerve. After arising from the sacral plexus (S2-4), the pudendal nerve exits the pelvis through Alcock's canal adjacent to the ischial tuberosity and traverses the ischiorectal fossa. From there it trifurcates into the hemorrhoidal, perineal, and penile or clitoral branches. The penile and clitoral branches provide sensory innervation to the penis and clitoris and motor innervation to the striated external urethral sphincter.

Physiology

Sexual response. Neurologic aspects of male sexual response are better understood than those of female sexual response and are more concretely impaired after rectal resection. Therefore the ensuing discussion is focused mainly on the male response. Perhaps future research will lead to a better understanding of the female sexual response and the defects that occur following pelvic resections.

Male sexual function encompasses erection, emission, ejaculation, and detumescence and is dependent on intact autonomic and, to a lesser degree, somatic nervous systems. Erection begins the process and can be initiated by either tactile or psychogenic stimulation. Erections originated by local tactile stimulation depend on sensory input carried by the genital branch of the pudendal nerve and efferent response mediated by the nervi erigentes (S2-4/parasympathetic fibers); psychogenic erections are mediated by the thoracolumbar sympathetic fibers, which in turn stimulate pelvic parasympathetic fibers of the nervi erigentes.

Ejaculation begins with emission, which delivers semen to the prostactic urethra, again in response to sympathetic stimulation. Sympathetic outflow causes contraction of the internal urethral sphincter to prevent retrograde ejaculation. Parasympathetic fibers then stimulate contraction of the ischiocavernosus and bulbocavernosus, creating expulsion of semen.

Micturition. For normal voiding, parasympathetic, sympathetic, and somatic innervation is necessary. Parasympathetic fibers are responsible for detrusor contraction. Sympathetic fibers control the internal urinary sphincter at the bladder neck, with stimulation causing contraction and lack of stimulation allowing relaxation. Somatic fibers, via the penile nerve, control the external urethral sphincter responsible for voluntary control of voiding. Visceral afferents that course with sympathetic nerve fibers carry the sensation of bladder fullness to the cerebral cortex to stimulate the voiding response.

Sexual Dysfunction

Sexual dysfunction is reported in 32% to 100% of patients after abdominoperineal resection.[72-75] Cunsolo et al.[76] found 59% of men and 50% of women had postoperative sexual dysfunction. Male dysfunction can be classified as erectile difficulty, retrograde ejaculation, and total impotence. Female complications included decreased libido, difficulty with orgasm, and most commonly, dyspareunia.[76] Sympathetic injury usually results in ejaculatory difficulty, including retrograde ejaculation, whereas parasympathetic denervation is associated with problems achieving and maintaining full erections.

Sexual dysfunction has been associated with increased age and resections for cancer versus inflammatory bowel disease.[15,77,78] Danzi et al.[77] found that 80% of men older than 57 years experience sexual difficulty, compared with 67% of those younger than 57 years. Fazio et al.[78] found an 11% rate of sexual dysfunction after proctectomy performed for inflammatory bowel disease versus 50% if proctectomy was performed for cancer. Fazio and colleagues attribute the low incidence of problems after resection for inflammatory bowel disease to dissection close to the rectal wall, as well as to performing the perineal excision in the intersphincteric plane. The young age of patients undergoing proctectomy for inflammatory bowel disease was also thought to be significant.[78]

Sexual dysfunction, particularly in male patients, depends on the nature of nervous injury and can be either temporary or permanent, partial or complete. In questioning 26 men 1 year after APR in which the surgeon specifically attempted to spare the pelvic nerve plexus, Danzi et al.[77] found 17% had ejaculatory dysfunction, 17% had partial or weak erections, and 26% had total impotence. Kinn and Ohman[79] evaluated voiding and sexual function after rectal resection in 26 patients. However, they questioned only men about postoperative sexual function. In 10 men alive 2 years after APR, they found 60% had total impotence and an additional 10% had ejaculatory dysfunction. Cunsolo et al.[76] evaluated long-term sexual function in 46 patients after proctectomy performed because of rectal neoplasia and found 76% of patients had some alteration in sexual activity related to the surgery. Twenty-four percent of men and 53% of women discontinued sexual relations altogether. Women most commonly reported dyspareunia (50%), but 25% reported decreased libido and 25% reported changes in orgasms. Fifty-nine percent of men described partial erections, 30% ejaculatory problems, and 14% total impotence.

Balslev and Harling[72] personally interviewed 110 men on average 3 years after low anterior or abdominoperineal resection performed because of cancer of the rectum. In 93 patients who underwent abdominoperineal resection, 32% complained of sexual dysfunction, 18% had reduced potency, 3% had retrograde ejaculation, and 11% complained of total impotence. After low anterior resection, however, there were no cases of total impotence, but 6% of men had partial dysfunction.[72] Fazio et al.[78] also compared sexual function after low anterior and abdominoperineal resections. In 21 male patients they discovered one with total impotence and two with partial dysfunction after APR and no complete impotence but two cases of partial dysfunction after low anterior resection.

Voiding Dysfunction

Genitourinary complications can be categorized as either early or late. Early complications usually appear on removal of the urinary catheter 4 or 5 days after surgery and include urinary retention, urinary tract infection, and incontinence. These are transient problems that respond to relatively simple therapy, such as bladder catheterization or antibiotic therapy. Rothenberger and Wong[3] reported a 6% incidence of urinary tract infection and a 4% incidence of urinary retention in 155 patients after APR. Petrelli et al.[15] examined 61 patients after APR and found urinary retention in 25% and incontinence in 9%. In reviewing the Mayo Clinic experience with 158 patients with carcinoma of the rectum treated with APR, Pollard et al.[16] reported no incontinence but a 22% rate of postoperative retention and a 16% rate of urinary tract infection. In a series of 230 patients from the Lahey Clinic, rates of urinary retention and urinary tract infection were 8% and 6%, respectively.[4]

Late or chronic genitourinary complaints are no different from early problems; however, they fail to respond to simple measures and often persist beyond 6 weeks after surgery. These are reported to occur in 3% to 33% of patients after rectal resection.[34,80] In an attempt to predict which patients are at risk for chronic voiding dysfunction after APR, Burgos et al.[81] performed preoperative urodynamic studies. Nineteen percent of 105 patients undergoing rectal resection for carcinoma developed chronic voiding problems after surgery. Fourteen had normal urodynamics before surgery, and six had symptoms of obstruction. Postoperative complaints included difficult voiding (13 patients), incontinence (five), and absence of sensation of a full bladder (two). Abnormal preoperative urodynamics did not predict postoperative voiding problems. However, male gender, tumors less than 10 cm from the anal verge, and extensive pelvic lymphadenectomy were associated with postoperative dysfunction.[81]

Micturition abnormalities after APR have been attributed to malalignment of the bladder, neurologic injury, or exacerbation of preexisting outlet obstruction. Marshall et al.,[82] in reviewing 600 cases, found displacement of the bladder from lack of posterior support as the most common cause. Posterior bladder displacement decreases the efficiency of bladder emptying and results in increased residual volume.[83] Ogiwara et al.[84] advocate placement of a tissue expander in the pelvic space to prevent this complication. In six patients undergoing abdominoperineal resection, a silicone tissue expander (330 ml) was left in the pelvic cavity for 3 to 8 weeks after surgery. It was then removed with the patient under local anesthesia. These patients had significantly lower postvoid residual urine (200 versus 700 ml) than did patients without pelvic tissue expanders. Use of a pelvic tissue expander may prevent posterior bladder displacement; however, its effects on perineal wound healing are unknown and should be carefully considered before use of this technique.

Neurologic sequelae are also common after pelvic dissection. In evaluating 13 patients with severe voiding difficulties after rectal resection, Blaivis and Barbalias[83] found the following abnormalities: decreased closing pressure at the bladder neck secondary to sympathetic denervation (100%), detrusor paralysis or weakness secondary to parasympathetic denervation (38%), and decreased external urethral sphincter pressure secondary to pudendal nerve injury (54%). Sympathetic denervation may often be asymptomatic but along with pudendal nerve injury may result in urgency or incontinence. Parasympathetic denervation, particularly in association with outlet obstruction, results in decreased bladder emptying, high postvoid residual urine, and symptoms similar to those of benign prostatic hypertrophy.

Cunsolo et al.[76] surveyed 104 patients after APR for rectal cancer. Forty-six questionnaires were returned. Urinary retention was found in 41% of male patients and 35% of female patients, and urinary incontinence in only 10% of male patients but 29% of female patients. Ten percent and 35%, respectively, had experienced urinary tract infections. Overall, 67% had some postoperative urinary complaints, but neither gender nor age correlated with symptoms.[76] Kinn and Ohman[79] compared preoperative and postoperative urodynamics in 27 patients after proctectomy, including both low anterior resection and APR. They found no increase in urinary complications after APR compared with low anterior resection or after preoperative radiation therapy. In contrast, Janu et al.[85] discovered permanent genitourinary sequelae in significantly more patients after APR (43%) than after low anterior resection (7%). In agreement with Burgos et al.,[81] Janu et al.[85] also found tumors less than 10 cm from the dentate line to be associated with an increased incidence of urinary complaints.

Because of the high frequency of micturition problems after pelvic surgery, Goldman et al.[86] have recommended prophylactic use of α-adrenergic blockers. Sympathetic stimulation is responsible for contraction of the internal urethral sphincter at the bladder neck and inhibition of detrusor infraction. Phenoxybenzamine, an α-adrenergic blocker, therefore will decrease sympathetic stimulation, allowing more effective detrusor function and relaxation of the bladder neck. In 153 patients determined to be at risk for urinary complications before rectal resection, Goldman et al. studied the effects of alpha blockage. Seventy-eight patients received phenoxybenzamine; 75 did not. Of the group receiving alpha blockade before surgery, urinary tract infections developed in 19% and urinary retention developed in 15%. In those not receiving alpha blockers, urinary tract infections and urinary retention developed in 65% and 55%, respectively. Goldman et al. concluded that alpha blockade significantly decreased the incidence of genitourinary complications after rectal resection.

• • •

In summary, both sexual dysfunction and voiding disturbances are common after rectal resection. Overall, these complications occur more frequently in men, after abdominoperineal resection versus lower anterior resection, and when surgery is performed because of cancer compared with inflammatory bowel disease. Although it will not eliminate these complications, attention to surgical technique will minimize lifestyle-altering dysfunction. There are several areas in which autonomic and somatic nerves are at risk. During high ligation of the inferior mesenteric artery, the superior hypogastric plexus, which lies anterior to the aorta and the left common iliac vein and supplies sympathetic fibers to the pelvis, is vulnerable. When performing this maneuver, particularly in resections to treat benign disease, care should be taken to avoid this plexus. Contrary to popular belief, once below the sacral promontory, posterior dissection is safe because sympathetic fibers have bifurcated and formed left and right hypogastric nerves that run along the pelvic side walls medial to the ureters. However, these fibers join with parasympathetic fibers from the nervi erigentes to form the inferior hypogastric plexus, which is at risk during wide ligation of the lateral stalks. The pelvic nerves then converge anteriorly in the area of the prostate gland or posterior vagina and again become vulnerable during anterior rectal mobilization.

Familiarizing oneself with pelvic neuroanatomy, performing appropriate resections for benign and malignant disease, and using caution in areas in which nervous structures are particularly vulnerable will minimize these postoperative complications and improve the quality of life for patients after proctectomy.

COLOSTOMY

Beck[87] has described the technique and complications related to end colostomy construction. Early complications are related to tension, ischemia, infection, or bleeding.

Adequate mobilization of the descending colon with division of the inferior mesenteric artery at its origin will usually allow a tension-free stoma. Ischemia with edema and mild discoloration of the mucosa may lead to superficial mucosal sloughing. Significant ischemia with dry, dark mucosa and often retraction leads to stenosis, separation, or infection. Early revision is mandatory if there is any question of the depth of ischemia or if it has extended below the fascia. A small-diameter sigmoidoscope or a glass test tube may help distinguish depth. Mild trauma or needle puncture of the mucosa may determine whether active bleeding is present.[87]

Peristomal infections require drainage and ultimately revision when the infection resolves. A minimal mucocutaneous abscess may be drained through the mucocutaneous junction, but most significant peristomal infections require a separate incision outside the faceplate of the stoma.

Late complications of stomas are numerous and include stenosis, fistula, prolapse, and peristomal hernia. Long-term acceptance depends on a well-placed stoma, good education, and support from the health care staff and family.[88]

BOWEL OBSTRUCTION

Differentiation of early small bowel obstruction from ileus is difficult. It is probably best defined as occurring between 7 and 30 days postoperatively.[89] Stewart et al.[90] stated its occurrence in rectal resection to be 3%. Most early obstructions resolve with nasogastric suctioning and continued intravenous nutritional support.[90]

Loops of small intestine may twist around the colostomy spur. Closure of the lateral gutter is difficult to accomplish and maintain, particularly posterolaterally. Extraperitoneal placement of the stoma has been advocated, without good controlled study, to prevent small bowel obstructions and to minimize peristomal hernia.[87]

Adherence of loops of intestine to the vascular pedicle, peritoneal closure, or herniation through the pelvic peritoneal closure are possible sites for obstruction. Although the evidence is conflicting, obstructive problems and perineal problems may be minimized when the pelvic peritoneum is left open.[59]

There is no good evidence[91] that routine nasogastric tube placement will shorten ileus or prevent obstructive symptoms. It is our practice to use nasogastric tubes only postoperatively when the patient has clinical obstruction or gastric dilatation or gastroparesis.

OTHER COMPLICATIONS

Constant perineal pain in the patient with cancer is usually related to pelvic recurrence of the cancer. When not related to cancer, the pain is difficult to explain. Pudendal nerve injury may cause pain with numbness of half or all of the penis or clitoris. The piriformis syndrome has been blamed for gluteal and perineal pain with entrapment as it crosses the sciatic notch. A physiotherapist familiar with such disorders may be able to offer some relief.

Phantom rectal sensations[59] of urgency or tenesmus may occur periodically. It has been reported to occur in as many as 65% of patients but is relatively rare as a continuing problem in our experience. Simple patient reassurance is usually enough to control the symptoms.

Ovaries trapped below the peritoneum with pain, cyst, or mass has been reported.[92] We have not seen this complication, perhaps because the peritoneum is left open and postmenopausal and advanced cancers in premenopausal women are usually treated with bilateral oophorectomy.

REFERENCES

1. Koenigs KP, McPhedran P, Spiro HM. Thrombosis in inflammatory bowel disease. J Clin Gastroenterol 9:627-631, 1987.
2. Miles WE. A method of performing abdominoperineal excision for carcinoma of the rectum and of the terminal portion of the pelvic colon. Lancet 2:1812, 1908.
3. Rothenberger DA, Wong WD. Abdominoperineal resection for adenocarcinoma of the low rectum. World J Surg 16:478-485, 1992.
4. Rosen L, Veidenheimer MC, Coller JA, Corman ML. Mortality, morbidity, and patterns of recurrence after abdominoperineal resection for cancer of the rectum. Dis Colon Rectum 25:202-208, 1982.
5. Irvin TT, Goligher JC. A controlled clinical trial of three different methods of perineal wound management following excision of the rectum. Br J Surg 62:287-291, 1975.
6. Altemeier WA, Culbertson WR, Alexander JW, Suturius D, Bossert J. Primary closure and healing of the perineal wound in abdominoperineal resection of the rectum for carcinoma. Am J Surg 127:215-219, 1974.
7. Elliott M, Todd IP. Primary suture of the perineal wound using constant suction and irrigation, following rectal excision for inflammatory bowel disease. Ann R Coll Surg Engl 67:6-7, 1985.

8. Oakley JR, Fazio VW, Jagelman DG, Lavery IC, Weakley FL, Easley K. Management of the perineal wound after rectal excision for ulcerative colitis. Dis Colon Rectum 28:885-888, 1985.
9. Tompkins RG, Warshaw AL. Improved management of the perineal wound after proctectomy. Ann Surg 202:760-765, 1985.
10. Silen W, Glotzer DJ. The prevention and treatment of the persistent perineal sinus. Surgery 75:535-542, 1974.
11. Campos RR, Ayllon, JG, Paricio PP, Tebar JC, Mompean JAL, Ruiz RL, Martinez JAT, Martinez JM. Management of the perineal wound following abdominoperineal resection: Prospective study of three methods. Br J Surg 79:29-31, 1992.
12. Lieberman RC, Feldman S. Primary closure of the perineal wound with closed continuous transabdominal pelvic irrigation after rectal excision. Dis Colon Rectum 27:526-528, 1984.
13. Page CP, Carlton PK, Becker DW. Closure of the pelvic and perineal wounds after removal of the rectum and anus. Dis Colon Rectum 23:2-9, 1980.
14. de Cannière L, Rosière A, Michel LA. Synchronous abdominoperineal resection without transfusion. Br J Surg 80:1194-1195, 1993.
15. Petrelli NJ, Nagel S, Rodriguez-Bigas M, Piedmonte M, Herrera L. Morbidity and mortality following abdominoperineal resection for rectal adenocarcinoma. Am Surg 59:400-404, 1993.
16. Pollard CW, Nivatvongs S, Rojanasakul A, Ilstrup DM. Carcinoma of the rectum. Profiles of intraoperative and early postoperative complications. Dis Colon Rectum 37:866-874, 1994.
17. Baudot PE, Keighley MRB, Alexander-Williams J. Perineal wound healing after proctectomy for carcinoma and inflammatory disease. Br J Surg 67:275-276, 1980.
18. Michalson AE, Brown BP, Warnock NG, Simonson TM. Presacral abscesses: Percutaneous transperineal drainage with use of bone landmarks and fluoroscopic guidance. Radiology 190:574-575, 1994.
19. Anthony JP, Mathes SJ. The recalcitrant perineal wound after rectal extirpation. Arch Surg 125:1371-1377, 1990.
20. Bacon HE, Nuguid TP. Problem of persistent perineal sinus following removal of the rectum for ulcerative colitis. Dis Colon Rectum 5:370-372, 1962.
21. Jalan KN, Smith AN, Ruckley CV, Falconer CWA, Small WP, Prescott RJ. Perineal wound healing in ulcerative colitis. Br J Surg 56:749-753, 1969.
22. Tolstedt GE, Bell JW, Harkins HN. Chronic perineal sinus following total colectomy for ulcerative colitis. Am J Surg 101:50, 1971.
23. Mathes SJ, Feng LJ, Hunt TK. Coverage of the infected wound. Ann Surg 198:420-429, 1983.
24. Ryan JA. Gracilis muscle flap for the persistent perineal sinus of inflammatory bowel disease. Am J Surg 148:64-69, 1994.
25. Baird WL, Hester TR, Nahai F, Bostwick J III. Management of perineal wounds following abdominoperineal resection with inferior gluteal flaps. Arch Surg 125:1486-1489, 1990.
26. McMullin ND, Johnson WR, Polglase AL, Hughes ESR. Post-proctectomy perineal hernia: Case report and discussion. Aust N Z J Surg 55:69, 1985.
27. Rutledge RN, Smith JP, Wharton JT, O'Quinn AG. Pelvic exenteration: An analysis of 296 patients. Am J Obstet Gynecol 129:881, 1977.
28. Brotschi E, Noe JM, Silen W. Perineal hernias after proctectomy. Am J Surg 149:301-305, 1985.
29. Bell JG, Weiser EB, Metz P, Hoskins WJ, Simons SA, Norris J. Instruments and methods. Gracilis muscle repair of perineal hernia following pelvic exenteration. Obstet Gynecol 58:377, 1980.

30. Sarr MG, Stewart JR, Cameron JC. Combined abdominoperineal approach to repair of postoperative perineal hernia. Dis Colon Rectum 25:597-599, 1982.
31. Beck DE, Fazio VW, Jagelman DG. Postoperative perineal hernia. Dis Colon Rectum 30:21-24, 1987.
32. Cass AS, Bubrick MP. Ureteral injuries in colonic surgery. Urology 18:359-364, 1981.
33. Higgins CC. Ureteral injuries during surgery. A review of 87 cases. JAMA 199:82-88, 1967.
34. Baumrucker GO, Shaw JW. Urological complications following abdominoperineal resection of the rectum. Arch Surg 67:502, 1953.
35. Colcock BP, Jarpa S. Complications of abdominoperineal resection. Dis Colon Rectum 1: 90, 1958.
36. Graham JW, Goligher, JC. The management of accidental injuries and deliberate resections of the ureter during excision of the rectum. Br J Surg 42:151, 1954.
37. Zinman LM, Libertino JA, Roth RA. Management of operative ureteral injury. Urology 12: 290-303, 1978.
38. McGinty DM, Mendez R. Traumatic ureteral injuries with delayed recognition. Urology 10: 115-117, 1977.
39. Bothwell WN, Bleicher RJ, Dent TL. Prophylactic ureteral catheterization in colon surgery: A five-year review. Dis Colon Rectum 37:330-334, 1994.
40. Leff EI, Groff W, Rubin RJ, Eisenstat TE, Salvati EP. Use of ureteral catheters in colonic and rectal surgery. Dis Colon Rectum 25:457-460, 1982.
41. Sakkas JL, Mandrekas A, Androulakis J, Pisidis A, Vezeridis M, Gray SA. Urologic complications in malignant disease of the rectosigmoid colon. South Med J 67:287-291, 1974.
42. Andersson A, Bergdahl L. Urologic complications following abdominoperineal resection of the rectum. Arch Surg 111:969, 1976.
43. Melick WF. Complications of colonic and rectal surgery—the causes and management of postoperative urologic complications. Dis Colon Rectum 16:7-11, 1973.
44. Sankey NE, Heller E. The urological complications of abdominoperineal resection. J Urol 97:367-370, 1967.
45. Tank ES, Ernst CB, Woolson ST, et al. Urinary tract complications of anorectal surgery. Am J Surg 123:118, 1972.
46. Presti JC, Carroll PR. Intraoperative management of the injured ureter. Perspect Colon Rectal Surg 1:98-106, 1988.
47. Zama N, Fazio VW, Jagelman DG, Lavery IC, Weakley FL, Church JM. Efficacy of pelvic packing in maintaining hemostasis after rectal excision for cancer. Dis Colon Rectum 31: 923-928, 1988.
48. Metzger PP. Modified packing technique for control of presacral pelvic bleeding. Dis Colon Rectum 31:981-982, 1988.
49. Wang O, Shi W, Zhaw Y, Zhou W, He Z. New concepts in severe presacral hemorrhage during proctectomy. Arch Surg 120:1013-1020, 1985.
50. Stolpi VM, et al. Newly designed occluder pin for presacral hemorrhage. Dis Colon Rectum 35:166-169, 1992.
51. Nivatvongs S, Fang DT. The use of thumbtacks to stop massive presacral hemorrhage. Dis Colon Rectum 29:589-590, 1986.
52. Nicholson MJ, McAlpine FS. Neural injuries associated with surgical positions and operations. In Martin JT, ed. Positioning in Anesthesia and Surgery. Philadelphia: WB Saunders, 1978, pp 193-224.
53. Dyke PJ, Thomas PK. Peripheral Neuropathy, vol 2, 3rd ed. Philadelphia: WB Saunders, 1993, pp 969-975.

54. Schaumburg HH, Spencer PS, Thomas PK. Disorders of Peripheral Nerves. Philadelphia: FA Davis, 1983.
55. Parks BJ. Postoperative peripheral neuropathies. Surgery 74:348-357, 1973.
56. Sunderland S. Nerves and Nerve Injuries. New York: Churchill Livingston, 1978.
57. Asbury AK, Johnson PC. Clinical aspects of peripheral neuropathies. Major Probl Pathol 9: 258-267, 1978.
58. Goldstein PJ. The lithotomy position. In Martin JT, ed. Positioning in Anesthesia and Surgery. Philadelphia: WB Saunders, 1978, pp 142-161.
59. Corman ML. Colon and Rectal Surgery, 3rd ed. Philadelphia: JB Lippincott, 1993, pp 632-645.
60. Haftek J, Thomas PK. Electron-microscope observations on the effects of localized crush injuries on the connective tissues of peripheral nerve. J Anat 103:233, 1968.
61. Britt BA, Joy N, Mackay MB. Positioning trauma. In Orkin FK, Cooperman LH, eds. Complications in Anesthesiology. Philadelphia: JB Lippincott, 1983, pp 647-670.
62. Lincoln JR, Sawyer JP Jr. Complications related to body positions during surgical procedures. Anesthesiology 22:800-809, 1961.
63. Leff RG, Shapiro SR. Lower extremity complications of the lithotomy position: Prevention and management. J Urol 122:138-139, 1979.
64. Glenn J. Neural damage resulting from dorsal lithotomy positioning. Surg Rounds 1:42-46, 1981.
65. Herrera-Ornelas L, Tolls RM, Petrelli NJ, Piver S, Miffelman A. Common peroneal nerve palsy associated with pelvic surgery for cancer: An analysis of 11 cases. Dis Colon Rectum 29:392-397, 1986.
66. Lyndon JC, Spielman FJ. Bilateral compartment syndrome following prolonged surgery in the lithotomy position. Anesthesiology 60:236-238, 1984.
67. Berry J, Richardson PM. Common peroneal nerve palsy: A clinical and electrophysiological review. J Neurol Neurosurg Psychiatry 39:1162, 1976.
68. Nivatvongs S. Complications of anorectal and colorectal operations. In Gordon PH, Nivatvongs, S, eds. Principles and Practice of Surgery for the Colon, Rectum, and Anus. St. Louis: Quality Medical Publishing, 1992, pp 1003-1021.
69. Masten FA III. Compartmental Syndromes. New York: Grune & Stratton, 1980, pp 1-162.
70. Masten FA, Winquist RA, Krugmire RB. Diagnosis and management of compartmental syndromes. J Bone Joint Surg [Am] 62:286-291, 1980.
71. Aichroth P, Rowe-Jones DC. Iliacus compartment compression syndrome. Br J Surg 58: 833, 1971.
72. Balslev I, Harling H. Sexual dysfunction following operation for carcinoma of the rectum. Dis Colon Rectum 26:785-788, 1983.
73. Weinstein M, Roberts M. Sexual potency following surgery for rectal carcinoma: A follow-up of 44 patients. Ann Surg 185:295-300, 1977.
74. Walsh PC, Schlegel PN. Radical pelvic surgery with preservation of sexual function. Ann Surg 208:391-400, 1988.
75. Aboseif SR, Matzel KE, Lue TE. Sexual dysfunction after rectal surgery. Perspect Colon Rectal Surg 3:157-172, 1990.
76. Cunsolo A, Bragaglia RB, Manara G, Poggioli G, Gozzetti G. Urogenital dysfunction after abdominoperineal resection for carcinoma of the rectum. Dis Colon Rectum 33:918-922, 1990.
77. Danzi M, Ferulano GP, Abate S, Califano G. Male sexual function after abdominoperineal resection for rectal cancer. Dis Colon Rectum 26:665-668, 1983.

78. Fazio VW, Fletcher J, Montague D. Prospective study of the effect of resection of the rectum on male sexual function. World J Surg 4:149-152, 1980.
79. Kinn AC, Ohman U. Bladder and sexual function after surgery for rectal cancer. Dis Colon Rectum 29:43-48, 1986.
80. Eickenberg HU, Amin M, Klompus W, Lich R. Urologic complications following abdominoperineal resection. J Urol 115:180, 1976.
81. Burgos FJ, Romero J, Fernandez E, Perales L, Tallada M. Risk factors for developing voiding dysfunction after abdominoperineal resection for adenocarcinoma of the rectum. Dis Colon Rectum 31:682-685, 1988.
82. Marshall VF, Pollack RS, Miller C. Observations on urinary dysfunction after excision of the rectum. J Urol 55:409, 1946.
83. Blaivas JG, Barbalias GA. Characteristics of neural injury after abdominoperineal resection. J Urol 129:83, 1983.
84. Ogiwara H, Nakai K, Kurahashi T, Baba S. Surgical trial for carcinoma of the rectum using a tissue expander in association with pelvic partition to prevent dysfunction of the bladder. J Am Coll Surg 178:301-302, 1994.
85. Janu NC, Bokey EL, Chapuis PH, Watters GR, Maher PO, Angstreich D. Bladder dysfunction following anterior resection for carcinoma of the rectum. Dis Colon Rectum 29:182-183, 1986.
86. Goldman G, Kahn PJ, Kashtan H, Stadler J, Wiznitzer T. Prevention and treatment of urinary retention and infection after surgical treatment of the colon and rectum with alpha adrenergic blockers. Surg Gynecol Obstet 166:447-450, 1988.
87. Beck DE. End sigmoid colostomy. In MacKeigan JM, Cataldo P, eds. Intestinal Stomas. St. Louis: Quality Medical Publishing, 1993, pp 97-106.
88. McLeod RS, Cohen Z. Quality of life with a stoma. In MacKeigan JM, Cataldo P, eds. Intestinal Stomas. St. Louis: Quality Medical Publishing, 1993, pp 85-94.
89. Pickleman J, Lee RM. The management of patients with suspected early postoperative small bowel obstruction. Ann Surg 210:216-219, 1989.
90. Stewart RM, Page CP, Brender J, Schwesinger W, Eisenhut D. The incidence and risk of early postoperative small bowel obstruction. A cohort study. Am J Surg 154:643-647, 1987.
91. Wolff BG, Pemberton JH, van Heerden JA, Beart RW Jr, Nivatvongs S, Devine RM, Dozois RR, Ilstrup DM. Elective colon and rectal surgery without nasogastric decompression: A prospective, randomized trial. Ann Surg 209:670-675, 1989.
92. Matthews JM, Kodner IJ, Fry RD, Fazio VW. Entrapped ovary syndrome. Dis Colon Rectum 29:341, 1986.

CHAPTER 22

Ileal Pouch–Anal Anastomosis

GREGORY A. DeLAURIER
HEIDI NELSON

The prototype for the ileal pouch–anal anastomosis (IPAA) was first performed by Nissen[1] in 1933 in a child with familial adenomatous polyposis (FAP). The procedure was reintroduced in 1947 by Ravitch and Sabiston,[2] who proposed mucosal proctectomy and straight ileoanal anastomosis to treat ulcerative colitis after performing the procedure in a dog model. The procedure was plagued, however, by unacceptable stool frequency, infection, and leakage rates and thus fell into disfavor. In 1955 Valiente and Bacon[3] fashioned a "pantaloon" pouch with a long efferent limb in dogs in an attempt to resolve the stool frequency problem. Two of seven dogs survived and were described as having stools of good consistency and frequency. Martin et al.[4] in 1977 successfully performed protocolectomy and straight ileoanal anastomosis in 17 patients with ulcerative colitis. In 1980 Parks et al.,[5] by creating a more distal reservoir (S pouch), demonstrated that total mucosal proctectomy and pouch–anal anastomosis was plausible in a group of 21 patients with ulcerative colitis and FAP. Since that time a number of pouch designs have been described, including the most popular J pouch devised by Utsunomiya et al.,[6] and acceptance of the IPAA has greatly advanced the surgical management of patients with ulcerative colitis and FAP. The procedure ensures that with mucosal proctectomy the entire diseased mucosa is removed, yet intestinal continuity is preserved and the need for a permanent stoma is averted. Because of the complexity of the procedure and the attendant learning curve for the surgeon, the complication rate following ileal pouch–anal anastomosis remains significant.

INDICATIONS

IPAA is indicated in patients with chronic ulcerative colitis, primarily when patients medical therapy has failed or intolerable complications have resulted from the disease or treatment. Patients who have had ulcerative colitis for longer than 10 years are also at risk for colorectal carcinoma, and surgical therapy should be offered, particularly when dysplasia is detected during colonoscopic surveillance. The second most common indication for IPAA is in patients with FAP. These patients have virtually a 100% chance of developing colorectal cancer if the large intestine is not removed and at least a 20% risk for rectal cancer if the colon but not the rectum is removed.[7]

PATIENT SELECTION

Several preoperative clinical features can be helpful in determining the feasibility of creation of an IPAA.

Body habitus is an important determinant as to whether the operation is technically feasible. Obese patients tend to have short, thick mesenteries that do not provide adequate mesenteric length for the pouch to reach the anus for a viable anastomosis.[8] The tall patient habitus similarly may create a challenge for pouch-to-anus reach. Finally, patients with FAP and an associated mesenteric desmoid may not have sufficient mesentery for ileoanal anastomosis.[9] It is advised that these considerations be explained to patients during the preoperative counseling session so that they are prepared for the consequences of a stoma if the pouch is not possible.

Even if the operation is technically feasible, certain patients should be advised of preexisting conditions that may adversely affect functional outcome. Patients with a history of anal sphincter injury or preexisting fecal incontinence likely will be significantly inconvenienced by unacceptable leakage or gross incontinence if ileoanal anastomosis is performed. Women with a poorly repaired episiotomy may be prone to incontinence, especially if the scar is located at the site of potential anastomosis.[10] A cautionary note: patients with active ulcerative colitis may report a history of incontinence when in fact their symptoms are the result of urgency associated with rectal inflammation and decreased rectal compliance. If such patients with chronic ulcerative colitis exhibit normal sphincter tone and anal manometry does not reveal gross deterioration of sphincter function, symptoms may actually improve after creation of an IPAA. It is also important to carefully inspect the anus for potential signs of Crohn's disease, such as nonmidline or multiple fissures or fistulas. Crohn's disease is an absolute contraindication to IPAA because of the well-known risks of recurrent inflammation, fistula formation, and pelvic sepsis.

Advanced age is an important preoperative factor to consider, particularly when counseling patients about anticipated functional results. An earlier report from the Mayo Clinic suggested that long-term continence and satisfaction with the pouch were suboptimal in older patients.[11] These problems were not significant in a group of patients older than 50 years reported by Lewis et al.[12] Although there is no specific age at which patients are refused the procedure at the Mayo Clinic, the oldest patient to undergo creation of an ileal pouch–anal anastomosis was 64 years old, and patients older than 50 years had previously been reported to have a significant increase in stool frequency after surgery.[11] It is hoped that ongoing studies will help in determination of the effects of age and the aging process on complication rates and pouch function.

Finally, the presence of a distal rectal carcinoma may contraindicate a pouch procedure, either because abdominoperineal resection is required to achieve appropriate margins or adjuvant radiation therapy and chemotherapy are required because of stage II or III disease. The extremely poor functional results of the pouch after pelvic radiation advises against the pouch in these cases. Patients who are otherwise debilitated are not candidates for this complex operation.

EARLY COMPLICATIONS

Vascular Compromise

One of the surgeon's primary concerns at operation is whether the pouch will reach the anal canal for a relatively tension-free anastomosis. This occasionally requires sacrifice of ileocolic vessels or even other ileal branches of the superior mesenteric artery for mesenteric lengthening. Even when these vessels are preserved, mucosal blood flow to the pouch is reduced to only 88% of normal.[13] If vascular division is required, the pouch mucosal blood flow can be decreased to approximately 60% of normal and only 30% at the anastomosis. This relative ischemia may contribute to the development of an anastomotic leak and pelvic sepsis or to subsequent anastomotic stricturing. It is rare that gross pouch ischemia requires pouch excision because of infarction. It has been postulated that relative ischemia may contribute to pouchitis, but there is little objective support for this concept.

Bleeding

Patients with chronic immunosuppression and those with protracted severe colonic inflammation may have particularly friable and fragile tissues, as often noted during mesenteric dissection. Gentle handling of the tissues is therefore necessary, especially during the delivery of the pouch to the anus, when mesenteric tension is most likely to be maximum and resulting tears irreparable. Presacral drains, placed at the time the IPAA is created, may provide an early sign of postoperative hemorrhage. Because rectal dissection is typically performed in a conservative manner close to the rectal wall, significant presacral plexus bleeding is uncommon. Suture- or staple-line bleeding may occur, leading to intrapouch hematoma, for up to 1 week postoperatively but does not usually require surgical intervention.

Pelvic or Intra-abdominal Sepsis

Pelvic sepsis, in most large series of ileal pouch–anal anastomosis, is variably reported as complicating the pouch procedure in 5% to 15% of cases.[8,14-19] Pelvic sepsis is most likely the result of an anastomotic or pouch suture-line leak but may also result from bacterial contamination of the peritoneal cavity during surgery. The overall incidence of this problem has generally declined as a result of increased surgical experience and technical refinements. This complication may become evident after the initial IPAA or after the ileostomy is reversed and GI continence is reestablished. In the case of sepsis after the initial pouch procedure, within the first several days postoperatively, typical symptoms include fever, lower quadrant or suprapubic pain, and leukocytosis, with or without perianal purulence. Lower abdominal tenderness and guarding may be present. A CT scan of the abdomen and pelvis may demonstrate a phlegmon, more common in the early stages, or a discrete abscess, more common in the late stages. Abscess may be amenable to CT-guided drainage. In the clinically stable patient with fecal diversion already in place, it may be prudent to administer intravenous antibiotic therapy and follow a course of close observation. If the patient does not respond clinically in the ensuing 24 to 48 hours, laparotomy should be performed for diagnosis and drainage. Thin, cloudy, peritoneal fluid and peripouch purulence are typical surgical findings. If a diverting ileostomy is not in place, one should be created.

Scott et al.[19] reviewed pouch outcome in 30 patients in whom intra-abdominal sepsis developed after IPAA. Among patients who did not undergo laparotomy because of pelvic sepsis, 92% ultimately had functional pouches and underwent ileostomy closure. If laparotomy was required, 41% had pouch excision and only 29% ultimately were able to undergo successful ileostomy closure. Although these findings are likely heavily biased against the group who underwent surgery as a more severely ill population, they do provide some evidence to support conservative treatment including a trial of nonsurgical management in clinically stable patients. If nonsurgical management is continued successfully, a repeat CT scan should be obtained 7 to 10 days later to ensure that no undrained fluid collections persist.

Even after what was considered to be a technically ideal procedure in an ideal candidate, pelvic sepsis may occur in the period immediately after ileostomy closure. This is one reason why acquisition of a pouchogram to detect a subclinical leak or fistula is recommended before ileostomy closure. If this complication does occur, the same principles apply as above. In general, the safest approach is to reestablish fecal diversion and delay another attempt at closure for 2 to 3 months.[20]

Pelvic sepsis may also have long-term sequelae. Previous pelvic sepsis predisposes the patient to pelvic fibrosis, which decreases pouch compliance with resulting suboptimal functional result.[18] Further, the anal sphincter mechanism may be affected, leading to imperfect continence. In female patients, pelvic sepsis can lead to infertility and in some cases has been thought to play a role in ill-defined chronic pelvic pain syndromes.

Overall, it is rewarding to know that the incidence of postoperative pelvic sepsis has declined as surgeons have gained experience and the techniques have been refined. At the Mayo Clinic, the frequency of pelvic sepsis declined from 15% in the first 200 patients who underwent IPAA to less than 4% in the last 400 patients (unpublished data). Experience from other institutions confirms an inverse relationship between experience and frequency of pelvic sepsis.[14,15]

Small Bowel Obstruction

The rate of small bowel obstruction ranges from 7% to 30% in reports of the IPAA procedure.[8,14-16,21,22] The rate is greater in patients with multiple previous abdominal operations. The frequency of small bowel obstruction, unlike pelvic sepsis, is not related to surgical experience and does not decline over time. Inasmuch as the reported rate of small bowel obstruction after proctocolectomy and Brooke ileostomy is 5% to 15%,[22] a similar incidence after IPAA would be anticipated. That the rate of small bowel obstruction is in some reports higher than expected for total proctocolectomy may in part be explained by the effect of a temporary diverting stoma and multiple (two) procedures. The contribution of the diverting ileostomy to small bowel obstruction was examined by Sagar et al.[18] In this report, a 29% incidence of small bowel obstruction was demonstrated in patients in whom a diverting loop ileostomy was performed, compared with a 7% rate in patients in whom no diverting stoma was created.[18] In a review of 460 patients, Marcello et al.[21] noted that the most common location of obstruction in patients who required surgery was at the site of ileostomy closure. It was also noted that most of these patients with obstruction at the closure site underwent 180-degree rotation of the stoma in an attempt to improve dependent drainage. As a result of the finding of increased risk of obstruction in patients with stomal rotation, this technical refinement has been abandoned. Other potential risk factors for obstruction, including age, sex, surgeon, previous colectomy, diagnosis, steroid use, previous obstruction, pouch type, and closure technique, have not been shown to influence the risk of small bowel obstruction.

In the Mayo Clinic series of more than 1600 patients, the 20% incidence of small bowel obstruction has not declined over a 12-year period, possibly because of inclusion of more patients with low-grade clinical obstruction. Three fourths of episodes of obstruction have occurred before loop closure, and previous operations were shown to increase risk. The causes of obstruction may include adhesions, internal hernia, or stenosis or may result from axial volvulus around the diverting loop. Fewer than half these patients require laparotomy, which suggests that initial conservative management is prudent. If the small bowel obstruction is thought to be related to the stoma, relief of obstruction may be accomplished by passing a soft rubber tube into the proximal stoma for decompression. Surgery is indicated in patients who do not respond clinically or who have evidence of intestinal ischemia or perforation. Bowel obstruction related to the stoma may be remedied by ileostomy takedown. In some cases this is performed before waiting the standard interval between pouch construction and ileostomy closure.

In addition to the more typical bowel obstructions that may develop after IPAA, as with any other abdominal surgery, three unique or pouch-specific forms of bowel obstruction deserve mention. The first involves the distal tip of the pouch. At the time of creation of the J pouch, two small bowel loops are stapled proximal and distal. If the distal end of the pouch is not completely divided, a mucosal bridge remains. Because the distal portion is sutured to the anus, the residual bridge can produce outlet obstruction. Sakanoue et al.[23] described a transanal technique of dividing the retained bridge to provide successful treatment of this unusual cause of obstruction. The second unique form of obstruction may result if the terminal ileum, which is folded back onto the more proximal ileum to create the J pouch, is not properly transfixed. The resulting "loose" J "appendage" may twist, causing obstruction and even perforation secondary to volvulus and ischemia.[24] Finally, a well-known complication associated with pouch design is obstructed defecation secondary to elongation of the efferent limb of the S pouch, a design used to allow an easier reach for pouch-anal anastomosis. Because of this problem, some centers have abandoned the S pouch in favor of the J pouch[21] except in cases where the J pouch would not reach. Others have stated that outlet obstruction is unlikely if the efferent limb of the S pouch does not exceed 2 cm.

Medically Related Complications

Many patients who require creation of an IPAA for ulcerative colitis are poor surgical candidates because of malnutrition resulting from chronic diarrhea and immunocompromise secondary to drug therapy. Patients who have been receiving chronic steroid therapy require perioperative stress doses of prednisone to prevent withdrawal and adrenal crisis. Signs and symptoms of insufficient steroid support may be subtle and include fever, myalgia, arthralgia, and malaise.[25] With more severe crisis, hyponatremia, hyperkalemia, and even cardiovascular collapse may result. It is for these reasons that steroid therapy should be withdrawn slowly over several weeks after surgery (see Chapter 3).

Patients with ulcerative colitis have an increased frequency of thromboembolic events[26] related to a hypercoagulation state characterized by increased levels of coagulation factors V, VIII, and IX and decreased levels of antithrombin III. These patients should therefore receive DVT prophylaxis such as sequential compression devices or subcutaneous low-dose heparin in the perioperative period.

In patients with a diverting ileostomy, output may be unacceptably increased and result in dehydration and metabolic complications.[27] Hyponatremia may occur as a result of loss of the usual colonic absorption. Prerenal azotemia with associated elevation in creatinine and blood urea nitrogen (BUN) concentrations may also occur if output is excessive, especially if the patient's intake is decreased during periods of illness. To minimize these complications, it is important to select the most distal portion of ileum possible for the diverting stoma. If high output develops in the postoperative period, medications that slow intestinal transit are usually successful in decreasing output.

LATE COMPLICATIONS

Fistula

Although pouch-related fistulas are generally rare (<2% in Mayo Clinic series), the rate may be as high as 16% in some series.[15,28] Fistulas may arise from a variety of sources. In a report of 168 patients with ileal pouches, 27 fistulas were identified. Thirteen enterocutaneous fistulas were found at different sites, including from the pouch (three), pouch–anal anastomosis (three) (for example, see Fig. 22-1), pouch appendage (three), loop ileostomy (two), and sites of iatrogenic bowel injury (two). Ten pouch-vaginal fistulas, three pouch-perineum fistulas, and one pouch-vesicle fistula developed. Factors considered important in the development of fistulas include ischemia with anastomotic breakdown, entrapment of adjacent organs such as the vagina by sutures or stapling devices, and development of postoperative pelvic sepsis. The presence of a fistula should always raise suspicion of Crohn's disease.

Pouch-vaginal fistulas are perhaps the most common, with a reported incidence of up to 10%.[29] Ten of the 27 fistulas reported by Keighley and Grobler[28] were of this variety. Groom et al.[29] reported on a series of 161 patients, of whom 17 had pouch-vaginal fistulas. Thirteen of the patients had either postoperative pelvic sepsis or documented anastomotic complications. It was noted that fistulas that developed before ileostomy closure were more likely to heal than those that developed after closure.

Several factors are crucial in determining the best treatment for pouch-related fistulas. Asymptomatic fistulas detected on routine radiographs of the pouch before planned ileostomy closure may resolve by simply delaying stoma closure. Simple perianal fistulas may be treated with fistulotomy with or without the use of a seton. In cases that do not respond to simple local measures, fecal diversion may be necessary.[30] More complex repairs are often required for fistulas that originate from the anastomosis or involve adjacent organs such as the vagina or bladder. Fistulas that arise at the anastomosis have been treated with dissection and elevation of the pouch with reanastomosis at the level of the dentate (Fig. 22-2). This is the most challenging and least often required corrective approach. Pouch excision is rarely required. Patients with a pouch-vesicle fis-

A

B

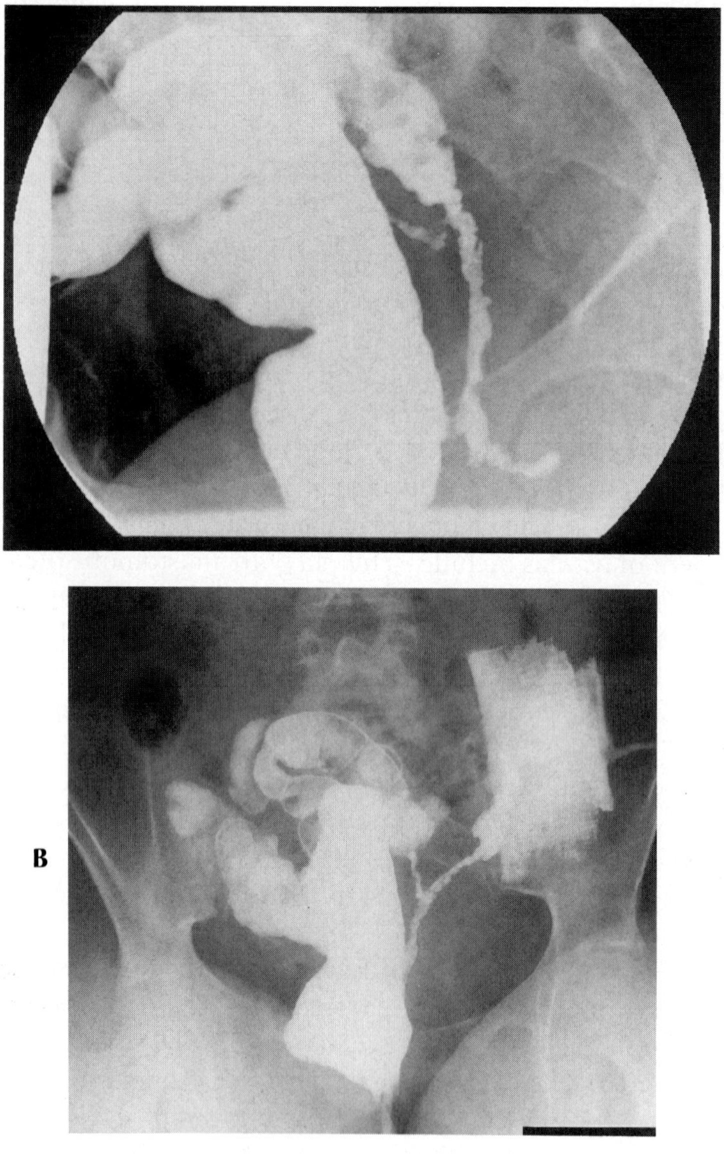

Fig. 22-1 Contrast radiograph of ileal pouch fistula. **A,** Oblique view demonstrating complex posterior fistula. **B,** Anteroposterior view demonstrating complex fistula with connection to the skin.

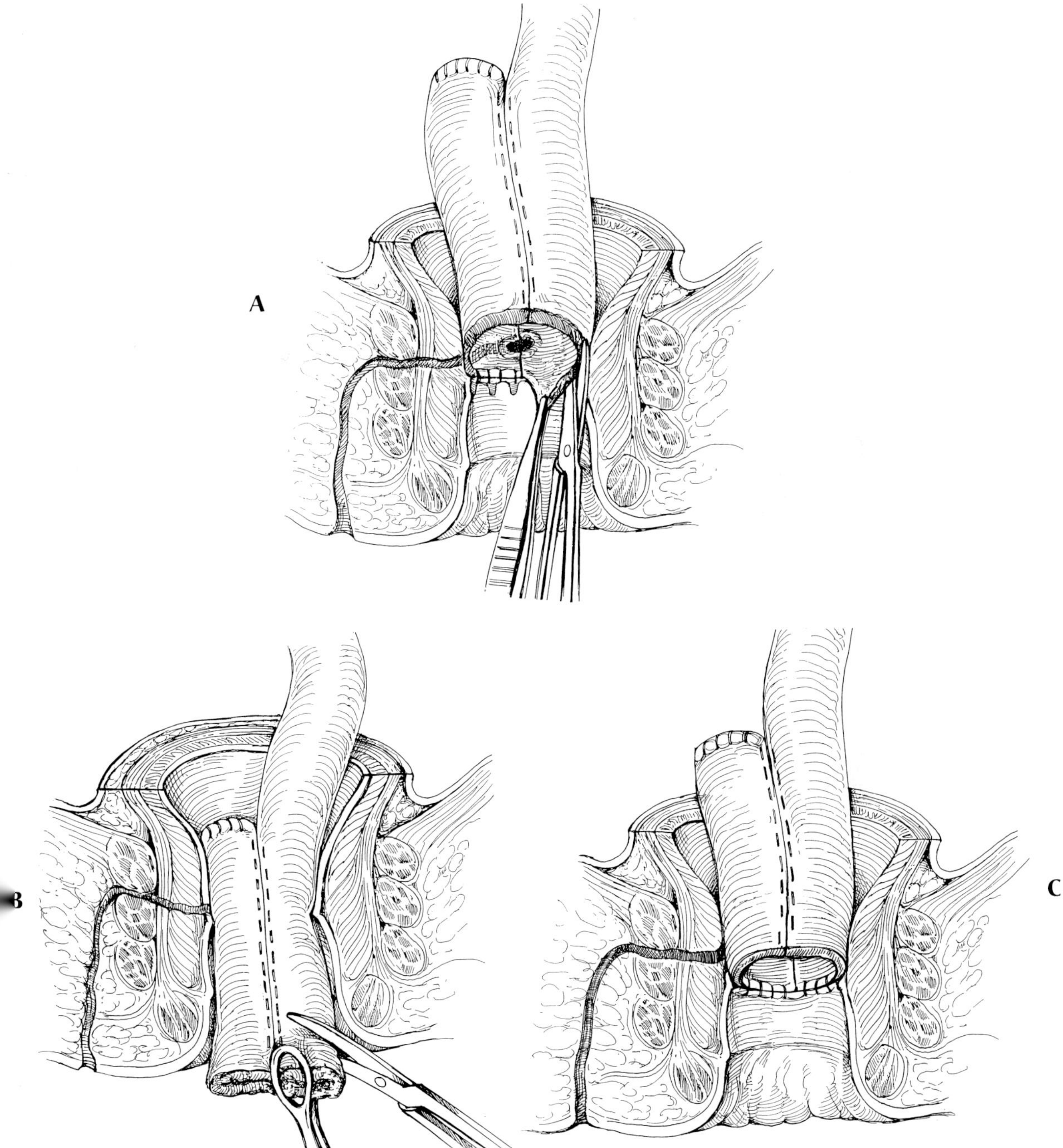

Fig. 22-2 Advancement flap repair of pouch anal fistula. **A**, Pouch anal anastomosis is divided via the anus and pouch rectal cuff adhesions are divided. **B**, Distal end of pouch (containing internal fistula opening) is divided. **C**, Fistula tract has been debrided and pouch anal anastomosis has been reconstructed (advanced pouch overlies fistula opening).

tula usually have pneumaturia or recurrent urinary tract infection. Cystoscopy is performed to locate the site of granulation tissue, which is characteristic of fistulas. Such fistulas may also be demonstrated on radiographs of the pouch. Laparotomy and direct repair with minimal bladder wall resection are generally necessary.

Two of the patients with fistulas in the series of Keighley and Grobler[28] were discovered to have Crohn's disease. The presence of a perianal fistula preoperatively should raise suspicion of Crohn's disease and therefore consideration of whether the pouch procedure is contraindicated. Similarly, postoperative development of a fistula, especially if late in onset, may be the first indication of Crohn's disease. Fortunately, this is a rare event.

Stricture

Anastomotic strictures are reported in 5% to 20% of ileal pouch–anal anastomoses.[8,15,31,32] It is relatively common for a soft stricture to develop before ileostomy closure. Such strictures, common during periods of fecal diversion, are thought to be secondary to disuse. It is therefore prudent to evaluate whether the patient will require anastomotic dilation at ileostomy closure. A radiograph of the pouch obtained in preparation for closure may reveal a stricture but is not as sensitive as physical examination in determining the character of the stricture. Tsao et al.,[20] in a study of 463 pouch radiographs obtained before ileostomy closure, reported that patients with an abnormal radiograph were more likely to require anastomotic dilation under anesthesia (33%) than were those with a normal radiograph (4%).

The contribution of surgical techniques to the risk of stricture development, specifically with reference to hand-sewn versus stapled anastomoses, is debatable. Wettergren et al.[32] reported a 23% rate of stricture formation with sewn anastomoses versus 6% for stapled anastomoses McIntyre et al.[31] reported no significant difference in the rate of stricture between sewn and stapled anastomoses. If stapled anastomosis is performed, it is prudent to use at least a 28 mm diameter stapler, because evidence shows that the frequency of stricture formation is increased with small-diameter staples.

Stricture is thought to result from tension or relative ischemia at the site of anastomosis. Pelvic sepsis may also lead to increased frequency of anastomotic stricture, possibly as a result of the surrounding fibrosis or interference with blood supply. Chronic outflow obstruction from a stricture may contribute to pouch stasis and may present symptoms attributed to pouchitis. These postsepsis strictures are more fibrotic and not easily dilated. Anal dilation or even pouch elevation and reanastomosis may be required.[30]

Pouchitis

Pouchitis as a clinical syndrome is typically characterized by a constellation of symptoms, including abdominal cramping, diarrhea, urgency, incontinence, malaise, and fever.[33,34] The initial episode usually occurs at a mean of 18 months after IPAA but may occur within days of the procedure. Although usually there are endoscopic findings of edema, friability, erythema, and mucopurulent exudate, there is no distinct correlation between endoscopic and clinical findings. Histologic analysis may demonstrate evidence of acute and chronic inflammation with villous atrophy,[35,36] but these findings are found in approximately 50% of asymptomatic patients as well. In severe cases crypt abscesses may be present. The rate of pouchitis, reported to be 10% to 30%,[33] has increased with longer periods of follow-up. The variability of reported rates among centers is probably attributable to differences in definitions of pouchitis, based on clinical, endoscopic, and histologic criteria.

Several theories regarding the cause of pouchitis have been proposed, including disease- and complication-related factors. The observation that pouchitis is relatively rare in patients with FAP and increasingly common in patients with chronic ulcerative colitis supports the idea that pouchitis is disease related.[37] Further support for this concept stems from the fact that pouchitis more commonly occurs in patients with chronic ulcerative colitis who experience extraintestinal manifestations.[33] Indeed, chronic pouchitis may represent a unique small bowel process related to the effects of "colonic" metaplasia[38,39] in patients with genetic or immunologic susceptibility.

In contrast, the possibility that pouchitis is related to technical or functional factors comes from both experimental and therapeutic observations. There is theoretic evidence that oxygen free radicals play a role in the cause of pouchitis.[40] It is postulated that pouch construction with ileocolic or distal ligation of the superior mesenteric artery or postoperative pouch dilation may produce relative mucosal ischemia. Such ischemia may result in production of oxygen free radicals. That a xanthine oxidase inhibitor, allopurinol, was effective in treatment of 11 of 22 cases of acute and chronic pouchitis[40] suggests that ischemia or at least oxygen free radicals may play a role in pouchitis.

Finally, although there is still no direct proof, it is widely believed that pouch stasis and/or bacterial overgrowth contributes to the clinical problem characterized as pouchitis. Pouch stasis may result from anastomotic stricture, excessive pouch capacity caused by technical factors, or poor contractility and inefficient emptying as a result of pelvic sepsis. Favorable response to antibiotic therapy, typically metronidazole (Flagyl), supports at least some measure of contribution from bacterial overgrowth or maldistribution of aerobic and anaerobic bacteria ratios. The true contribution of bacterial overgrowth to pouchitis remains elusive because correlative studies between culture results and clinical condition have not been established.

Regardless of possible causes, patients with clinical findings suggestive of pouchitis should undergo thorough anal examination to ensure that strictures that require dilation are not present. In most of these patients the episodes are short lived and readily treated with a 5- to 7-day course of oral metronidazole

(Flagyl). However, approximately 3% of patients with an ileoanal pouch require long-term maintenance therapy with metronidazole. Pemberton[10] reported that 16% of patients with pouchitis have chronic recurrence. In resistant cases, ciprofloxacin is effective. In persistent cases, 5-ASA compounds have been used. In the few patients who will have debilitating recurrent or persistent pouchitis, diversion and/or pouch excision is required.

SPECIAL CONSIDERATIONS

Ulcerative Colitis Compared With Familial Adenomatous Polyposis

As might be anticipated, patients who undergo IPAA for FAP tend to have fewer postoperative complications and better functional results than do patients with chronic ulcerative colitis. In 1989, Dozois et al.[37] compared 758 consecutive patients with chronic ulcerative colitis and 94 consecutive patients with FAP who underwent ileal pouch–anal anastomosis. Postoperative sepsis developed in 6% of patients with chronic ulcerative colitis compared with none of the patients with FAP. The FAP group also had better functional results, with less daytime stool frequency and nocturnal incontinence. The overall postoperative complication rate, however, was not significantly different. It is noteworthy that despite "good" functional results the overall quality of life from the patients' point of view was not improved in patients with FAP compared with those with chronic ulcerative colitis. The incongruity between pouch functional results and satisfaction with the pouch for patients with FAP versus chronic ulcerative colitis likely reflects the different preoperative status of these patients. While most patients with chronic ulcerative colitis will experience a reduction in bowel movement frequency after creation of the pouch, the opposite is true for patients with FAP.

Staged Procedures

The pouch may be created in one, two, or three stages, depending on the clinical status of the patient. Whereas most patients are currently treated in two stages, first with colectomy, pouch anastomosis, and fecal diversion, and second by delayed ileostomy closure, the three-stage procedure was more common in the early years of IPAA development and remains an important option for patients with acute colitis. Penna et al.[41] reported that patients with acute colitis had fewer complications when the colectomy was performed before the pouch procedure (16%) rather than at the same time (38%). However, there was a 20% complication rate after previous subtotal colectomy. Scott et al.[19] reported that previous subtotal colectomy did not protect against pelvic sepsis, and Galandiuk et al.[42] reported that when the IPAA was delayed after subtotal colectomy there was a higher rate of sepsis but a lower rate of postoperative obstruction. The three-stage approach remains a useful option for patients who are acutely and/or chronically compromised from severe disease and immunosuppressive therapies, those in whom the diagnosis of Crohn's is being considered, and young male patients who are concerned about their future ability to father children. Because normal childbearing is feasible after IPAA,[43] the role of the three-stage procedure in young women is less certain.

Even though the two-stage procedure remains the standard, one-stage IPAA without fecal diversion is gaining in popularity. Tjandra et al.[44] compared outcomes in 50 patients without fecal diversion to matched controls with diversion. Anastomotic leak and pelvic abscess rates were higher in patients without diversion (14%) than in patients with diversion (4%). Six percent of patients who had undergone the one-stage procedure required a repeat operation because of septic complications, compared with none of the patients with initial diversion. In this same report, patients receiving more than 20 mg of prednisone per day were noted to have more complications; therefore diversion was recommended in these patients. This point remains debatable, because not all reports confirm a risk with steroid therapy.[18] In contrast to the reduced risk of sepsis with diversion, the risk of small bowel obstruction is reported more frequently with ileostomy (29%) compared with no diversion (7%). Anastomotic stricture was increased in patients who underwent the one-stage procedure (33% versus 14%). Preconditions for considering a one-stage procedure should include the absence of urgent surgery; absence of systemic toxicity; a tension-free watertight anastomosis; and absence of gross contamination during surgery. Because of the potential risk of infertility in female patients in whom pelvic sepsis develops, it is suggested that diversion be performed in those patients with future childbearing potential.

Stapled Versus Hand-Sewn Anastomosis

Perhaps the most controversial pouch-related issue is the manner and site of the anastomosis. The stapled ileoanal anastomosis, which is generally easier to perform than mucosectomy with hand-sewn anastomosis, has become increasingly popular in recent years. Because of retained cuff length, this technique allows the pouch to reach the anus in the unusual case where a tension-free anastomosis at the dentate is not possible. Wettergren et al.[32] compared 96 patients with hand-sewn anastomoses with 48 patients with stapled anastomoses and found that rates of anastomotic breakdown and stenosis were significantly higher in the group with hand-sewn anastomoses. Comparing functional outcomes, McIntyre et al.[31] found no significant difference in pouchitis, incontinence, or stool frequency associated with stapled versus hand-sewn anastomoses. They felt that complication rates might be related more to surgical "familiarity" and experience rather than the technique itself. Of note, a mucosectomy is preferred by the authors in patients with FAP because of the risk of carcinoma in the retained segment.[45,46]

Indeterminate Colitis

Indeterminate colitis, the inability to histologically distinguish between chronic ulcerative colitis and Crohn's disease, may occur in as many as 20% of patients for whom IPAA is considered. Atkinson et al.[47] reported on a pathologic review of 175 patients who underwent IPAA and found indeterminate colitis in 16. Reports on pouch results with the diagnosis of indeterminate colitis are variable and probably reflect differences in definition or inclusion criteria. In the Mayo Clinic series, in which indeterminate colitis was defined as a perioperative clinical diagnosis of chronic ulcerative colitis, followed by a pathologic result that cannot be used as the basis on which to confidently confirm chronic ulcerative colitis, functional results were very similar to those described for chronic ulcerative colitis.[48] In this series, however, failure was more frequent for indeterminate colitis (19% versus 8%). In contrast, some authors have documented that patients with indeterminate colitis are more likely to develop fistulas and infections.[48] In a retrospective analysis by Koltun,[49] the risk of pouch excision or permanent ileostomy because of complications was 28% in patients with indeterminate colitis. Grobler et al.[50] also found an increased complication rate in patients with indeterminate colitis compared with patients with pathologic ulcerative colitis. Thus patients classified with indeterminate colitis had overall outcomes similar to those in patients in whom Crohn's disease was detected after IPAA. By contrast, Pezim et al.[51] noted that only those patients with some other preoperative suggestion of Crohn's disease, such as perianal fistulas, had more complications than did patients with documented ulcerative colitis. It appears that preoperative clinical impressions together with the surgical pathologic findings are most predictive of outcome. Whereas a clinical impression of chronic ulcerative colitis and pathologic diagnosis of indeterminate colitis yields favorable results, a clinical suspicion of Crohn's disease should provide concern. In these cases it is advised that a pathologic diagnosis of chronic ulcerative colitis be confidently established before a pouch procedure is performed.

Genitourinary Function

Sexual dysfunction is known to occur in rare cases and is most likely the result of injury to parasympathetic and sympathetic nerves associated with the presacral plexus. Injury may result from trauma if a conservative rectal resection is not done, particularly, at the sacral promontory. Postoperative sepsis and subsequent pelvic scarring may also lead to nerve injury. Erectile impotence in men results from parasympathetic damage and has been shown to occur in approximately 4% of men after IPAA.[10,15] Retrograde ejaculation also occurs in approximately 4% of men and is caused primarily by sympathetic nerve injury.[10] Although less is known about female sexual function, dyspareunia has been reported in 5% to 8% of cases.[10,15] Normal childbearing, including vaginal delivery, is possible after the pouch procedure.[43] Finally, although early postoperative urinary retention may occur in approximately 5% of patients after IPAA, chronic urinary retention is extremely rare.

Miscellaneous Complications

An unusual complication that may complicate the IPAA in patients with FAP is formation of intra-abdominal (mesenteric) desmoid tumors. These tumors, which may be present at the pouch procedure, may technically compromise or contraindicate construction of a pouch or may develop after the pouch procedure, as has occurred in at least 10 patients at the Mayo Clinic. Bowel obstruction or pouch complications may result from mechanical compression. These tumors tend to recur if excised or subjected to radiation therapy, and anti-inflammatory drugs (e.g., sulindac) and hormonal agents (e.g., tamoxifen) have only inconsistently generated tumor-shrinking effects.

An unusual complication of ileal pouch–anal anastomosis that may affect chronic ulcerative colitis is primary sclerosing cholangitis. Forty patients with primary sclerosing cholangitis were identified through 1990,[52] which represents approximately 5% of patients with chronic ulcerative colitis who underwent the pouch procedure. Although early postoperative complications in these patients are similar to those reported for patients with chronic ulcerative colitis without primary sclerosing cholangitis, patients with primary sclerosing cholangitis, have a greater than 50% rate of long-term complications, primarily related to liver disease. Although peristomal varices occur in approximately 50% of patients with primary sclerosing cholangitis, no patient in the Mayo Clinic series has developed anastomotic variceal bleeding after the IPAA procedure.[53]

POUCH FAILURE

In approximately 3% to 6% of patients, ileal pouch–anal anastomosis ultimately fails and pouch excision or permanent diversion is necessary.[10,54] The usual reasons for failure are septic complications, poor function with incontinence or increased stool frequency, unrecognized Crohn's disease, and stricture.[10,14,42,54,55] With longer follow-up, chronic pouchitis may play an increasing role in this complication.

REFERENCES

1. Nissen R. Berlin Chirurgical Society. Chirurg 15:888-890, 1933.
2. Ravitch MM, Sabiston DC. Anal ileostomy with preservation of the sphincter: A proposed operation in patients requiring total colectomy for benign lesions. Surg Gynecol Obstet 84:1095-1099, 1947.
3. Valiente MA, Bacon HE. Construction of pouch using "pantaloon" technique for pull-through of ileum following total colectomy: Report of experimental work and results. Am J Surg 90:742-750, 1955.

4. Martin LW, LeCoultre C, Schubert WK. Total colectomy and mucosal proctectomy with preservation of continence in ulcerative colitis. Ann Surg 186:477-480, 1977.
5. Parks AG, Nicholls RJ, Belliveau P. Proctocolectomy with ileal reservoir and anal anastomosis. Br J Surg 67:533-538, 1980.
6. Utsunomiya J, Iwama T, Imajo M, Matsuo S, Sawai S, Yaegashi K, Hirayama R. Total colectomy, mucosal proctectomy, and ileoanal anastomosis. Dis Colon Rectum 23:459-466, 1980.
7. Bess MA, Adson MA, Elveback LR, Moertel CG. Rectal cancer following colectomy for polyposis. Arch Surg 115:460-467, 1980.
8. Poppen B, Svenberg T, Bark T, Sjogren B, Rubio C, Drakenberg B, Slezak P. Colectomy-proctomucosectomy with S-pouch: Operative procedures, complications, and functional outcome in 69 consecutive patients. Dis Colon Rectum 35:40-47, 1992.
9. Penna C, Tiret E, Parc R, Sfairi A, Kartheuser A, Hannoun L, Nordlinger B. Operation and abdominal desmoid tumors in familial adenomatous polyposis. Surg Gynecol Obstet 177:263-268, 1993.
10. Pemberton JH. Complications, management, failure, and revisions. In Nicholls J, Bartolo D, Mortensen N, eds. Restorative Proctocolectomy. Cambridge, England: Blackwell Scientific, 1993, pp 34-52.
11. Metcalf AM, Dozois RR, Kelly KA, Beart RW, Wolff BG. Ileal "J" pouch–anal anastomosis. Clinical outcome. Ann Surg 202:735-739, 1985.
12. Lewis WG, Sagar PM, Holdsworth PJ, Axon ATR, Johnston J. Restorative proctocolectomy with end to end pouch–anal anastomosis in patients over the age fifty. Gut 34:948-952, 1993.
13. Perbeck L, Lindquist K, Liljequist L. The mucosal blood flow in pelvic pouches in man: A methodologic study of fluorescine flowmetry. Dis Colon Rectum 28:931-936, 1985.
14. McMullen K, Hicks TC, Ray JE, Gathright JB, Timmcke AE. Complications associated with ileal pouch–anal anastomosis. World J Surg 15:763-776, 1991.
15. Keighley MRB, Grobler S, Bain I. An audit of restorative proctocolectomy. Gut 34:680-684, 1993.
16. Pescatori M, Mattana C, Castagneto M. Clinical and functional results after restorative proctocolectomy. Br J Surg 75:321-324, 1988.
17. Gemlo BT, Wong WD, Rothenberger DA, Goldberg SM. Ileal pouch–anal anastomosis—patterns of failure. Arch Surg 127:784-787, 1992.
18. Sagar PM, Lewis W, Holdsworth PJ, Johnston DJ. One-stage restorative proctocolectomy without temporary defunctioning ileostomy. Dis Colon Rectum 35:582-588, 1992.
19. Scott NA, Dozois RR, Beart RW, Pemberton JH, Wolff BG, Ilstrup DM. Postoperative intra-abdominal and pelvic sepsis complicating ileal pouch–anal anastomosis. Int J Colorect Dis 3:149-152, 1988.
20. Tsao JI, Galandiuk S, Pemberton JH. Pouchogram: Predictor of clinical outcome following ileal pouch–anal anastomosis. Dis Colon Rectum 35:547-551, 1992.
21. Marcello PW, Roberts PL, Schoetz DJ, Coller JA, Murray JJ, Veidenheimer MC. Obstruction after ileal pouch–anal anastomosis: A preventable complication? Dis Colon Rectum 36:1105-1111, 1993.
22. Francois Y, Dozois RR, Kelly KA, Beart RW, Wolff BG, Pemberton JH, Ilstrup DM. Small intestinal obstruction complicating ileal pouch–anal anastomosis. Ann Surg 209:46-50, 1989.
23. Sakanoue Y, Shoji Y, Kusunoki M, Utsunomiya J. Transanal division of an apical pouch bridge after restorative proctocolectomy with a J shaped reservoir. Br J Surg 80:248, 1993.
24. Pezim ME, Taylor BA, Davis CJ, Beart RW. Perforation of terminal ileal appendage of J-pelvic ileal reservoir. Dis Colon Rectum 30:161-163, 1987.

25. Kusunoki M, Moeslein G, Shoji Y, Fujita S, Yanagi H, Sakanoue Y, Saito N, Utsunomiya J. Steroid complications in patients with ulcerative colitis. Dis Colon Rectum 35:1003-1009, 1992.
26. Talbot RW, Heppell J, Dozois RR, Beart RW. Vascular complications of inflammatory bowel disease. Mayo Clin Proc 61:140-145, 1986.
27. Max E, Trabanino G, Reznick RK, Bailey HR, Smith KW. Metabolic changes during the defunctionalized stage after ileal pouch–anal anastomosis. Dis Colon Rectum 30:508-512, 1987.
28. Keighley MRB, Grobler SP. Fistula complicating restorative proctocolectomy. Br J Surg 80:1065-1067, 1993.
29. Groom JS, Nicholls RJ, Hawley PR, Phillips RKS. Pouch-vaginal fistula. Br J Surg 80:936-940, 1993.
30. Galandiuk S, Scott NA, Dozois RR, Kelly KA, Ilstrup DM, Beart RW, Wolff BG, Pemberton JH, Nivatvongs S, Devine RM. Ileal pouch–anal anastomosis—reoperation for pouch-related complications. Ann Surg 212:446-454, 1990.
31. McIntyre PB, Pemberton JH, Beart RW, Devine RM, Nivatvongs S. Double-stapled vs handsewn ileal pouch–anal anastomosis in patients with chronic ulcerative colitis. Dis Colon Rectum 37:430-433, 1994.
32. Wettergren A, Gyrtrup HJ, Grosmann E, Svendsen LB, Hjortrup A, Stadil F, Kirkegraard P. Complications after J-pouch ileoanal anastomosis: Stapled compared with handsewn anastomosis. Eur J Surg 159:121-124, 1993.
33. Fozard BJ, Pemberton JH. Results of pouch surgery after ileo-anal anastomosis: The implications of pouchitis. World J Surg 16:880-884, 1992.
34. Sandborn WJ, Tremaine WJ, Batts KP, Pemberton JH, Phillips SF. Pouchitis after ileal pouch–anal anastomosis: A pouchitis disease activity index. Mayo Clin Proc 69:409-415, 1994.
35. Kmiot WA, Youngs D, Tudor R, Thompson H, Keighley MRB. Mucosal morphology, cell proliferation and faecal bacteriology in acute pouchitis. Br J Surg 80:1445-1449, 1993.
36. McLeod RS, Antonioli D, Cullen J, Dvorak A, Onderdonk A, Silen W, Blair JE, Monahan-Earley R, Cisneros R, Cohen Z. Histologic and microbiologic features of biopsy samples from patients with normal and inflamed pouches. Dis Colon Rectum 37:26-31, 1994.
37. Dozois RR, Kelly KA, Welling DR, Gordon H, Beart RW, Wolff BG, Pemberton JH, Ilstrup DM. Ileal pouch–anal anastomosis: Comparison of results in familial adenomatous polyposis and chronic ulcerative colitis. Ann Surg 210:268-273, 1989.
38. Banerjee AK. Hypothesis: Pouchitis represents a useful clinical model of ulcerative colitis. Med Hypotheses 42:36-38, 1994.
39. Subramani K, Harpaz N, Bilotta J, Bodian C, Rubin PH, Janowitz HD, Gelernt IM, Sachar DB. Refractory pouchitis: Does it reflect underlying Crohn's disease? Gut 34:1539-1542, 1993.
40. Levin KE, Pemberton JH, Phillips SF, Zinsmeister AR, Pezim ME. Role of oxygen free radicals in the etiology of pouchitis. Dis Colon Rectum 35:452-456, 1992.
41. Penna C, Daude F, Parc R, Tiret E, Frileux P, Hannoun L, Nordlinger B, Levy E. Previous subtotal colectomy with ileostomy and sigmoidostomy improves the morbidity and early functional results after ileal pouch–anal anastomosis in ulcerative colitis. Dis Colon Rectum 36:343-348, 1993.
42. Galandiuk S, Pemberton JH, Tsao J, Ilstrup DM, Wolff BG. Delayed ileal pouch–anal anastomosis—Complications and functional results. Dis Colon Rectum 34:755-758, 1991.
43. Juhasz ES, Fozard B, Dozois RR, Ilstrup DM, Nelson H. Ileal pouch–anal anastomosis function following childbirth: An extended evaluation. Dis Colon Rectum 38:159-165, 1995.

44. Tjandra JJ, Fazio VW, Milsom JW, Lavery IC, Oakley JR, Fabre JM. Omission of temporary diversion in restorative proctocolectomy—is it safe? Dis Colon Rectum 36:1007-1014, 1993.
45. Hoehner JC, Metcalf AM. Development of invasive adenocarcinoma following colectomy with ileoanal anastomosis for familial polyposis coli—report of a case. Dis Colon Rectum 37:824-828, 1994.
46. Puthu D, Rajan N, Rao R, Rao L, Venugopal P. Carcinoma of the rectal pouch following restorative proctocolectomy—report of a case. Dis Colon Rectum 35:257-260, 1992.
47. Atkinson KG, Owen DA, Wankling G. Restorative proctocolectomy and indeterminate colitis. Am J Surg 167:516-518, 1994.
48. McIntyre PB, Pemberton JH, Wolff BG, Dozois RR, Beart RW Jr. Indeterminate colitis: Long-term outcome in patients after ileal pouch-anal anastomosis. Dis Colon Rectum 38:51-54, 1995.
49. Koltun WA, Schoetz DJ, Roberts PL, Murray JJ, Coller JA, Veidenheimer MC. Indeterminate colitis predisposes to perineal complications after ileal pouch–anal anastomosis. Dis Colon Rectum 34:857-860, 1991
50. Grobler SP, Hosie KB, Affie E, Thompson H, Keighley MRB. Outcome of restorative proctocolectomy when the diagnosis is suggestive of Crohn's disease. Gut 34:1384-1388, 1993.
51. Pezim ME, Pemberton JH, Beart RW, Wolff BG, Dozois RR, Nivatvongs S, Devine R, Ilstrup DM. Outcome of "indeterminate" colitis following ileal pouch–anal anastomosis. Dis Colon Rectum 32:653-658, 1989.
52. Kartheuser AH, Dozois RR, Wiesner RH, LaRusso NF, Ilstrup DM, Schleck CD. Complications and risk factors after ileal pouch–anal anastomosis for ulcerative colitis associated with primary sclerosing cholangitis. Ann Surg 217:314-320, 1993.
53. Fucini C, Wolff BG, Dozois RR. Bleeding from peristomal varices: Perspectives on prevention and treatment. Dis Colon Rectum 34:1073-1078, 1991.
54. Poggioli G, Marchetti F, Selleri S, Laureti S, Stocchi L, Gozzetti G. Redo pouches: Salvaging of failed ileal pouch–anal anastomosis. Dis Colon Rectum 36:492-496, 1993.
55. Schoetz DJ, Coller JA, Veidenheimer MC. Can the pouch be saved? Dis Colon Rectum 31:671-675, 1988.

CHAPTER 23

Ostomies

JAMES W. FLESHMAN, Jr.

The construction of ostomies in the treatment of colorectal disease dates to the late nineteenth century for colostomy and as recently as 1952 for ileostomy. The techniques to create a well-functioning stoma and the appliances used to collect ostomy effluent have evolved over the years to provide a good quality of life for patients in whom an ostomy is necessary as part of the treatment of their disease. Alternatives to ostomy construction have been discovered in the treatment of several diseases, and surgical techniques have improved to reduce the use of stomas to a minimum. However, when a stoma is required, the surgeon must make every effort to create an ostomy that allows good function, minimal interference with the patient's lifestyle, and maximal reintegration into society for the patient. These efforts involve preoperative marking of the stoma site, the intraoperative aspects of stoma construction, and care of any early and late complications of the ostomy.

GENERAL CONSIDERATIONS

The development of complications after stoma surgery is influenced by several general principles that should be considered first as we review complications related to ostomy surgery. Most late complications tend to increase in frequency over long-term follow-up.[1] Patients with a tendency toward hernia development have an increased incidence of parastomal hernias.[2] Elderly patients also seem to have more late complications after stoma surgery.[2] Complications occur at a higher rate in patients who undergo unplanned ostomy construction.[3,4] Obese patients are at higher risk for early complications such as necrosis.[5] Apparently, the disease process, segment of bowel, or stoma location does not affect the development of complications.[4] Improper siting of the stoma (e.g., near a bony prominence) does affect the incidence of complications from ostomies, especially the skin problems that result from a poorly fitting appliance.[3,6] It is possible that stoma position also affects the development of late complications such as hernia and prolapse.[1]

Preoperative stoma marking is important to avert skin and appliance problems (Fig. 23-1). Selection of a stoma site is best accomplished before surgery with the patient sitting, standing, and supine while wearing clothes typical of his or her

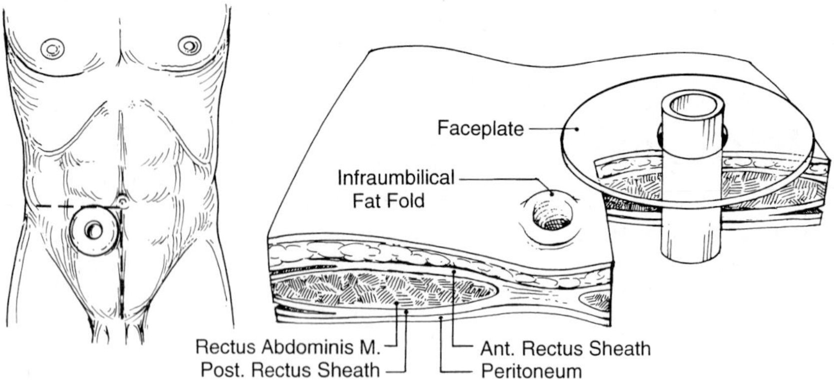

Fig. 23-1 Location for ileostomy.

lifestyle. This allows the enterostomal therapist or other trained professional to select potential sites that are visible to the patient, do not interfere with clothes, belts, bony prominences, or scars, and coincide with the apex of any fat fold.[7] Visibility should be the primary concern.[6] A scar can be used to site the stoma if it is flat and narrow or can be flattened with reconstructive surgery. Positioning the site above the umbilicus is an option if visibility is poor inferior to the umbilicus. The least critical consideration is location within the rectus muscle sheath.[6] Several authors have suggested that the incidence of complications of hernia or prolapse may not be affected by transrectus placement of the stoma.[2,8]

COMPLICATIONS

Complications of ostomies can be classified by stoma type and time of occurrence, that is, early or late. It is more difficult to categorize complications as major or minor, because a seemingly insignificant skin irritation may affect the life of the ostomate as much as a hernia that requires surgical management. It is always important to remember the patient's perception of the problem in these circumstances, because ostomy surgery has a major effect on quality of life. Any negative factor may alter the patient's ability to cope.

CONVENTIONAL ILEOSTOMY

Altered Physiology

The typical ileostomy excretes 1000 to 1500 mL in a 24-hour period immediately after construction. As the stoma matures, the volume of stoma effluent decreases to 500 to 800 mL over 24 hours. Output greater than 1000 mL in a mature stoma may result in sodium and water depletion that may eventually produce clinically significant dehydration that requires parenteral replacement of fluid and electrolytes. Circumstances that predispose to high output include ileus, bacterial overgrowth, gastroenteritis, radiation enteritis, partial small bowel obstruction, short bowel syndrome, Crohn's disease, and intra-abdominal abscess.[6] The risk of dehydration in a proximal ileostomy, such as a diverting loop ileostomy for a pelvic pouch procedure, may be as high as 20%.[9] The chronic dehydration and acid urine may lead to formation of uric acid renal calculi, which are the most common stones associated with an ileostomy.[10] The simple addition of 4 g of $NaHco_3$ to the diet and adequate fluid intake may prevent uric acid stone formation.[11]

The number of bacteria within the effluent of the ileostomy increase to a level 80 times that of the normal terminal ileum. These are mostly coliform bacteria.[10] Bile acid excretion is usually higher if more than 10 cm of terminal ileum is resected. Ileostomy effluent is also rich in proteolytic enzymes that attack the keratin layer of the epidermis. The result is an increase in odor and skin irritation if the effluent comes in contact with the skin. A significant deficit in vitamin B_{12} absorption is unusual if less than 10 cm of ileum is resected. In fact, B_{12} levels have been shown to be normal even in patients with 30 to 40 cm of terminal ileum used to create a reservoir.

Ileostomy dysfunction was common after ileostomy construction before the 1950s. The stoma was brought through the abdominal wall and amputated several centimeters above the level of the skin, exposing serosa to the extra-abdominal environment. The process of mucosa growing down from the lumen at the cut edge of the bowel along the serosa to the skin was called *delayed maturation* and required 6 to 8 weeks. Initially serositis occurred that produced partial obstruction of the ileostomy and high output. This dysfunction resolved as the granulation tissue supported growth of mucosa to cover the serosa. Variable success was obtained by grafting skin to the exposed serosa. However, it was not until Brooke[12] described the "evagination of the ileal end at the time of operation and suturing the mucosa to the skin" that the problem of ileostomy dysfunction was completely resolved.

Skin Problems

Peristomal skin irritation has been reported in a significant number of patients (15% to 79%) in most series.[9,13] Although severe skin irritation occurs more frequently in patients with a colostomy (23% vs. 11%), bacterial or fungal infection of the skin occurs more commonly (11% vs. 2%) in patients with an ileostomy.[13] The most common stoma-related infection in the immediate postoperative period is *Candida albicans* (monilia).

Skin problems are usually the result of poor adherence of the appliance and exposure of the skin to the stoma effluent. Conditions that predispose to skin irritation include a flush or retracted stoma, improperly placed stoma (near a bony promontory, through a dimpling scar, in a fold, under a belt), inadequate

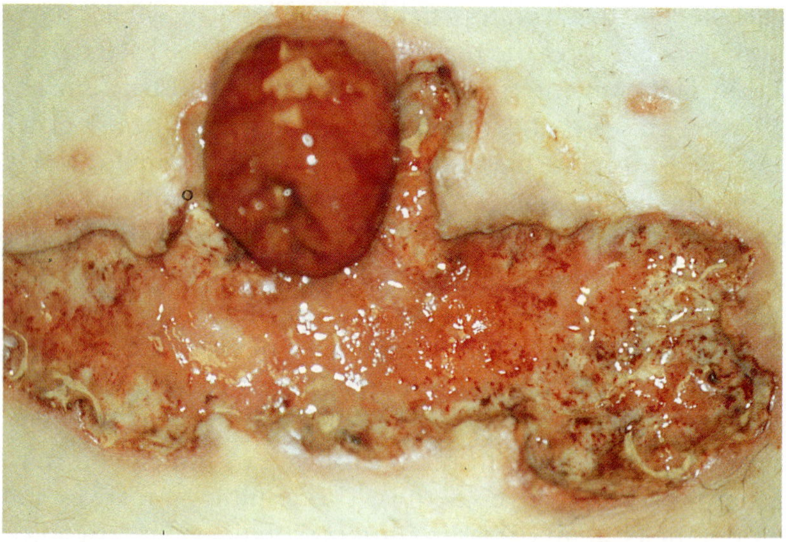

Fig. 23-2 Pyoderma surrounding a right lower quadrant ileostomy.

care of a well-made stoma (improper fitting of an appliance, infrequent appliance change), and allergy to adhesive materials on the bag.[3,6,14] Skin irritation, the most common stoma-related complication, is the most preventable.[13] Proper stoma siting and construction and appliance maintenance can eliminate the majority of significant skin problems in patients with an ileostomy.

Unavoidable problems arise as a result of the patient's disease state. Pyoderma gangrenosum in patients with inflammatory bowel disease often occurs around the ileostomy (Fig. 23-2) and prevents placement of an appliance. This most commonly occurs in patients after colectomy who have active disease elsewhere. In the majority of these patients, pyoderma will respond to steroids with 5-ASA or cyclosporine; however, it is sometimes necessary to remove the active disease to control the pyoderma.[15]

Early Complications

Stoma necrosis. Ischemic necrosis of the stoma has been reported in 2.3% to 17% of patients who undergo ileostomy construction.[3] Skeletonization of the terminal ileum may be the most frequent cause of the acute problem. Ileostomy necrosis may also result when the abdominal wall is thickened from subcutaneous fat, the mesentery is thickened from inflammation or fat, and the abdominal opening is inadequate (Fig. 23-3).

Ileostomy necrosis should be evaluated to determine the level of necrosis.

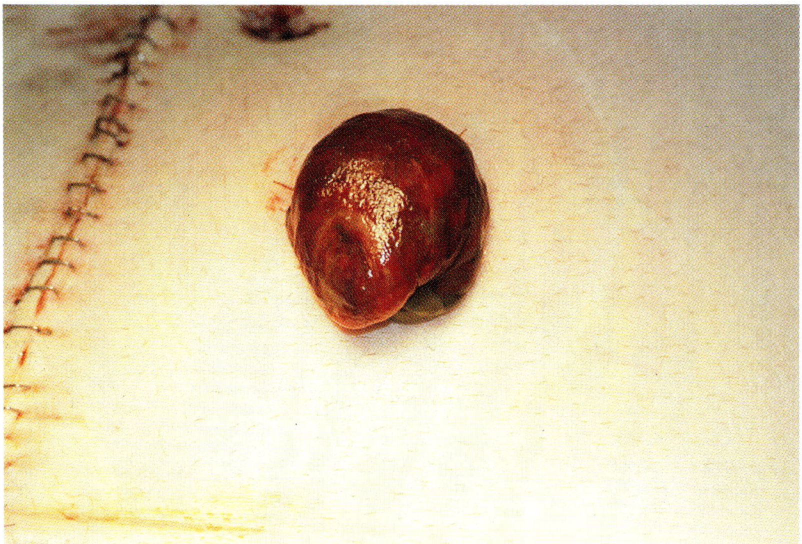

Fig. 23-3 Ileostomy necrosis that required immediate repeat exploration.

Pin-prick testing may help differentiate between venous engorgement and discoloration and ischemia from inadequate arterial flow. Another method is to place a small, clear test tube into the stoma and with flashlight illumination look for pink mucosa. Better visualization of the stoma is possible with use of a pediatric (10 mm) proctoscope. If viable tissue is present above the fascial level, conservative therapy is usually possible. Good pouching techniques, dietary manipulation, and even bowel rest and TPN may allow the surgeon to temporize in the unstable or immediately postoperative patient until the stoma can be revised at local exploration.

Necrosis below the level of the fascia requires immediate exploratory laparotomy. If conditions exist that predispose the patient to repeat stoma necrosis, a loop ileostomy should be considered. This prevents skeletonization of the distal ileum and maintains adequate vasculature to the body of the stoma. Techniques for constructing loop-end and divided-end-loop stomas may also be useful. The loop-end ileostomy can be constructed to provide an adequate spigot and a minimal blind pouch (Fig. 23-4). The stapled end of the loop may be left below the fascia if necessary as long as a proximal opening is maintained at skin level in the nonfunctional (distal) limb.

Retraction. Stoma retraction occurs in as many as 15% of patients.[3,5,10] Tension on the stoma, obesity, improper construction or siting, and ischemia are predisposing

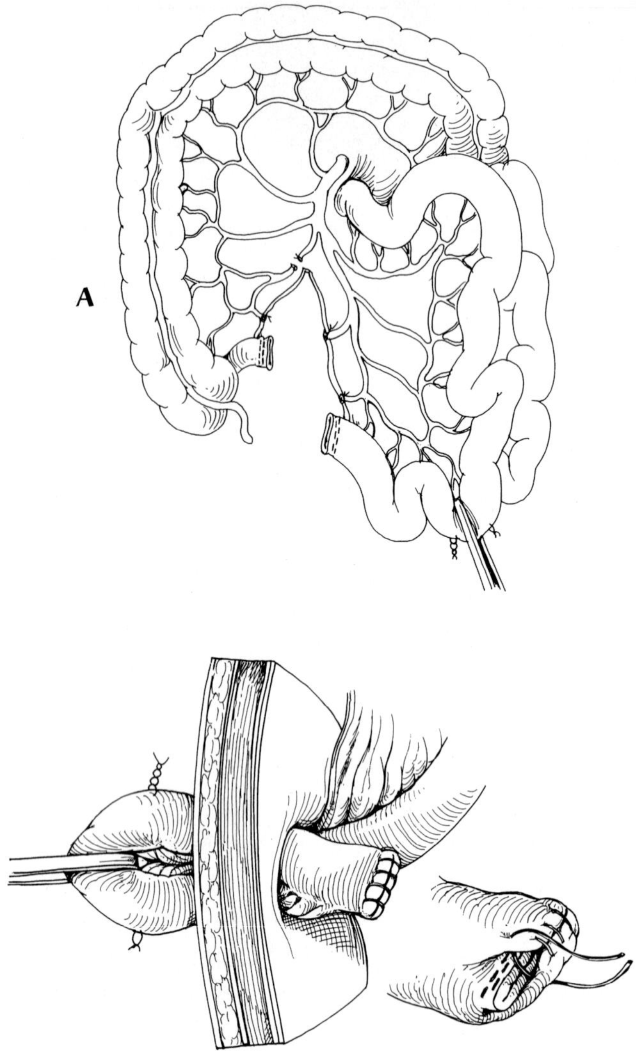

Fig. 23-4 Construction of a loop-end ileostomy. **A**, Tracheostomy tape is placed around the loop of intestine, with the mesentery mobilized but completely preserved. **B**, The end of the ileum is closed. The intestine is pulled through the abdominal wall so that the functional limb is in the inferior position and the closed end is allowed to reside just within the abdominal cavity.

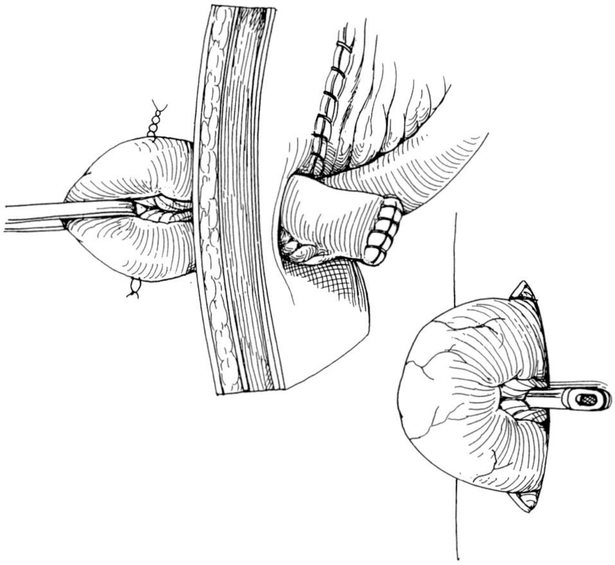

C

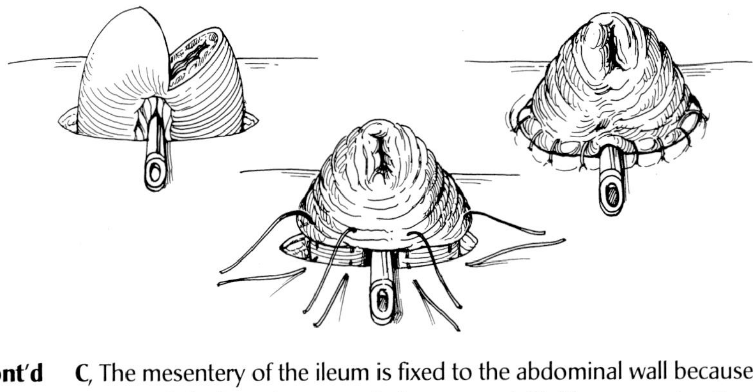

D

Fig. 23-4, cont'd **C**, The mesentery of the ileum is fixed to the abdominal wall because this is meant to be a permanent stoma, and the loop is suspended over a rod. **D**, Stoma construction is completed as for a standard loop ileostomy.

A

B

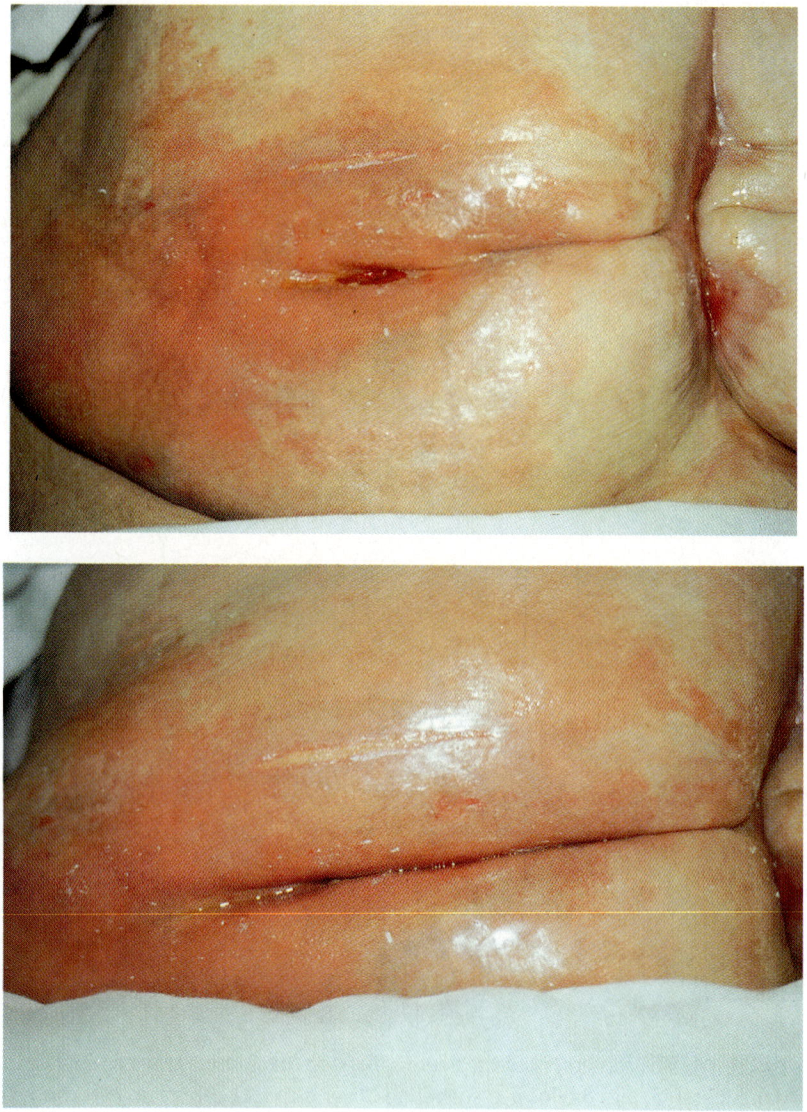

Fig. 23-5 Ileostomy retraction in an obese patient. **A**, Supine position. **B**, Sitting position.

factors.[6] Stoma retraction may occur as a late complication if a patient gains excessive weight or an adequate scar fails to form in the everted stoma. Recurrent Crohn's disease may cause retraction of an ileostomy.[16] The impetus to revise the stoma is usually the severe skin excoriation that results from poor appliance adherence to a flush stoma (Fig. 23-5). Local revision to reconstruct a protruding 2.5-cm spigot is usually possible. Bidirectional seromyotomies placed 1 cm apart on the surface of the bowel from skin level upward may induce adequate scarring to prevent unfolding of the spigot (Fig. 23-6). Suspension of the cut edge of the mesentery of the ileum from the anterior abdominal wall peritoneum may prevent tension on the stoma. Use of four tripartite sutures (bowel edge, serosa at skin level, and dermal layer) or separate sutures from serosa to Scarpa's fascia around the stoma may also maintain eversion of the stoma until the normal fibrosis of healing can occur to prevent retraction. Recurrent retraction may require more drastic measures such as placing a serosal strip within the stoma or stapling the stoma in its everted position with a bladeless linear cutting stapling instrument.[16,17]

Obstruction. Ileostomy obstruction within the first 6 months after construction is usually caused by high residue food lodging behind the stoma.[6] Small bowel obstruction is a frequent (6% to 11%) complication related to the loop ileostomy constructed for temporary diversion after pelvic pouch construction.[9,18] Early food bolus obstruction proximal to an edematous new ileostomy usually resolves with gentle saline solution irrigation of the ileostomy through a Foley catheter or a Hypaque stoma injection.[6]

Late obstruction of an ileostomy is most likely caused by an adhesive band or stenosis at the stoma.[5] Food bolus obstruction is also possible but less common.

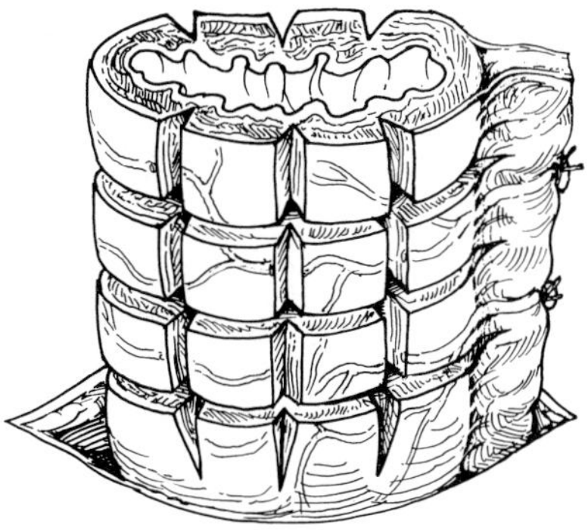

Fig. 23-6 Two-directional myotomy. Incisions are made through the muscular layers but not the mucosa of the exteriorized ileum. The ileostomy is then fashioned as described to prevent retraction of the stoma. (From Fry RD. End ileostomy: Techniques for construction and management of complications. Semin Colon Rectal Surg 2:86-92, 1991. With permission.)

Recurrent inflammatory bowel disease may cause stoma obstruction. Again, a stoma injection of water-soluble contrast medium is helpful in diagnosis and to provide relief of the blockage without surgery or excessive manipulation. Stenosis is usually caused by ischemia of the stoma or separation of the mucocutaneous junction and serositis-induced scarring after the initial procedure (Fig. 23-7). Stenosis is best treated with local revision or relocation of the stoma. Chronic

A

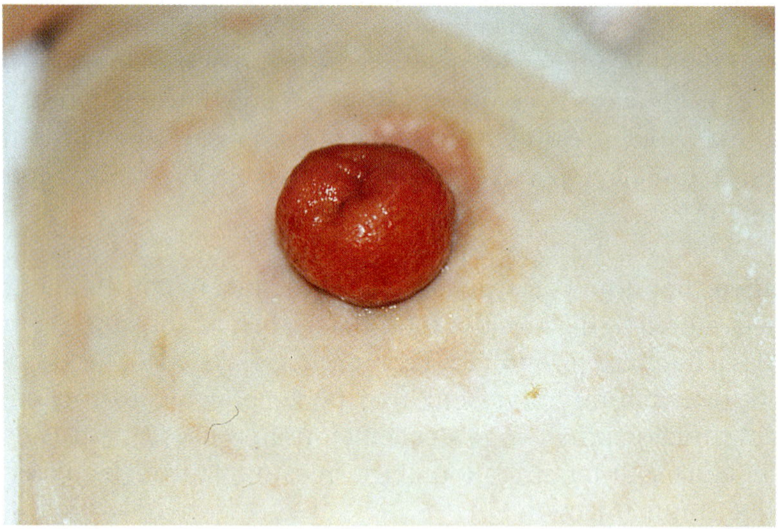

B

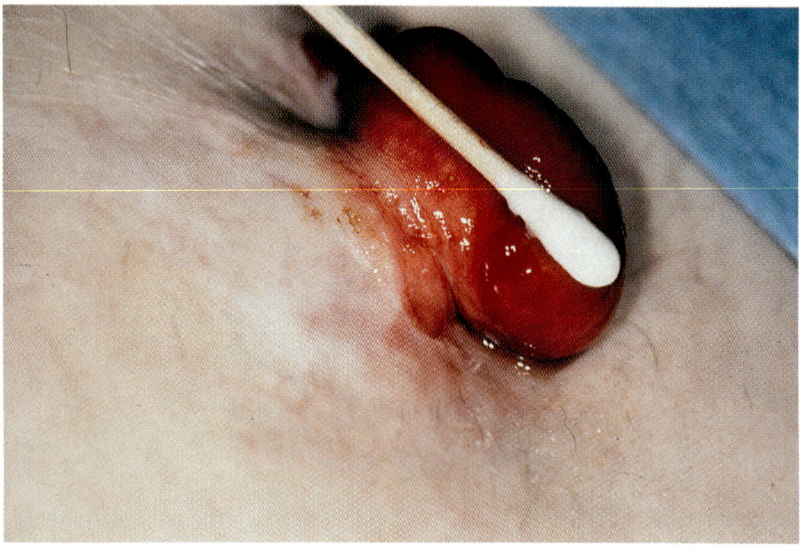

Fig. 23-7 **A**, Ileostomy stenosis with scar at the base of the stoma caused a button deformity 1 month after mucosal necrosis had resolved. **B**, Side view of stenotic ileostomy.

partial small bowel obstruction at the stoma may result in intermittent high ileostomy output, dehydration, and complete obstruction.

Recurrent stenosis that causes obstruction or ileostomy retraction may occasionally require revision of the stoma site with a square or modified elliptical opening to prevent recurrence of the stenosis. A double Z-plasty of the peristomal skin also provides excellent long-term results (Fig. 23-8).[19]

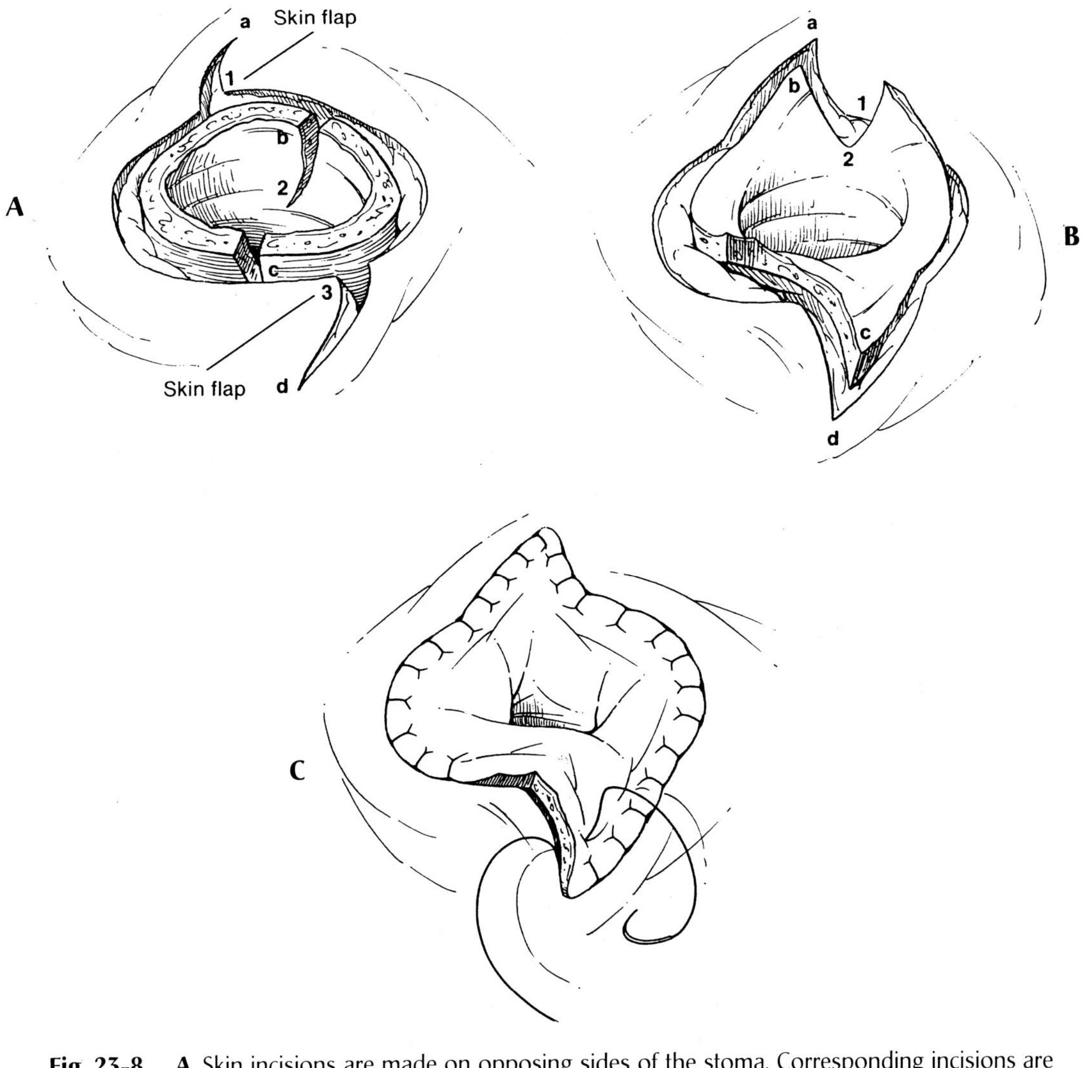

Fig. 23-8 **A**, Skin incisions are made on opposing sides of the stoma. Corresponding incisions are made in the ileum. Skin between *a* and *1* and *d* and *3* is mobilized to create two flaps. **B**, Skin flaps are rotated into the grooves cut in the ileum; *b* is brought to *a*, and *1* is brought to *2*; similarly, *c* is brought to *d*. **C**, New mucocutaneous junction is sewn with interrupted 3-0 absorbable sutures. (From Gorfine SR, Bauer JJ, Gelernt IM. Continent stomas. In MacKeigan JM, Cataldo PA, eds. Intestinal Stomas. Principles, Techniques, and Management. St. Louis: Quality Medical Publishing, 1993, pp 154-187. With permission.)

Late Complications

Prolapse. Ileostomy prolapse is an unusual complication (6%) of a Brooke ileostomy[20] (Fig. 23-9). Several factors have been suggested as contributing to stoma prolapse. The prolapse is usually associated with a parastomal hernia. Prolapse is more common in the obese patient, when the stoma site is placed outside the rectus sheath or in a part of the abdominal wall with previous incisions. Prolapse may be prevented by suspending the mesentery of the ileum from the abdominal wall along the cut edge of the mesentery; this is not always successful, however.

Repair of a prolapsed ileum usually requires repair of the associated parastomal hernia. Local revision is rarely successful over long-term follow-up but is a reasonable first effort when trying to avoid a full exploratory laparotomy and stoma relocation.[6] The prolapsing ileum should not be excised, because the terminal ileum is all physiologically important. Reduction of the prolapse, suture repair of the abdominal wall hernia, and revision of the ostomy are the major components of the local approach to this problem. The use of bidirectional seromyotomies and tripartite sutures around the ileostomy may provide adequate scarring to prevent future prolapse.

The ultimate method of repair involves relocation of the stoma, suspension of the ileal mesentery from the abdominal wall, wrapping the inner aspect of the ileostomy with a strip of fascia, and primary maturation as usual.

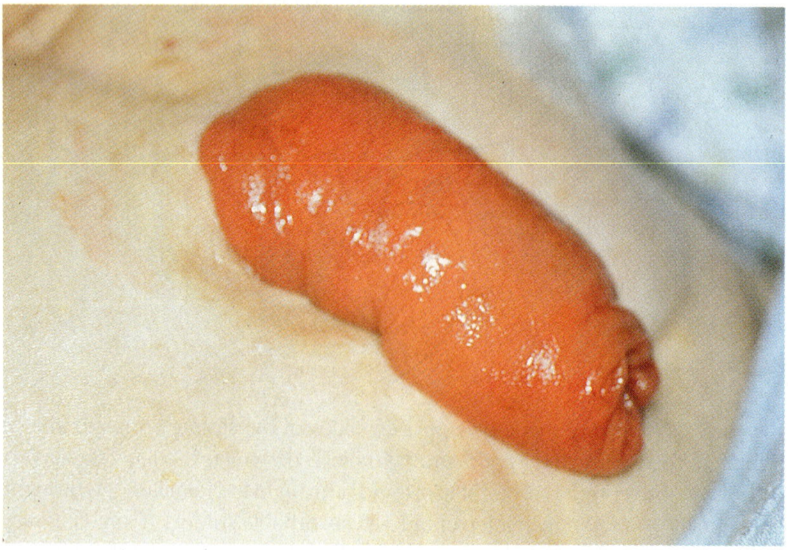

Fig. 23-9 Brooke ileostomy demonstrates ileostomy prolapse.

Hernia. Parastomal hernia is not so common after ileostomy (3%) as after colostomy (1% to 58%).[21-23] Factors that predispose to parastomal herniation include obesity, chronic obstructive pulmonary disease, and a previous repair.[21] A predilection to an abdominal hernia other than the stoma has been reported.[21] Placement of the stoma outside the rectus muscle may also influence the development of parastomal hernias,[1,24] although this has not been confirmed by all authors.[2,25] A CT scan of the abdomen is helpful in evaluation of the patient with symptoms but no obvious hernia.[23]

Paraileostomy hernias are a clinical problem only if the hernia prevents adherence of the appliance, causes pain from intestinal incarceration or partial or complete obstruction, or is associated with prolapse. As with prolapse, local fascial repair is rarely successful and usually requires relocation of the stoma to achieve success. This can sometimes be done through the existing stoma site if adhesions are not prohibitive. However, when relocation is not possible because of body habitus or previous incisions, Marlex mesh underlay or overlay repair of the fascia at the existing site may be successful in nearly two thirds of patients.[21] Care is needed when placing the mesh to avoid contact of the cut edge of the mesh with the stoma. Special care to avert gross fecal contamination of the mesh is also prudent.

Stenosis. Stenosis of the ileostomy was a much more frequent problem before the concept of everting the protruding end of the ileum to create a spigot was developed.[12] However, more recent series note stenosis of the ileostomy in 6% to 10% of patients,[1,10,26] and the United Ostomy Association registry reports 2%.[24] Stoma revision is the best method of treatment, with relocation as necessary. The problem of clinical obstruction due to ostomy stenosis is best managed by decompression with a nasogastric tube, evaluation of the entire GI tract with an ileostomy injection, marking a new ostomy site, and revision of the stoma. If local revision is not possible, the stoma should be moved.

Inadequate diversion. The use of a loop ileostomy to divert the fecal stream after ileal pouch anal anastomosis has become commonplace. The problems associated with the loop ileostomy are significant enough to cause surgeons who perform large numbers of pouch operations to attempt the procedure without a diverting ileostomy.[9] The complications associated with a loop ileostomy include obstruction, parastomal herniation, skin irritation, and retraction. Complications also occur after loop ileostomy closure and include anastomotic leak and small bowel obstruction.[9,18] All of these result in a higher complication rate than is associated with a Brooke ileostomy. The most significant problem is inadequate diversion, which occurs in 6% of cases.[18] Since the stoma is constructed specifically for diversion, a means to accomplish the goal must be identified. Converting the ileostomy to a divided end-loop ileolostomy should provide adequate diversion

(Fig. 23-10). A staple line is placed across the defunctionalized end, and the antimesenteric corner of the staple line is tacked to the dermis at the inferior aspect of the stoma as the proximal functioning limb is matured as a Brooke ileostomy. Rotating the ileostomy to place the defunctionalized distal opening superiorly in the stoma site has not improved the diverting properties of the stoma and has caused increased obstruction at the stoma.

A

B

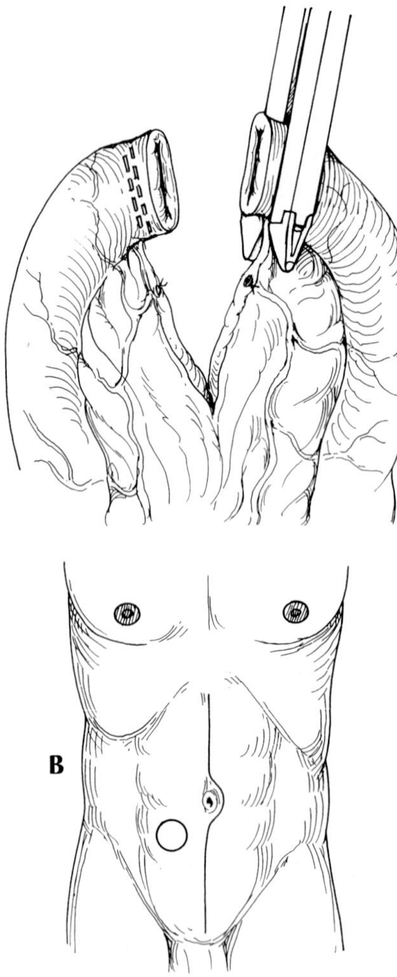

Fig. 23-10 End-loop ileostomy. **A**, Ileum is divided with the linear cutting stapler at a point where the proximal and distal limbs can be drawn through the abdominal wall without tension. **B**, Ileostomy incision is placed in the right lower quadrant overlying the rectus muscle.

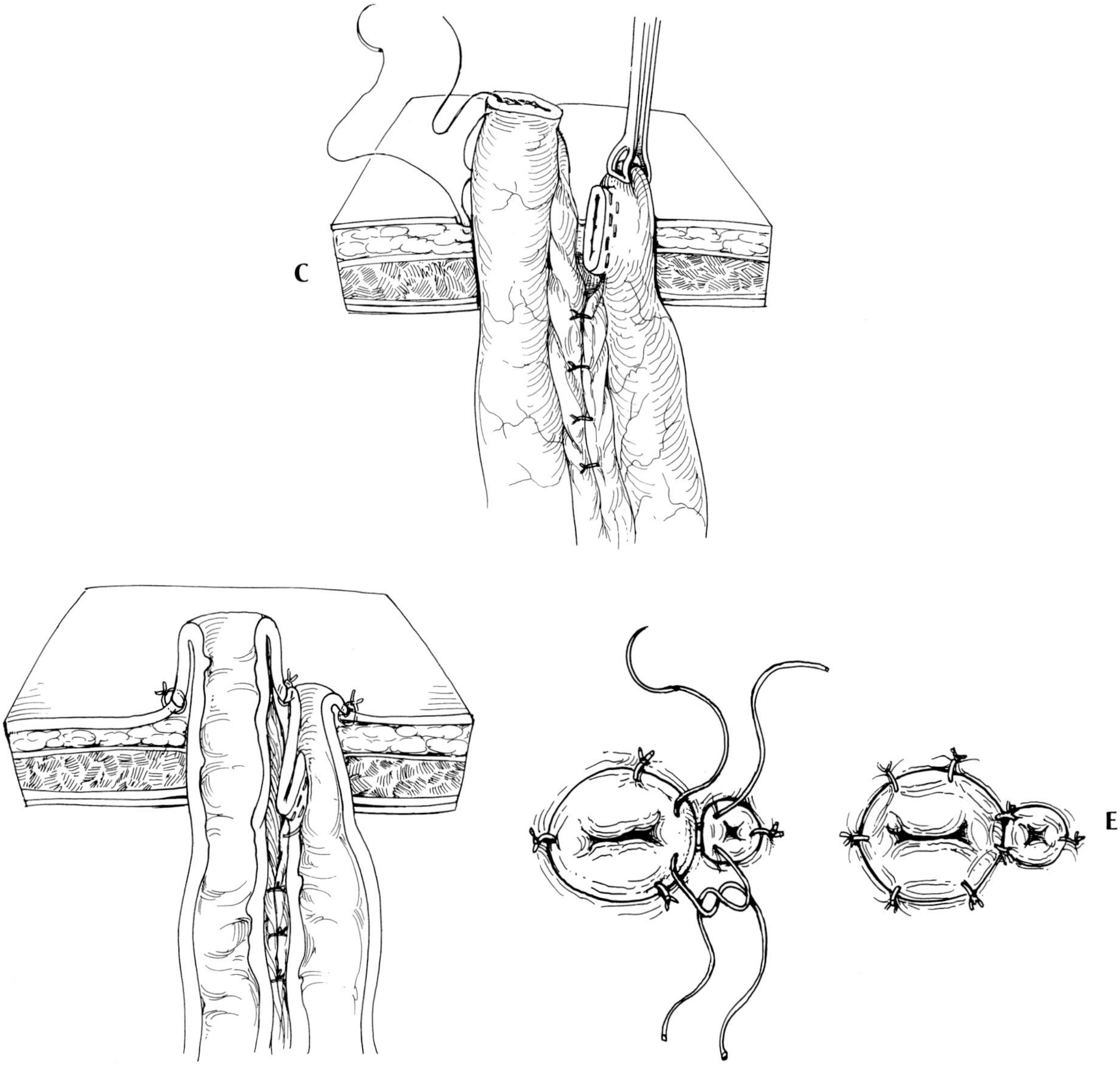

Fig. 23-10, cont'd C, Divided end of the proximal ileum and the antimesenteric corner of the distal ileum are gently drawn through the opening in the rectus muscle. The mesenteric defect is closed. **D**, Sagittal view of the completed end-loop ileostomy. **E**, Two transition sutures are placed to help mature the distal "mini-stoma."

COLOSTOMY

Altered Physiology

It is rare that a colostomy alters the patient's physiologic state enough to cause complications. Occasionally, loss of the distal colon is sufficient to cause diarrhea in a patient who has had a significant amount of colon and small bowel previously resected. A colostomy usually functions with the same bowel pattern as before the operation. A left-sided colostomy will result in excretion of solid stool, because the right colon is responsible for the absorption of the 1000 mL of liquid, which passes from the ileum to the colon. The left colon is primarily a transportation conduit with daily routine peristaltic motions that result in delivery of stool to the rectum or, after colostomy, to an ostomy appliance. Only a right-sided colostomy produces liquid stool and risk for dehydration.

Skin Problems

Parastomal skin irritation is less common (6% to 14%) around a colostomy than around an ileostomy.[4,13,26] A colostomy is usually constructed as a flush stoma. The skin around a left-sided stoma that is irrigated daily will rarely become irritated. However, liquid stool from a right-sided or transverse colostomy will cause local skin irritation because the appliance does not allow a watertight seal around the flat stoma. Malpositioning of the stoma on a scar, within a crease, or near a bony prominence will also contribute to skin irritation. Irritation of the skin consists mainly of minor excoriation and redness and rarely is due to fungal or bacterial skin infection.[13] The majority of skin problems can be managed with aggressive hygiene, enterostomal therapy consultation, and local antimicrobial application. A malpositioned stoma may require relocation.

Early Complications

Ischemia and gangrene. Colostomy necrosis is fairly common (2% to 17%) and is influenced by the same factors that predispose to necrosis of an ileostomy: obesity or skeletonization of the terminal portion of the bowel.[3,5] Necrosis of the colostomy above the fascia may be due to an inadequate abdominal wall opening or skeletonization of the terminal portion of the bowel. This problem is readily recognized by changes in the color of the mucosa from purple to black to gray. An effort should be made to document the level of necrosis or viability. Cotton-tipped swabs as retractors to expose the lumen, a glass test tube with pen light, or a flexible sigmoidoscope are all helpful to look within the stoma. If the necrosis is above the fascia, a conservative, watchful approach is possible. Incision of the mucosa may confirm a submucosal or muscle blood supply. The long-term result of superficial necrosis (Fig. 23-11) of a colostomy is stenosis, which can be treated locally in most cases.

The problem of ostomy necrosis that extends below the fascia and therefore intraperitoneally can be managed only by immediate reexploration and revision

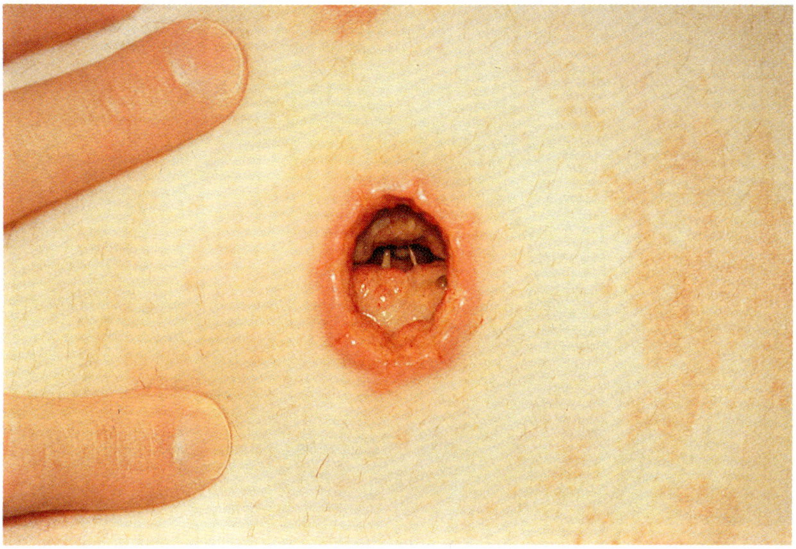

Fig. 23-11 Colostomy necrosis above the fascia treated conservatively.

of the colostomy. If the blood supply is difficult to maintain because of tension or body wall thickness, a loop-end colostomy may be helpful.

Retraction. Colostomy retraction is not so clinically significant as retraction of an ileostomy. Only when the stoma separates from the skin and releases into the peritoneum does the problem demand urgent surgical intervention. Retraction occurs in 1.5% to 10% of cases in most series.[2,3,5,27] Lateral space closure does not prevent retraction of the colostomy.[2] Revision of the stoma with both fascial sutures and mucocutaneous sutures may help prevent recurrence. Complete freedom from tension is essential and probably the most significant factor. This may require mobilization of the splenic flexure of the colon or even division of the inferior mesenteric artery at its origin in the extremely obese patient.

Obstruction. Acute obstruction of the colostomy early after construction is unusual. Obstruction is most commonly caused by the late formation of a paracolostomy hernia or stenosis at the skin level; treatment of these is discussed later. Fecal impaction is easily treated with injection of a water-soluble contrast medium into the stoma during fluoroscopy to control distention of the colon. The contrast material acts as a laxative and stool softener.

Late Complications

Prolapse. Colostomy prolapse occurs in most reported series in 2% to 5% of cases.[2,4,24,27] If prolapse occurs in the immediate postoperative period, the cause

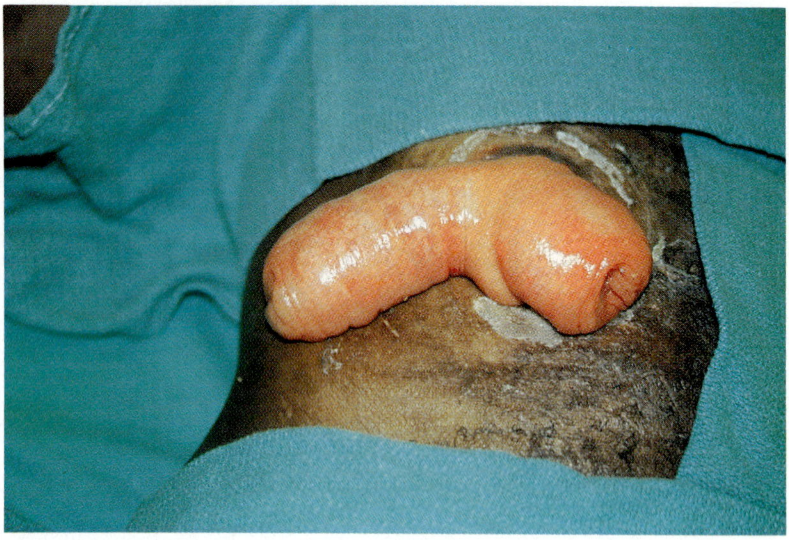

Fig. 23-12 Transverse loop colostomy with prolapse of both proximal and distal limbs.

may be improper construction.[3] Colostomy prolapse usually occurs in conjunction with parastomal hernia but has also been shown to occur more frequently in stomas sited in the exploratory laparotomy incision.[4]

The treatment of colostomy prolapse is usually not urgently required. Loss of blood supply to the prolapsed segment is unusual. Colostomy prolapse causes patient discomfort, anxiety about the protrusion, and concern about appearance. An elective procedure to excise the redundant segment and fix the colon laterally should be the initial effort. This is successful in approximately one third of cases.[22] If the prolapse recurs, resiting the stoma or eventual colectomy with ileostomy will eventually be successful (33% and 67%, respectively).[22]

Ostomy prolapse is a special problem in paraplegic patients who have had a colostomy placed because of constipation, rectal prolapse, or incontinence. Prolapsed right-sided or transverse colostomies have been noted after long-term follow-up in a high percentage of cases[28] (Fig. 23-12). Colectomy with construction of an ileostomy is eventually required if prolapse recurs. The best colostomy in these patients is an end sigmoid colostomy.

Stenosis. Colostomy stenosis or stricture occurs in 2% to 9% of patients after colostomy construction.[2-5] The scar from early ischemia or separation at the skin is the cause of the stricture. It is rarely significant. In the majority of cases (96%), local excision of the scar is sufficient, and resiting is only rarely required.[21] Multiple operations to revise the scarred stoma may be required, however, before the problem is resolved.[22]

Hernia. The most common complication experienced by patients with a colostomy is paracolostomy hernia. The risk of a colostomy hernia over the patient's lifetime varies from 1% to 58%.[2,21,27] The significance of a parastomal hernia is manifested clinically by inability to maintain an ostomy appliance, pain in the parastomal area, or intestinal incarceration and obstruction. The majority of paracolostomy hernias occur within the first 2 years after construction.[1,27] The risk of hernia increases with age, duration of follow-up, obesity, chronic pulmonary disease, and the existence of other abdominal wall hernias.[2,21] There is some controversy about the effect of the stoma site on the development of hernia. Popular teaching and retrospective reviews suggest that development of parastomal hernia is less likely with stomas that pass through the rectus muscle.[1] More recent data (also retrospective) however, suggest that herniation does not occur more frequently when the stoma is placed outside the rectus muscle or in the incision itself.[2,4,8] The determining factor for placement of the stoma (when marked preoperatively) should therefore be the best site for patient accessibility, visibility, and comfort.

Only 10% to 20% of paracolostomy hernias require repair. The vast majority are operated on because of psychological stress, pain, or difficulty with irrigation.[1] A small group of patients (16%) undergo surgery because of incarceration or obstruction.[21] Local repair of the paracolostomy hernia can be successful (53%).[22] Permanent sutures placed in the fascia to approximate the edges of the herniated fascia with or without mesh reinforcement on the anterior surface of the fascia is the simplest method. It is prudent to place a closed-suction drain in the subcutaneous pocket if mesh is placed. If the local repair fails and the hernia recurs, the stoma should be resited; the lower quadrants, either right or left, and the midline at the umbilicus seem to be the best choices.[22] An upper quadrant stoma, however, should function well if properly constructed, and the risk of recurrent hernia is affected more by the previously mentioned factors than the upper quadrant site.

Other complications. There have been reports of complications related to colostomy irrigation. Irrigation of the colostomy for bowel control is usually quite safe: 90% in elderly patients, with continence achieved in 97.8% of patients. Stenosis, prolapse, bleeding, hernia, and displacement of the colostomy loop occurred in 10% of a large Italian series.[29] Perforation of the colostomy with a red rubber catheter was a frequent complication in the past when irrigation was not performed with an irrigation cone. A recent case report documented a hot water burn to the colostomy as a result of inattention on the part of the person irrigating the colostomy.[30] Perforation of the colostomy has also been caused by a bone caught behind the relative stenosis of the colostomy with a subcutaneous paracolostomy abscess.[31]

Fistula formation due to suture placement occurs occasionally.[2] Elimination of tacking of the serosa to the fascia can prevent the perioperative subcutaneous infection and fistula formation.[3]

CONTINENT ILEOSTOMY

The institution of the continent ileal reservoir in 1967 by Dr. Nils Kock changed the lives of many patients with ulcerative colitis. Continence was possible for many patients who would have otherwise been treated with total proctocolectomy and end ileostomy. The tradeoff for bowel control was having to deal with the complications (as many as two thirds required repeat surgery). Complication rates vary from 20% to 52% in recent reports.[26,32] The indications for the continent ileostomy have essentially decreased to use in those patients who have already had a Brooke ileostomy for ulcerative colitis and FAP, urinary reservoir construction after cystectomy, or incompetent sphincters who require colectomy because of ulcerative colitis or FAP. Patients with Crohn's disease are not candidates for a continent ileal reservoir because pouch complications have been noted to occur in 100% of these patients over long-term follow-up and the majority will require pouch excision.[32]

Continence is achieved by placing a nipple valve of intussuscepted intestine at the outlet of the pouch. The pouch itself is constructed from two or three folded loops of intestine, which are opened along their antimesenteric borders and sewn together as a single 250- to 300-mL unit. The pouch fills with intestinal contents, and pressure develops not only on the walls of the pouch but also on the mucosal surface of the intussuscepted nipple valve. The pressure collapses the nipple valve proximal to the flush ileostomy and provides outlet obstruction to the pouch. Only by passing a flexible tube through the ileostomy and the nipple valve (usually four times per day) can the pouch be emptied. The pouch itself is suspended from the anterior abdominal wall beneath the ileostomy site.

Nipple Valve Problems

Continence is achieved in 90% of patients with a Kock pouch.[26] This may require several operations if there are problems with the pouch or the nipple valve. More than half of the initial series of patients who underwent the Kock procedure have required nipple valve revisions (13 patients required 25 revisions) in long-term follow-up.[33] The majority of late pouch complications involved nipple valve slippage (12.5%) or valve angulation and prolapse (8%).[25] Radiologic studies have shown that a nipple valve shorter than 2.5 cm results in incontinence.[34] Careful contrast-enhanced studies of the pouch by an experienced radiologist are usually accurate in defining the problem with the pouch: nipple valve prolapse (96%), pouch detached from wall (40%), Crohn's disease (60%), fistulas (100%), afferent limb stenosis (25%), and pouchitis (80%).[34] Endoscopy of the pouch often aids in evaluation of pouch dysfunction.

New techniques have been developed to prevent slippage of the nipple valve. The valve is stapled to the anterior pouch wall with a linear stapler without a cutting blade or a transverse stapler.[35] Other methods of pouch and nipple valve construction show no clear advantage over these techniques.[36]

Obstruction

Pouch obstruction may be secondary to blockage of the nipple valve by pouch contents or alteration of the outlet at the ileostomy or nipple valve.

Obstruction of the pouch due to nipple valve angulation, stenosis, or prolapse requires urgent attention by an experienced surgeon to reestablish an outlet to the pouch. A technique for intubating the pouch with a longitudinally split Medina catheter over a flexible ileoscope has been reported.[37] The split catheter is changed to an intact Medina catheter over a stent by means of the Seldinger technique. The catheter is secured in the pouch until definitive repair is possible. Unusual causes of pouch obstruction have been reported. Medication with a non-digestible vehicle has caused intrapouch concretions that require endoscopic removal.[38] Food bezoars and undissolved tablets have also caused pouch obstruction.

Minor revisions to the pouch outflow tract may be necessary to keep the pouch functioning. Stenosis at the flush ileostomy due to intense scarring can usually be managed by excising the stricture and placing interdigitating skin flaps to revise the stoma (see Fig. 23-8).[39] A prolapsing or angulating valve may require stapling of the valve to the anterior pouch wall or stiffening of the nipple valve with cautery and 0-chromic catgut sutures.[39]

The nipple valve is not always repairable and must be replaced. It is possible to reverse the pouch, excise the old nipple valve, use the old pouch inlet (15 cm) to construct a new nipple valve, and reconnect the small intestine to the base of the reversed pouch[40] (Fig. 23-13). The most common reason for pouch reversal

A

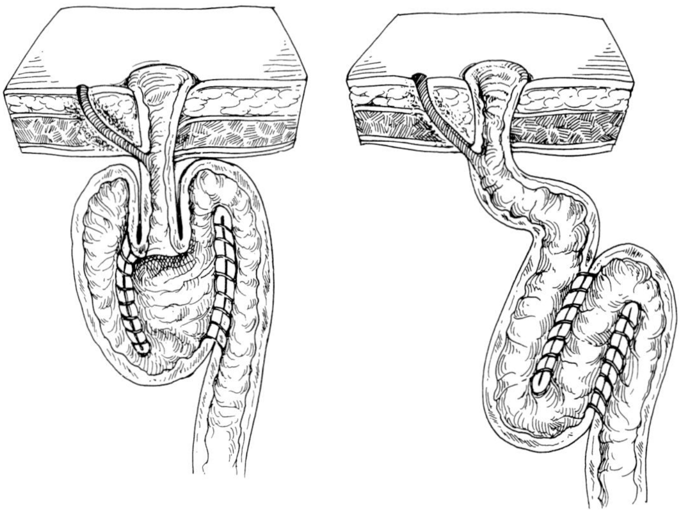

Fig. 23-13 Preservation of the continent ileostomy after fistula formation or loss of the nipple configuration. **A**, Fistula between skin and nipple valve *(left)* and slipped nipple valve *(right)*.

Continued.

B 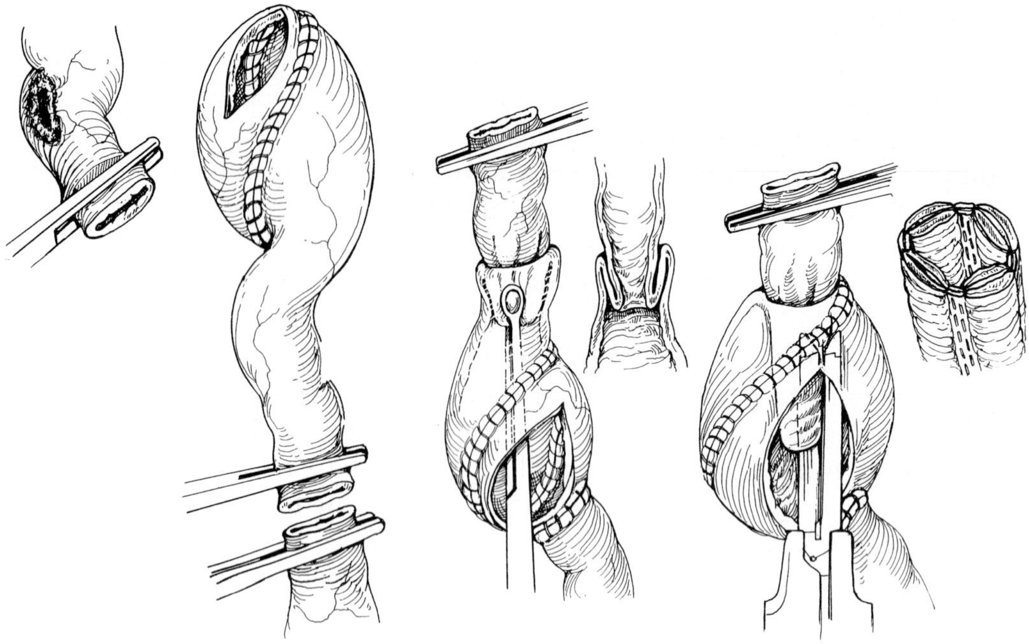 C

Fig. 23-13, cont'd **B**, Faulty nipple valve and outlet are excised. Distal ileum is transected 15 cm proximal to the pouch, leaving enough intestine to reconstruct the valve and stoma. **C**, Pouch is rotated 180 degrees, and the intestine is anastomosed to the pouch by means of a second enterostomy. Nipple valve is reconstructed as before through the enterostomy made by resecting the old valve. (From Kodner IJ, Fleshman JW, Fry RD. Intestinal stomas.

and valve replacement is formation of a fistula between the valve and the pouch from catheter trauma.[41] A fistula due to Crohn's disease should be treated medically, and usually the pouch will have to be excised.[32]

Altered Physiology

The mucosa of the ileal reservoir undergoes transition. There is mild chronic inflammation, villous hypotrophy, and reduction in mucosa surface area by 20%.[41] This conversion of the ileal mucosa to resemble the colon is not associated with dysplasia.[41] The change in mucosa of the pouch does not usually have a clinically significant effect. Vitamin B_{12} deficiency is noted only if other areas of the intestine have been removed or become involved with Crohn's disease. Gallstones were found in 8% of patients followed up for 20 years, and renal calculi developed in 17% (all men) as a result of chronic dehydration.[33]

Pouchitis occurs in a significant number of patients (19% to 50%).[26,33] The majority of patients report mild symptoms of cramping, high output, and lower abdominal fullness. In only 4% to 6%, severe pouchitis develops that requires chronic treatment with metronidazole.[26]

QUALITY OF LIFE ISSUES

Comparison of lifestyle and perceived quality of life in patients in whom a Brooke ileostomy was converted to a Kock pouch showed that patients perceived that life was better with a Kock pouch in all categories.[26] However, only travel was shown to increase after Kock pouch construction. Of interest, the quality of life experienced with either ileostomy or Kock pouch was better than that with active ulcerative colitis. Most patients (80%) reported no limitations in their lifestyle, and only minor limits affected the remainder (20%).[33] There are thus some advantages to conversion to a continent ileal reservoir for certain patients with a Brooke ileostomy. Medical centers with a large experience with Kock pouch construction should maintain those skills, even as the pelvic pouch procedure continues to gain favor with most surgeons who treat ulcerative colitis.

REFERENCES

1. Pearl RK. Parastomal hernias. World J Surg 13:569-572, 1989.
2. Londono-Schimmer EE, Leong APK, Phillips RKS. Life table analysis of stomal complications following colostomy. Dis Colon Rectum 37:916-920, 1994.
3. Pearl RK, Prasad L, Orsay CP, Abcarian H, Tan AB, Melzl MT. Early local complications from intestinal stomas. Arch Surg 120:1145-1147, 1985.
4. Porter JA, Salvati EP, Rubin RJ, Eisenstat TE. Complications of colostomies. Dis Colon Rectum 32:299-303, 1989.
5. Leenen LPH, Kuypers JHC. Some factors influencing the outcome of stoma surgery. Dis Colon Rectum 32:500-504, 1989.
6. Fazio VW, Tjandra JJ. Prevention and management of ileostomy complications. J ET Nurs 19:48-53, 1992.
7. Kodner IJ, Fry RD, Fleshman JW, Birnbaum EH. Colon, rectum and anus. In Schwartz SI, ed. Principles of Surgery, 6th ed. New York: McGraw-Hill, 1993, pp 1191-1306.
8. Oritz H, Sara MJ, Armendariz P, deMiguel M, Marti J, Chocarro C. Does the frequency of paracolostomy hernias depend on the position of the colostomy in the abdominal wall? Int J Colorect Dis 9:65-67, 1994.
9. Feinberg SM, McLeod RS, Cohen Z. Complications of loop ileostomy. Am J Surg 153:102-107, 1987.
10. Pemberton JH. Management of conventional ileostomies. World J Surg 12:203-210, 1988.
11. Fukushima T, Sugita A, Masuzawa S, Yamazaki Y, Takemura H, Tsuchiya S. Prevention of uric acid stone formation by sodium bicarbonate in an ileostomy patient: A case report. Jap J Surg 18:465-468, 1988.
12. Brooke BN. The management of an ileostomy including its complications. Dis Colon Rectum 36:512-516, 1993.
13. Hellman J, Lago CP. Dermatologic complications in colostomy and ileostomy patients. Int J Dermatol 29:129-133, 1990.
14. Nordstrom GM, Borglund E, Nyman CR. Local status of the urinary stoma—The relation to peristomal skin complications. Scand J Urol Nephrol 24:117-122, 1990.
15. Tjandra JJ, Hughes LE. Parastomal pyoderma gangrenosum in inflammatory bowel disease. Dis Colon Rectum 37:938-942, 1994.

16. Speakman CTM, Parker MC, Northover JMA. Outcome of stapled revision of retracted ileostomy. Br J Surg 78:935-936, 1991.
17. Truedson H, Press V. A new method of stomal reconstruction in patients with retraction of conventional ileostomy. Surg Gynecol Obstet 162:60-61, 1986.
18. Metcalf AM, Dozois RR, Beart RW Jr, Kelly KA, Wolff BG. Temporary ileostomy for ileal pouch–anal anastomosis. Dis Colon Rectum 29:300-303, 1986.
19. Gorfine SR, Bauer JJ, Gelernt IM. Continent stomas. In MacKeigan JM, Cataldo PA, eds. Intestinal Stomas. Principles, Techniques, and Management. St. Louis: Quality Medical Publishing, 1993, pp 154-187. (With permission.)
20. Carlstedt A, Fasth S, Hulten L, Nordgren S, Palselius I. Long-term ileostomy complications in patients with ulcerative colitis and Crohn's disease. Int J Colorect Dis 2:22-25, 1987.
21. Rubin MS, Schoetz DJ Jr, Matthews JB. Parastomal hernia: Is stoma relocation superior to fascial repair? Arch Surg 129:413-419, 1994.
22. Allen-Mersh TG, Thomson JPS. Surgical treatment of colostomy complications. Br J Surg 75:416-418, 1988.
23. Etherington RJ, Williams JG, Hayward WJ, Hughes LE. Demonstration of para-ileostomy herniation using computed tomography. Clin Radiol 41:333-336, 1990.
24. Wiliams JG, Etherington R, Hayward MWJ, Hughes LE. Paraileostomy hernia: A clinical and radiological study. Br J Surg 77:1355-1357, 1990.
25. Sjodahl R, Lemon E, Nystrom PO, Olaison G. Complications, surgical revision and quality of life with conventional and continent ileostomy. Acta Chir Scand 156:403-407, 1990.
26. Von Smitten K, Husa A, Kyllonen L. Long-term results of sigmoidostomy in patients with anorectal malignancy. Acta Chir Scand 152:211-213, 1986.
27. Fleshman JW, Lewis MG. Complications and quality of life after stoma surgery: A review of 16,470 patients in the UOA data registry. Semin Colon Rectal Surg 2:66-72, 1991.
28. Arun H, Ledgerwood A, Lucas CE. Ostomy prolapse in paraplegic patients: Etiology, prevention, and treatment. J Am Paraplegia Soc 13:7-9, 1990.
29. Venturini M, Bertelli G, Forno G, Grandi G, Dini D. Colostomy irrigation in the elderly: Effective recovery regardless of age. Dis Colon Rectum 33:1031-1033, 1990.
30. Giunchi F, Cacciaguerra G, Drudi G. Burn and stricture of the ostomy due to colostomy irrigation: Report of a case. Dis Colon Rectum 28:873-874, 1985.
31. Haiart DC. An unusual complication of stenosis of a colostomy. Postgrad Med J 61:549-550, 1985.
32. Handelsman JC, Gottlieb LM, Hamilton SR. Crohn's disease as a contraindication to Kock pouch (continent ileostomy). Dis Colon Rectum 36:840-843, 1993.
33. Ojerskog B, Kock NG, Nilsson LO, Philipson BM, Ahren C. Long-term follow-up of patients with continent ileostomies. Dis Colon Rectum 33:184-189, 1990.
34. Lycke KG, Gothlin JH, Jensen JK, Philipson BM, Kock NG. Radiology of the continent ileostomy reservoir. II. Findings in patients with late complications. Abdom Imag 19:124-131, 1994.
35. Fazio VW, Tjandra JJ. Technique for nipple valve fixation to prevent valve slippage in continent ileostomy. Dis Colon Rectum 35:1177-1179, 1992.
36. Barnett WO. Current experiences with the continent intestinal reservoir. Surg Gynecol Obstet 168:1-5, 1989.
37. Tichenor GA, Orkin BA, Lavery IC. A technique for decompression of the obstructed Kock continent ileostomy. Surg Gynecol Obstet 170:75-76, 1990.

38. Haynes HS, Wang KK, Ahlquist DA. Ileal Kock pouch obstruction secondary to retained medicoliths. Gastrointest Endosc 38:613-614, 1992.
39. Gottlieb LM, Handelsman JC. Treatment of outflow tract problems associated with continent ileostomy (Kock pouch). Dis Colon Rectum 34:936-940, 1991.
40. Kodner IJ, Fleshman JW, Fry RD. Intestinal stomas. In Schwartz SI, ed. Maingot's Abdominal Operations, 9th ed. Norwalk, Conn.: Appleton & Lange, 1989, pp 1169-1170.
41. Helander KG, Ahren C, Philipson BM, Samuelsson BM, Ojerskog B. Structure of mucosa in continent ileal reservoirs 15 to 19 years after construction. Hum Pathol 21:1235-1238, 1990.

CHAPTER 24

Acute and Late Toxicity of Radiation Therapy in Rectal Cancer

ROBERT R. KUSKE, Jr.

THE ROLE OF AND RATIONALE FOR RADIATION THERAPY IN RECTAL CANCER

Ionizing radiation has been used as a weapon against cancer for 100 years. Three years after Roentgen discovered X rays in 1895, Pierre and Marie Curie reported their discovery of radium to the French Academy of Science. The tumoricidal potential of ionizing radiation was immediately recognized and used in the treatment of cancer, although the methodology was crude, unreliable, and even dangerous. Not until the mid-1960s did megavoltage radiation therapy become the predominant treatment modality at radiation oncology centers throughout the world. In the late 1960s cobalt-60 teletherapy units were used, which exposed a 2 cm lump of radioactive cobalt metal through collimating shields onto the patient's body. Four to 6 MeV linear accelerators were then developed, which led to the current 18 MeV linear accelerator that is now state of the art. Technologic advances allowed the radiation oncologist to increase the tumor dose delivered to deep-seated tumors such as rectal carcinomas while reducing the dose to adjacent organs such as skin, femoral heads, bladder, and small bowel. At most institutions before 1970, skin toxicity limited the dose that could be delivered, and fractures of the femoral head were common because the bone dose was high. Today, except after postoperative treatment following abdominoperineal resection, acute skin toxicity is rarely found. Improvements in precision and dosimetry in new machines that permit multiple-field techniques allow quality control measures involving reproducible treatment techniques that can be tested accurately in prospective and retrospective clinical trials.

The frequency of locoregional relapse after surgery to treat rectal carcinoma prompted clinicians to add pelvic irradiation. Numerous studies demonstrated that the pelvic failure rate after surgery alone increased from 20% to 50% or more if tumor penetrated the muscle wall of the rectum or pelvic lymph nodes contained metastatic carcinoma.[1-3] Furthermore, the consequences of uncontrolled pelvic tumor are extremely debilitating, negatively affect the patient's quality of life, and frequently become the patient's chief complaint until death.

Table 24-1 Rationale for irradiation: patterns of failure after potentially curative surgery

Stage	Local failure (%)
T1-2N0M0	<10
T3N0 to T1-2N1M0	15 to 35
T3-4N1-2M0	45 to 65

Data from Massachusetts General Hospital and Rich T, Gunderson LL, Lew R, et al. Patterns of recurrence of rectal cancer after potentially curative surgery.

A study carried out at Massachusetts General Hospital found that if there was gross penetration through the bowel wall (stage T3N0M0) (Table 24-1), the local regional recurrence rate was 25%.[1] The rationale for radiation therapy is provided by the pattern of local failure after surgery alone, ranging from a recurrence rate of only 17% with microscopic penetration (T3N0M0) to 67% for node-positive tumors that penetrate through the bowel wall and invade adjacent organs (T4N1M0).[2]

Improvement in both local control and 5-year survival has been demonstrated by stage-by-stage comparisons of nonrandomized patients treated with surgery alone with patients treated with surgery and adjuvant radiation therapy (Table 24-2). Use of postoperative radiation therapy for T3-4N1-2M0 rectal cancer was examined in four randomized trials (Table 24-3).[2,4,6] Three of these trials are seriously flawed conceptually. The National Surgical Adjuvant Breast Project (NSABP) randomized trial found that postoperative radiation therapy decreases the local failure rates ($p < 0.05$).[6] The NSABP was the only trial of the four in which radiation therapy was delivered with "modern" technique in a continuous course with full curative doses. Three major randomized trials of postoperative combined-method therapy have been reported (Table 24-4).[3,6,21]

Radiation therapy has clear limitations in its ability to affect survival, as demonstrated in Fig. 24-1. However, patients with residual microscopic disease within the pelvis only after surgery or chemotherapy may have improved survival (Table 24-2).[6] Radiation therapy may be indicated in other subgroups to prevent the consequences of uncontrolled local regional tumor.

INDICATIONS FOR ADJUVANT RADIATION THERAPY IN RECTAL CANCER

Several randomized prospective clinical trials now in progress may produce changes in treatment policies. Participation in formal clinical trials will help to answer the seminal questions that still perplex us.

The choice of any adjuvant therapy and how aggressive it should be must be made after taking into account the age and medical and functional status of

Table 24-2 Adjuvant postoperative radiation therapy for resectable rectal cancer selected by nonrandomized trials

Investigator	Dose (cGy)	Stage	Local failure* (%)				5-year survival (%)	
			No. of patients	Surgery	No. of patients	Surgery plus postoperative radiation therapy	Surgery	Surgery plus postoperative radiation therapy
Massachusetts General Hospital[1]	4500-5040 +boost†	T3N0	44	23	53	9	47	76‡
		T4N0	15	53	7	0	27	69
		T1-2N1-2	4	50	10	20	25	69
		T3N1-2	34	17	77	21	27	34
		T4N1-2	6	67	15	53	0	13
M.D. Anderson Cancer Center[3]	4000-5000 +boost†	T3N0		13	24	4		65
		T4N0		26	13	21		48
		T1-2N1-2			12	8		65
		T3N1-2		30	45	18		48
		T4N1-2		49	5	20		60

*Cumulative failure as a component of failure.
†Fourteen patients received chemotherapy.
‡No evidence of disease.

Table 24-3 Randomized trials of postoperative radiation therapy

Study (year)	No. of patients	Treatment	Results	Comments
Gastrointestinal Tumor Study Group[2] (1985)	58	Surgery only	NSD	39% Radiation therapy protocol deviations
	50	Postoperative radiation therapy (40 to 48 Gy)		8 Gy dose range too broad
National Surgical Adjuvant Breast Project[6] (1986)	184	Surgery only	25% Local failure	Survival = NSD
	184	Surgery+radiation therapy	16% Local failure ($p = 0.06$)	
Odense, Denmark[4] (1986)	250	Surgery only	9% Local failure Time to failure, 19 mo	Short median follow-up (3 yr)
	244	Surgery+radiation therapy	6% Local failure (NSD) Time to failure, 6 mo	43% Not randomized
				20 patients in radiation therapy arm of study received <45 Gy
				Failure rate in surgery alone arm of study unusually low

NSD = no significant difference.

Table 24-4 Randomized trials of postoperative chemotherapy–radiation therapy

Study	No. of patients	Treatment	Results: Survival (%)		Results: Failure (%)		Comments
Gastrointestinal Tumor Study Group[21]	202	Surgery alone	27				
		Postoperative radiation therapy	NSD				
		Radiation therapy + 5-FU/MeCCNU	54 ($p = 0.005$)				
			5-year	**Overall**	**Local**	**Distant**	
Mayo Clinic–North Central Cancer Treatment Group[3]	204	Postoperative radiation therapy + 5-FU/MeCCNU	42	48	25	46	
			63	57	14	29	
			($p = 0.0016$)	($p = 0.025$)	($p = 0.036$)	($p = 0.011$)	
			Disease free				**Subset analysis**
National Surgical Adjuvant Breast Project[6]	528	Surgery alone	30	43	25	26	Only node-negative patients benefited
		Postoperative radiation therapy	NSD	NSD	16		Only male patients benefited
		Postoperative MOF	42	53	21	24	Only male patients younger than 65 years benefited
			($p = 0.006$)	($p = 0.05$)		($p = 0.06$)	

5-FU/MeCCNU = 5-fluorouracil–methylchloroethylcyclohexylnitrosurea [semustine]; MOF = methotrexate, Oncovin, and fluorouracil; NSD = no significant difference.

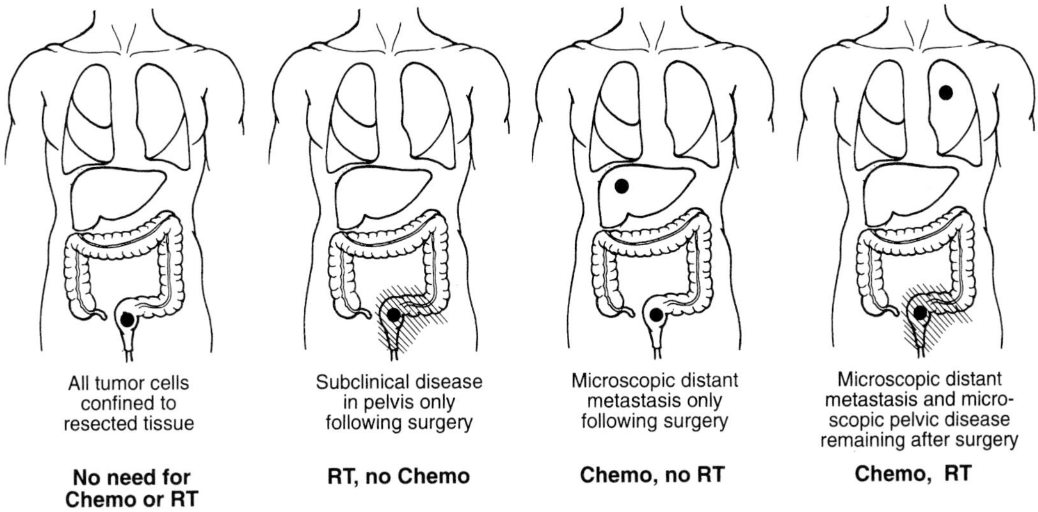

Fig. 24-1 Extent of subclinical malignant cells potentially remaining following definitive surgery defines optimal treatment strategies.

the patient, as well as psychologic and financial factors. Diagnostic transrectal ultrasound, CT scans, or MR images that reveal transmural penetration of the tumor or suspicious nodes may call for preoperative chemoradiotherapy. Patients with T3, T4, or N1 disease should be considered for adjuvant chemoradiotherapy. For patients with locally advanced or even metastatic disease, radiation therapy with or without systemic chemotherapy can be successful in alleviating pelvic pain, rectal bleeding, or other sequelae of uncontrolled local and regional tumor growth.

PREOPERATIVE, POSTOPERATIVE, SANDWICH, AND RADICAL PELVIC IRRADIATION METHODS

Preoperative Pelvic Irradiation

Advantages of preoperative pelvic irradiation in the treatment of T3, T4, or N1 rectal cancer include the following:

1. Risk of subsequent pelvic failure is reduced from 20% to 35% overall with surgery alone to less than 5% with appropriate preoperative radiation therapy.
2. The potential for spread of clonogenic cells during pelvic dissection is decreased as a result of shrinking overall tumor volume and lethal damage to remaining cells.
3. Potential for sphincter preservation and fecal continence is increased because abdominoperineal resection can be avoided.

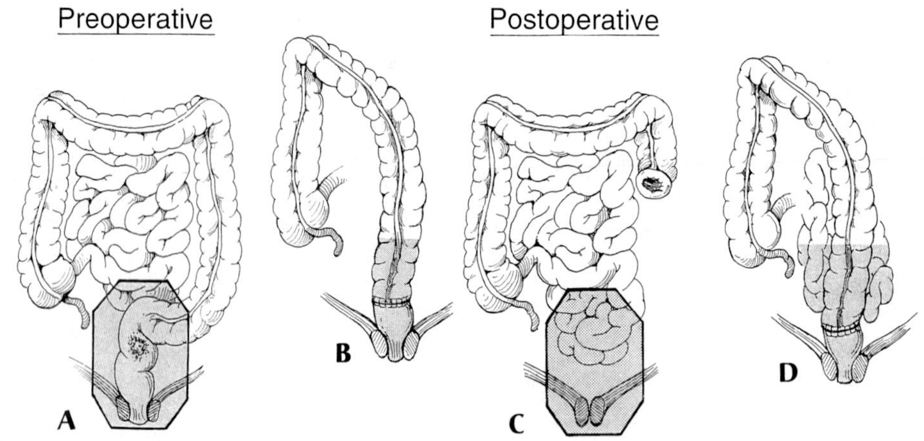

Fig. 24-2 **A**, There is less small bowel in the preoperative RT fields. **B**, The proximal portion of the large bowel above the anastomosis is not irradiated, reducing the risk or dehiscence or fistula formation. **C**, Small bowel descends into the pelvis and may become fixed after surgery, increasing the risk of radiation enteritis. **D**, Postoperative radiotherapy irradiates both sides of the anastomosis, increasing the risk of complications.

4. Surgery is technically less complex because of tumor volume reduction.
5. Sterilization of cancer within pelvic lymphatic vessels is possible.
6. Cancer is downstaged, potentially improving prognosis.
7. Decreased risk of anastomotic dehiscense exists after low anterior resection, because only the distal bowel beyond the suture line is irradiated (Fig. 24-2).
8. Better oxygenation of pelvic tissues leads to improved radiosensitivity and better local regional control rates.
9. Small bowel fixation within the pelvis is prevented, which can potentially lower the complication rate.
10. Higher doses of chemotherapy can be delivered with preoperative radiation therapy than with postoperative radiation therapy.[7]
11. Improvements in the technology and imaging quality of transrectal ultrasound permit more accurate staging of cancer before surgery, eliminating radiation therapy to cancers confined to the bowel wall (T1-2) and reducing the likelihood of overtreatment.

Disadvantages of preoperative pelvic irradiation for rectal cancer include the following:

1. Definitive pathologic staging cannot be determined by transrectal ultrasound or CT scans or MR images only.

2. Patients with T1-2N0M0-1 disease who will not benefit may receive irradiation.
3. The results of postoperative pelvic irradiation with or without chemotherapy have not been definitively proved inferior to results with preoperative radiation therapy.

Postoperative Pelvic Irradiation

Advantages of postoperative radiotherapy in the treatment of rectal cancer include the following:

1. A thorough pathologic assessment of the resected tissue specimen can be made.
2. Potentially valuable prognostic histologic features are not lost.
3. Pelvic irradiation can be reserved for stages T3, T4, or N1 lesions, for which benefits in local control and survival are proven.
4. Patients who have T1-2N0M0 disease are spared undergoing any unnecessary treatment.
5. Clips can be placed during surgery at sites of close margins or areas of particular concern; permitting improved treatment planning, delivery of higher doses to the tumor bed, and potentially improving pelvic tumor control.

The disadvantages of postoperative pelvic irradiation in rectal cancer include the following:

1. Intraoperative spread of cancer is not prevented.
2. The colon proximal to the anastomotic suture line is not protected from irradiation, thereby increasing the possibility of long-term adverse effects such as proctitis, stricture, and fistulas (see Fig. 24-2).
3. After surgery, the small bowel descends into the pelvis and adheres to the bladder, other soft tissues, and the pelvic side wall, increasing the risk of enteritis with hemorrhage, small bowel obstruction, and fistula formation (see Fig. 24-2).
4. Hypoxic postsurgical tissue in the irradiation fields decreases radiation sensitivity and potentially reduces pelvic tumor control rates.
5. Because the number of abdominoperineal resections may be increased using postoperative irradiation rather than preoperative radiation, patient quality of life may be inferior.
6. When an abdominoperineal resection is performed, the inferior aspect of the field is extended, sometimes increasing acute skin toxicity to such a degree that treatment may have to be stopped before the prescribed dose is achieved (Fig. 24-3).

A

B

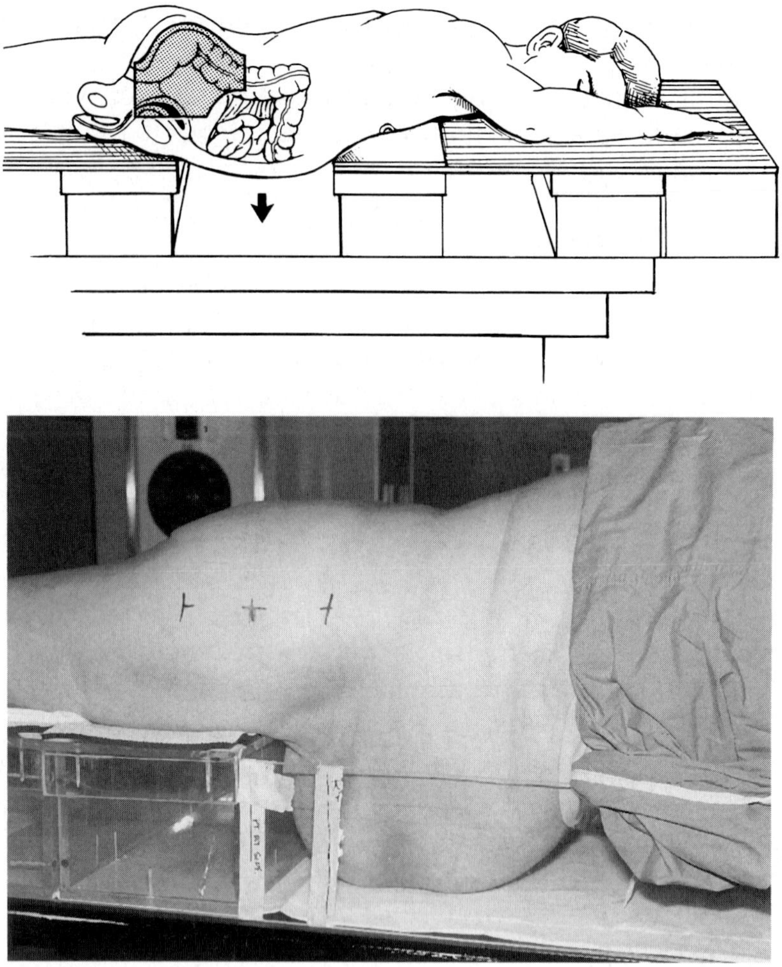

Fig. 24-3 Open-table technique. **A**, "Belly board." **B**, Patient set up on belly board.

Sandwich Technique

The sandwich technique of adjuvant pelvic irradiation usually consists of a single preoperative fraction of 500 cGy followed immediately by surgery and postoperative pelvic irradiation (if the tumor is confirmed to penetrate the bowel wall or pelvic lymph nodes are involved). This technique has the theoretical advantage of reducing the risk of intraoperative spread of clonogenic tumor cells, with all the advantages of postoperative irradiation in terms of patient selection. All the disadvantages of postoperative irradiation remain. In addition, presurgical downstaging of tumor and recovery of normal tissues from the acute effects of irradiation are lost with this technique, because there is no 4- to 6-week rest interval after preoperative irradiation.

Radical Pelvic Irradiation

Radical radiation therapy is reserved for use in patients who are medically unfit or who refuse surgery. Although survival and local disease control are clearly inferior to that after combined therapy, with a sustained tumor control rate for moderately bulky tumors of approximately 30%, this treatment does prevent therapeutic nihilism for these patients.[8] At Princess Margaret Hospital, 52 Gy in 20 fractions was delivered to such patients over 4 weeks.[9] Papillon[10] gave 30 Gy in 10 fractions over 2 weeks to the whole pelvis, followed by an 8-week rest interval, then 25 Gy of intracavitary irradiation, followed by a 20 to 30 Gy boost with interstitial iridium-192. With these high doses, Papillon reported a 5-year disease-free survival rate of 65% in 71 patients with clinical stage T2 and T3 disease. Thirty patients at Washington University in St. Louis with fixed tumors greater than 3 cm in diameter (clinical T2 or pathologic T3) received 45 Gy in 25 fractions over 5 weeks, followed by a 6-week rest interval, followed by 30 to 90 Gy with intracavitary superficial irradiation. The local failure rate was only 30% with 2-year median follow-up, with a 42% disease-free survival rate, which improved to 55% after salvage therapy.[11]

LESS COMMON METHODS OF PELVIC TUMOR IRRADIATION

Delivery of short-course preoperative irradiation followed immediately by surgery has been investigated at some institutions. Selection criteria include patients with early lesions not selected for downstaging to improve resectability and patients who are not ideal candidates for conservative nonsurgical endocavitary irradiation. A typical regimen is the Washington University protocol of 20 Gy delivered in five fractions followed immediately by surgery. Although 24 of 41 patients proved to have pathologic stage B2 or C disease, the local control rate was 92%.[11] In the Stockholm trial, 25 Gy in five fractions was administered to the pelvis through simple anterior and posterior opposed fields.[12]

Minsky et al.[13] selected patients on the basis of favorable tumor size, mobility, location, circumference, grade, and negative histologic assessment of margins for local excision followed by postoperative pelvic irradiation. T1 tumors with adverse histologic features and all T2 tumors received post-operative pelvic irradiation to 45 to 50 Gy, with or without a boost. An advantage of this technique is that it allows for pathologic evaluation of surgical margins, size, grade, and location of the tumor.[13,14]

Another approach is preoperative radiotherapy followed by local excision or proctectomy with coloanal anastomosis. Otmezguine et al.[15] treated lesions in 25 patients with 34.95 Gy in 233 cGy fractions, followed by transanal excision after a 6- to 8-week rest interval. Marks et al.[16] reported a 23% pelvic failure rate and 61% survival at 2 years after treatment with 40 to 45 Gy followed by local excisions.

Intraoperative radiation therapy delivers a focused electron beam boost to the tumor bed during the surgical procedure. Typically, 50.40 Gy of preoperative irradiation is followed by surgical resection after 4 to 6 weeks, with an intraoperative boost of 10 to 15 Gy for microscopic residual disease or a 15 to 20 Gy boost for gross residual disease. With direct visualization of the tumor bed, small bowel retracted, and thin lead strips placed by the radiation oncologist to protect other normal tissues, a plastic cylinder attached to the linear accelerator is placed directly on the surface at risk either in the surgical suite (when the institution has a dedicated intraoperative radiation therapy machine) or in the accelerator vault after the patient is transferred to the radiation oncology department. The Massachusetts General Hospital experience after complete resection with negative margins, including more patients than any other study worldwide, reported an actuarial 5-year local failure rate (LFR) of 12% with intraoperative radiation therapy compared with 29% in historical control groups. Where patients had positive margins, the LFR was 40% even with intraoperative radiation therapy, and 50% with gross residual disease.[17]

For facilities with a short focal distance (contact) x-ray unit with 50 kVp photons, endocavitary radiation therapy can be useful to treat (1) lesions located 10 cm or less from the anal verge, (2) tumors confined to the bowel wall on digital rectal examination or preferably transrectal ultrasound evaluation, (3) tumors less than 3 by 5 cm, (4) tumors with no significant extension to the anal canal, and (5) preferably grade 1 or 2 lesions with exophytic architecture.[18] Four 30 Gy treatments separated by 2 weeks each are delivered with an endocavitary device, typically by a colorectal surgeon–radiation oncologist team. Papillon[18] reported a local failure rate of 11% at 5 years, and only 3% of these patients developed distant metastases.

A technique more readily available but underutilized is intraoperative placement of interstitial brachytherapy catheters with ^{192}Ir seeds. An alternative to afterloading ^{192}Ir sources is permanent ^{125}I or palladium-103 seeds, which can be implanted directly into the tissues or sutured into absorbable mesh laid over the tumor bed.[19] Harrison et al.[20] reported the use of high-dose ^{192}Ir as a source for this technique. Patients with primary unresectable disease were treated with 45 to 50.40 Gy before surgery, in addition to chemotherapy, and, after a 4- to 6-week rest, received a brachytherapy dose of 12 Gy at 1 cm. For pelvic recurrence, patients are treated with 12 Gy at 1 cm at the time of surgical debulking, followed by postoperative external beam pelvic irradiation to 45 Gy over 5 weeks. If the patient has had previous pelvic radiation therapy, 15 Gy at 1 cm delivered at the time of surgical debulking is recommended, and no further treatment.

ACUTE TOXICITY AND COMPLICATIONS OF PELVIC IRRADIATION

Host Factors

Well-documented host factors influence the risk of acute and chronic toxicity after radiation therapy. Patients with diabetes mellitus, hypertension, and collagen vascular disease generally have poor tolerance to treatment, no doubt related to impaired microvasculature patency. Morbidly obese patients also are at higher risk of toxicity, in part because they frequently have poor general health but also because of dosimetric inhomogeneity resulting from the large skin surface to prescription point distances along the central axis of the radiation beam. A history of prior pelvic or abdominal surgery also carries increased risk for the development of acute and chronic toxicity, because adhesions can fix the small bowel in the pelvis, resulting in daily irradiation of one segment of bowel throughout the course of therapy. Finally, for unknown and unpredictable reasons, some patients have innate sensitivity to ionizing radiation that will not be detected until the planned course is well underway.

Treatment Factors

The type of linear accelerator and simulator, its maintenance and quality assurance, and the skill and knowledge of the radiation oncologist can influence treatment effects. A facility with an 18 MeV photon beam from a reputable manufacturer of linear accelerators can be expected to have fewer complications in a cohort of patients undergoing adjuvant pelvic irradiation than a radiation oncology department with a ^{60}Co unit that produces 1.25 MeV gamma rays. A radiation oncologist using three- or four-field techniques, with each field treated daily, and a cGy fraction of 180 to 200 will have lower complication rates than one who treats just anterior and posterior fields or one field daily or who prescribes fraction sizes larger than 200 cGy/day.

Late effects of irradiation are related to the daily fraction size, with higher doses per fraction resulting in damage to the microvasculature appearing 4 months to 2 years after treatment. The acute toxicity of irradiation is related to the total dose, even when administered in smaller fractions.

Systemic chemotherapy administered concommitantly with pelvic irradiation can substantially increase both acute and late toxicity over that with radiation therapy alone. In the Mayo Clinic–North Central Cancer Treatment Group (NCCTG) study,[5] patients who received chemoradiotherapy had significantly increased toxicity compared with those treated with concurrent radiation therapy alone. A Memorial Sloan-Kettering Cancer Center pilot study of preoperative chemoradiotherapy in 20 patients produced seven postoperative complications (35%).[7] This represents a significant increase in postoperative complications compared with historical control studies of patients who received radiation therapy alone. Sequential treatment for surgical stage T2, T3, T4, or N1 with preoperative radiation therapy and postoperative chemotherapy may reduce toxicity. With postoperative chemoradiotherapy, there can also be substantial toxicity. In the Gastrointestinal Tumor Study Group (GITSG) trial, 26% of patients experienced hematologic toxicity and 35% had nonhematologic toxicity of grade 3 or higher (Table 24-5). Thirty-five percent of these patients did not complete all planned cycles of chemotherapy because of toxicity.[21] In the Mayo Clinic/NCCTG trial, 41% of patients had severe diarrhea and 33% had leuko-

Table 24-5 LENT SOMA* scale

	Grade 1	Grade 2	Grade 3	Grade 4
Small intestine/colon				
Subjective				
Stool frequency	2-4/day	5-8/day	>8/day	Refractory diarrhea
Stool consistency	Bulky	Loose	Mucous, dark, watery	
Pain	Minimal/ occasional	Intermittent/ tolerable	Persistent/ intense	Refractory/ rebound
Constipation	3-4/wk	Only 2/wk	Only 1/wk	No stool in 10 days
Objective				
Melena	Occult/ occasional	Intermittent/ tolerable, normal hemoglobin	Persistent, 10%-20% decrease in hemoglobin	Refractory or frank blood, >20% decrease in hemoglobin
Weight loss from time of treatment	≥5%-10%	>10%-20%	>20%-30%	>30%
Stricture	>2/3 normal diameter with dilation	1/3-2/3 normal diameter with dilation	<1/3 normal diamater	Complete obstruction
Ulceration	Superficial ≤1 cm	Superficial >1 cm	Deep ulcer	Perforation, fistulas
Management				
Pain	Occasional nonnarcotic	Regular nonnarcotic	Regular narcotic	Surgical intervention
Stool consistency/ frequency	Diet modification	Regular use of nonnarcotic antidiarrheal	Continuous use of narcotic antidiarrheal	
Bleeding	Iron therapy	Occasional transfusion	Frequent transfusions	Surgical intervention
Stricture	Diet adaptation (occasional)	Diet adaptation required	Medical intervention, NG suction	Surgical intervention
Ulceration			Medical intervention	Surgical intervention

From Late Effects of Normal Tissues (LENT) Consensus Conference, Rubin P, Constine LS, Fajardo LF, Phillips TL, Wasserman TH, eds. LENT SOMA scales for all anatomic sites. Int J Radiat Oncol Biol Phys 31:1049-1091, 1995.

*SOMA = subjective objective management analytic.

Table 24-5 LENT SOMA scale–cont'd

	Grade 1	Grade 2	Grade 3	Grade 4
Rectum				
Subjective				
Tenesmus	Occasional urgency	Intermittent urgency	Persistent urgency	Refractory
Mucosal loss	Occasional	Intermittent	Persistent	Refractory
Sphincter control	Occasional	Intermittent	Persistent	Refractory
Stool frequency	2-4/day	4-8/day	>8/day	Uncontrolled diarrhea
Pain	Occasional/ minimal	Intermittent/ tolerable	Persistent/ intense	Refractory/ excruciating
Objective				
Bleeding	Occult	Occasionally >2/week	Persistent/ daily	Gross hemorrhage
Ulceration	Superficial ≤1 cm^2	Superficial >1 cm^2	Deep ulcer	Perforation, fistulas
Stricture	>2/3 normal diameter with dilation	1/3-2/3 normal diameter with dilation	<1/3 normal diameter	Complete obstruction
Management				
Tenesmus/stool frequency	Occasional, ≤2 antidiarrheal agent/wk	Regular, >2 antidiarrheal agent/wk	Multiple, >2 antidiarrheal agent/day	Surgical intervention/ permanent colostomy
Pain	Occasional nonnarcotic	Regular nonnarcotic	Regular narcotic	Surgical intervention
Bleeding	Stool softener, iron therapy	Occasional transfusion	Frequent transfusions	Surgical intervention/ permanent colostomy
Ulcerations	Diet modification, stool softeners	Occasional steroids	Steroids per enema, hyperbaric oxygen	Surgical intervention/ permanent colostomy
Stricture	Diet modification	Occasional dilation	Regular dilation	Surgical intervention/ permanent colostomy
Sphincter control	Occasional use of incontinence pads	Intermittent use of incontinence pads	Persistent use of incontinence pads	Surgical intervention/ permanent colostomy

Continued.

Table 24-5 LENT SOMA scale—cont'd

	Grade 1	Grade 2	Grade 3	Grade 4
Bladder				
Subjective				
Dysuria	Occasional/ minimal	Intermittent/ tolerable	Persistent/ intense	Refractory/ excruciating
Frequency	3-4 hr intervals	2-3 hr intervals	1-2 hr intervals	Hourly
Hematuria	Occasional	Intermittent	Persistent with clot	Refractory
Incontinence	<weekly	<daily	>1 pad/under-garments per day	Refractory
Decreased stream	Occasionally weak	Intermittent	Persistent but incomplete obstruction	Complete obstruction
Objective				
Hematuria	Microscopic, normal hemoglobin	Intermittent, macroscopic, <10% decrease in hemoglobin	Persistent macroscopic, 10%-20% decrease in hemoglobin	Refractory, >20% decrease in hemoglobin
Endoscopy	Patchy atrophy, telangi-ectasia, no bleeding	Confluent atrophy or telangi-ectasia, gross bleeding	Ulcerations into muscle	Perforation, fistula
Maximum volume	>300-400 ml	>200-300 ml	>100-200 ml	≤100 ml
Residual volume	25 ml	>25-100 ml	>100 ml	
Management				
Dysuria	Occasional nonnarcotic	Regular nonnarcotic	Regular narcotic	Surgical intervention
Frequency	Alkalinization	Occasional anti-spasmodic agent	Regular narcotic	Cystectomy
Hematuria/ telangiectasia	Iron therapy	Occasional transfusion or single cautery	Frequent transfusion or coagulation	Surgical intervention
Incontinence	Occasional use of pads	Intermittent use of pads	Regular use of pad or self-catheteri-zation	Permanent catheter
Decreased stream		1×/day cath-eterization	Dilation, >1×/day catheteri-zation	Permanent catheter, surgery

Table 24-5 LENT SOMA scale–cont'd

Scoring systems					
Colon		*Rectum*		*Bladder*	
______	Score the	______	Score the	______	Score the
______	13 SOMA	______	14 SOMA	______	14 SOMA
______	parameters	______	parameters	______	parameters
______	with 1-4	______	with 1-4	______	with 1-4
______	Score = 0 if	______	Score = 0 if	______	Score = 0 if
______	no toxicities	______	no toxicities	______	no toxicities
______		______		______	
______	Total the	______	Total the	______	Total the
______	scores and	______	scores and	______	scores and
______	divide by 13	______	divide by 14	______	divide by 14
______	LENT score:	______	LENT score:	______	LENT score:
______		______		______	
______	______	______	______	______	______
______		______		______	

penia, compared with 5% of patients who received radiation therapy alone.[5] Twenty-five percent of patients refused to complete chemotherapy.

The skill and experience of the surgeon also has an impact on complication rates after radiation therapy. At Washington University, the incidence of grade 3 or higher sequellae was 4% for colorectal surgeons and 12% for nonspecialists (significant on multivariate analysis, $p = 0.015$). The experience of the surgeon was the only significant predictor of sequellae of treatment. Radiation dose, technique, and timing were not statistically correlated with complications, which probably reflects consistent treatment policies and excellent technique at this prestigious radiation oncology department. The third most significant predictor of disease-free survival on multivariate analysis was the experience of the surgeon.[11]

Attention to technical details is critical in treatment with adjuvant pelvic irradiation, in both successful treatment outcome and reduction of complication rates. The volume of tissue irradiated also significantly influences the toxicity rate. For example, after abdominoperineal resection, it is standard practice for the radiation field to include the perineal scar. This results in inferior and posterior extension of the radiation fields, with a dramatic increase in subsequent skin toxicity, primarily erythema and moist desquamation.

TOXICITY SCORING

With modern megavoltage radiation therapy, the normal tissues most at risk for early and late toxicity are the small bowel, large bowel, and bladder, and after abdominoperineal resection, the perineal skin.

A standard scoring system for late effects will be of significant value in comparing treatment regimens and evaluating the relationship between dose and complications.

At the Late Effects of Normal Tissues (LENT) Consensus Conference held in San Francisco in 1992, the Radiation Therapy Oncology Group (RTOG) and European Organization for Research and Treatment of Cancer (EORTC) SOMA scales, a simplified and reproducible evaluation of acute and late toxicity end points was developed, along with a description of pathogenesis, clinical findings, management, and potential interventions (Table 24-5). Acute injury to the small and large intestine is found primarily in the mucosa, as opposed to late radiation effects, which appear in the bowel wall. The symptoms associated with late effects include fecal frequency or urgency, bleeding, pain, fistula formation, and small bowel obstruction. Late radiation injury to the intestine is attributable to vascular insufficiency resulting in chronic ischemia, and fibrosis.[22-25] Chronic intestinal radiation injury appears mottled and fibrotic with adhesions. Focal areas of stenosis, ulceration, or both can be seen, frequently with pale mucosa and telangiectasia. Ulcers and fistulas may be present.

Stigmata of late effects are seen microscopically in the submucosa, in contrast to the mucosal alterations characteristic of early effects. Late injury is manifested by submucosal atypical fibroblasts and collagen proliferation, along with atypical vascular changes that include small arteries with hyalinized wall thickening and intimal foam cell proliferation. The mucosal layer may show little abnormality.

The most common clinical symptom is frequency and urgency of bowel movements. Diarrhea without tenesmus, frank blood, or mucus discharge may be a manifestation of injury from more proximal segments of bowel. Other symptoms include hematochezia, lower abdominal cramping, rectal pain from chronic proctitis, or anal canal ulceration.[26,27] Most major medical and surgical interventions result from small bowel obstruction, severe bleeding, fistula formation, and intractable diarrhea. Clinically apparent malabsorption syndrome is unlikely unless there has been extensive small bowel resection.

The radiologic signs of late radiation injury relate to fibrosis and ischemia. Contrast-enhanced studies may show spasm with either increased or decreased transit times, as well as thickened folds or ulceration.

The tolerance dose of small bowel is considered to be 45 to 50 Gy. The incidence of small bowel complications increases rapidly with doses above 50 to 55 Gy when a substantial volume of small bowel is irradiated.

The rectum generally tolerates higher doses of radiation than the small intestine. In the treatment of cervical cancer, when the maximum rectal dose is less than 80 Gy, severe proctitis is seen in less than 4% of patients, compared with 7% to 8% with 80 to 95 Gy and 13% with greater than 95 Gy.[28,29]

Endocavitary irradiation of rectal cancer produces no major toxicity despite doses in excess of 100 Gy and a small number of fractions. This is the result of limited treatment volume, typically a circular surface area 3 cm in diameter or smaller, with rapid dose falloff through the submucosa and muscularis propria as a result of low-energy photons with short source-to-skin distance.[30-32]

Management of late bowel injury depends on the severity of the symptoms. Mild cases are managed with a low-residue diet and stool softeners and occasional loperimide or diphenoxylate with atropine. Fiber laxatives can be helpful if there is reduced rectal compliance because they give form and consistency to the stool. Hydrocortisone acetate (0.25 mg) in a hydrogenated coccoglyceride base suppository or steroid foam preparation (10% hydrocortisone) can alleviate symptoms of proctitis. Cholestyramine controls chronic diarrhea from small bowel injury by reducing the level of intraluminal biosalts.[33,34] Sodium pentosanpolysulfate is a synthetic sulfated polysaccharide that has been demonstrated in a phase II trial to reduce proctitis and cystitis.[35] Gastrointestinal bleeding from radiation-induced ulcers may require endoscopic laser treatment or suction cautery. Small bowel obstruction can be managed with bowel rest and decompression followed by dietary modification.[20] An aggressive surgical approach with lysis of all adhesions, freeing up the full length of small bowel and resecting all severely involved segments, is preferred by some surgeons,[36,37] but the reported mortality rates range from 0% to 44%.[22,36-39]

SUGGESTED TECHNIQUES

Suggested techniques of pelvic irradiation to minimize acute and late toxicity while maximizing tumor control include the following.

Place the patient in a prone position for treatment. In the prone position, the angulation of the pelvis is such that the small bowel tends to fall toward the umbilicus and away from the pelvis. This position also facilitates exposure of the anus, which is helpful for inserting contrast medium and marking the anal verge at the time of simulation. This position can be uncomfortable and awkward for patients with especially large abdominal girth, but the "belly board" reduces this problem.[40]

Use the open-table (belly board) technique. A belly board (Fig. 24-3, *A*) can be used, as well as other immobilization devices such as an alpha-cradle, if needed. When the patient is lying on a flat, hard table, the increased intra-abdominal pressure can prevent the small bowel from fully escaping the pelvis in the prone position. Shanahan et al.[41] reported that the use of an open table top allows the anterior abdominal wall to fall into the hole in the table, decreasing intra-abdominal pressure and permitting the small bowel to fall away from the pelvic cavity. With this device, the small bowel can be frequently shielded on lateral simulation films.

Use small bowel follow-through contrast medium. A dilute solution of meglumine ditrizoate (Gastrografin) or a similar contrast medium given ½ to 1 hour before simulation will allow visualization of the small bowel on the simulator films.

This occasionally creates a problem in visualization of the bottom of the L5 vertebra, a landmark for the superior border of the field. To prevent this problem, the posteroanterior field is simulated first, before administration of the contrast medium. Drawing the blocks with a crayon on the simulator films can sometimes be aided by small bowel contrast, particularly in minimizing the amount of small bowel within the lateral fields.[42]

Insert a rectal marker. A rectal marker may be inserted approximately 10 cm past the anal verge, with an additional metallic ring or marker at the anal verge. Some radiation oncologists use contrast medium at this step of the procedure, but this also can obscure some helpful details on the simulator films; the rectal marker is preferred. The principal benefit is the ability to shield a portion of the anus within the lateral fields, thereby reducing acute anal toxicity.

Wire the perineum. If the patient has undergone an abdominoperineal resection, the perineum may be wired to ensure coverage of the perineal scar, which cannot otherwise be visualized.

Use a three-field technique. The three-field technique (one posterior and two lateral) is preferred to the two-field technique, which delivers unnecessary irradiation to the small bowel located anteriorly in the superior aspect of the field. The small bowel can be shielded with lateral beams, and omission of the anterior field also reduces small bowel irradiation. In some situations, a four-field technique may be preferred, which restores the anterior field to the treatment plan. This is best determined after careful review of multiple isodose plans created by the dosimetrist.[43]

Have the surgeon routinely place surgical clips near the tumor bed. This mea sure is especially effective when the gross surgical margin is close. This allows the radiation oncologist to use the "shrinking field" technique. Small-field boost to the area at greatest risk for residual microscopic disease can be given without large margins, reducing the risk of toxicity.

Treat all radiation fields each day. Although inconvenient for an extremely busy radiation oncology department, treating all three or four fields daily improves the homogeneity of the dose distribution during each treatment. If one field is treated per day, the dose to a designated point within the pelvis will be high one day and low the next.

Make certain the patient has a full bladder before treatment. This also decreases the volume of small bowel within the pelvis, sometimes a small improvement and at other times rather dramatic.

Use computerized dosimetry. Because patients vary in shape and size, inhomogeneities can be created within the target volume. Use of wedges or altering the beam weights can frequently correct these inhomogeneities.

Use three-dimensional treatment planning. Although this is not standard practice at most facilities, research protocols are underway to investigate the applications and usefulness of this innovation in computerized treatment planning are now underway. A CT scan is obtained with the patient in an immobilization device on a flat table in the treatment position. The sections are digitized, and the computer presents a three-dimensional "beam's eye" view of the tumor volume, as well as the bladder, small bowel, large bowel, skin, bone, and other critical structures. Potentially, this technology could improve the therapeutic ratio by selectively allowing higher doses to gross tumor and lower doses to normal tissues.[44]

Consider using preoperative irradiation. I prefer treatment with preoperative pelvic irradiation. This is controversial, and many reputable centers (e.g., the Mayo Clinic) prefer postoperative irradiation. For the reasons described earlier, I find the risk for acute and late toxicity lower with preoperative pelvic irradiation.

Explore special surgical techniques. In difficult cases, special surgical techniques may be required. In patients with small bowel adhesions deep in the pelvis, surgical exploration with adhesiolysis followed by the use of absorbable mesh to temporarily retract the small bowel from the pelvis can be beneficial.[45] Other techniques include an omental pedicle flap to prevent the small bowel from falling into the pelvis, retroversion of the uterus, and reperitonealization of the pelvic floor.

Prescribe an elemental diet. Elemental diets significantly decrease the frequency and severity of diarrhea, nausea, vomiting, abdominal cramps, and time to recovery of small bowel function.[46]

CONCLUSION

Radiation therapy can be an effective adjuvant therapy for treatment of patients with transmural tumor extension or positive pelvic lymph nodes and assists in sphincter and other function-preserving procedures. As with any treatment capable of erradicating cancer, early and late toxicity is associated with the delivery of cancericidal doses of pelvic irradiation. Host and treatment factors, including the skill of the radiation oncologist and the quality of the equipment and support personnel, remain major determinants of successful tumor control and minimal toxicity.

In offering adjuvant or definitive radiation therapy for rectal cancer, the risk of life-threatening subacute or chronic injuries must be kept to an acceptable minimum (5% or less). To achieve this minimum complication rate in carcinoma of the rectum, most radiation oncologists treat with 45 Gy to the pelvis followed by a boost to the tumor bed of an additional 5 to 9 Gy.

REFERENCES

1. Rich T, Gunderson LL, Lew R, et al. Patterns of recurrence of rectal cancer after potentially curative surgery. Cancer 52:1317-1329, 1983.
2. Gastrointestinal Tumor Study Group (GITSG). Prolongation of the disease-free interval and surgically treated rectal carcinoma. N Engl J Med 312:1465-1472, 1985.
3. Douglass HO, Moertel CG, Mayer RJ, et al. Survival after postoperative combination treatment of rectal cancer. N Engl J Med 315:1294-1295, 1986.
4. Balslev I, Pedersen M, Teglbjaerg PS, et al. Postoperative radiotherapy in Dukes' B and C carcinoma of the rectum and rectosigmoid: A randomized multicenter study. Cancer 58: 22-28, 1986.
5. Krook JE, Moertel CG, Gunderson LL, et al. Effective surgical adjuvant therapy for high-risk rectal carcinoma. N Engl J Med 324:709-715, 1991.
6. Fisher B, Wolmark N, Rockette HE, et al. Adjuvant chemotherapy or postoperative radiation for rectal cancer: Five-year results of NSABP protocol. In Salmon SE, ed. Adjuvant Therapy of Cancer. New York: Grune & Stratton, 1987, pp 547-554.
7. Minsky BD, Cohen AM, Kemeny N, et al. Phase I trial of postoperative 5-FU, radiation therapy, and high-dose leukovorin for resectable rectal cancer. Int J Radiat Oncol Biol Phys 22: 139-145, 1991.
8. Minsky BD, Kemeny N, Cohen AM, et al. Preoperative high-dose leukovorin/5-fluorouracil and radiation therapy for unresectable rectal cancer. Cancer 67:2859-2866, 1991.
9. Brierley JD, Cummings BJ, Wong CS, et al. Adenocarcinoma of the rectum treated by radical external radiation therapy. Int J Radiat Oncol Biol Phys 31:255-259, 1995.
10. Papillon J. Present status of radiation therapy and the conservative management of rectal cancer. Radiother Oncol 17:275-283, 1990.
11. Myerson RJ, Michalski JM, King ML, et al. Adjuvant radiation therapy for rectal carcinoma: Predictors of outcome. Int J Radiat Oncol Biol Phys 32:41-50, 1995.
12. Cedermark B, Johansson H, Rutqvist LE, et al. The Stockholm I trial of preoperative short term radiotherapy in operable rectal carcinoma: A prospective randomized trial. Cancer 75: 2269-2275, 1995.
13. Minsky BD, Cohen AM, Enker WE, et al. Sphincter preservation in rectal cancer by local excision and postoperative radiation therapy. Cancer 67:908-914, 1991.
14. Willet CG, Tepper JE, Donnelly S, et al. Patterns of failure following local excision and postoperative radiation therapy for invasive rectal adenocarcinoma. J Clin Oncol 7:1003-1008, 1989.
15. Otmezguine Y, Grimard L, Calitchi E, et al. A new combined approach in the conservative management of rectal cancer. Int J Radiat Oncol Biol Phys 17:539-545, 1989.
16. Marks LB, Carroll PR, Dugan TC, et al. The response of the urinary bladder, urethra, and ureter to radiation and chemotherapy. Int J Radiat Oncol Biol Phys 31:1257-1280, 1995.
17. Willet CG, Shellito PG, Tepper JE, et al. Intraoperative electron beam radiation therapy for primary locally advanced rectal and rectosigmoid carcinoma. J Clin Oncol 9:843-849, 1991.
18. Papillon J. Rectal and Anal Cancers: Conservative Treatment by Irradiation—an Alternative to Radical Surgery. Berlin: Springer-Verlag, 1982.

19. Minsky BD, Cohen AM, Enker WE, et al. Intraoperative brachytherapy alone in incompletely resected recurrent rectal cancer. Radiother Oncol 21:115-120, 1991.
20. Harrison LB, Enker WE, Anderson LL. High-dose-rate intraoperative radiation therapy for colorectal cancer. Oncology 9:737-741, 1995.
21. Gastrointestinal Tumor Study Group. Adjuvant therapy of colon cancer: Results of a prospectively randomized trial. N Engl J Med 310:737-743, 1984.
22. Coia LR, Myerson RJ, Tepper JE. Late effects of radiation therapy on the gastrointestinal tract. Int J Radiat Oncol Biol Phys 31:1213-1236, 1995.
23. Berthrong M. Pathologic changes secondary to radiation. World J Surg 10:155-170, 1986.
24. Fajardo L. Pathology of radiation injury. In Sternberg SS, ed. Masson Monographs in Diagnostic Pathology. Chicago: Year Book Medical Publishers, 1982, pp 47-76.
25. Rubin P, Casarett G. Alimentary tract: Esophagus and stomach. Clin Radiat Pathol 5:193-230, 1968.
26. Cox JD, Byhardt RW, Wilson JF, et al. Complications of radiation therapy and factors in their prevention. World J Surg 10:171-188, 1986.
27. Yeoh EK, Horowitz M. Radiation enteritis. Surg Gynecol Obstet 165:373-379, 1987.
28. Perez CA, Fox S, Lockett MA, et al. Impact of dose in outcome of irradiation alone in carcinoma of the uterine cervix: Analysis of two different methods. Int J Radiat Oncol Biol Phys 21:885-898, 1991.
29. Pourquier H, Bubois JB, Delard R. Cancer of the uterine cervix: Dosimetric guidelines for prevention of late rectal and rectosigmoid complications as a result of radiotherapeutic treatment. Int J Radiat Oncol Biol Phys 8:1887-1895, 1982.
30. Myerson RJ, Walz BJ, Kodner IJ, et al. Endocavitary radiation therapy for rectal carcinoma: Results with and without external beam. Endocuriether/Hypertherm Oncol 5:195-200, 1989.
31. Papillon J. Intracavitary irradiation of early rectal cancer for cures: A series of 186 cases. Cancer 36:696-701, 1975.
32. Sischy G. The use of endocavitary irradiation for selected carcinomas of the rectum: Ten years' experience. Radiother Oncol 4:97-101, 1985.
33. Chary S, Thomson DH. A clinical trial evaluating cholestyramine to prevent diarrhea in patients maintained on low-fat diets during pelvic radiation therapy. Int J Radiat Oncol Biol Phys 10:1885-1890, 1984.
34. Newman A, Katsaris J, Blendis LM, et al. Small-intestinal injury in women who have had pelvic radiotherapy. Lancet 2:1471-1473, 1973.
35. Grigsby PW, Pilepich MV, Parsons CL. Preliminary results of a Phase I/II study of sodium pentosanpolysulfate in the treatment of chronic radiation-induced proctitis. Am J Clin Oncol 13:28-31, 1990.
36. Lucarotti ME, Mountford RA, Bartolo DCC. Surgical management of intestinal radiation injury. Dis Colon Rectum 34:865-869, 1991.
37. Marks GF, Mohiuddin M. The surgical management of the radiation-injured intestine. Surg Clin North Am 63:81-96, 1983.
38. Lillemoe KD, Brigham A, Harmon JW, et al. Surgical management of small-bowel radiation enteritis. Arch Surg 118:905-907, 1983.
39. Schmitt EH, Symmonds RE. Surgical treatment of radiation induced injuries of the intestine. Surg Gynecol Obstet 153:896-900, 1981.
40. Gallagher MJ, Brereton HD, Rostock RA, et al. A prospective study of treatment techniques to minimize the volume of pelvic small bowel with reduction of acute and late effects associated with pelvic irradiation. Int J Radiat Oncol Biol Phys 12:1565-1573, 1986.

40. Gallagher MJ, Brereton HD, Rostock RA, et al. A prospective study of treatment techniques to minimize the volume of pelvic small bowel with reduction of acute and late effects associated with pelvic irradiation. Int J Radiat Oncol Biol Phys 12:1565-1573, 1986.
41. Shanahan TG, Mehta MP, Bertelrud KL, et al. Minimization of small bowel volume within treatment fields utilizing customized "belly boards." Int J Radiat Oncol Biol Phys 19:469-476, 1990.
42. Herbert SH, Curran WJ, Solin LJ, et al. Decreasing gastrointestinal morbidity with the use of small bowel contrast during treatment planning for pelvic irradiation. Int J Radiat Oncol Biol Phys 20:835-842, 1991.
43. Vigliotti A, Rich TA, Romsdahl MM, et al. Postoperative adjuvant radiotherapy for adenocarcinoma of the rectum and rectosigmoid. Int J Radiat Oncol Biol Phys 13:999-1006, 1987.
44. Shank B, LoSasso T, Brewster L, et al. Three-dimensional treatment planning for postoperative treatment of rectal carcinoma. Int J Radiat Oncol Biol Phys 21:253-265, 1991.
45. Gunderson LL, Russell AH, Llewellyn HJ, et al. Treatment planning for colorectal cancer: Radiation and surgical techniques and value of small bowel films. Int J Radiat Oncol Biol Phys 11:1379-1393, 1985.
46. McArdle AH, Reid EC, Laplante MP, et al. Prophylaxis against radiation injury: The use of elemental diet prior and during radiotherapy for invasive bladder cancer and in early postoperative feeding following radical cystectomy and ileal conduit. Arch Surg 121:879-885, 1986.

CHAPTER 25

Chemotherapy for Colorectal Cancer

GEORGE M. FUHRMAN
JOHN S. BOLTON

Historically, surgeons have had the ability to solely provide care for patients with nonmetastatic colorectal carcinoma. The surgeon could provide colonoscopic identification of disease, organize an appropriate metastatic evaluation, perform surgery, and provide surveillance and occasionally repeat surgery to treat recurrent disease. The management of nonmetastatic colorectal carcinoma has become more complicated in recent years because of the development of effective forms of adjuvant chemotherapy and radiation therapy. Appropriate management of colorectal carcinoma can no longer be provided by a single physician representing one specialty; a multidisciplinary team of physicians is required. It is imperative that surgeons become knowledgeable about the potential benefits and risks of adjuvant therapies to maintain their central role in the evolving multidisciplinary team.

We will discuss current indications for and uses of systemic agents in the management of nonmetastatic colorectal carcinoma and provide detailed information regarding the complications associated with chemotherapy.

INDICATIONS FOR CHEMOTHERAPY

Colon

The National Institutes of Health (NIH) Consensus Conference[1] statement on adjuvant therapy for patients with carcinoma of the colon and rectum has led to the use of multimodality treatment in the majority of patients with colorectal cancer. The Conference concluded that sufficient data exist to justify the use of 5-fluorouracil (5-FU) and levamisole in patients with resected node-positive colon carcinoma and to support the use of combined chemotherapy and radiation therapy after resection of stage II and III rectal carcinoma (Table 25-1). Although the Conference concluded that additional adjuvant therapy trials were required to better define the optimal systemic agents and sequence of treatment modali-

Table 25-1 Colorectal cancer staging

TNM*	Definition	Staging system: AJCC/UICC†	Staging system: Dukes (1932)	Staging system: Astler-Coller (1954)
T1	Tumor invades submucosa			A
T2	Tumor invades muscularis propria	Stage I	A	B_1
T3	Tumor invades through muscularis propria into subserosa	Stage II	B	B_2
T4	Tumor directly invades other organs or structures			
N0	No lymph node metastasis			
N1	Metastasis in one to three pericolic or perirectal lymph nodes	Stage III	C	C_1, C_2
N2	Metastasis in four or more pericolic or perirectal lymph nodes			
N3	Metastasis in any lymph node along named vascular trunk or apical node			
M0	No distant metastasis	Stage IV	—	D
M1	Distant metastasis			

*Tumor-node-metastasis staging system of the American Cancer Society.
†American Joint Committee on Cancer and Union Internationale Control le Cancer.

ties, the above recommendations have become the standard of care for cancer treated outside ongoing clinical trials.

The Conference conclusions were based on findings from well-designed randomized prospective trials. Data from retrospective studies and prospective trials that included comparisons with historic controls were ignored. Retrospective studies were considered flawed because of the potential for selection bias often associated with nonprospective studies. Prospective studies that compare current multimodality-treated cancer with historic control groups with cancer treated with surgery alone have been criticized because of the potential for stage shifting.[2] Stage shifting implies that patients who received treatment in the 1950s and 1960s, those most often used as historic control groups, demonstrate lower survival rates stage for stage than the survival rates noted in prospective trials of current patient groups with colorectal carcinoma treated with surgical resection alone. The lower survival rate noted in historic control groups is attributed to inadequate mesenteric lymph node excision for histologic analysis and inaccurate pathologic staging of surgical specimens. For example, cancer staged as node negative in a previous era might now be correctly staged as node positive as a result of more thorough and accurate surgical and pathologic techniques. The shifting of cancer from a node-negative stage to a node-positive stage (stage shifting) by more accurate assessment is a theoretic explanation for the weakness noted in the prospective trials that used historic control groups.

The Consensus Conference recommendations regarding adjuvant chemotherapy in patients with resected colon carcinoma were largely based on two well-designed randomized trials. The North Central Cancer Treatment Group (NCCTG) reported improved disease-free and overall survival rates for node-positive cancer treated with surgery and postoperative 5-FU and levamisole compared with surgery alone and surgery combined with levamisole only.[3] A larger, confirmatory intergroup trial again demonstrated improved disease-free and overall survival for patients with resected node-positive colon cancer treated with postoperative adjuvant 5-FU and levamisole.[4] An updated analysis with a median follow-up of 5 years was reported in 1992.[5] Patients in the node-positive group treated with adjuvant 5-FU and levamisole demonstrated a 39% reduction in recurrence rate and a 31% reduction in mortality.

The rationale for use of levamisole, an agent whose biologic effect is poorly understood, in the therapy of colon carcinoma is unclear. Levamisole has not demonstrated efficacy as a single agent in the treatment of metastatic colon cancer.[6] In addition, the adjuvant levamisole-alone arms of the NCCTG and intergroup trials did not demonstrate a survival advantage compared with the surgery-alone arms.[3,4] Yet, levamisole clearly has a synergistic effect with 5-FU, because 5-FU alone has been used in several adjuvant trials without evidence of a significant survival benefit.[7-10] The improved survival rate noted with the combination of two agents that alone have no beneficial effect in the adjuvant setting is difficult to explain without a clear understanding of the biologic effects associated with levamisole.

A clearer understanding exists of the biologic effects of folinic acid, an agent that has more recently been used in combination with 5-FU for treatment of metastatic colon carcinoma.[11-13] Folinic acid enhances the binding of 5-FU to thymidylate synthase, resulting in enhanced suppression of DNA synthesis through depletion of thymidine and thereby increasing the cytotoxic potential of 5-FU. A meta-analysis of three randomized series of patients who received treatment with adjuvant 5-FU and folinic acid demonstrated a survival benefit for those given the drug combination.[14] Ongoing trials evaluating the dose and schedule for adjuvant 5-FU and folinic acid with and without levamisole should help clarify the optimal adjuvant approach for treatment of colon carcinoma.

Mitomycin C and the chloroethylnitrosureas have demonstrated activity in the treatment of disseminated colorectal carcinoma.[15-17] In a trial of 5-FU versus 5-FU, methyl-CCNU, (*N*-[2-chloroethyl]-*N*'-cyclohexyl-*N*-nitrosurea) and vincristine (Oncovin) demonstrated a slightly higher response rate for the multidrug combination.[18] This limited increased efficacy of the adjuvant drug combination was overshadowed by the leukemogenic effect of methyl-CCNU.

Rectum

The treatment of rectal carcinoma must be discussed separately from the treatment of colon carcinoma. Tumors arising from below the peritoneal reflection have similar ability to metastasize as do tumors arising from above the peritoneal reflection, and therefore patients with advanced stages of disease should benefit from adjuvant systemic therapies. The difference in considering adjuvant therapies for rectal carcinoma compared with colon carcinoma is the propensity for local recurrence below the peritoneal reflection.[19-22] The surgeon is limited by the confines of the bony pelvis and cannot achieve wide radial margins in removal of rectal cancers. Therefore higher rates of local recurrence are noted for rectal cancers that demonstrate node positivity (N1) or penetration into the mesorectum (T3), compared with node-negative tumors and those confined to the bowel wall.[23,24] Radiation therapy is a logical treatment method to enhance local control rates.

Three randomized prospective studies of adjuvant therapy for rectal cancer were considered by the NIH Consensus Conference in the development of their conclusions regarding adjuvant therapy for rectal cancer. The Gastrointestinal Tumor Study Group (GITSG) rectal cancer adjuvant study,[25] the National Surgical Adjuvant Breast and Bowel Project (NSABP) R-01 trial,[26] and an NCCTG trial[27] all demonstrated improved local control rates for surgery and radiation therapy compared with surgery alone. The addition of chemotherapy was necessary in all three trials to have an effect on survival rates.

Several questions were not answered by these trials. First, all three trials used postoperative radiation therapy. The potential for enhanced local control with preoperative radiation therapy has been advocated to minimize viable tumor cell spillage at the time of resection and allow for radiation therapy to be used in a well-oxygenated field, where it will be more effective.[28] The chemotherapy used in all three trials included methyl-CCNU. Additional studies will be required to identify the optimal chemotherapeutic agents to be used in the treatment of rectal carcinoma, because the nephrotoxicity and leukemogenic potential of methyl-CCNU does not justify its continued use in the adjuvant setting. The elimination of methyl-CCNU in the adjuvant treatment of rectal cancer is further supported by the ability of less toxic agents such as levamisole and folinic acid to enhance the efficacy of 5-FU.

Metastasis

The optimal treatment for metastatic colorectal carcinoma, unlike most other solid tumors, must account for the difference between results in patients with hepatic metastasis only and patients with extrahepatic disease. The unique biology of colorectal metastasis confined to the liver has allowed the use of regional, rather than systemic, treatment strategies that can be curative. Two large series of unselected patients with colorectal metastases treated with hepatic resection demonstrated a 5-year survival rate of 33% and a median survival of more than 3 years.[29,30] If strict selection criteria for resection are used, a 5-year survival rate of 44% can be anticipated.[31] Clearly, those patients amenable to hepatic resection of colorectal metastasis should be considered for liver surgery. Patients who have undergone successful liver resection remain at high risk for recurrence in both the liver and extrahepatic sites. The use of adjuvant chemotherapy in patients after hepatic resection of colorectal metastasis has not been demonstrated to provide a survival benefit in retrospective analysis.[32] Prospective trials evaluating the potential benefit for adjuvant therapy after liver resection are ongoing and should help clarify the indications for chemotherapy in this subset of patients.

COMPLICATIONS

Chemotherapeutic Agents

The mechanism of action for the three agents (5-FU, levamisole, and folinic acid) most commonly used in the treatment of colorectal carcinoma is as follows.

5-FU is an antimetabolite that creates a thymidine deficiency resulting in cell death. The cytotoxic effect of 5-FU is achieved by blockade of the methylation reaction of deoxyuridilic acid to thymidylic acid. The inhibition of this reaction blocks DNA synthesis, which is most pronounced in rapidly dividing cells such as neoplastic cells, GI epithelium, and bone marrow. Adverse reactions to 5-FU include stomatitis, esophagopharyngitis, diarrhea, thrombocytopenia, and alopecia. The usual dose of 5-FU is 500 mg/kg/m^2/day given for 3 or 4 days over a 30-day cycle. Floxuridine (FUDR) has a mechanism of action similar to that of 5-FU and is administered through the hepatic artery at a dose of 0.1 to 0.2 mg/kg/day. Higher doses infused directly into the hepatic artery are associated with unacceptable rates of biliary sclerosis.

The antineoplastic effect of levamisole, if one exists, remains unknown. Levamisole enhances immune function. The drug stimulates antibody formation and T cell activation and proliferation, potentiates phagocytosis and chemotaxis, and increases neutrophil mobility, adherence, and chemotaxis. The usual dose of levamisole is 50 mg/day orally given in conjunction with 5-FU.

The action of folinic acid (leucovorin) to potentiate the effect of 5-FU was discussed earlier. The drug can be administered orally or parenterally. The parenteral route is preferred because of altered GI absorption secondary to the toxic effects of 5-FU. The usual dose of folinic acid is 10 to 20 mg/m^2/day in conjunction with 5-FU. Adverse effects are limited to allergy.

Regional Chemotherapy

Regional chemotherapy (hepatic arterial infusion) has been used in the treatment of hepatic metastases from colorectal carcinoma that are not amenable to surgical resection but where metastases are confined to the liver. Regional chemotherapy is associated with response rates of 50% to 83%, but with an unproved effect on survival.[33-38] Several randomized trials of regional chemotherapy vs. systemic chemotherapy failed to demonstrate a survival difference.[34-38] The design of these trials, which used crossover arms for patients failing to respond to either treatment, and other questions regarding the quality of the surgical technique used for hepatic arterial catheter insertion justify additional evaluation of regional chemotherapy in patients with metastatic disease strictly confined to the liver.[39] The chemotherapeutic agent commonly administered by hepatic arterial infusion is FUDR, an antimetabolite similar in action to 5-FU. FUDR is an attractive agent for regional administration through the hepatic artery because 95% to 99% of the drug is metabolized during the first pass through the liver, resulting in high hepatic levels of chemotherapy but negligible systemic exposure. Therefore, the complications associated with systemic administration of 5-FU are not seen with hepatic arterial infusion of FUDR. Regional toxicity of FUDR includes chemical cholecystitis, gastroduodenitis, and biliary arteritis. Cholecystitis and gastroduodenitis can be prevented with prophylactic cholecystectomy and ligation of the right gastric artery and other small arterial branches from the common hepatic artery distal to the gastroduodenal artery and proximal to the hepatic artery bifurcation at the time of pump insertion.[40] Gastric and duodenal misperfusion can be further evaluated with intraoperative injection of fluorescein through the pump and evaluation of the stomach and duodenum with a Wood's lamp to ensure that perfusion of drug is limited to the hepatic parenchyma.[41] The complication of biliary arteritis is dose dependent and can be diagnosed before permanent liver damage occurs by monitoring serum alkaline phosphatase levels.[42] If elevation of alkaline phosphatase concentration occurs and therapy is continued without dose reduction, biliary sclerosis and hepatic failure can occur. Other complications associated with hepatic arterial infusion include infectious complications with the pump device and bleeding secondary to catheter dislodgment.[43]

Systemic Chemotherapy

The use of systemic cytotoxic chemotherapy can result in complications that may require surgical intervention. Other complications could necessitate dose reduction or discontinuation of chemotherapy and should be recognized by the surgeon. Finally, other complications are amenable to medical treatment and will not require reduction in the dosage of chemotherapy.

Complications of colorectal carcinoma chemotherapy that may require surgical intervention include intestinal perforation, obstruction, hemorrhage, neutropenic enterocolitis, colonic pseudo-obstruction, and central venous access catheter complications. Intestinal perforation can occur as a result of benign disease, from tumor involvement, or as a consequence of chemotherapy. The diagnosis is generally clinically apparent on the basis of development of peritonitis with associated intravascular hypovolemia. Once adequate volume restoration has been achieved, urgent laparotomy to save the patient is generally required. The surgical management of intestinal perforation in patients with malignancy should not differ from the principles of management in patients without malignancy. Resection of the perforated GI segment, when feasible, is desirable. A conservative approach should be used in debilitated patients, especially when the surgeon must make an intraoperative decision to restore or divert intestinal continuity. Ostomies can be reversed after the patient's condition improves. Enteral feeding tubes should be used liberally to facilitate postoperative nutritional management in these patients. Fascial retention sutures can help limit postoperative complications associated with dehiscence.

Intestinal obstruction is not a direct result of chemotherapy but may occur in the patient with colorectal carcinoma who is receiving chemotherapy. The surgeon must be aware of the myelosuppressive effects of chemotherapy when planning surgical intervention for intestinal obstruction. Unless complete intestinal obstruction or bowel ischemia is suspected, conservative treatment with nasogastric suction and intravenous hydration should allow most patients an opportunity to recover from the myelosuppressive effects of chemotherapy before surgical intervention. The cause of intestinal obstruction in the patient with colorectal carcinoma is not always disease recurrence; in fact, in as many as one third of patients with intestinal obstruction after resection of colorectal carcinoma, the cause of obstruction is benign.[44-46] Surgical intervention should be considered in all patients with a history of colorectal carcinoma and intestinal obstruction that does not resolve with conservative therapy unless advanced disease is demonstrated and anticipated survival is limited. Most patients with obstructed bowel from recurrence of malignancy still benefit from surgical intervention to resect or bypass segments of obstructed bowel to restore intestinal continuity. Placement of a gastrostomy tube can avert prolonged use of uncomfortable nasogastric tubes in patients with extensive obstructing disease that cannot be resected or bypassed. The palliative benefit of restoring the ability to eat or averting prolonged use of a nasogastric tube has tremendous benefit for quality of life in patients with advanced colorectal carcinoma.

The complication of hemorrhage as a direct result of malignancy is uncommon. The cause of GI bleeding in the patient with cancer is more likely secondary to benign disease (e.g., peptic ulcer disease, gastritis) than to a bleeding tumor.[47] Chemotherapy can predispose a patient to bleeding problems secondary to its myelosuppressive effects on platelet formation. Thrombocytopenia as a result of chemotherapy is usually most profound during the second week after treatment. Thrombocytopenia should be anticipated after chemotherapy and invasive procedures not done until platelet counts have recovered from the myelosuppressive effects of treatment. An occasional patient with unresectable rectal cancer may have significant hemorrhage from the pelvic tumor. Electrocautery or an intraluminal laser (e.g., yttrium aluminum garnet [YAG]) has been used successfully to reduce the hemorrhage. Several treatments with anesthesia are often required.

Neutropenic enterocolitis, sometimes referred to as typhlitis, is a complication associated with chemotherapy and may require surgical intervention for diagnosis and treatment. The clinical characteristics of neutropenic enterocolitis include right-sided abdominal pain, fever, neutropenia, tenderness, and diarrhea. Neutropenic enterocolitis is usually associated with chemotherapy for hematologic malignancy, but it has occurred in patients undergoing treatment of solid tumors.[48] The diagnosis of neutropenic enterocolitis must be differentiated from the more common causes of abdominal pain (e.g., appendicitis, cholecystitis, diverticulitis). The presence of diarrhea requires consideration of the diagnosis of pseudomembranous colitis. Stool examination for *Clostridium difficile* toxin should be included in the diagnostic evaluation of neutropenia. The diagnostic study of choice to evaluate patients with neutropenia with abdominal pain is CT. Edematous and thickened intestine in the distal ileum, cecum, or both may suggest the diagnosis of neutropenic enterocolitis at CT.[49] Treatment of neutropenic enterocolitis consists of bowel rest, nasogastric suction, and broad-spectrum antibiotics.[50,51] Surgical intervention is limited to patients whose condition deteriorates with medical treatment. Surgery may also be required when the cause of abdominal pain in a patient with neutropenia is in doubt, and laparotomy is required to exclude other potentially correctable causes of the patient's symptoms.

Intestinal pseudo-obstruction, or ileus, is a complication that may occur in the patient with colorectal carcinoma undergoing chemotherapy. Patients receiving chemotherapy are susceptible to dehydration and serum electrolyte disturbances secondary to fluid losses associated with vomiting and diarrhea or poor oral intake. The metabolic derangements associated with volume and electrolyte abnormalities are considered causal for intestinal ileus. Ileus of the small intestine or colon can also occur in a well-hydrated patient with normal serum electrolyte balance. The diagnosis of intestinal ileus can usually be made with plain supine and upright abdominal radiographs. Rarely, a contrast material–enhanced study will be required to differentiate intestinal obstruction from ileus. Treatment of intestinal ileus consists of rehydration and correction of serum electrolyte abnormalities.[52] In patients with a functional ileocecal valve and colonic ileus, severe dilatation can develop and lead to cecal perforation.[53-55] Patients with colonic ileus should be monitored with daily abdominal radiographs to follow the progression of colon dilation. The actual dimensions of the cecum are less important than the rate of dilation.[56] Patients who demonstrate a rapid rate of colonic dilation should be considered for colonoscopic decompression.[57,58] Surgical intervention for intestinal ileus is not warranted unless the diagnosis of mechanical obstruction cannot be excluded radiographically or perforation develops.

Patients receiving chemotherapy may require a long-term central venous access device to facilitate prolonged drug administration. These devices are associated with the complications of thrombosis and infection.[59-61] The diagnosis of catheter-related thrombosis can be made clinically on the basis of signs of venous obstruction that affect the upper extremity on the side of catheter insertion. Thrombolytic therapy through the catheter may be effective in recanalizing the thrombosed vein and salvaging the catheter.[62] If thrombolytic therapy fails, the catheter must be removed, and systemic anticoagulation will be required. The diagnosis of catheter-related infection depends on the documentation of blood cultures drawn from the catheter. Coagulase-negative staphylococci are documented in a majority of cases of catheter-related infection. Infected catheters can be salvaged in most cases with use of antibiotic therapy administered through the venous access device.[63] In catheters with multilumen ports, antibiotics should be administered through each port in rotation. In patients with neutropenia or sepsis with an infected venous catheter, the catheter must be emergently removed.

Complications of colorectal carcinoma chemotherapy that may require dose reduction or medical treatment include GI toxicity and bone marrow suppression. Severe GI toxicity associated with chemotherapy for colorectal carcinoma includes mucositis or inflammation of any part of the GI tract from mouth to anus. Mucositis occurs as a result of direct toxicity to the rapidly dividing cells that line the GI tract. Mucositis occurs during the first week after administration of cytotoxic chemotherapeutic agents; healing is rapid during the week after drug administration unless ulceration develops. Mucositis in the mouth, or stomatitis, is the most frequent type of mucositis and is dose related. Stomatitis can be treated with a variety of topical agents. Agents such as 2% viscous lidocaine reduce the pain associated with mucositis. Topical antibacterial and antifungal agents can be used to treat secondary infection of inflamed or ulcerated oral mucosa. Finally, because mucositis is dose dependent, patients refractory to topical agents may require reduction of chemotherapy dosage to avert this potentially severe form of toxicity.

Nausea and vomiting are common complications of chemotherapy. Cytotoxic drugs are powerful emetic agents. Once a patient experiences chemotherapy-related nausea and vomiting, anticipatory vomiting on the scheduled day of chemotherapy may develop.[64] The optimal method to prevent anticipatory vomiting is to avert severe nausea and vomiting associated with the initial dose of chemotherapy. Standard antiemetics are ineffective in treating chemotherapy-induced nausea and vomiting. Metoclopramide and dexamethasone can prevent nausea and vomiting in 63% of patients and markedly reduce the severity of this complication in an additional 20% of patients.[65] Cannabinoids, the active ingredient in marijuana, have been used in cases of refractory chemotherapy-induced nausea and vomiting.[66] The newest antiemetic is the serotonin antagonist ondansetron. Ondansetron in early clinical experience appears to be the most potent and promising antiemetic agent available.[67-69] Currently, ondansetron is considered a second-line agent for patients with refractory chemotherapy-induced nausea and vomiting; the expense of this new agent has limited its use as a first-line antiemetic.

Myelosuppression is associated with most cytotoxic chemotherapeutic agents. The rapidly dividing precursor bone marrow cells are a target for the nonspecific cytotoxic effects of chemotherapy. Susceptibility to infection is dramatically increased when the absolute granulocyte count falls below 1000. Life-threatening neutropenia was the dose-limiting side effect of most chemotherapeutic agents until hematopoietic growth factors became available. Granulocyte-macrophage colony–stimulating factor (GM-CSF) stimulates the pleuripotential lymphoblast-like cells to produce colonies of granulocytes and macrophages.[70,71] Rapid increases in absolute neutrophil count are noted after administration of GM-CSF. GM-CSF is rarely required in patients receiving systemic treatment of colorectal carcinoma because of the less severe myelosuppressive effect of 5-FU compared with that of other standard chemotherapeutic agents. The ability to prevent neutropenia with GM-CSF has led to thrombocytopenia as the most common dose-limiting myelosuppressive complication of chemotherapy. Platelet counts reach a nadir during the second week after chemotherapy administration. Platelet transfusions may be needed in patients who require emergency surgery during the second week after receiving chemotherapy.

CONCLUSION

Surgeons should continue to play a central role in the multidisciplinary management of colorectal carcinoma. A thorough knowledge of the indications for and complications associated with chemotherapy is critical. Failure to maintain a central role could result in the surgeon's being reduced to a simple technician called on to perform surgery at the discretion of a nonsurgical member of the multidisciplinary team. A reduced role would negatively affect the quality of surgical practice by denying surgeons the opportunity to contribute to treatment-related decisions and, more important, would have a negative effect on the quality of medical care by denying patients the benefit of a surgical opinion about the management of their cancer. Finally, all providers are encouraged to participate in well-designed, controlled trials to assist in expanding our knowledge of this developing field.

REFERENCES

1. NIH Consensus Conference. Adjuvant therapy for patients with colon and rectal cancer. JAMA 264:1444-1450, 1990.
2. Steele G. Advances in the treatment of early-to-late stage colorectal cancer: 20 years of progress. Ann Surg Oncol 2:77-88, 1995.
3. Laurie JA, Moertel CG, Fleming TR, et al. Surgical adjuvant therapy of large bowel carcinoma: An evaluation of levamisole and the combination of levamisole and 5-fluorouracil. J Clin Oncol 7:1447-1456, 1989.
4. Moertel CG, Fleming TR, Macdonald JS, et al. Levamisole and fluorouracil for adjuvant therapy of resected colon carcinoma. N Engl J Med 322:352-358, 1990.
5. Moertel CG, Fleming TR, Macdonald JS, et al. The intergroup study of fluorouracil (5-FU) plus levamisole (LEV) and levamisole alone as adjuvant therapy for stage C colon cancer: A final report. Clin Oncol 11(P):161, 1992.
6. Mayer RJ. Does adjuvant therapy work in colon cancer? N Engl J Med 322:399-401, 1990.
7. Hafstrom L, Rudenstam CM, Domellof L, et al. A randomized trial of oral 5-fluorouracil versus placebo as adjuvant therapy in colorectal cancer Duke's B and C; Results after 5 years observation time. Br J Surg 72:138-141, 1985.
8. Higgins GA, Humphrey E, Juler GL, et al. Adjuvant chemotherapy in the surgical treatment of large bowel cancer. Cancer 38:1461-1467, 1976.
9. Lawrence W, Terz JJ, Horsely JS III, et al. Chemotherapy as an adjuvant to surgery for colorectal cancer. Arch Surg 113:164-168, 1978.
10. Buyse M, Zeleniuch-Jacquotte A, Chalmers TC. Adjuvant therapy of colorectal cancer. Why we still don't know. JAMA 259:3571-3578, 1988.
11. Erlichman C, Fine S, Wong A, et al. A randomized trial of fluorouracil and folinic acid in patients with metastatic colorectal carcinoma. J Clin Oncol 6:469-475, 1988.
12. Poon MA, O'Connell MJ, Moertel CG, et al. Biochemical modulation of fluorouracil: Evidence of significant improvement of survival in quality of life with advanced colorectal carcinoma. J Clin Oncol 7:1407-1417, 1989.
13. Petrelli N, Douglass HO, Herrera L, et al. The modulation of fluorouracil with leucovorin in metastatic colorectal carcinoma: A prospective randomized phase III trial. J Clin Oncol 67:257-267, 1989.
14. Advanced colorectal cancer meta-analysis project. Modulation of fluorouracil by leucovorin in patients with advanced colorectal cancer: Evidence in terms of response rates. J Clin Oncol 10:896-903, 1992.
15. Carter SK. Large bowel cancer: The current status of treatment. J Natl Cancer Inst 56:3-10, 1976.
16. Moertel CG. Therapy of advanced gastrointestinal cancer with nitrosureas. Cancer Chemother Rep 4:27-34, 1973.
17. Macdonald JS, Neefe J. Chemotherapy in the management of gastrointestinal cancer. Abdom Surg 21:126-131, 1979.
18. Moertel CG, Schutt AJ, Hahn RG, et al. Therapy of advanced colorectal carcinoma with a combination of 5-fluorouracil, methyl CCNU, and vincristine. J Natl Cancer Inst 54:69-71, 1975.
19. Rich T, Gunderson LL, Lew R, et al. Patterns of recurrence of rectal cancer after potentially curative surgery. Cancer 52:1317-1329, 1983.
20. Pilipshen SJ, Heilweil M, Quan SHQ, et al. Patterns of pelvic recurrence following definitive resection of rectal cancer. Cancer 53:1354-1362, 1984.

21. Phillips RKS, Hittinger, R, Blesovsky L, et al. Local recurrence following curative surgery for large bowel cancer. Br J Surg 71:17-20, 1984.
22. McDermott FT, Hughes ESR, Pihl E, et al. Local recurrence after potentially curative resection for rectal cancer in a series of 1,008 patients. Br J Surg 72:34-37, 1985.
23. Moosa AR, Ree PC, Marks JE, et al. Factors influencing local recurrence after abdominoperineal resection for cancer of the rectum and rectosigmoid. Br J Surg 62:727-730, 1975.
24. Rich T, Gunderson LL, Galdabini J, et al. Clinical and pathologic factors influencing local failure after curative resection of carcinoma of the rectum and rectosigmoid. Cancer 52: 1317-1329, 1983.
25. Gastrointestinal Tumor Study Group. Prolongation of the disease-free interval in surgically resected rectal cancer. N Engl J Med 312:1465-1472, 1985.
26. Fisher B, Wolmark N, Rockette H, et al. Postoperative adjuvant chemotherapy or radiation therapy for rectal cancer: Results from NSABP Protocol R-01. J Natl Cancer Inst 80:21-29, 1988.
27. Krook J, Moertel CG, Gunderson LL, et al. Effective surgical adjuvant therapy for high risk rectal carcinoma. N Engl J Med 324:709-715, 1991.
28. Metzger U. Adjuvant therapy for colorectal carcinoma. World J Surg 15:576-582, 1991.
29. Hughes KS, Simon R, Songhorabodi S, et al. Resection of the liver for colorectal carcinoma metastases: A multi-institutional study of indication for resection. Surgery 103:278-288, 1988.
30. Steele G, Bleday R, Mayer RJ, et al. A prospective evaluation of hepatic resection for colorectal carcinoma metastases to the liver. Gastrointestinal Tumor Study Group Protocol 6584. J Clin Oncol 9:1105-1112, 1991.
31. Fuhrman GM, Curley SA, Hohn DC, et al. improved staging with intraoperative ultrasound and portal lymph node assessment improves survival following resection of colorectal liver metastases. Ann Surg Oncol 2:537-541, 1995.
32. Kemeny MM, Goldberg D, Metter GE, et al. Hepatic resection and regional perfusion: A randomized protocol on the treatment of hepatic metastases. Contr Oncol 29:143-156, 1988.
33. Ensminger W, Neiderhuber J, Dakill S, et al. Totally implanted drug delivery system for hepatic arterial chemotherapy. Cancer Treat Rep 65:393-398, 1981.
34. Kemeny N, Daly J, Reichman B, et al. Intrahepatic or systemic infusion of fluorodeoxyuridine in patients with liver metastases from colorectal carcinoma. Ann Intern Med 107:459-465, 1987.
35. Chang AE, Schneider PD, Sugarbaker PH, et al. A prospective randomized trial of regional versus systemic continuous 5-fluorodeoxyuridine chemotherapy in the treatment of colorectal liver metastases. Ann Surg 206:685-693, 1989.
36. Hohn DC, Stagg RJ, Friedman MA, et al. A randomized trial for continuous intravenous versus hepatic intra-arterial floxuridine in patients with colorectal cancer metastatic to the liver. The Northern California Oncology Group Trial. J Clin Oncol 7:1646-1654, 1989.
37. Martin LK, O'Connell MJ, Wieand HS, et al. Intra-arterial floxuridine versus system fluorouracil for hepatic metastases from colorectal cancer. Arch Surg 125:1022-1027, 1990.
38. Rougier P, Laplanche A, Hugier M, et al. Hepatic arterial infusion of floxuridine in patients with liver metastases from colorectal carcinoma: Long-term results of a prospective randomized trial. J Clin Oncol 10:1112-1118, 1992.
39. Stagg RJ, Venook AP, Chase JL, et al. Alternating hepatic intra-arterial floxuridine and fluorouracil: A less toxic regimen for treatment of liver metastases from colorectal cancer. J Natl Cancer Inst 83:423-428, 1991.

40. Hohn DC, Stagg RJ, Price DC, et al. Avoidance of gastroduodenal toxicity in patients receiving hepatic arterial 5-fluoro-2 deoxyuridine. J Clin Oncol 3:1257-1260, 1985.
41. Curley SA, Hohn DC, Roh MS. Hepatic artery infusion pumps: Cannulation techniques and other surgical considerations. Langenbecks Arch Chir 375:119-124, 1990.
42. Ludwig J, Kim CH, Weisner RH, et al. Floxuridine-induced sclerosing cholangitis: An ischemic cholangiopathy? Hepatology 9:215-218, 1989.
43. Curley SA, Chase JL, Roh MS, et al. Technical considerations and complications associated with the placement of 180 implantable hepatic arterial infusion devices. Surgery 114: 928-935, 1993.
44. Ketcham AS, Hoye RC, Pilch YH, et al. Delayed intestinal obstruction following treatment for cancer. Cancer 25:406-410, 1970.
45. Osteen RT, Guyton S, Steele G, et al. Malignant intestinal obstruction. Surgery 87:611-615, 1980.
46. Spears H, Petrelli NJ, Herrera L, et al. Treatment of bowel obstruction after operation for colorectal carcinoma. Am J Surg 155:383-386, 1988.
47. Lightdale CJ, Kurtz RC, Boyle CC, et al. Cancer and upper gastrointestinal tract hemorrhage: Benign causes of bleeding demonstrated by endoscopy. JAMA 226:139-141, 1973.
48. Wade DS, Douglass H, Nava HR, et al. Abdominal pain in neutropenic patients. Arch Surg 125:1119-1127, 1990.
49. Vas WG, Seelig R, Mahanta B, et al. Neutropenic colitis: Evaluation with computed tomography. J Comput Tomogr 12:211-215, 1988.
50. Alt B, Glass NR, Sollinger H. Neutropenic enterocolitis in adults. Review of the literature and assessment of surgical intervention. Am J Surg 149:405-408, 1985.
51. Mower WJ, Hawkins JA, Nelson EW. Neutropenic enterocolitis in adults with acute leukemia. Arch Surg 121:571-574, 1986.
52. Vanek VW, Al-Salti M. Acute pseudoobstruction of the colon (Oglivie's syndrome). An analysis of 400 cases. Dis Colon Rectum 29:203-310, 1986.
53. Wojtalik RS, Lindenauer SM, Kahn SS. Perforation of the colon associated with adynamic ileus. Am J Surg 125:601-606, 1973.
54. Dudley HAG, Patterson-Brown S. Pseudoobstruction. Br Med J 292:1157-1158, 1986.
55. Spira IA, Wolff WI. Gangrene and spontaneous perforation of the cecum as a complication of pseudoobstruction of the colon. Dis Colon Rectum 19:557-562, 1976.
56. Geelhoed GW. Colonic pseudoobstruction in surgical patients. Am J Surg 149:258-265, 1985.
57. Nano D, Prindiville T, Pauly M, et al. Colonoscopic therapy of acute pseudoobstruction of the colon. Am J Gastroenterol 82:145-148, 1987.
58. Martin FM, Robinson AM, Thompson WR. Therapeutic colonoscopy in the treatment of colonic pseudoobstruction. Am Surg 54:519-522, 1988.
59. Sariego J, Bootorabi B, Matsumoto T, et al. Major long-term complications in 1,422 permanent venous access devices. Am J Surg 165:249-251, 1993.
60. Henriques HF, Karmy-Jones R, Knoll SM, et al. Avoiding complications of long-term venous access. Am Surg 59:555-558, 1993.
61. Puel V, Caudry M, Le Metayer P, et al. Superior vena cava thrombosis related to catheter malposition in cancer chemotherapy given through implanted ports. Cancer 72:2248-2252, 1993.
62. Weinstein SM. Thrombolytic therapy. NITA 9:31-35, 1986.
63. Pizzo PA, Ladisch SL, Robichaud K. Treatment of gram-positive septicemia in cancer patients. Cancer 45:206-207, 1980.

64. Morow GR. Prevalence and correlates of anticipatory nausea and vomiting in chemotherapy patients. J Natl Cancer Inst 66:1601-1604, 1982.
65. Sridhar KS, Donnelly E. Combination antiemetics for cisplatin chemotherapy. Cancer 61: 1508-1517, 1988.
66. Carey MP, Burish TG, Brenner DE. Delta-9-tetrahydrocannabinol in cancer chemotherapy: Research problems and issues. Ann Intern Med 99:106-114, 1983.
67. Marty M, Pouillart P, Scholl S, et al. Comparison of the 5-hydroxytryptamine (serotonin) antagonist ondansetron (GR 38032F) with high-dose metoclopramide in the control of cisplatin-induced emesis. N Engl J Med 322:816-821, 1990.
68. DeMulder PHM, Seynaeve C, Vermorker JB, et al. Ondansetron compared with high-dose metoclopramide in prophylaxis of acute and delayed cisplatin-induced nausea and vomiting: A multicenter, randomized, double-blinded, crossover study. Ann Intern Med 113:834-840, 1990.
69. Hainsworth J, Harvey W, Pendergrass K, et al. A single-blinded comparison of intravenous ondansetron, a selective serotonin antagonist, with intravenous metoclopramide in the prevention of nausea and vomiting associated with high-dose cisplatin chemotherapy. J Clin Oncol 9:721-728, 1991.
70. Cebon JS, Lieschke GJ. Granulocyte-macrophage colony-stimulating factor for cancer treatment. Oncology 51:177-188, 1994.
71. Gulati SC, Gopal R, Prowda JB, et al. Growth factors and hematopoietic recovery. Med Oncol 11:1-6, 1994.

CHAPTER 26

Limitations of Anal Physiologic Testing

ALAN E. TIMMCKE

Anorectal physiologic testing consists of techniques to objectively evaluate primarily the mechanisms of fecal continence. The tests used most frequently are anorectal manometry, pudendal nerve terminal motor latency, concentric needle EMG, single-fiber EMG, cine defecography, and colonic transit studies.[1] As time progresses, additional studies may be added or these core studies refined, but for now these tests represent the foundation on which most of our understanding of the physiologic mechanism of fecal continence is based. The following is a summary of current understanding of the mechanisms of fecal continence, commonly used methods for performing each of the above listed studies, observations concerning their limitations, and indications for their use.

MECHANISMS OF FECAL CONTINENCE

Fecal continence is defined as the ability to limit the passage of stool or flatus to a socially acceptable time and place. This definition implies a certain learned voluntary behavior. Physiologic testing is of limited usefulness in evaluating impairment of continence due to dementia or behavioral abnormalities. Perhaps only in those instances when a concomitant physiologic abnormality is suspected is physiologic testing warranted.

Learned voluntary control is primarily the function of the striated muscles of the anal canal, the external anal sphincter, and the puborectalis muscle. In addition to a degree of tonic activity, the external sphincter can be voluntarily contracted. Contraction of the external sphincter and puborectalis muscles results in a transient increase in the pressure required to open the anal canal, increasing the resistance to passage of stool or flatus.

Voluntary muscle contraction is necessary only when the involuntary or tonic anal canal resistance is threatened.[2] This tonic resistance is the opening pressure of the anal canal at rest, or the so-called resting pressure. The smooth muscle internal anal sphincter is responsible for approximately 70% to 85% of the resting pressure.[3-6] When the rectal wall is stretched, as occurs in rectal filling or inflation of a rectal balloon, the internal anal sphincter relaxes (Fig. 26-1, *D*). The greater the volume distending the rectum, the greater the amplitude and

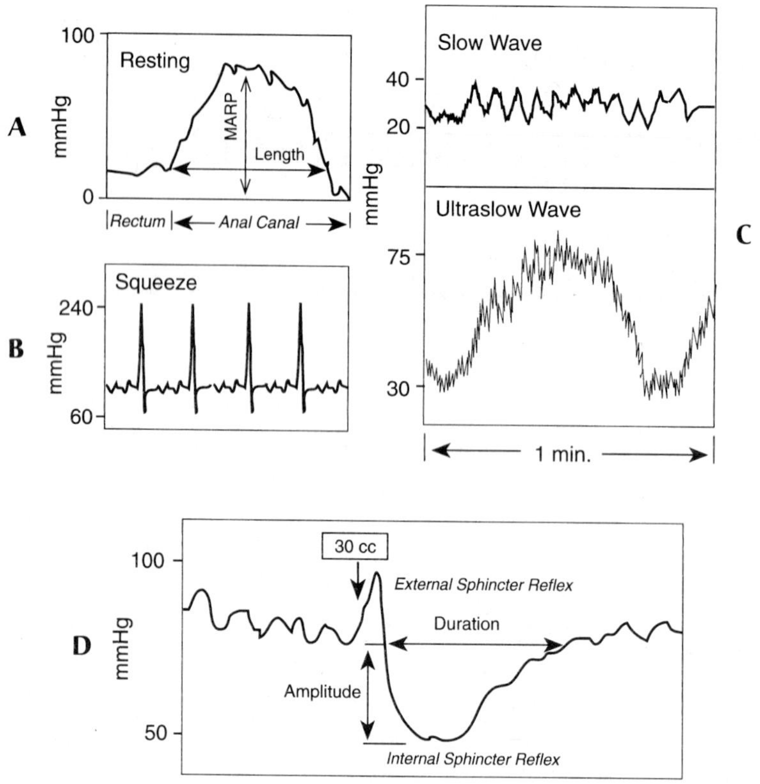

Fig. 26-1 **A**, Resting anal sphincter profile produced by continuous constant-speed pullout. **B**, Example of multiple squeeze pressures determined with the catheter stationary. **C**, Examples of the normal internal anal sphincter motility patterns measured with the catheter stationary within the anal high-pressure zone. Note the lower amplitude high-frequency slow waves and the higher amplitude low-frequency ultraslow waves. **D**, Typical rectoanal inhibitory reflex.

duration of internal sphincter relaxation. This phenomenon is known as the rectosphincteric reflex or rectoanal inhibitory reflex. In patients with normal fecal continence, the minimum volume producing rectal sensation corresponds closely with the volume necessary to produce detectable sphincter relaxation.[7,8] These characteristics have led to the rectosphincteric reflex being referred to teleologically as the "sampling reflex," or means by which the rectal contents can be allowed to descend into the more sensitive proximal anal canal where their nature, gas or otherwise, can be ascertained and a socially appropriate decision concerning expulsion rendered.

In addition, the contribution of the abdominal and diaphragmatic muscles, which voluntarily control intra-abdominal pressure, must be considered. Intrarectal pressure varies directly with intra-abdominal pressure. For normal defecation to occur, the internal anal sphincter must reflexly relax; the sensation of stool or gas within the rectum and anal canal must be perceived; the voluntary muscles of the anal canal must be inhibited; and the intrarectal pressure must be raised to exceed anal canal opening pressure by contraction of abdominal muscles.

ANORECTAL MANOMETRY

Various catheters, probes, and recording devices are used to perform anorectal manometry. Because of the variability of equipment and technique, the data obtained from different laboratories are not easily compared. Indeed, efforts to standardize measurement and reporting of anorectal physiologic indices have thus far been to no avail.[9] This has resulted in some confusion about the ability of anorectal manometry to objectively and consistently demonstrate physiologically significant abnormalities of the sphincter mechanism and to thus aid in decision making concerning treatment options. It is clear that over the last 30 years many refinements of manometric techniques have ensued, and a large number of studies have been performed in both healthy volunteers and patients with anorectal disorders. These findings, for the most part, have resulted in our current understanding of anorectal function in health and disease and will likely contribute to the development of future treatment options.

Methods

Hill et al.[10] in 1960 were the first to compare a water-filled, nonperfused, open-tipped catheter with microballoon probes for the measurement of the resting anal pressure profile. They found that lower pressures were recorded with the open-tipped catheter than with the balloon probes and that increasing the diameter of the microballoon increased the recorded pressure. The open-tipped, water-filled catheter described in their publication actually had a single side opening.

Harris et al.[11] in 1966 demonstrated the importance of perfusing the catheter with water to keep the small openings from being occluded by the tissues of the anal canal. They demonstrated that lack of perfusion resulted in measurement of pressures that were too low. In 1976, Hancock[12] demonstrated that the rate of perfusion was also important. If the catheter was perfused too slowly, the measured pressures were too low. Too rapid perfusion of the catheter can result in collection of water within the rectum and inadvertent lowering of anal resting pressure because of the rectoanal inhibitory reflex. In general, perfusion rates between 0.2 and 1.0 ml per channel per minute are considered optimal; most investigators select 0.5 or 0.6 ml per channel per minute.[12,13] Perfused catheters can have a single lumen with multiple radiating side holes attached to a single transducer or they can have multiple lumens with each channel having its own side opening and a separate transducer. These multichannel catheters usually have from 2 to 8 channels arranged radially, either concentrically or longitudinally. In addition to the perfusion rate, the diameter of the catheter affects the measured pressure during both resting and squeeze. Using regression analysis, Rasmussen[14] demonstrated a positive correlation between the diameter of the probe and the maximum resting pressure. His data were taken from 20 published studies from 16 different centers involving a total of 693 control subjects. By analyzing data from 14 published studies from 10 different centers involving a total of 530 control subjects, he was able to demonstrate a similar but less significant finding for the maximum squeezing pressure. In general, the optimum catheter diameter is considered to be less than 0.5 cm.

Resting anal sphincter pressure profiles can be obtained by either continuous pull-through technique at rates of 1 to 8 mm/sec or station pull-through technique at intervals of 0.5 to 1.0 cm. The continuous pull-through technique using synchronized rates of withdrawal and recording, generally 1.0 mm/sec or greater, offers the advantage of producing a real-time recording of the anal high-pressure zone[13] (see Fig. 26-1, *A*). Although any movement of measurement devices within the anal canal may produce elevations in the recorded pressure by stimulating the reflex contraction of the external sphincter, continuous pull-through techniques have not been shown to substantially increase measured pressures.[13] Station pull-through techniques produce artifactual elevations of pressure that require a delay at each station before initiating recording.[15] These delays, unless perfectly uniform, make accurate determination of anal sphincter length impossible.

In the additional method of determining anal sphincter pressures, water-filled microballoons 2 to 10 mm in diameter are generally withdrawn with a station pull-through technique. As with catheters and probes, a correlation with the diameter of the balloon and the magnitude of the measured resting pressure would be expected. In his review, Rasmussen[14] was unable to demonstrate any such relationship. Perhaps the deformability of the balloon reduces the variability over the narrow range of balloon diameters used. The disadvantage of balloon catheters is that they have no directionality and their deformability causes asymmetry to be ignored within the anal canal. Also the distensibility and compliance of the balloon itself contributes to the total pressure measurement and must be taken into account.[13]

More recently, microtransducer catheters have been advocated for the study of anal canal pressures. Multiple transducers can be mounted radially, either concentrically or longitudinally, similar to perfused catheters, and have the theoretical advantage of being able to measure the pressure directly within the anal canal without having to transmit the pressure through a water-filled tube, which by its resistance may reduce the recorded pressure. An advantage is that microtransducers have enabled continuous ambulatory pressure recordings. Their disadvantages are that they are expensive, fragile, and of a larger diameter than a perfused catheter with a comparable number of channels.

Krogh-Pedersen and Christiansen,[16] in a study of 78 healthy volunteers, demonstrated that the intraindividual variation in the length of the high-pressure zone, resting pressure, and squeeze pressure was 10 mm, 26 mm Hg, and 65 mm Hg, respectively. They believed that most of the intraindividual variation could be accounted for by the effects of "slow waves" or "ultraslow waves," that is, the normal variations of anal pressure observed during measurements of anal motility (see Fig. 26-1, *C*). These normal variations in resting pressure from one measurement to the next may account for some of the lack of agreement between investigators and should be controlled for by obtaining a sufficient number of measurements. Krogh-Pedersen and Christiansen, as well as others,[17-20] have also demonstrated gender, parity, and age-related variations. In general, maximal resting and squeeze pressures are greater in men than in women and tend to decrease with aging in both. In women, maximal resting and squeeze pressures also tend to decrease with increasing parity. Taylor et al.[21] demonstrated in 18 healthy volunteers consistent radial and longitudinal variations in pressure along the anal canal. They found lower pressures anteriorly in the proximal anal canal and posteriorly in the distal anal canal. In an anal manometry study of patients with fecal incontinence, nearly 40% of patients had maximum resting pressures and maximum squeeze pressures within the normal range.[18] These findings only underscore that fecal continence is not related only to anal sphincter pressures. Thus, for anorectal manometric studies to have any degree of comparability, these variables must be anticipated in both study design and results reporting.

Our preference is to use continuous pull-through to determine the resting sphincter pressure profile and anal sphincter length, station pull-through to measure the maximal squeeze pressure, and a stationary catheter to determine the rectoanal inhibitory reflex and minimum rectal sensory volume (Fig. 26-2). We use two catheters, both four-channel perfused with side ports arranged radially at 90 degrees to one another (Fig. 26-3). The 3.6 mm catheter, with its side ports located 5 cm from the tip, is used for continuous pull-through to measure resting pressure and sphincter length and for station pull-through to measure squeeze pressure. Absence of a balloon on this catheter eliminates the tendency of the deflated balloon to torque the catheter and displace the measurement orifices. The 4.6 mm catheter, with a 150 ml balloon at its tip and the side ports located 10 cm from the tip, is used to demonstrate the rectoanal inhibitory reflex and to determine the minimum rectal sensory volume.

Indications

Indications for anorectal manometry include the following:

1. To evaluate patients with chronic constipation, particularly children and young adults, for absence of the rectoanal inhibitory reflex, which suggests the presence of Hirschsprung's disease

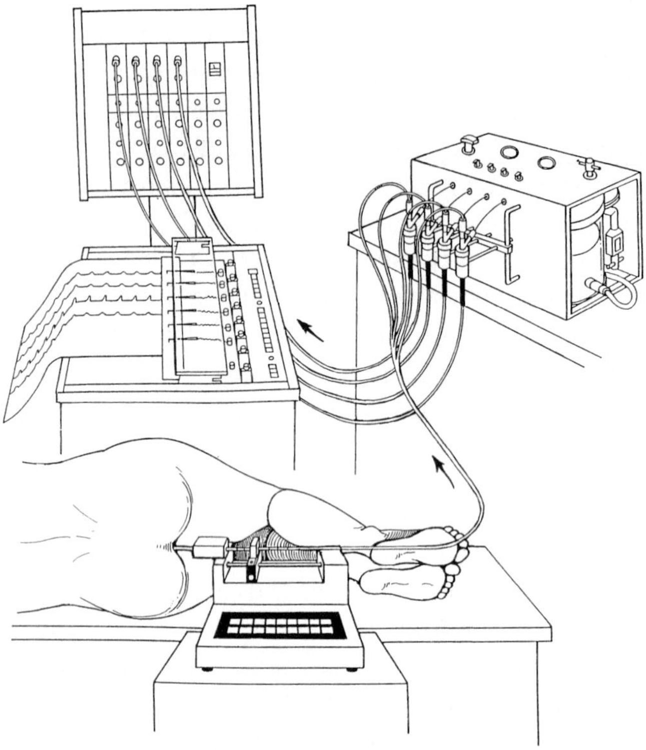

Fig. 26-2 Anal manometry system consisting of a catheter withdrawn by a small motor, perfused by a water perfusion device, and attached to multiple transducers that transmit to a recording device. (Redrawn from Smith LE. Practical Guide to Anorectal Testing, 2nd ed. New York: Igaku-Shoin, 1995.)

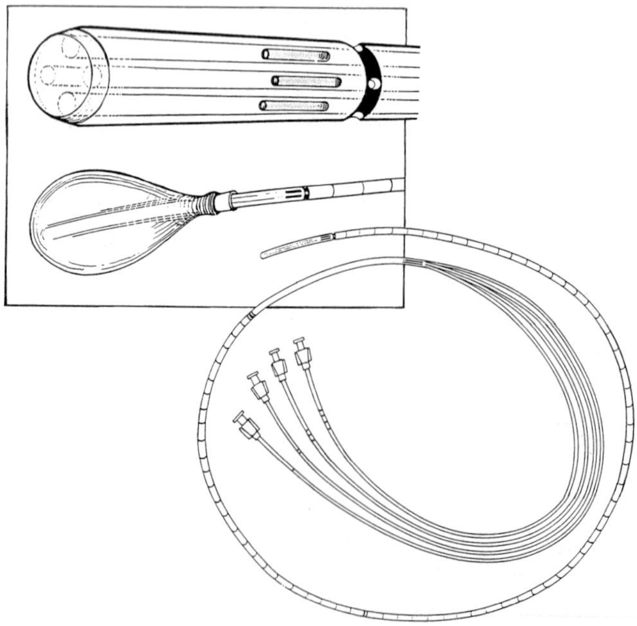

Fig. 26-3 Typical four-channeled water perfusion catheter. *Inset:* Catheters with and without a balloon tip. (Redrawn from Smith LE. Practical Guide to Anorectal Testing, 2nd ed. New York: Igaku-Shoin, 1995.)

2. To document the level of anorectal function before performance of procedures that affect continence or in which the outcome would be adversely affected by less than perfect continence
3. To locate and quantify a sphincter defect after injury, whether obstetric, surgical, or traumatic (probably more accurately determined by endoanal ultrasonography)
4. To assess the contribution of the neural and muscular components necessary for fecal continence, to determine the most effective treatment for incontinence

ELECTROMYOGRAPHY

Anal sphincter EMG was first reported by Beck in 1930.[22] EMG is the recording of electrical activity generated by muscle fibers. Electrical activity can be measured either during voluntary contraction or at rest (Fig. 26-5). Specifically, EMG is used to evaluate muscles whose nerve supply may have been damaged. In pelvic floor disorders and disorders of fecal continence, EMG can be performed on the external sphincter or the puborectalis muscles. The electrical activity within the muscle can be recorded with surface electrodes, concentric needle electrodes, or single-fiber electrodes. Measurement of the amplitude, duration, and number of phases of motor unit action potentials generates information about the innervation and functional state of the motor units within a particular muscle. A motor unit is all of the individual muscle fibers innervated by a single axon or anterior horn cell. In gravitational muscles the number of muscle fibers per motor unit is large (e.g., 100 to 200), and in muscles necessary for precise motor functions the number of fibers per motor unit is small (e.g., 6 to 10).

Surface Electromyography

Measurement of muscle electrical activity with a surface electrode is a rather crude and imprecise method to assess the integrity of motor units. Surface electrodes are usually applied in pairs overlying the muscle to be studied, with a ground electrode placed at some distance. With surface EMG, because the electrodes are at a distance from the muscle activity, it is not always possible to be sure the electrical activity being measured is occurring within the muscle closest to the electrodes. This lack of sensitivity makes surface EMG less accurate than conventional needle EMG. Surface EMG is particularly useful to determine nerve conduction velocity, as in pudendal nerve terminal motor latency, when the nerve to the muscle being studied is being directly stimulated. Also, surface EMG techniques, because of their simplicity and painlessness, are useful in continuous ambulatory monitoring and biofeedback therapy.

Pudendal Nerve Terminal Motor Latency

Pudendal nerve terminal motor latency is a technique by which the innervation of the perianal and periurethral striated muscles can be evaluated. The pudendal nerve originates from the ventral roots of S_2 through S_4 and gives rise to terminal branches, the inferior rectal nerve and the perineal nerve, which innervate the external anal and periurethral sphincters, respectively. With an electrode placed over a gloved finger, the examiner can stimulate the pudendal nerve transrectally as it passes the ischial spine, penetrates the pelvic floor, and passes into Alcock's canal (Fig. 26-4). The length of time in milliseconds from stimulation of the nerve to contraction of the sphincter muscle can be measured by means of surface electrodes mounted at the base of the intra-anal finger. Normal pudendal nerve terminal motor latency is 2.1 ± 0.2 msec and increases with age, as does motor unit potential duration and fiber density.[23] Prolonged pudendal nerve terminal motor latency indicates the pudendal nerve is intact but has sustained some form of injury such as traction, degeneration, or compression. Snooks et al.,[24] using both pudendal nerve terminal motor latency and single fiber EMG showed that routine vaginal delivery injured the innervation of the external sphincter (pudendal nerves) that was both persistent and may worsen over time. Recently a disposable one-piece stimulating and recording electrode has been made commercially available (Dantec Medical, Inc., Houston, Tx.). It is as effective[25] and causes less discomfort[26] than the original St. Mark's reusable electrode. Still, the technique requires considerable practice to produce consistent results, and the occasional obese or muscular patient may be impossible to study because of anatomic constraints.

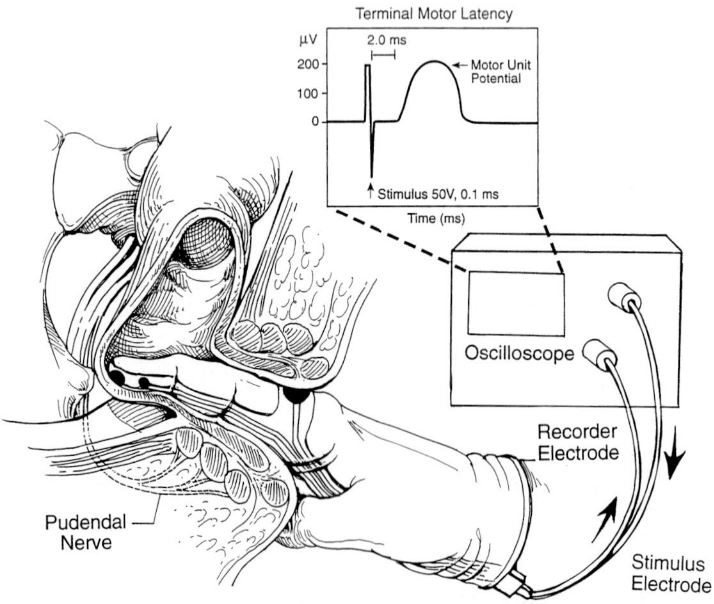

Fig. 26-4 Determination of pudendal nerve terminal motor latency.

Indications

Indications for pudendal nerve terminal motor latency include the following:

1. To evaluate anal sphincter injury secondary to parturition, trauma, or surgery before attempts at repair
2. To evaluate idiopathic fecal incontinence or idiopathic urinary incontinence to aid in selection of therapeutic options
3. To evaluate pelvic floor abnormalities such as rectal prolapse, perineal descent, and solitary rectal ulcer to determine the likelihood of incontinence after surgical treatment

Concentric Needle Electromyography

Needle electrodes allow selective recording within the muscle of interest. In concentric needle EMG, the electrode consists of a fine 0.1-mm steel wire within a larger beveled needle from which it is insulated by a nonconducting material. The inner wire has a small surface area at its tip that ensures that the electrical activity being measured is from the muscle into which the needle has been inserted. In concentric needle EMG, the important parameters are amplitude, duration, number of phases, and firing rate. These parameters vary with electrode position and depend on the filtering settings of the amplifier (Fig. 26-5). Bartolo et al.,[27] using trigger and delay techniques and changing filter characteristics, identified individual motor unit potentials. In general, the longer the duration and the greater the number of phases in the action potential, the more likely the muscle has undergone denervation and reinnervation. The motor unit potential duration varies greatly in healthy persons and increases gradually with age. Insertion of the needles is painful, the necessary equipment is expensive, and the technique requires a great deal of patience and experience to master. The denervation and reinnervation characteristics of the anal sphincter muscle can probably be more accurately measured with single-fiber EMG when it is available.[23]

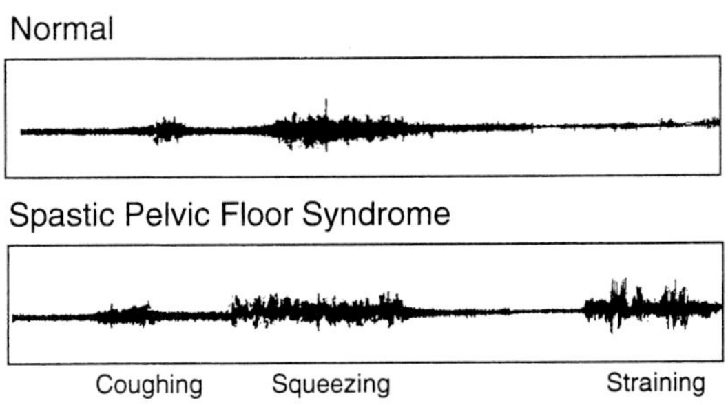

Fig. 26-5 Conventional concentric needle EMG of the puborectalis muscle in a healthy volunteer and a patient with nonrelaxing puborectalis form of disordered defecation.

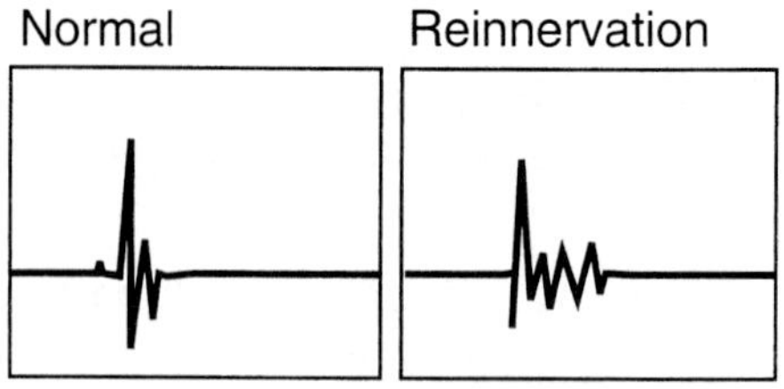

Fig. 26-6 Single-fiber EMG shows normal and reinnervation patterns.

Single-Fiber Electromyography

With a much smaller recording surface area (25 μm) located on the side of the recording needle, single-fiber EMG can record individual muscle fiber action potentials. During muscle reinnervation, the muscle fibers that have lost their axon are recruited by surviving axons, thereby increasing the number of individual muscle fibers per motor unit and the density of muscle fibers within the electrode uptake area (270 μm). This results in increased fiber density, which is manifested by an increased number of components or phases in the recorded motor unit potentials (Fig. 26-6). Each component represents the electrical activity of a nearby muscle fiber. Increased fiber density is a useful indicator of muscle reinnervation. Increased fiber density in the external anal sphincter is seen in some patients with fecal incontinence and is indicative of nerve injury, suggestive of a poor result from muscle repair.[28] The technique of single-fiber EMG is highly demanding in both time and fastidiousness. The mean fiber density is derived from 20 recordings, which requires frequent repositioning of the needle and approximately four or five skin puncture sites. All potentials containing any component of amplitude greater than 100 μV must be included in the calculation. As with concentric needle EMG, the equipment is expensive, and results are related to the patience and experience of the examiner.

Indications

Indications for EMG include the following:

1. To provide information about the denervation and reinnervation of the muscles of continence in patients with fecal incontinence, urinary incontinence, or both
2. To map the anal sphincter in children with atresia and in adults undergoing reconstruction after trauma
3. To investigate pelvic floor disorders such as rectal prolapse, solitary rectal ulcer syndrome, perineal descent, anal pain, and functional outlet obstruction

DEFECOGRAPHY

Defecography is a radiologic study popularized by Mahieu et al.[29] in which thickened barium is introduced into the rectum and the patient is seated on a radiolucent commode and instructed to evacuate the contrast material. A video recording of the fluoroscopic monitor taken in the lateral projection is then made. Defecography is particularly useful in the evaluation of tenesmus, feelings of anal blockage, incomplete evacuation, or in patients requiring digital pressure or manipulation to defecate. Features such as rectocele, enterocele, excessive perineal descent, internal intussusception, occult rectal prolapse, prominent puborectalis impression, and inability to evacuate can be identified. A number of these findings have been reported in persons without defecation disorders.[30,31] Presently the significance of many of the "abnormal" findings seen at defecography is unclear.

COLONIC TRANSIT STUDIES

Colonic transit studies require patients to ingest radiopaque markers while receiving a normal diet, without using laxatives. Serial radiographs are taken at specified intervals to determine the speed with which the markers traverse the colon.[32-34] Marker transit techniques have been used to determine parameters of bowel motility in healthy persons.[33] Even techniques that allow calculation of normal rates of colonic transit in various segments of the colon have been described.[34] Despite the seeming ease with which such studies can be performed, their interpretation is subject to a number of errors. If patients are not viewed swallowing the markers, their subsequent absence from abdominal radiographs cannot be interpreted to mean the patient has passed them. Variations in the size, shape, and specific gravity of the markers affect their rate of colonic transit.[32] Even with a standard marker, a great deal of intraindividual variation, ranging from 14 to 51 hours, has been described.[32] Other patient-related factors that occur during the study, such as whether laxatives are used, the amount of fiber ingested, or the patient's level of activity, affect the measurement of transit times.[32-34]

CONCLUSION

Manometric, electrophysiologic, and radiologic techniques used in combination provide important basic information necessary to understand anorectal and pelvic floor disorders. Whether any of these tests are mandatory and under what circumstances is a contentious issue. Indeed, an experienced colorectal surgeon can obtain as much information about anorectal sphincter function from a digital examination as from anorectal manometry.[35] What is equally true is that not every clinician's digit is connected to the same objective recording device. Despite whatever shortcomings today's anorectal physiologic tests appear to exhibit in terms of sensitivity, specificity, ability to predict the natural history of a disorder, and the likely outcome of surgery,[36] they currently represent the only means by which objective information about coloanal function can be obtained. Physiologic tests provide objective data that can confirm the clinical impression of an experienced clinician, occasionally alter treatment, and produce important medicolegal documentation. Recognition of the limitations of physiologic testing allows for more precise indications and a better understanding of the usefulness of the results.[37] Combined manometric, electrophysiologic, radiographic, and functional studies of anorectal physiology will eventually achieve great clinical importance in the management of fecal incontinence and disorders of defecation.

REFERENCES

1. Karulf RE, Coller JA, Bartolo DCC, Bowden DO, Roberts PL, Murray JJ, Schoetz DJ Jr, Veidenheimer MC. Anorectal physiology testing; A survey of availability and use. Dis Colon Rectum 34:464-468, 1991.
2. Dalley AF II. The riddle of the sphincters: The morphophysiology of the anorectal mechanism reviewed. Am Surg 53:298-306, 1987.
3. Lestar B, Penninckx F, Kerremans RP. The composition of anal basal pressure. An in vivo and in vitro study in man. Int J Colorectal Dis 4:118-122, 1989.
4. Duthie HL, Watts JM. Contribution of the external anal sphincter to the pressure zone in the anal canal. Gut 6:64-68, 1965.
5. Frenckner B, Euler C. Influence of pudendal block on the function of the anal sphincters. Gut 16:482-489, 1975.
6. Schweiger M. Method for determining individual contributions of voluntary and involuntary anal sphincters to resting tone. Dis Colon Rectum 22:415-416, 1979.
7. Hoffmann BA, Timmcke AE, Gathright JB Jr, Hicks TC, Opelka FG, Beck DE. Fecal seepage and soiling: A problem of rectal sensation. Dis Colon Rectum 38:746-748, 1995.
8. Sun WM, Read NW, Miner PB. Relation between rectal sensation and anal function in normal subjects and patients with faecal incontinence. Gut 31:1056-1061, 1990.
9. Keighley MRB, Henry MM, Bartolo DC, Mortensen NJ. Anorectal physiology measurement: Report of a working party. Br J Surg 76:356-357, 1989.
10. Hill JR, Kelley ML, Schlegel JF, Code CF. Pressure profile of the rectum and anus of healthy persons. Dis Colon Rectum 3:203-209, 1960.
11. Harris LD, Winans CS, Pope CE II. Determination of yield pressures: A method for measuring anal sphincter competence. Gastroenterology 50:754-760, 1966.
12. Hancock BD. Measurement of anal pressure and motility. Gut 17:645-651, 1976.
13. Coller JA. Clinical application of anorectal manometry. Gastroenterol Clin North Am 16: 17-33, 1987.
14. Rasmussen OO. Anorectal function. Dis Colon Rectum 37:386-403, 1994.
15. Read NW, Bannister JJ. Anorectal manometry techniques in health and anorectal disease. In Henry M, Swash M, eds. Coloproctology and the Pelvic Floor: Pathophysiology and Management. London: Butterworth, 1985, pp 70-71.

16. Krogh-Pedersen I, Christiansen J. A study of the physiological variation in anal manometry. Br J Surg 76:69-70, 1989.
17. Leoning-Baucke V, Anuras S. Effects of age and sex on anorectal manometry. Am J Gastroenterol 80:50-53, 1985.
18. McHugh SM, Diamant NE. Effects of age, gender, and parity on anal canal pressures. Dig Dis Sci 32:726-736, 1987.
19. Eckardt VF, Elmer T. Reliability of anal pressure measurements. Dis Colon Rectum 34:72-77, 1991.
20. Cali RL, Blatchford GJ, Perry RE, Pitsch RM, Thorson AG, Christensen MA. Normal variation in anorectal manometry. Dis Colon Rectum 35:1161-1164, 1992.
21. Taylor BM, Beart RW Jr, Phillips SF. Longitudinal and radial variations in pressure in the human anal sphincter. Gastroenterology 86:693-697, 1984.
22. Beck A. Electromyographische untersuchungen am Sphincter ani. Pflugers Arch 224:278-292, 1930.
23. Swash M, Snooks SJ. Electromyography in pelvic floor disorders. In Henry M, Swash M, eds. Coloproctology and the Pelvic Floor: Pathophysiology and Management. London: Butterworth, 1985, pp 94-95.
24. Snooks SJ, Swash M, Mathers SE, Henry MM. Effect of vaginal delivery on the pelvic floor: A 5-year follow-up. Br J Surg 77:1358-1360, 1990.
25. Rogers J, Henry MM, Misiewicz JJ. Disposable pudendal nerve stimulator: Evaluation of the standard instrument and new device. Gut 29:1131-1133, 1988.
26. Parks TG. The usefulness of tests in anorectal disease. World J Surg 16:804-810, 1992.
27. Bartolo DCC, Jarratt JA, Read NW. The use of conventional electromyography to assess external anal sphincter neuropathy in man. J Neurol Neurosurg Psychiatry 46:1115-1118, 1983.
28. Neill ME, Swash M. Increased motor unit fibre density in the external anal sphincter muscle in ano-rectal incontinence: A single fibre EMG study. J Neurol Neurosurg Psychiatry 43:343-347, 1980.
29. Mahieu P, Pringot J, Bodart P. Defecography. II. Contribution to the diagnosis of defecation disorders. Gastrointest Radiol 9:253-261, 1984.
30. Jones PN, Lubowski DZ, Henry MM, Swash M. Is paradoxical contraction of puborectalis muscle of functional importance? Dis Colon Rectum 30:667-670, 1987.
31. Stevenson GW, Shorvon PJ. Proctography [symposium]. Int J Colorectal Dis 3:67-89, 1988.
32. Hinton JM, Lennard-Jones JE, Young AC. A new method for studying gut transit times using radioopaque markers. Gut 10:842-847, 1969.
33. Martelli H, Devroede G, Arhan P, Duguay C, Dornic C, Faverdin C. Some parameters of large bowel motility in normal man. Gastroenterology 75:612-618, 1978.
34. Metcalf AM, Phillips SF, Zinsmeister AR, MacCarty RL, Beart RW, Wolff BG. Simplified assessment of segmental colonic transit. Gastroenterology 92:40-47, 1987.
35. Hallan RI, Marzouk DEM, Waldron DJ, Womack NR, Williams NS. Comparison of digital and manometric assessment of anal sphincter function. Br J Surg 76:973-975, 1989.
36. O'Kelly TJ, Mortensen NJ. Tests of anorectal function [editorial]. Br J Surg 79:988-989, 1992.
37. Wexner SD, Jorge JMN. Colorectal physiological tests: Use or abuse of technology? Eur J Surg 160:167-174, 1994.

CHAPTER 27

Surgery for Constipation

MICHAEL P. SPENCER
DAVID A. ROTHENBERGER

Constipation remains a complex, variably defined condition for which the cause and pathophysiology are poorly understood. Despite advances in our understanding of gastrointestinal physiology and the availability of more sophisticated studies such as transit time and intestinal motility, our ability to characterize specific disorders remains limited. Surgical management is often a last resort and is based more often on our inability to effect change with medical intervention than our understanding of the disease process itself. Thus it should not be surprising that the success of surgical management remains variable, regardless of the procedure used.

Timely surgical intervention, on the other hand, should not be denied to the small subset of patients with incapacitating constipation refractory to conservative measures but amenable to surgical intervention. These highly symptomatic patients are vulnerable to the complications of chronic constipation, including dilatation of proximal bowel, occasionally resulting in volvulus; chronic straining that predisposes to procidentia of the rectum; and stercoral ulceration with potential perforation with peritonitis.

INCIDENCE

It is estimated that more than 4 million persons in the United States have chronic constipation and that nearly one third of the healthy population experiences occasional difficulty, making constipation the most common digestive disorder.[1,2] Constipation is two to three times more common in women than in men, and it increases in frequency in the sixth and seventh decades of life. The current demographic trend of an aging population suggests this is likely to become a more common health concern.

More than half of patients with chronic constipation are prescribed cathartics and laxatives annually. According to the National Hospital Discharge Survey, nearly 1000 patients die each year of diseases associated with or related to constipation.[3] These statistics provide some insight into the personal and economic burden of this disease process.

DEFINITION

Constipation is a subjective condition that may be defined as having fewer than three bowel movements per week[4] or straining with defecation more than 25% of the time.[5] Stool volume and frequency are altered by a number of factors, including age, gender, personality, and diet. Stool weight, transit time, and frequency of defecation correlate strongly with dietary fiber. Because the average daily consumption of fiber in the United States is less than 20 g, the prevalence of constipation is not surprising.[6,7]

CAUSES

Mechanical causes of constipation are usually easy to diagnose, but more often constipation is associated with other factors, including a wide variety of pharmacologic agents and numerous endocrine, neurologic, and systemic diseases (see the box). After eliminating these specific causes, one is left with a group of patients with constipation of unclear cause, or idiopathic constipation (Table 27-1). Five subgroups have been increasingly recognized as clinically and physiologically distinct: normal transit or functional constipation, pelvic floor dysfunction or outlet obstruction, colonic inertia or slow-transit constipation, generalized intestinal dysmotility, and idiopathic megabowel.[8-11] Differentiating these subtypes is diagnostically feasible in most patients and likely to have therapeutic implications (Table 27-1). The remainder of this chapter is restricted to discussion of the diagnosis and management of idiopathic constipation.

Normal-transit constipation is most often diagnosed in patients with poor dietary habits or a psychological profile as yet poorly defined that results in functional constipation. There may be some underlying lack of coordination of gut motility, as observed in patients with irritable bowel syndrome, but these patients have no demonstrable transit delay or pelvic floor dysfunction. Despite the lack of objective abnormalities, they remain clinically symptomatic. In the vast majority of these patients, constipation can be managed with dietary alterations, counseling, and bowel regimens. This group should undergo surgical intervention only as a last resort, because they generally will fail to achieve satisfactory long-term success.

Outlet obstruction is associated with both physiologic and anatomic factors that create a functional blockage of stool in the distal rectum or anal canal and alter evacuation. Anorectal manometry and cinedefecography have greatly facilitated the diagnosis of occult and overt procidentia of the rectum, paradoxic puborectalis activity, and the associated pelvic floor problems of rectocele, cystocele,

EXTRACOLONIC CAUSES OF CONSTIPATION

Mechanical

Neoplasm
Stricture (iatrogenic, inflammatory, ischemic)
Volvulus
Hernia
Endometriosis

Pharmacologic

Narcotic agents
Anticholinergic agents
Antidepressant drugs
Antacids
Iron
Barium
Metallic intoxication
Antiparkinsonian agents
Alpha-adrenergic agonists
Calcium channel blockers
Anesthetics
Paralytic agents

Endocrine

Hypothyroidism
Hypopituitarism
Pheochromocytoma
Pregnancy
Diabetes mellitus
Parathyroid dysfunction

Neurologic

CNS
Alzheimer's disease
Stroke
Tumors
Parkinson's disease

Spinal
Iatrogenic
Tumors
Trauma
Multiple sclerosis
Myelocele
Damage to nervi erigentes

Peripheral
Chagas' disease
Autonomic neuropathy
Aganglionosis
von Recklinghausen's disease
Hirschsprung's disease

Systemic

Systemic lupus
Amyloidosis
Scleroderma
Uremia
Hypokalemia
Hypercalcemia
Porphyria

Table 27-1 Idiopathic constipation

Category	Characteristics	Treatment options
1. Normal transit or functional constipation	No pathophysiologic characteristics	Diet alterations (increased fiber and water) Counseling (e.g., stress control, exercise) Bowel regimens
2. Pelvic floor dysfunction or outlet obstruction	Procidentia of rectum Paradoxic puborectalis Rectocele Cystocele Enterocele Hypertonia of anal sphincter	Biofeedback Specific operations for diagnosed conditions (e.g., procidentia repair, rectocele repair, sphincterotomy)
3. Colonic inertia or slow-transit constipation	Delayed colonic transit Normal pelvic floor function Normal upper GI motility	Same as category 1 Total colectomy with ileorectal anastomosis Ileostomy Ileal pouch–anal anastomosis
4. Generalized intestinal dysmotility	Delayed colonic and GI transit Normal pelvic floor	Same as category 1 Total colectomy with ileorectal anastomosis
5. Idiopathic megabowel	Dilated rectum Dilated colon Dilated colorectum Dolichocolon ±Delayed transit ±Pelvic floor dysfunction	Segmental colectomy with coloanal anastomosis

and enterocele (Fig. 27-1). An occasional patient has severe hypertonia characterized by extremely high resting pressures and a long anal canal high-pressure zone. Some of these conditions are amenable to medical treatment such as biofeedback; others require surgical intervention.

Colonic inertia or slow-transit constipation is the result of altered colonic motility, which may be due to colonic atony and/or excessive smooth muscle activity. The latter could explain the occasional retrograde movement of feces typically observed in such cases. Colonic atony results in increased water absorption, leading to the formation of hard stool, which exacerbates the already delayed transit. This group of patients has generally responded favorably to resection, provided no other abnormalities are present.

Redmond et al.[11] recently identified a subgroup of patients with generalized intestinal dysmotility. They reported that fewer than half the patients with generalized intestinal dysmotility had long-term success following abdominal colectomy. This was significantly less than the success achieved after colectomy in patients with isolated colonic inertia. They recommended that patients identified with colonic inertia undergo complete examination of upper GI motility before surgical intervention. Generalized intestinal dysmotility is often not suspected, because colonic dysfunction typically dominates the clinical features. Occasionally patients will have clinically apparent esophageal or gastric symptoms, but unless manometric or myoelectric activity is assessed, the diffuse abnormality is easily overlooked. Esophageal, gastric, and small bowel motility is well characterized and can be assessed with commercially available devices, if suspected. The clinical relevance of these studies and their precise role in treatment selection remain controversial. It is conceivable that proximal gut motility is adversely affected by colonic resection, accounting for the apparent increase in symptoms after surgery. Alternatively, the underlying motility abnormality may simply continue to progress. To date, the cause of generalized intestinal dysmotility is poorly understood and remains a focus of investigation.

A final subset of patients with chronic constipation have megabowel, an uncommon condition in which a segment or occasionally the entire colon and rectum are dilated (Fig. 27-2). Megarectum is defined as a rectum exceeding 6.5 cm in diameter at the pelvic brim, whereas megacolon is defined as a colon with a diameter exceeding 10 cm in the sigmoid colon or 7 to 8 cm in the proximal colon. Megabowel may be associated with other disease processes, such as Hirschsprung's or Chagas' disease, a cauda equina lesion, and occasionally strictures, or may be idiopathic. To date, no specific physiologic or pathologic process has been identified to account for this condition; however, it is likely an acquired abnormality of neuromuscular origin.[13-15] Although symptoms may develop later in life, most patients have symptoms and seek attention in the first and second decades of life.

Another anatomic variant of megabowel is dolichocolon, a markedly redundant colon. No specific definition is available, and the surgeon must be cautioned

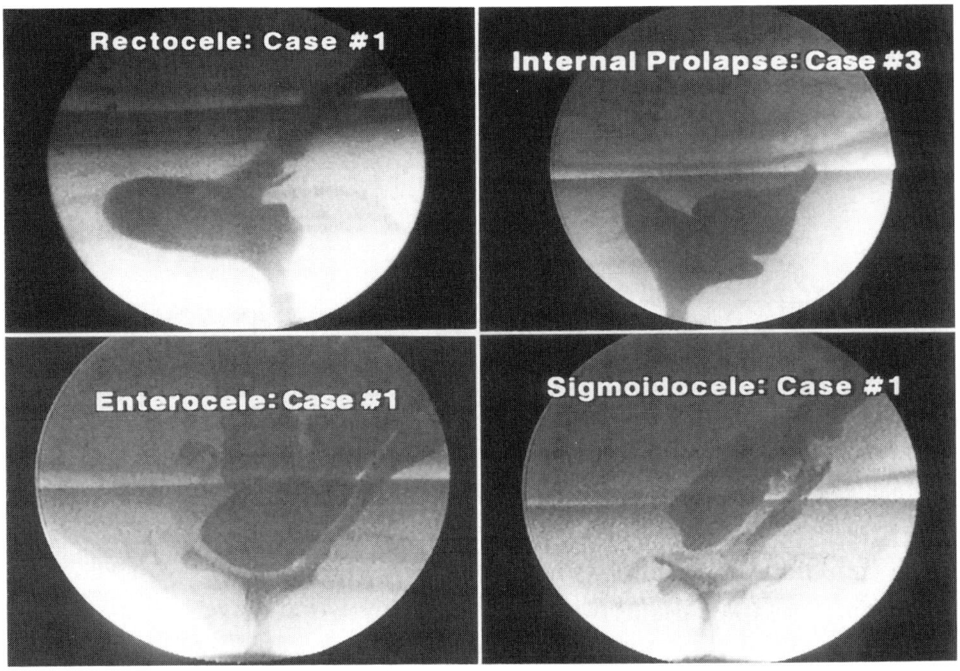

Fig. 27-1 Cine defecography can differentiate specific causes of constipation resulting from outlet obstruction. Four examples are shown: rectocele, internal prolapse, enterocele, and sigmoidocele.

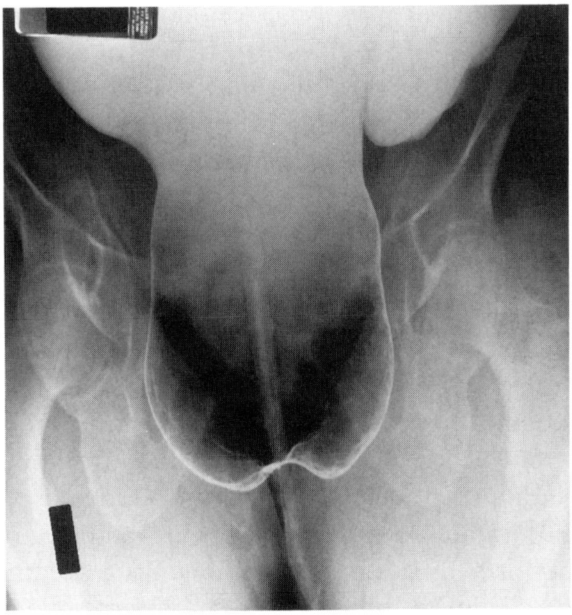

Fig. 27-2 Barium enema reveals a megarectum in a patient with severe constipation.

not to assume that a redundant colon is necessarily responsible for symptoms of constipation. Many patients have a markedly redundant colon but normal bowel function. Little has been published on this condition, but it is possible that prolonged transit through a long, redundant colon could alter stool consistency, leading to evacuation difficulties.

EVALUATION

Patients who fail to respond to the usual dietary measures for presumed idiopathic constipation should undergo a complete examination. It is imperative to consider both colonic and extracolonic causes (see the box) before extensive investigations are undertaken. Selective use of transit and motility studies, endoscopy, cinedefecography, and contrast-enhanced radiography are extremely helpful in differentiating the five subgroups of idiopathic constipation. Patients not infrequently have multiple causes of constipation and may require resolution of pelvic floor dysfunction before colonic inertia can be adequately assessed. The use of an algorithm to guide an appropriate and timely workup is useful not only for the physician and staff but also for the patient. Visualization of the complex interactions and course of events often assures the patient and provides a sense of direction in dealing with this frustrating problem. We generally follow an algorithm (Fig. 27-3) similar to that published by Pemberton and Levin.[17]

SURGICAL INTERVENTION AND COMPLICATIONS

The literature on surgery for constipation is generally nonspecific and difficult to interpret, in part because of lack of clarity about the definition of constipation and indications for surgery and also because of lack of uniformity of operations performed to treat constipation. A review of 13 series with 200 patients who underwent total colectomy and ileorectal anastomosis to treat constipation revealed a success rate of 84%.[18] The patients averaged 40 years in age, and 93% were female. Follow-up ranged from 1.2 to 5.7 years, and the prevalence of postoperative small bowel obstruction ranged from 8% to 44%, with surgical intervention required in 41% to 100%. The author concluded that in appropriately selected patients colonic inertia could be successfully treated surgically.[18] In a general sense, there is no documented increase in complications after surgery to treat constipation compared with the same procedure used for different indications. For example, the frequency of wound infections; intra-abdominal abscesses; anastomotic leaks, strictures, or bleeding; thrombophlebitis; urinary tract infections; cardiopulmonary complications; and subsequent small bowel obstructions appears to be the same whether a total colectomy and ileorectal anastomosis are performed because of colonic inertia or familial adenomatous polyposis. We have a clinical impression that patients operated on for severe

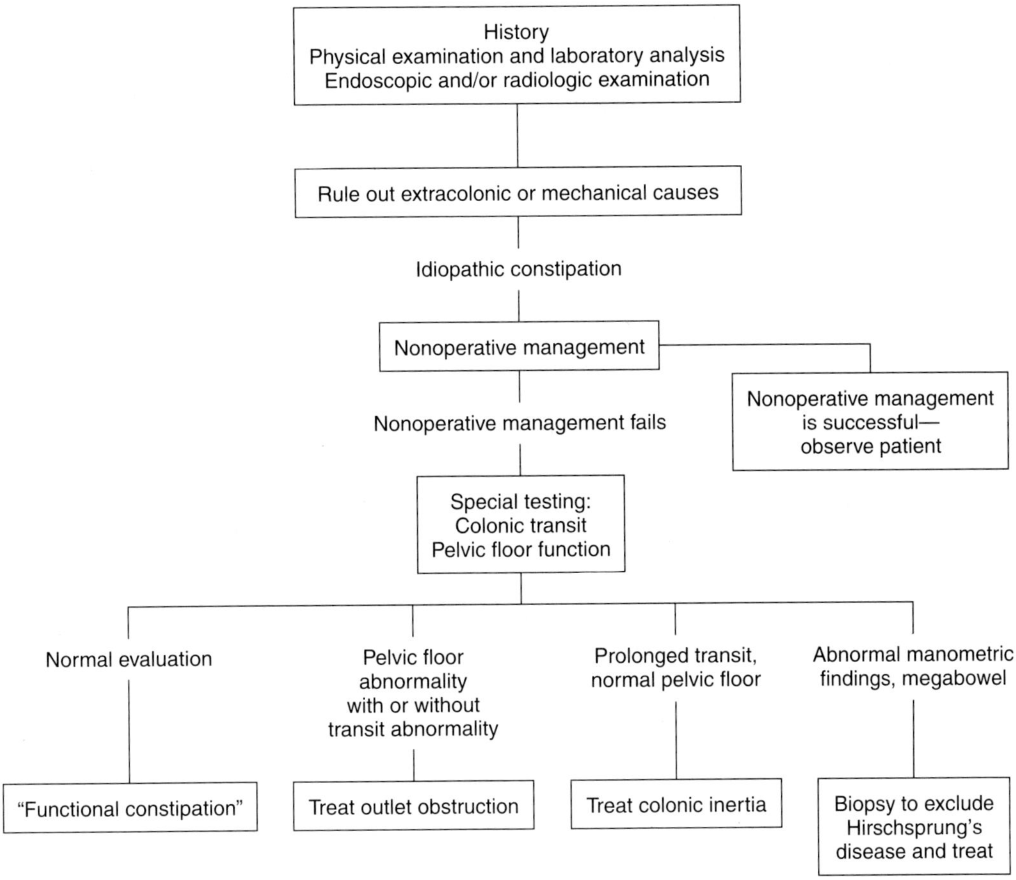

Fig. 27-3 Algorithm for clinical assessment and treatment of chronic constipation.

constipation often have more prolonged ileus than do those undergoing the identical operation for a different disease process. We also have a clinical impression that anastomoses performed to megacolon or megarectum segments or proximal to pelvic outlet obstruction are more prone to problems than other anastomoses. No documentation of these impressions is available, however.

Rectal mobilization, whether to facilitate an ileorectal anastomosis, perform an ileal pouch–anal anastomosis, or correct some form of outlet obstruction, increases the potential for autonomic nerve dysfunction, which can alter bladder and sexual functions. Care must be taken to minimize this risk. Thus, for the most part, morbidity of surgery for constipation is dictated by the procedure itself, not by the indication for the procedure.

Inappropriate operative intervention to treat constipation results in recurrence or persistence of constipation, replacing the misery of chronic constipation with other equally disabling conditions such as excess stool frequency, urgency, or fecal incontinence. In our experience, inappropriate surgical intervention is the most common complication related to surgery for constipation. Thus, one cannot review complications of surgery for constipation without addressing the issues related to appropriate operative intervention. Several principles, discussed below, should guide the surgeon's decision making.

1. Operative intervention for constipation is rarely necessary. In most patients referred for consideration of surgery, constipation can be managed conservatively. Mechanical and pharmacologic causes and treatable endocrine, neurologic, and systemic diseases must be excluded. The surgeon should be especially wary of considering surgical intervention for constipation in patients who have undergone previous operations because of vague problems such as pain or nonobstructing adhesions. Only patients with significant and prolonged alteration of lifestyle because of constipation are potential candidates for surgery.

2. Understand what the patient means by constipation and document its existence. This is critical to success in treating the condition. The objective criteria described earlier to define the medical term "constipation" often do not correlate with the layman's use of the term. Patient education is a key element in the treatment of constipation. Patients must understand that it is not essential to have a bowel movement at the same time each day. Similarly, having a bowel movement only every 2 or 3 days is not considered constipation, despite a patient's use of the term. Although diaries are not encouraged, the physician often gains insight into the problem by having the patient keep a log of diet and bowel function for a short time. With such a diary coupled with a transit-time study, true constipation can objectively be documented and, more important, one can rule out other functional disorders.

3. Constipation is rarely cause for urgent or emergent intervention. With the exceptions of stercoral ulceration with hemorrhage or perforation or obstruction that produces proximal bowel dilation, urgent or emergent intervention is not needed for constipation. The surgeon should not allow the patient to push the decision-making process but should insist on an orderly review of the patient's condition and trials of dietary and other interventions over several months. This time allows the surgeon and patient to better understand the extent of the problem and consider nonoperative options, as well as develop a trust relationship often essential to success in these cases.

4. Suggest patients obtain a second opinion before undertaking surgical intervention. This principle serves two purposes. First, it forces the surgeon to be prepared for a peer review of the workup and recommended operative intervention. This will help prevent a haphazard or incomplete evaluation and an overly aggressive approach to surgery to treat constipation. Second, it builds patient-physician trust that may be useful to long-term success.

5. Use objective testing to determine which operation is best suited to the patient's problem. Segregation of the five subgroups is useful in selecting therapy. Various approaches to these problems are available; however, it is critical that the surgeon understand that many patients have a mixed condition and surgical intervention must be tailored accordingly. For example, although incapacitating colonic inertia is best treated with total colectomy, this surgery would not be advised for a patient with significant sphincter dysfunction.

6. *Carefully obtain informed consent for any surgical intervention.* The proposed surgery should be discussed in detail with the patient in the context that the condition is benign and almost never life threatening, and thus nonintervention is a viable alternative. The surgeon should indicate that the surgery is being performed with the hope of improving the patient's lifestyle, but serious complications may occur during or after the procedure, in both the immediate postoperative period and over the long term.

NORMAL TRANSIT CONSTIPATION

Most patients evaluated for constipation have no demonstrable pathophysiologic findings. In a small group of patients their constipation remains refractory to medical management and they are referred for surgical treatment. These patients should undergo reevaluation with attention to underlying medical disorders and consideration for discontinuation or alteration of medications, especially psychiatric drugs. Psychopathologic findings are not uncommon. Whether this is a primary psychiatric disorder or a consequence of chronic constipation is occasionally difficult to assess.

A trial of dietary and lifestyle changes should be instituted, with emphasis on increased water intake. Bulking agents are helpful in some patients but actually worsen constipation for many others. Flexibility in bowel regimens, including use of stool softeners, mild stimulant laxatives, enemas, and suppositories, is essential in finding a successful routine. Some patients gain partial relief by increasing exercise in their daily routine. Underlying depression or life stresses can greatly affect bowel function in some persons and cannot be ignored. Psychologic intervention may be necessary. Close observation and frequent follow-up to evaluate progress and ensure compliance are essential.

Occasionally these patients have undergone a previous segmental resection that may have produced a favorable response for at least a short time. They return even more convinced of the need for additional surgery. The physician must again rule out obstruction as the cause and institute conservative measures. Although conservative management of constipation in this group of patients is challenging, more extensive resection will likely result in only temporary improvement and may create new problems, with increased stool frequency, urgency, and occasionally incontinence.

PELVIC FLOOR DYSFUNCTION

The availability of anorectal physiologic evaluation has greatly facilitated our ability to document causes of pelvic outlet obstruction. Although controversies regarding the significance and interpretation of selected findings persist, there is increasing documentation of anismus, rectocele, internal intussusception, rectal prolapse, enterocele, and descending perineum. Less obvious strictures and obstructing lesions are also recognized occasionally at defecography.

Anismus, or paradoxic puborectalis contraction, deserves particular attention because not infrequently it may be associated with other evacuation disorders. In an attempt, often forceful, to evacuate, a paradoxic response can develop that contracts pelvic and perineal muscles during defecation. If this abnormal response is not recognized, resection, rectopexy, or other corrective measures for constipation will likely fail because of outlet obstruction. In extreme cases, severe outlet obstruction could jeopardize an anastomosis by creating undue tension on the suture line, leading to disruption. The incidence of paradoxic activity in chronic constipation is unknown, but it should be evaluated before surgical intervention because it often responds favorably to biofeedback.

COLONIC INERTIA AND GENERALIZED INTESTINAL DYSMOTILITY

Although transit studies have occasionally suggested segmental delay, the results of segmental resection for constipation, particularly over the long term, have been poor.[21,22] Frequently patients respond favorably for short periods after segmental resection, but then the preoperative status returns, eventually requiring a completion colectomy with ileorectostomy or end ileostomy. Preservation of the ileocecal valve and cecorectal anastomosis were at one time advocated; this too failed to provide satisfactory function because the retained cecum became distended, creating pain, obstruction, and occasionally overflow incontinence.[23] Today most surgeons agree that for those patients with documented severe colonic inertia, a total abdominal colectomy and ileorectal anastomosis is the operation of choice.

The treatment for slow transit constipation continues to evolve with our increased ability to distinguish primary colonic abnormalities from pelvic outlet obstruction and generalized intestinal dysmotility. Pelvic outlet obstruction often responds to biofeedback or surgery to correct a specific disorder, such as procidentia, and should thus be excluded before subjecting patients to total colectomy and ileorectostomy.

Redmond et al.[11] reported that 90% of patients with isolated colonic inertia and 88% of patients with generalized intestinal dysmotility initially responded favorably to total colectomy and ileorectal anastomosis. Although the results in the latter group deteriorated over time, many patients would prefer several years of good function to the alternative of generalized dysfunction for which there is no good treatment. Pemberton and Levin[17] failed to show any functional difference in a review from the Mayo Clinic for patients with colonic inertia and generalized intestinal dysmotility. One possible explanation for the discrepancy in this review and others is the short follow-up of only 20 months in the Mayo series. Long-term results and greater numbers of patients will certainly aid in our understanding of the role of generalized intestinal dysmotility and constipation. Given the overall favorable outcome after ileorectostomy for slow transit constipation, one could argue that, rather than evaluating all patients to exclude generalized intestinal dysmotility before surgery, as suggested by Redmond et al.,[11] only those patients in whom ileorectostomy failed should undergo examination for upper intestinal motility disorders. Presently, a total abdominal colectomy with ileorectostomy remains the procedure of choice for severe colonic inertia or generalized intestinal dysmotility after medical management has failed. Ileostomy, although not a popular option for many patients, has the lowest reported complication rate and remains an acceptable alternative, especially if the patient's overall fitness is poor or when the diagnosis remains questionable. The surgeon must be aware that for those patients who have generalized intestinal dysmotility and fail to achieve long-term success after total colectomy and ileorectostomy, conversion to an end ileostomy has produced inconsistent results.

Hosie et al.[24] suggested that proctocolectomy and ileoanal anastomosis is an acceptable treatment alternative for severe colonic inertia. Although the procedure may improve short-term function in selected patients, long-term functional results are pending. Because the complication rate after proctocolectomy and ileoanal anastomosis exceeds that for ileorectal anastomosis and because most surgeons use a two-stage approach with a temporary diverting ileostomy, ileoanal anastomosis should be reserved for those patients in whom ileorectostomy fails and who adamantly oppose undergoing an end ileostomy. It is essential that pelvic outlet obstruction be excluded before creating an ileoanal anastomosis to treat constipation.

IDIOPATHIC MEGABOWEL

Megarectum, megacolon, and dolicholcolon are unusual causes of constipation. Even in those patients with documented colonic inertia, it is rare to find abnormally dilated or elongated colon. Of no surprise, many of the reviews of idiopathic constipation fail to identify this subset of patients as a unique group. As opposed to colonic inertia, segmental transit delay associated with megacolon or megarectum appears to respond favorably to segmental resection.[15] Pancolonic involvement should be treated with abdominal colectomy because the remaining dilated segment is not likely to regain function. Occasionally after diversion the previously dilated bowel will return to normal caliber. Although the bowel may appear normal, it has been our experience that after reestablishment of intestinal continuity the bowel quickly returns to its dilated and dysfunctional state.

Isolated megarectum is likewise amenable to segmental resection. Proctectomy with coloanal anastomosis has generally been regarded as superior to low anterior resection because of the difficulties in dealing with the dilated distal segment. Perhaps because of the similarity to Hirschsprung's disease, a number of reports have advocated myectomy. The results of myectomy, however, are inconsistent at best and associated with a higher frequency of incontinence than is coloanal anastomosis. Before consideration of surgical intervention, Hirschsprung's disease must be excluded. As the rectal-anal inhibitory reflex is often difficult to elicit or is absent in patients with megarectum, rectal biopsy should be considered to exclude the diagnosis. Patients with both megacolon and megarectum should undergo proctocolectomy with ileostomy or ileal pouch–anal anastomosis.

Dolichocolon is not well classified but appears to respond to subtotal colectomy in those rare patients truly incapacitated with colonic inertia. Distinguishing this entity from other forms of constipation is difficult without appropriate use of manometry and transit studies.

CONCLUSION

No longer is the indiscriminate use of segmental colectomy acceptable for the treatment of constipation. If we are to continue improving our results with surgical intervention from those reported at the turn of the century, it is imperative we use and refine current diagnostic and therapeutic methods. Failure to exclude an extracolonic cause or institute appropriate medical intervention before subjecting the patient to surgery remains the most common complication. A thorough and coordinated approach with selected investigation will not only identify those few patients who require surgery because of constipation but should provide a means to tailor the procedure to address the pathophysiologic process that accounts for the problem. This should help prevent needless surgery and complications associated with inappropriate procedures and help eliminate a frequent source of frustration for patient and surgeon alike.

REFERENCES

1. National Center for Health Statistics. Interviewing methods in the Health Interview Survey. Vital and Health Statistics, Series 2, No. 48. DHEW Publ. No. HSM 72-1048. Health Services and Mental Health Administration. Washington, DC: US Government Printing Office, 1972.
2. Wyman JB, Heaton KW, Manning AP, Wicks ACP. Variability of colonic function in healthy subjects. Gut 19:146-150, 1978.

3. National Center for Health Statistics, Simmons WR. Development of the design of the NCHS Hospital Discharge Survey. Vital and Health Statistics. Series 2, No. 39. DHEW Publ. No. (HRA) 77-1199. Public Health Service. Washington, DC: US Government Printing Office, 1977.
4. Connell AM, Hilton C, Irvine G. Variation of bowel habit in two population samples. Br Med J 2:1095-1099, 1965.
5. Drossman DA, Sandler RS, Mekes DC, et al. Bowel patterns among subjects not seeking health care. Gastroenterology 83:529-534, 1982.
6. Davis GJ, Crowder M, Reid B, et al. Bowel function measurements of individuals with different eating patterns. Gut 27:164-169, 1986.
7. Rendtorf RC, Kashgarian M. Stool patterns of healthy adult males. Dis Colon Rectum 10: 222-228, 1967.
8. Shouter P, Keighley MRB. Changes in colorectal function in severe idiopathic chronic constipation: Outlet obstruction. Gastroenterology 75:623-631, 1978.
9. Martelli H, Devroede G, Arhan P, et al. Mechanisms of idiopathic constipation: Outlet obstruction. Gastroenterology 75:623-631, 1978.
10. Pemberton JH, Rath DM, Ilstrup DM. Evaluation and surgical treatment of severe chronic constipation. Ann Surg 214:403-411, 1991.
11. Redmond JM, Smith GW, Barofsky I, et al. Physiological tests to predict long-term outcome of total abdominal colectomy for intractable constipation. Am J Gastroenterol 90:748-753, 1995.
12. Stanghellini V, Camilleri M, Malogelada JR. Chronic idiopathic intestinal pseudo-obstruction: Clinical and intestinal manometric findings. Gut 28:5-12, 1987.
13. Lane RHS, Todd IP. Idiopathic megacolon: A review of 42 cases. Br J Surg 64:305-310, 1977.
14. Stewart J, Kumar D, Keighley MRB. Results of anal or low rectal anastomosis and pouch construction for megarectum and megacolon. Br J Surg 81:1051-1053, 1994.
15. Kamm MA, Stabile G. Management of idiopathic megarectum and megacolon. Br J Surg 78: 899-900, 1991.
16. Belliveau P, Goldberg SM, Rothenberger DA, et al. Idiopathic acquired megacolon: The value of subtotal colectomy. Dis Colon Rectum 25:118-121, 1982.
17. Pemberton JH, Levin KE. Current practice in surgery. Surg Clin North Am 2:118, 1990.
18. Beck DE. Colectomy for colonic inertia. Semin Colon Rectal Surg 3:115-119, 1992.
19. Preston DM, Lennard-Jones JE, Thomas BM. Towards a radiologic definition of idiopathic megacolon. Gastrointest Radiol 10:167-169, 1985.
20. Hughes ESR, McDermott FT, Johnson WR, et al. Surgery for constipation. Aust N Z J Surg 51:144-148, 1981.
21. Preston DM, Rees LH, Lennard-Jones JE, et al. Results of colectomy for severe idiopathic constipation in women. Br J Surg 71:547-552, 1984.
22. Walsh PV, Peebles-Brown G, Watkinson G. Colectomy for slow transit constipation. Ann R Coll Surg 69:71-75, 1987.
23. Todd IP. Adult Hirschsprung's disease. Br J Surg 64:311-312, 1977.
24. Hosie KB, Kmiot WA, Keighley MRB. Constipation: Another indication for restorative proctocolectomy. Br J Surg 77:801-802, 1990.

CHAPTER 28

Colorectal Trauma

FRANK G. OPELKA
DAVID E. BECK

Trauma remains a major cause of death and major morbidity.[1] The economic and social consequences to the community are even more acutely felt when the patient survives the initial traumatic insult but dies hours or days later from complications of the injury or the surgery. Although colorectal injuries may be visually impressive, they are rarely immediately life threatening. However, prompt detection and management are crucial to preserving function and reducing morbidity. It is therefore critical that all life-threatening injuries are identified and managed initially, followed by a systematic evaluation to identify any colorectal trauma. This chapter briefly reviews the causes of colorectal trauma, discusses management of colorectal trauma, and reviews principles to minimize complications.

ETIOLOGIC FACTORS

Colorectal trauma can occur from a variety of causes. The history obtained from the patient or emergency personnel often provides information about the cause and timing of injury. The frequency of injuries to each organ is related to the mechanism of injury, and classically, colorectal trauma has been categorized as blunt or penetrating.

Blunt Trauma

Blunt trauma accounts for only 4% of colorectal injuries, with motor vehicle accidents being the most frequent cause.[2] Because of the protected location of the anus and rectum, anorectal injuries are infrequent with blunt trauma and usually are associated with pelvic fractures. Seat belts reduce lethal injuries and allow increased survival of patients with blunt GI injuries, including injuries to the colon and rectum.[3] Falls and crush injuries account for most of the remaining blunt injuries. Injuries significant enough to injure the anorectum usually have multiple associated injuries. Therefore, patients with major injuries should undergo a complete diagnostic evaluation.

Penetrating Trauma

Most colorectal injuries (96%) are caused by penetrating injuries.[1,4,5] Although stab wounds may penetrate the bowel, projectile injuries (e.g., gunshot wounds) are most commonly seen.[6] Projectiles may cause injury by direct penetration of the bowel, blast effect, or secondary penetration from fragmented bone.[7] The latter two mechanisms are especially important in wounds associated with high-velocity military-type weapons. Rectal impalement injuries result when a patient falls on a penetrating object.[8]

Iatrogenic injuries of the rectum and anus are uncommon. Colorectal perforation during barium contrast studies occurs in approximately 0.02% to 0.04% of patients, usually in the rectum above the peritoneal reflection.[9] Four mechanisms of injury have been suggested: trauma from the enema tip, overinflation of the balloon, recent colonic instrumentation, and presence of rectal disease.[10] The majority of rectal perforations from enema tips are on the anterior rectal wall, and most are identified at the time of examination.[11] Other iatrogenic anorectal injuries result from cleansing enemas, thermometers, proctosigmoidoscopy, colonoscopy (see Chapter 9), and surgical procedures.

Several unusual and unfortunate causes of rectal trauma also exist. Sexually related trauma can cause significant injury to the anorectum.[12] A great variety of rectal foreign bodies are used for sexual gratification and have the potential to cause serious injuries. Most causes of anorectal trauma in children are related to child abuse.[13]

The majority of ingested foreign bodies will pass through uneventfully. However, perforation, hemorrhage, abscess, bowel obstruction, and death have been reported.[14] The sigmoid colon is the most common site of these complications. Other causes of anorectal injuries include pneumatic and suction perforations, radiation necrosis, and chemical burns.

Injuries that result from warfare deserve special comment. Combat conditions produce a spectrum of injuries that are rarely encountered in civilian practice. High-velocity weapons deliver significantly more kinetic energy to the pelvis than do handguns or blunt injuries. The resulting blast injuries mandate an aggressive evaluation. Transportation and logistic limitations frequently cause delay in evaluation, and the transport of patients according to military evacuation policies often prevents continuity of care. Experience with combat injuries led to development of guidelines that may not be required in all civilian injuries but are essential to optimize management of combat casualties.

The Organ Injury Scaling Committee of the American Association for Surgery

Table 28-1 Severity score for colorectal injuries

Grade	Injury	ICD-9
I	Contusion or hematoma without devascularization or partial-thickness laceration	863.45
II	Laceration <50% of circumference	863.55
III	Laceration ≥50% of circumference	863.55
IV	Full-thickness laceration with extension into the perineum	863.55
V	Devascularized segment	863.55

From Moore EE, Cogbill TH, Malangoni MA, et al. Organ injury scaling. II. Pancreas, duodenum, small bowel, colon, and rectum. J Trauma 30:1427-1429, 1990.
ICD = International Classification of Diseases, 9th rev.

of Trauma (AAST)[15] has developed a severity score classification for colorectal injuries (Table 28-1). The AAST supports this system to facilitate clinical research and assist in comparing outcomes of different management strategies. Although this system classifies colorectal injuries, it does not take into account associated injuries that are common in pelvic trauma and does not quantify any delay in diagnosis or treatment.

Traumatic injuries to the colorectum usually occur in a bowel filled with feces and are potentially lethal. Complications of colorectal injury can be divided into undiagnosed injuries and incorrect treatment. Undiagnosed injuries may be the result of associated extra-abdominal injuries that are ignored, misdiagnosed, or inappropriately managed. Intra-abdominal injuries are overlooked because of inadequate exploration, failure to fully explore the tract of the penetrating implement, failure to explore hematomas, or inadequate mobilization and inspection of suspect areas of the colon. Rectal injuries are particularly likely to be missed, because these injuries frequently cannot be recognized from within the abdomen during laparotomy. Correct management of rectal injuries therefore depends largely on preoperative diagnosis.

EVALUATION AND MANAGEMENT

A systematic approach with simultaneous evaluation and resuscitation is recommended by the American College of Surgeons Advanced Trauma Life Support Program.[16] Their recommendations include four phases of management. During the initial *primary survey,* all life-threatening injuries are identified. This includes recognition of airway problems and difficulties with breathing resulting from tension pneumothorax, sucking chest wounds, flail chest, or massive hemothorax. Cardiac tamponade, arrhythmias, and external hemorrhage should also be immediately recognized. The primary survey should lead to the *resuscitation*

Table 28-2 Approach to multiple-trauma patients

Phase	Identify	Diagnostic or therapeutic techniques
Primary survey	Airway patency Cervical spine control in all patients with suspected cervical spine injury	Oxygen administration Chin lift (oral airway) Intubation Cricothyroidotomy
	Breathing difficulties	
	Tension pneumothorax	Needle decompression or chest tube
	Flail chest	Intubate and volume ventilate
	Circulation problems	
	Cardiac arrhythmia	Monitor, treat
	Cardiac tamponade	Pericardiocentesis, thoracotomy
	External hemorrhage	Control with direct pressure
Resuscitation	Shock	Airway maintenance Oxygen administration IV lactaged Ringer's solution via large-bore tubes
Secondary survey	Abdominal injury	Insert nasogastric tube (contraindicated in cribriform plate fracture)
	Rectal injury Presence of blood High-riding prostate Anal sphincter tone	Proctoscopic examination for pelvic trauma
	Vaginal injury	Speculum examination for pelvic trauma
	Urethral injury Blood at meatus High-riding prostate Perineal hematoma	Insert Foley catheter (contraindicated in transected urethra)
Definitive care	Need for exploratory laparotomy Positive peritoneal lavage Penetrating gunshot wound Specific stab wound	Exploratory laparotomy Management of specific organ injuries

phase, during which the life-threatening injuries are managed. This includes tracheal intubation or cricothyroidotomy, chest tube insertion, pericardiocentesis, control of hemorrhage, and establishment of large-bore intravenous lines. Once the patient's condition is stabilized, the physician proceeds with a more definitive *secondary survey.* During this phase, occult injuries are identified, radiographs are obtained and laboratory tests are performed, and all of the patient's injuries are evaluated. At the conclusion of the secondary survey, the final *definitive care* phase is initiated (Table 28-2).

Abdominal injuries are assessed in the secondary survey because these injuries are rarely immediately life-threatening. This assessment includes "a finger or a tube in every orifice." A nasogastric tube allows removal of gastric contents, which reduces the risk of aspiration during anesthesia, and permits examination of the stomach contents for blood suggestive of a gastric injury. It also prevents gastric dilation and reduces the effects of the ileus that inevitably follows any serious abdominal injury. Passage of a nasogastric tube, however, is contraindicated in the presence of a cribriform plate fracture. Although rare, this injury occurs with head or facial trauma and is suggested by leakage of cerebrospinal fluid from the nose. Attempts to pass a nasogastric tube in this situation may result in the tube passing through the cribriform plate fracture into the cranial vault.

A Foley catheter should also be inserted into the bladder to measure urinary output, examine the urine for blood, and allow cystography if required. The passage of a Foley catheter is contraindicated if the urethra is injured. Such injuries, which occur almost exclusively in male patients, are generally caused by blunt trauma with associated pelvic fractures. A urethral injury is suggested by the presence of blood at the external urinary meatus, extravasation of blood or urine into the perineum, and the presence of a high-riding prostate gland on rectal examination. The urethra tends to tear posteriorly, and the extravasation of blood and urine creates local collections that cause displacement of the prostate and bladder. The examining finger in the rectum then fails to feel the prostate but instead feels a soft boggy mass of extravasated blood and urine. If a urethral injury is suspected, no attempt should be made to pass the Foley catheter, but a retrograde ureterogram should be obtained to evaluate the status of the urethra.

An inexperienced provider may not appreciate these subtleties or may overlook the need for a rectal examination in a traumatized patient. However, the importance of this examination cannot be overemphasized for evaluating the prostate and determining the presence of blood in the rectum, which indicates a penetrating injury to the rectum or lower colon. The degree of anal sphincter tone is also important, especially in patients with apparent spinal cord transections. The presence of anal sphincter tone in such patients indicates a degree of sacral neuronal sparing and a better prognosis.

INDICATIONS FOR SURGERY

Intra-abdominal Injury

In patients with abdominal trauma it is not necessary to diagnose a specific intra-abdominal organ injury but only that an indication for surgical intervention exists. All abdominal injuries should be discovered during laparotomy to assess the extent of trauma. The surgical indications in abdominal trauma are considered emergent when the patient must be operated on immediately, without any delay, and urgent when the patient should be operated on as soon as possible but there is enough time to obtain some diagnostic radiographs or laboratory tests before the exploration. Indications for immediate exploration are rare and include the unresponsive patient in shock. Trauma patients in shock should receive 3 to 4 L of an isotonic crystalloid solution over 10 to 15 minutes. If the vital signs fail to respond, the patient should be moved immediately to the operating room, where definitive control of the intra-abdominal bleeding can be accomplished. Blood loss in these patients requires definitive control of the hemorrhage as part of the resuscitation. A second indication for immediate laparotomy is the patient who initially responds to resuscitation but relapses into shock when the intravenous fluids are tapered to a slower rate. This signifies that the patient is continuing to bleed at a rate that cannot be tolerated and demands definitive management in the operating room. Fewer than 5% of all patients with abdominal trauma fall into either of these emergent categories. In general, there is time for diagnostic or therapeutic steps to determine the need for operative intervention.

The indications for surgery in abdominal trauma largely are related to the mechanism of injury. In blunt abdominal trauma, the presence of peritonitis, free air on abdominal radiographs (Fig. 28-1) or a positive peritoneal lavage re-

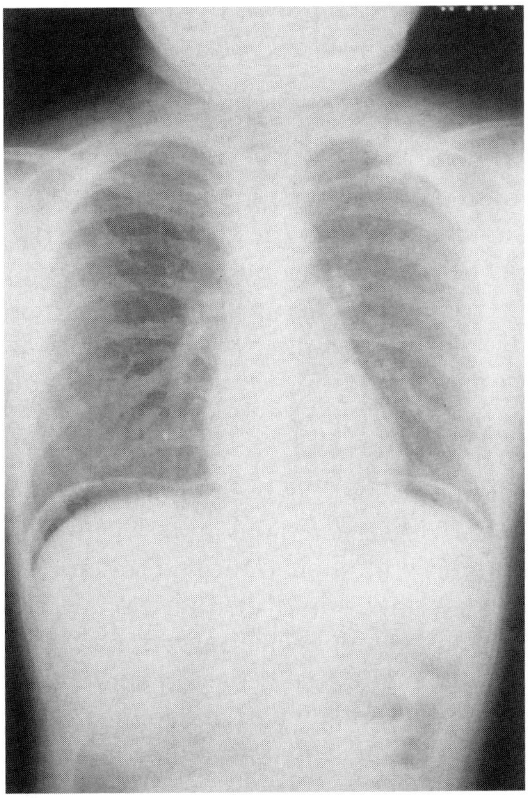

Fig. 28-1 Upright radiograph of chest demonstrates free intra-abdominal air.

turn is an indication for surgery. Diagnostic peritoneal lavage is useful to identify intraperitoneal hemorrhage or gross intraperitoneal contamination.[17] This test is helpful in evaluating patients in whom an accurate abdominal examination is not possible (e.g., patients with head injuries, spinal cord damage, or lower chest injuries; those under the influence of drugs or alcohol; and those who will require operative intervention for other injuries, generally orthopedic). Diagnostic peritoneal lavage is contraindicated in patients who already manifest indications for abdominal exploration (e.g., penetrating abdominal wounds or acute abdomen). An open or closed technique may be used for diagnostic peritoneal lavage catheter placement, and a supraumbilical approach is preferred if pelvic injuries are suspected. An abnormal lavage return (>100,000 RBCs/mm^3, >500 WBCs/mm^3, or gross food or fecal matter) strongly suggests significant intraperitoneal injury and usually mandates exploratory laparotomy. Diagnostic peritoneal lavage is an exquisitely sensitive test with a low rate of false positive and false negative results; however, a negative result does not exclude injuries to the retroperitoneal structures.[18,19]

Most surgeons will explore any gunshot wound that penetrates the abdominal cavity, because 98% of these wounds produce significant intra-abdominal injury.[20] However, tangential gunshot wounds of the abdominal wall that do not appear to enter the abdominal cavity are controversial. Although some authors[21] have advocated the routine exploration of all such wounds because of the possibility that the "blast effect" may have caused an intra-abdominal injury, this consequence is rare in civilian injuries.[1,20] Should doubt exist as to whether the bullet has penetrated the abdominal cavity, a diagnostic perineal lavage may resolve the question.

Pelvic gunshot wounds also present problems. First, it may also be difficult to ascertain whether the bullet entered the abdominal cavity. Again, a diagnostic peritoneal lavage may be helpful. Second, penetrating wounds of the buttocks and pelvis may injure one of the perineal structures. Injuries to the bladder, urethra, rectum, and vagina must be discovered during the assessment phase, because they may not be apparent during the course of an exploratory laparotomy. This is particularly true of rectal injuries. Therefore, any patient who has a penetrating pelvic injury, particularly injuries that cross the midline, and patients with blood in the rectum should undergo a careful proctoscopic examination. Proctoscopic examinations are frequently tedious and difficult to perform, because the patient who has experienced multiple traumas is often difficult to position and the bowel is unprepared. A slow, careful examination with frequent irrigation to remove retained feces allows complete visualization of the entire rectal mucosa for at least 20 cm proximal to the anal verge.[2] In addition to rectal injuries, suspected lesions of the bladder should be excluded by means of cystography that includes anteroposterior, oblique, and postvoiding views of the bladder. Vaginal injuries are evaluated with a careful speculum examination.

The management of abdominal stab wounds remains controversial. One viewpoint holds that all stab wounds that penetrate the abdominal cavity should be explored.[22,23] If this attitude is accepted, the examiner has only to ascertain whether the implement has penetrated the abdominal cavity. Methods for determining penetration have included "stabograms" (in which contrast material is injected into the tract),[24,25] local wound exploration, and diagnostic peritoneal lavage. Of these, lavage is the most sensitive. A policy of exploring all stab wounds that penetrate the abdominal cavity results in a high percentage (30% to 50%) of negative laparotomy results.[26] The Cook County Hospital experience demonstrated that a negative laparotomy for trauma was not a benign procedure. In their review of 178 patients with negative laparotomies, Lowe et al.[27] reported that this institution had a mortality rate of 1.6% and a complication rate of 19%. These patients also had a 4% incidence of intestinal obstruction within 6 months after the negative laparotomy for trauma.[27] Based on this experience, the Cook County surgeons adopted a policy of selective management of abdominal stab wounds. Their indications for exploration of abdominal stab wounds included shock; the presence of peritonitis; the presence of free air on abdominal radiographs; blood in the nasogastric tube, rectum, or urine; evisceration of abdominal contents; an abnormal intravenous pyelogram or cystogram; an abnormal arteriogram or scan; and a retained stabbing implement. Penetrating injuries of the retroperitoneum were explored because of failure of peritoneal lavage to adequately evaluate this area. This policy lowered the rate of negative laparotomy without missed injuries.[1,26]

Genitourinary Injury

Intravenous pyelography (IVP) is necessary for evaluation of gross or microscopic (>5 RBCs per high-powered field) hematuria. Patients with penetrating or blunt perinephric trauma (flank swelling, fractures of the lower ribs or the vertebral bodies, external bruises, abrasions, penetrations, or perinephric tenderness) or who require an exploratory laparotomy for trauma should also be evaluated with an intravenous pyelogram. Intraoperative decisions regarding nephrectomy are simplified if the surgeon is assured that a functioning contralateral kidney exists. An IVP can be obtained in the emergency department or operating room with administration of diatrazoate sodium (Renografin), 1 to 2 ml/kg, as an intravenous bolus. One flat abdominal radiograph is obtained within 5 minutes after the contrast material is administered. Adequate blood pressure and perfusion of the kidneys (as evidenced by good urinary output) are necessary for adequate IVP. The infusion IVP is inspected to ensure that both kidneys are present and functioning and there is no extravasation from the ureters. Although the IVP may also show some contrast material in the bladder, lack of extravasation of contrast material from the bladder on this film cannot be interpreted as an intact bladder. A cystogram is required to exclude an injured bladder.

Before cystography, it is important to rule out injury to the urethra (indicated by blood at the external meatus, extravasation of blood or urine into the perineum, or a high-riding prostate at rectal examination). A retrograde urethrogram can easily be obtained in the emergency department by inserting the tip of a large syringe filled with contrast material into the external urinary meatus and injecting the contrast material retrograde. A plain lateral radiograph will demonstrate whether the urethra is injured, as judged by extravasation of the contrast material. If the urethra is intact, a Foley catheter can be inserted in the bladder and a cystogram obtained by attaching the barrel of a 50 ml syringe to the end of the catheter and holding both above the bladder. Contrast material poured into the syringe barrel will fill the bladder by means of gravity. The bladder is filled until the contrast material backs up into the syringe. Injection of an additional 50 ml of contrast material will dislodge any omentum that may be tamponading a bladder injury. Anteroposterior, lateral, oblique, and evacuation films of the bladder are examined for extravasation of contrast material.

ANTIBIOTIC THERAPY

All patients with abdominal trauma who are to undergo exploratory laparotomy should receive preoperative antibiotics against colorectal bacterial flora (aerobes and anaerobes). Single-agent antimicrobial therapy with broad-spectrum coverage (e.g., cefoxitin, cefotetan) is appropriate, although some surgeons prefer multiple-drug therapy (e.g., an aminoglycoside such as gentamycin or tobramycin combined with clindamicin, metronidazole, timentin, or ampicillin). A colonic or rectal injury is the most important determinant of infectious complications.[28]

The duration of therapy is determined by the patient's clinical condition. Patients at lower risk (without GI perforation) may require only 24-hour antibiotic therapy after surgery, whereas those at high risk (e.g., with colorectal injury, multiple-organ injuries, incomplete hemostasis, shock) may receive postoperative antibiotic therapy for 48 to 72 hours.[28] If the half-life of the drugs used is not longer than the operative procedure, additional doses may be required during surgery.[29] Jones et al.[30] at Parkland Memorial Hospital in Dallas observed an infection rate of 36% in 96 patients with penetrating colonic injuries.

LAPAROTOMY

Before surgery, potential stoma sites are marked. The patient should be cleansed from the neck to the knees with a topical antimicrobial skin preparation. If an intra-abdominal vascular injury is suspected, access to the femoral and saphenous vessels is maintained. The patient is draped widely to allow for extension of incisions into the chest and placement of stomas. A long midline incision affords quick and easy access to all of the intra-abdominal organs, may be easily extended into the chest, and does not compromise any stoma sites.

Once the abdomen is entered, exploration should proceed by giving preference to the most-life-threatening injuries. The primary goal is to control the intra-abdominal bleeding. Hepatic and splenic hemorrhage can be temporarily controlled by packing the injured organ. After bleeding is controlled, the next step is to control the intra-abdominal contamination. Holes in the colon may be temporarily controlled by quickly closing them with running sutures or skin staples or by excluding the injured segment with noncrushing clamps. Once the bleeding is controlled and temporary control of spillage has been achieved, the abdomen can be thoroughly explored. The tract of the knife or the bullet is determined and pursued vigorously for its entire length. The entire small bowel and its mesentery are carefully examined, and holes in the diaphragm are repaired early to reduce the risk of contamination of the pleural cavities. The entire colon is carefully examined, which may require mobilizing the ascending or descending colon and the flexures.

With the exception of a stable perinephric hematoma around a functioning kidney, hematomas due to penetrating trauma should be explored. For hematomas in the retroperitoneum, the major vascular structures below the renal vessels can be explored after mobilization of the right half of the colon and the small bowel upward and to the right, as described by Catell and Braash.[31] Suspected injuries to the suprarenal aorta can be discerned by mobilizing the entire contents of the left upper quadrant (spleen, kidney, pancreas, splenic flexure, and descending colon) to the right. It should again be emphasized that wide mobilization of the colon and careful inspection of any suspect areas are mandatory to identify injuries of the retroperitoneal colon.

SURGICAL TREATMENT

Colonic Injury

Various methods of treatment of colonic injuries include exteriorization of the injured segment, resection with or without anastomosis, closure of the injured segment with a proximal protecting colostomy, or primary closure of the colonic injury. Major controversy centers on the choice between primary repair and exteriorization.

Primary closure. Although it is true that some colonic injuries may be primarily closed, it is also true that there are many that should not.[32] The following guidelines suggest circumstances in which primary closure is not indicated:

1. The patient is or has been in shock (systolic blood pressure <80 mm Hg).
2. The interval between the original colonic injury and its discovery at laparotomy is >8 hours.
3. More than one organ system has sustained significant injury.
4. There is massive colonic destruction (>2 cm defect in the colonic wall after adequate debridement.

5. There is massive contamination (presence of gross fecal soilage >5 cm from the colonic defect).
6. Associated injuries will require the use of prosthetic materials for repair.
7. The colon is injured in two anatomic locations (e.g., hepatic flexure and sigmoid).

No distinction is made between injuries to the right or left colon[32-35] or between mesenteric and antimesenteric injuries. These injuries are closed in one or two layers. Should any of the criteria that contraindicate primary closure exist, an alternate method of treatment should be used. Because "the anastomosis that is not made cannot leak," the injured segment must be removed from the abdominal cavity by exteriorization, resection of the injured segment, or closure with a diverting proximal colostomy.

Exteriorization. Simple exteriorization of the injury as a colostomy commits the patient to a second surgical procedure, and colostomy closure is not a procedure completely without risks. Major complications (leakage, sepsis, evisceration, and peristomal hernia) have been reported in 8% to 50% of patients after colostomy closure.[36-42] Few bowel injuries are small enough or located in appropriate sections of the colon to accommodate this option.

To circumvent this problem, it has been suggested that the injured colon be repaired and then exteriorized.[43,44] Theoretically this would allow the exteriorized repair to be returned to the abdomen during the same hospitalization (generally at 10 to 14 days after the original repair). Lou et al.[44] reported such management in 50 patients. The repaired, exteriorized loop was covered with occlusive petrolatum gauze and inspected daily. In this series 60% of the injuries healed, but 34% leaked between the third and tenth postoperative days and required formal conversion to a colostomy. In the Cook County experience, 50% of the injuries treated in this manner either leaked or became obstructed.[1] Although it is appealing to return the segment early to the abdomen, at 10 to 14 days after surgery there is still a great deal of inflammatory reaction around the exteriorized loop and the procedure can be technically difficult and complicated. The technique is also unsuitable for extensive injuries to the colon or injured segments that cannot be exteriorized. For all these reasons, this technique is seldom used.

Suture closure with proximal colostomy. Injuries to the low sigmoid colon that do not fulfill the criteria for primary closure present a special problem. Frequently these injuries cannot be brought up to the abdominal wall for exteriorization as a colostomy despite adequate mobilization of the sigmoid colon. In these cases the injury is repaired in one or in two layers and is protected by a proximal colostomy or loop ileostomy. Although some would advocate a double-barrel split colostomy in these cases to ensure complete diversion of the fecal stream, we have had very satisfactory results with use of a loop stoma.

Resection with ostomy and fistula. In colonic injuries in which there is extensive loss of tissue (e.g., gunshot wounds), the entire injured and devitalized segment should be resected and the proximal colon brought out as a colostomy and the distal segment managed as a mucous fistula. In creating these end colostomies, great care is taken to maintain a small fascial opening around the colon to prevent parastomal herniation. The proximal bowel is matured as a colostomy and the distal bowel as a mucous fistula, or the closed end may be implanted in the subcutaneous tissue.

Cecal injury. Simple injuries to the cecum that fulfill the criteria for primary closure can be closed in two layers. With more complex injuries, cecal resection is advocated. Once the cecum is resected, a primary anastomosis can be accomplished or an ileostomy and long Hartmann's closure of the distal bowel can be performed.

Primary closure of the injury with protection of the repair with a proximal diverting loop ileostomy is another option. We do not advocate this approach, because it does not remove the necessity for a second operation to close the stoma and has none of the advantages of a well-created end ileostomy.

Rectal Injury

The mortality rate for rectal injuries decreased from 67% during World War I to 23% during World War II with the addition of routine diverting colostomies, presacral drainage, antibiotic therapy, and blood transfusions.[6,45,46] During the Vietnam era, surgeons added distal rectal washouts to limit further contamination of the pelvis through the rectal injury site.[47] These advances, along with improved antibiotic therapy and rapid evacuation, reduced the mortality rate to 14%.[48] The lessons learned from wartime surgery, in concert with civilian experience with low- and high-velocity injuries to the rectum, have shaped the treatment of rectal injuries. The reported morbidity and mortality for civilian rectal trauma have been much lower (Table 28-3).

Table 28-3 Morbidity and mortality of civilian rectal injuries*

Author	Year	No. of patients	Morbidity (%)	Mortality (%)
Vitale et al.[49]	1983	32	16	3
Grasberger and Hirsch[50]	1983	20	40	10
Tuggle and Huber[51]	1984	47	36	0
Mangiante et al.[52]	1986	43	37	0
Shannon et al.[53]	1988	26	60	4
Burch et al.[5]	1989	100	11	4
Thomas et al.[54]	1990	52	10	0

*Mechanisms of injury and methods of reporting varied considerably.

Critical in the management of rectal injuries is to recognize the presence of the injury before embarking on an exploratory laparotomy. Careful proctoscopic examination to at least 20 cm must be carried out in every patient with penetrating pelvic trauma, complex pelvic fractures, and blood noted on rectal examination. The procedure is performed in the left lateral or Lloyd-Davies position, and retained feces are removed by irrigation through the proctoscope. A meticulous detailed examination of the entire rectal mucosa is carried out by the surgeon, who will decide whether laparotomy is necessary. This prevents confusion as to whether bruises on the mucosa are in fact rectal injuries or were iatrogenically produced during the initial proctoscopic examination.

An aggressive approach is warranted for any rectal injuries above the dentate line. Middle or high rectal injuries require surgical intervention with a diverting proximal sigmoid colostomy. If the injury is in the upper rectum, the pelvic peritoneum is opened and an attempt made to close the injury from within the abdomen. The presacral space is dissected from within the abdomen, and a large Silastic sump drain is placed in the presacral space. A diverting stoma (colostomy) is created and the abdomen closed. For lower injuries, wide drainage of the presacral spaces is established with an incision made midway between the anus and the tip of the coccyx. Penrose drains are inserted into the presacral space through this perineal skin incision (Fig. 28-2). This technique ensures wide presacral drainage

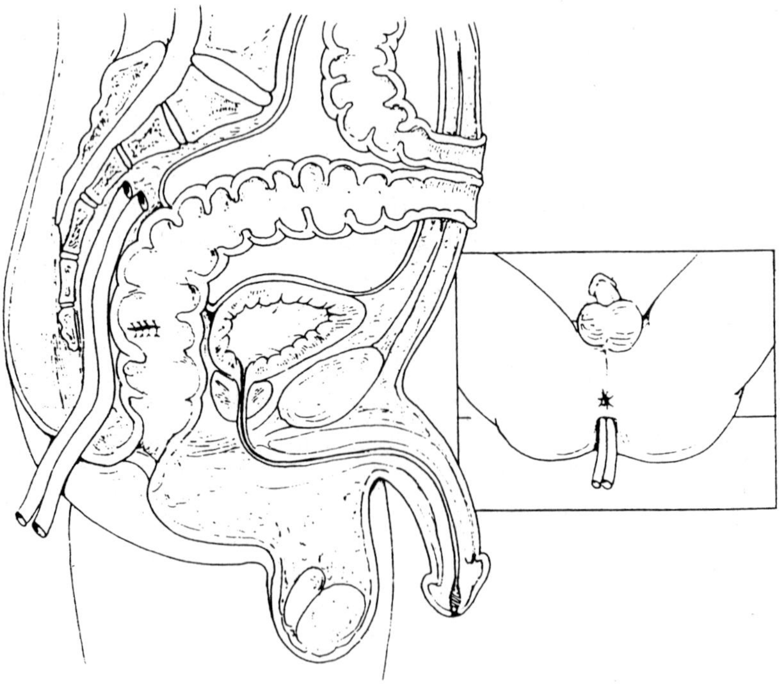

Fig. 28-2 Penrose drains in presacral space.

of the rectal injury. The final maneuver is removal of any retained feces in the rectum and the sigmoid colon distal to the colostomy. Most of the feces will have been removed during the proctoscopic examination. Should there be any retained feces, however, it is important to remove them with irrigation through the distal limb of the colostomy or a transrectal approach.[27] If the rectal injury is the result of penetrating trauma (e.g., a bullet), it should be remembered that the wound tract is contaminated. It is therefore wise to debride the skin edges of both entry and exit wounds (especially the exit wound) and to provide for external drainage of the wound tract to reduce the chances of infection and abscess formation. Fecal diversion is the cornerstone for the treatment of high-velocity penetrating rectal injuries, because failure to drain the presacral space is associated with a statistically significant increase in infectious complications.[5,42] Coccygectomy is not necessary to improve drainage of most rectal wounds.[4,5,54]

Patients with iatrogenic rectal injuries represent a unique subset of patients. Many patients in this group have undergone mechanical bowel preparation before the injury, which reduces the risks of fecal contamination and associated complications. A primary repair without colostomy is an option in patients at good risk if the iatrogenic injuries are quickly discovered and treated. As described in Chapter 9, patients with sealed colonoscopic perforations or transmural thermal injuries (postpolypectomy syndrome) may have mild to moderate abdominal pain, free intraperitoneal air, and localized tenderness. In selected patients who lack evidence of sepsis or diffuse peritonitis, management with close observation, bowel rest, and antibiotic therapy has been successful.[55]

Unlike colonoscopic perforations, perforations from barium contrast studies are associated with significant morbidity and mortality. The synergy of barium and stool has been described earlier.[56] This complicated injury has an associated mortality as high as 50% in older studies.[57] The recommended management of these injuries includes adequate intravenous fluids, early surgery with complete cleansing with antibiotic irrigation and mechanical debridement of the abdominal cavity, excision of the perforated segment of bowel, and establishment of an end colostomy or ileostomy and distal mucous fistula if possible.[58]

The reported morbidity and mortality of rectal injuries depends on the cause of the trauma and associated injuries. In modern military conflicts the mortality rate from rectal injuries has varied from 3% to 17% compared with 0% to 10% in civilian series.[6] The range of values reflects a spectrum of causes and associated injuries in each individual series.

Wound Closure

Before closure the abdominal cavity is irrigated with a copious amount of warm saline solution. Although some may claim this spreads the contamination, ample evidence shows a decreased frequency of complications after abdominal irrigation.[33,59] Antibiotic irrigation has been recommended by some authors.[60] The midline fascia is then closed with monofilament sutures. The incision is irrigated again, and the wound is packed open or closed, depending on the status of the abdomen. Skin closure after significant contamination in patients with traumatic injuries has produced a 40% to 50% prevalence of wound infection.[32] Open wounds are managed with sterile dressing changes three time daily. The majority of these wounds remain clean and lend themselves nicely to delayed primary closure in 4 or 5 days.

Drains

Colonic injuries per se—whether closed or not—need not be drained. Ample evidence in the literature shows that although drains are useful to remove infectious material from the wound, they may well serve to increase the incidence of infection and intra-abdominal abscess formation.[61] Associated intra-abdominal injuries to other viscera (pancreas, kidney, liver, duodenum, and bladder) may, however, require drainage. When the surgeon is presented with the problem of creating a colostomy and draining an associated visceral injury, a degree of ingenuity is required. The stoma and the drain should be kept as far apart as possible, ideally on opposite sides of the abdomen. To accomplish this it may be necessary to mobilize the colon so that the stoma can be optimally sited. Sterile wound drainage bags are now available and have proved helpful in isolating the drains in a "sterile" environment. In addition, these bags facilitate collection, measurement, and analysis of the drainage material.

Anal Injury

Traumatic anal injuries are uncommon. The gluteal muscles and ischiorectal soft tissues protect the anal sphincter muscles and pelvic nerves from significant blunt or penetrating trauma. However, certain sexual practices result in more unusual injuries of the anorectum. Frequently these injuries involve the anal sphincters[62]; the excellent blood supply to the perineum, however, promotes healing in repaired anal sphincters and lessens the chance of ischemic necrosis.

A variety of traumatic events lead to anal and perineal trauma. The most common injury is iatrogenic obstetric trauma.[63] An extensive episiotomy or puerperal anal injuries from third- and fourth-degree tears (e.g., traumatic cloaca) create anal sphincter damage.[64] These injuries are often identified and repaired immediately. If the initial repair does not adequately approximate the sphincters or the repair breaks down from infection, the patient is left with a rectovaginal postpartum anal incontinence.

Other less common causes include lacerations, impalements, and straddle injuries. Gunshot or blast injuries, foreign body anorectal trauma, and fist fornication are more unusual and infrequent causes of anal injury.

A detailed history and physical examination provide appreciation of present sphincter function and define the extent of perineal trauma and associated injuries. With obstetric trauma, the history may entail the location of an episiotomy or a complicated forceps delivery. In penetrating or blunt trauma, the history may reveal associated pelvic injuries that require further evaluation. Undetected sphincter injuries frequently lead to a delay in diagnosis of incontinence; therefore, sphincter function should be documented at initial evaluation in all patients. The history should include assessment of the extent of continence for gas, liquid, and solid feces. The physician should detail how well the patient copes with urgency, seepage and soiling, and diarrhea. It is also important to obtain a past history of anorectal surgery including hemorrhoidectomy, fistulotomy, sphincter repair, and abscess drainage. Digital examination should be performed to assess the extent of the injury and the presence of a defect. In acute trauma, other studies such as manometry, saline solution retention, balloon expulsion, EMG, or other tests of anal sensation are often unavailable. After the acute phase, these studies and intra-anal ultrasound studies help to categorize the injury and provide important prognostic information.

The primary goal of therapy is debridement of necrotic tissue and open drainage to prevent perineal sepsis. After this, attempts are made to restore the contractile competence of the sphincter by means of identification, mobilization, and reapproximation of the severed muscular components, with re-creation of the perineal body. Superficial lacerations in the perineum are easily debrided and left open for drainage. Small internal sphincter lacerations or isolated sphincteric injuries may be repaired in selected cases without a colostomy. Antibiotics are used to assist in control of local wound infections.

Larger perineal wounds are treated when the patient's medical condition is stabilized. Sphincter injuries are rarely life threatening and in unstable patients are best managed with a diverting stoma, drainage, and delayed repair. In stable patients significant sphincter injuries are managed with patient and meticulous reapproximation of tissue without tension.[64] Closure of easily identifiable layers such as the anal mucosa assists in orienting the other perineal structures. Because of the acute nature of the injury, requirement for debridement, and lack of supporting scar tissue, an overlapping sphincter repair is not possible. Use of slowly absorbing sutures such as polyglycolic acid or polyglactin 910 reduces the risk of chronic suture sinuses.[65] Proximal diversion and adequate drainage are critical in these complex injuries.

Combat blast injuries to the sphincter are extremely difficult wounds to treat. Lung et al.[7] found that during the Vietnam War,[24] soldiers with this injury were hospitalized on average for 207 days and required on average 3.2 operations.

POSTOPERATIVE COMPLICATIONS

The postoperative complications from surgery to treat trauma to the colorectum are essentially similar to those from other types of colonic surgery: anastomotic leakage, infection, abscess, fistulas, and stoma complications.

FOREIGN BODY IN THE RECTUM AND COLON

Foreign bodies may be introduced into the rectum and colon for a variety of reasons: diagnostic and therapeutic procedures (e.g., administration of enemas in which the enema tip may become dislodged, misplacement of a rectal thermometer),[59] or criminal assault,[66] or, by far the most common cause of foreign bodies in the colorectum, autoeroticism.[67,68]

In patients who have retained a rectal foreign body, a careful history and physical examination should be followed by a biplanar radiograph of the abdomen to determine not only the exact position of the foreign body (or bodies) but also whether there is free air in the abdomen. This is particularly important if the patient has already removed the foreign body but the abdomen is tender and peritoneal signs are present.[67]

Once the foreign body is located, it can be classified as low lying (palpable in the rectum) or high lying (in or proximal to the rectosigmoid junction). Treatment goals include transanal removal whenever possible, removal of the object intact (especially glass objects), prevention of colorectal lacerations (and subsequent bleeding and perforation), and avoidance of a colotomy in unprepared bowel (with the associated septic complications). Appropriate relaxation and sedation are essential for removal of retained rectal foreign bodies.[69] Local anal anesthesia provides both sphincter relaxation and analgesia and allows the examiner to insert instruments for examination and removal of the object. An awake patient can also assist extraction with the Valsalva maneuver. It is often possible to remove the object through the anus and maintain an intact anal sphincter. If a sphincterotomy is performed or created, the muscles must be repaired.

Multiple and new approaches have been described to remove a wide variety of objects while minimizing morbidity.[42,70] Techniques that have been used to remove foreign bodies through the anus include inserting a Foley catheter above the object, inflating the balloon, and using it to pull the object down; inserting a taneculum, snare, or forceps through a proctoscope or anoscope to grasp the object; and, in the case of hollow objects, inserting plaster of paris along with a string or handle to pull the object out after the plaster hardens.[69] Nehme-Kingsley and Abcarian[71] noted no severe injuries in more than 50 cases of rectal foreign body removal. After the foreign body is removed, it is essential to evaluate the anorectum with endoscopy and contrast-enhanced studies to exclude perforations.

Laparotomy is used only as a last resort after failure of anal manipulations. With the patient under general anesthesia and receiving systemic antibiotics, a combined abdominal and transanal approach is used. The foreign body can often be "milked down" to the middle or lower rectum and subsequently removed by the perineal surgeon.[69] If this fails, a generous colotomy may be necessary to remove the object. Complications may include abdominal abscesses, wound infection, and ventral hernia.[67] Foreign body perforations are managed as previously described for other penetrating injuries.

Table 28-4 Iatrogenic perforation of the colon

Study	No. of studies	No. of perforations (%)	Mortality (%)
Barium (lower GI)	42,000	7 (0.016)	7 (100)
Protosigmoidoscopy	16,325	3 (0.018)	1 (33)
Colonoscopy	1,207	3 (0.24)	0 (0)

From Nelson RL, Abcarian H, Prasad ML. Iatrogenic perforation of the colon and rectum. Dis Colon Rectum 25:305-308, 1982.

After the foreign body is removed, proctosigmoidoscopy is performed to ensure that there has been no laceration or perforation of the rectum and there are no other radiolucent foreign bodies proximal to the one already removed. It is not unusual to observe minor mucosal contusions and submucosal hematoma after extraction of foreign bodies. All patients with such contusions and hematomas should be hospitalized and observed for delayed bleeding or perforation for at least 24 hours.[67] If signs and symptoms of peritoneal irritation are present or the abdominal films reveal free air, an emergency laparotomy is indicated. Often, the foreign body may already have been removed by the patient.

IATROGENIC PERFORATION OF THE COLON

Iatrogenic perforation of the colon is an unfortunate and, for the most part, avoidable complication of diagnostic tests of the colon. The frequency of this complication is related not only to the integrity of the colon examined but also, to a great extent, to the experience of the examiner.

An 8-year experience with iatrogenic perforation of the colon at Cook County Hospital is summarized in Table 28-4.[72] The most frequent cause of endoscopic perforation is the use of excessive force. Complications and principles of management of these perforations are described in Chapter 9. These perforations, if detected early and treated appropriately, will heal completely with minor septic complications. This is not true of perforations from lower GI barium studies, because barium sulfate acts synergistically with blood, feces, or bile to accelerate the inflammatory and septic processes.[68-75] Even with early diagnosis, immediate resuscitation, and surgery, the mortality rate may exceed 50%.[76]

CONCLUSION

Traumatic injuries to the colon or rectum have the potential for serious morbidity. Reduction in morbidity and prevention of complications depend on a systematic team approach prioritized to deal first with life-threatening injuries. After the patient's vital signs have been stabilized, a decision about the need for abdominal exploration must be made. Injuries to the rectum must be recognized before decisions are made to explore the abdomen. A systematic approach to the injured abdominal viscera must be used during laparotomy for trauma. Decisions about primary closure of colonic injuries depend largely on the anatomic nature of the injury, associated injuries, degree of contamination, and stability of the patient's condition. If the injury is unsuitable for primary closure, it should be either repaired or resected with proximal diversion. Use of these principles will reduce the degree and magnitude of complications after surgery to treat trauma to the colon and rectum.

REFERENCES

1. Abcarian H, Barrett JA. Complications of surgery for trauma to colon and rectum. In Gathright JB, Ferrari BT, Ray JE, eds. Complications in Colon and Rectal Surgery. Philadelphia: WB Saunders, 1985, pp 143-155.
2. Abcarian H, Lowe R. Colon and rectal trauma. Surg Clin North Am 58:519-537, 1978.
3. Rutledge R, Thomason M, Oller D, et al. The spectrum of abdominal injuries associated with the use of seat belts. J Trauma 31:820-826, 1991.
4. Ivatury RR, Licata J, Gunduz Y, et al. Management options in penetrating rectal injuries. Am Surg 57:50-55, 1991.
5. Burch JM, Feliciano DV, Mattox KL. Colostomy and drainage for civilian rectal injuries: Is that all? Ann Surg 209:600-611, 1989.
6. Marcet JE, Gottesman L. Anorectal trauma and necrotizing infections. In Beck DE, Wexner SD, eds. Fundamentals of Anorectal Surgery. New York: McGraw-Hill, 1992, pp 440-452.
7. Lung JA, Turk RP, Miller RE, et al. Wounds of the rectum. Ann Surg 172:985-990, 1970.
8. Nance FC. Injuries to colon and rectum. In Moore EE, Mattox KL, Feliciano DV, eds. Trauma. Norwalk, Conn.: Appleton & Lange, 1991, pp 521-532.
9. Williams SM, Harned RK. Recognition and prevention of barium enema complications. Curr Probl Diagn Radiol 20:123-151, 1991.
10. Tadros S, Watters JM. Retroperitoneal perforation of the rectum during barium enema examinations. Can J Surg 31:49-50, 1988.
11. Hool GJ, Bokey EL, Pheils MT. Enema-nozzle injury of the rectum. Med J Aust 1:364, 381, 1980.
12. Sohn N, Weinstein MA, Gonchar J. Social injuries of the rectum. Am J Surg 134:611-612, 1977.
13. Black CT, Pokorny WJ, McGill CW, et al. Ano-rectal trauma in children. J Pediatr Surg 17: 501-504, 1982.
14. Schwartz GF, Polsky HS. Ingested foreign bodies of the gastrointestinal tract. Am Surg 42: 236-238, 1976.
15. Moore EE, Cogbill TH, Malangoni MA, et al. Organ injury scaling. II. Pancreas, duodenum, small bowel, colon, and rectum. J Trauma 30:1427-1429, 1990.
16. Committee on Trauma, American College of Surgeons. Advanced Trauma Life Support. Chicago: The College, 1981.
17. Root HD, Hauser CW, McKinley CR, et al. Diagnostic peritoneal lavage. Surgery 57:633, 1965.

18. Fischer RP, Beverlin BC, Engrav LH, et al. Diagnostic peritoneal lavage: Fourteen years and 2,586 patients later. Am J Surg 136:701-704, 1978.
19. Pachter HL, Hofstetter SR. Open and percutaneous paracentesis and lavage for abdominal trauma. A randomized prospective study. Arch Surg 116:318-319, 1981.
20. Lowe RJ, Saletta JD, Read DR, et al. Should laparotomy be mandatory or selective in gunshot wounds of the abdomen? J Trauma 17:903-907, 1977.
21. Edwards J, Gaspard DJ. Visceral injury due to extraperitoneal gunshot wounds. Arch Surg 108:865, 1974.
22. Bull JC Jr, Mathewson C Jr. Exploratory laparotomy in patients with penetrating wounds of the abdomen. Am J Surg 116:223-228, 1968.
23. Forde KA, Ganepola GA. Is mandatory exploration for penetrating abdominal trauma extinct? The morbidity and mortality of negative exploration in a large municipal hospital. J Trauma 14:764-766, 1974.
24. Bowerman JW, Smithwick W III. Contrast examination of abdominal stab wounds. Radiology 97:619-624, 1970.
25. Trimble C. Stab wound sinography. Surg Clin North Am 49:1217-1221, 1969.
26. Nance FC, Wennar MH, Johnson LW, et al. Surgical judgement in the management of penetrating wounds of the abdomen—experience with 2,212 patients. Ann Surg 179:639-646, 1974.
27. Lowe RJ, Boyd DR, Folk FA, et al. The negative laparotomy for abdominal trauma. J Trauma 12:853-861, 1972.
28. Rowlands BJ, Ericsson CD, Fischer RP. Penetrating abdominal trauma: The use of operative findings to determine length of antibiotic therapy. J Trauma 27:250-255, 1987.
29. Wexner SD, Beck DE. Sepsis prevention in colorectal surgery. In Operative Surgery, 5th ed. London: Butterworth-Heinemann, 1993, pp 41-46.
30. Jones RC, Thal ER, Johnson NA, et al. Evaluation of antibiotic therapy following penetrating abdominal trauma. Ann Surg 201:576-585, 1985.
31. Catell RB, Braash JW. A technique for the exposure of the third and fourth portions of the duodenum. Surg Gynecol Obstet 111:379, 1960.
32. Stone HH, Fabian TC. Management of perforating colon trauma. Randomization between primary closure and exteriorization. Ann Surg 190:430-436, 1979.
33. Polk HC Jr. Generalized peritonitis: A continuing challenge [editorial]. Surgery 88:777, 1979.
34. Flint LM, Vitale GC, Richardson JD, et al. The injured colon. The relationship of management to complications. Ann Surg 193:619-623, 1981.
35. Thompson JS, Moore EE, Moore JB. Comparison of penetrating injuries of the right and left colon. Ann Surg 193:414-448, 1981.
36. Mollett DL, Malangoni MA, Ballatine TV, et al. Colostomy complications in children: An analysis of 146 cases. Arch Surg 115:455-458, 1980.
37. Dolan PA, Caldwell FT, Thompson CH, et al. Problems of colostomy closure. Am J Surg 137: 188-191, 1979.
38. Khoury D, Beck DE, Opelka FG. Colostomy closure: The Ochsner experience (submitted for publication).
39. Sullivan WG, Miller RE, Eiseman B. Closure of colonic stomas in patients injured in combat. Surg Gynecol Obstet 131:1045-1051, 1970.
40. Thal ER, Yeary EC. Morbidity of colostomy closure following colon trauma. J Trauma 20: 287-291, 1980.
41. Mirelman D, Corman ML, Veidenheimer MC, et al. Colostomies—indications and contraindications. Lahey Clinic experience, 1963-1974. Dis Colon Rectum 21:172-176, 1978.

42. Beck DE, Opelka FG. Pelvic and perineal trauma. Perspect Colon Rectal Surg 6:134-156, 1993.
43. Dang CV, Peter ET, Parks SN, et al. Trauma of the colon: Early drop-back of exteriorized repair. Arch Surg 117:652-656, 1982.
44. Lou MA, Johnson AP, Atk M, et al. Exteriorized repair in the management of colon injuries. Arch Surg 116:926-929, 1981.
45. Trunkey D, Hays RJ, Shires GT. Management of rectal trauma. J Trauma 13:411-415, 1973.
46. Chunn CF, Hauver RV. Wounds of the colon and rectum (1,222 casualties). In General Surgery, vol 2. Surgery in World War II. Washington, DC: Office of the Surgeon General, Department of the Army, 1953, pp 255-274.
47. Ganchrow MI, Laverson GS Jr, McNamara JJ. Surgical management of traumatic injuries of the colon and rectum. Arch Surg 100:515-520, 1970.
48. Laverson GS Jr, Cohen A. Management of rectal injuries. Am J Surg 122:226-230, 1971.
49. Vitale GC, Richardson JD, Flint LM. Successful management of injuries to the extraperitoneal rectum. Am Surg 49:159-162, 1983.
50. Grasberger RC, Hirsch EF. Rectal trauma—a retrospective analysis and guidelines for therapy. Am J Surg 145:795-799, 1983.
51. Tuggle D, Huber PJ. Management of rectal trauma. Am J Surg 148:806-808, 1984.
52. Mangiante EC, Graham AD, Fabian TC. Rectal gunshot wounds—Management of civilian injuries. Am Surg 52:37-40, 1986.
53. Shannon FL, Moore EE, Moore FA, et al. Value of distal colon washout in civilian rectal trauma-reducing gut bacterial translocation. J Trauma 28:989-994, 1988.
54. Thomas DD, Levison MA, Dykstra BJ, et al. Management of rectal injuries. Dogma versus practice. Am Surg 56:507-510, 1990.
55. Opelka FG, Hicks TC, Beck DE. Management of colonoscopic perforations (submitted for publication).
56. Sisel RJ, Donovan AJ, Yellin AE. Experimental fecal peritonitis: Influence of barium sulfate or water-soluble radiologic contrast material on survival. Arch Surg 104:765-768, 1972.
57. Zhuetlin N, Lasse JC, Riler LG. Clinical studies on effect of barium in the peritoneal cavity following rupture of the colon. Surgery 32:967-979, 1952.
58. Hardy TG Jr, Hartmann RF, Aguilar PS, et al. Survival after colonic perforation during barium-enema examination. Modified radical surgical debridement. Dis Colon Rectum 26: 116-118, 1983.
59. Hunt J. Generalized peritonitis. To irrigate or not to irrigate the abdominal cavity. Arch Surg 117:209-212, 1982.
60. Anderson B, Korner B, Osrergaard AH. Topical ampicillin against wound infection after colorectal surgery. Ann Surg 176:129, 1972.
61. Bartizal JF, Boyd DR, Folk FA, et al. A critical review of management of 392 colonic and rectal injuries. Dis Colon Rectum 17:313-318, 1974.
62. Critchlow JF, Houlihan MJ, Landolt CC, et al. Primary sphincter repair in anorectal trauma. Dis Colon Rectum 28:945-947, 1985.
63. Tancer ML, Lasser D, Rosenblum N. Rectovaginal fistula or perineal and anal sphincter disruption, or both, after vaginal delivery. Surg Gynecol Obstet 171:43-46, 1990.
64. Hambrick E. Sphincteroplasty/perineoplasty for traumatic anal sphincter injuries. Perspect Colon Rectal Surg 2:91-98, 1989.
65. Rebell FG. Problems of foreign bodies of the colon and rectum. Am J Surg 76:678, 1948.
66. Macht SH. Foreign body (bottle) in the rectum. Radiology 42:500, 1944.
67. Barone JE, Sohn N, Nealon TF. Perforation and foreign bodies of the rectum. Ann Surg 184: 601-604, 1976.

68. Eftaiha M, Hambrick E, Abcarian H. Principles of management of colorectal foreign bodies. Arch Surg 112:691-695, 1977.
69. Smith LE. Traumatic injuries. In Gordon PH, Natvatvongs S, eds. Principles and Practice of Surgery for the Colon, Rectum and Anus. St. Louis: Quality Medical Publishing, 1992, pp 958-980.
70. Koplatadze AM, Bondarev Iu A. Injuries and foreign bodies of the rectum [Russian]. Khirurgiia 9:53-56, 1990.
71. Nehme-Kingsley A, Abcarian H. Colorectal foreign bodies—management update. Dis Colon Rectum 28:941-944, 1985.
72. Nelson RL, Abcarian H, Prasad ML. Iatrogenic perforation of the colon and rectum. Dis Colon Rectum 25:305-308, 1982.
73. Kay S, Choy SH. Results of intraperitoneal injection of barium sulfate contrast medium: Experimental study. Arch Pathol 59:388, 1955.
74. Hau T, Ahrenholz DH, Simmons RL. Secondary bacterial peritonitis: The biologic basis of treatment. Curr Probl Surg 16:1-65, 1979.
75. Foley MJ, Ghahremani GG, Rogers LF. Reappraisal of contrast media used to detect upper gastrointestinal perforations: Comparison of ionic water-soluble media with barium sulfate. Radiology 144:231-237, 1982.
76. Grodsky L. Perforations of the colon and rectum during administration of barium enema. Dis Colon Rectum 2:216, 1959.

CHAPTER 29

Medicolegal Issues

CHARLES F. GAY, Jr.

This chapter addresses some risk-prevention techniques for colorectal surgeons. It endeavors to provide physicians with a general overview of the legal process pertaining to medical malpractice issues and tips to help prevent and defend such cases. It is intended to provide practical information that can be used, not a comprehensive scholarly discussion of medicolegal issues.

In today's litigious society, physicians who practice good medicine, exercise effective communications skills, establish rapport with the patient, and accurately document care have the best chance of averting malpractice claims. Even when physicians do all of these, however, a bad outcome may still result in the patient's filing a claim for malpractice.[1] Research appears to support the position that a patient who perceives the physician as having good interpersonal skills and communication is less likely to sue.[2]

There are ways to conduct a medical practice that deter patients from making claims and, even after one is made, can enhance the chances of winning the case.

PHYSICIAN-PATIENT RELATIONSHIP

Medicine has changed dramatically in the last few decades because of extraordinary technologic advances that have resulted in specialization, such as colorectal surgery. This fragmentation often decreases the opportunity to communicate effectively with patients, who have also become much more demanding consumers, increasingly aware of their "rights" through media and lawyer advertising. Health insurers contribute to the problem, not only by creating incentives that discourage referrals to a specialist but also by placing restrictions on the specialist, once referral is made, that can impede opportunities to establish rapport with the patient. Under such circumstances, it is important to make the most of each opportunity to listen to the patient, remember and use the patient's name, explain procedures in lay terms (avoid medical terminology), and take the time necessary to answer any and all questions. Remember that listening to a patient's questions and complaints will be much less time consuming than defending a malpractice claim.

Still one of the best books for improving communication and relationships is Dale Carnegie's *How to Win Friends and Influence People.*[3] For a more practical guide with a medical orientation one should read *Malpractice Prevention and Liability Control for Hospitals,* by Orlikoff and Vanagunas.[4]

The frequency of medical malpractice claims has been on the rise since the early 1970's.[5] As long as the contingency fee system exists and there is not a loser pay provision, the rise in suits against physicians will likely continue. Accordingly, it is incumbent on the well-educated and well-trained specialist to be aware of areas of treatment in colorectal disease that present an increased risk of malpractice claims.[6]

HIGH-RISK AREAS IN COLORECTAL TREATMENT

The following circumstances associated with increased risk for malpractice claims in colorectal disease have been identified[6]:

1. Delay in diagnosis of colon and rectal cancer and appendicitis
2. Iatrogenic colon injury (e.g., colon perforation)
3. Iatrogenic medical complications during diagnosis or treatment
4. Sphincter injury with fecal incontinence resulting from anorectal surgery
5. Lack of informed consent

The colorectal physician who is aware of these potential high-risk conditions can use risk-prevention strategies to avoid litigation.

INFORMED CONSENT

Physicians should be mindful that consent and informed consent are quite different concepts. Consent implies permission. Informed consent is assent given based on information provided or knowledge of the procedure and its inherent risks, benefits, and alternatives.

Courts have long recognized that "Every human being of adult years and sound mind has a right to determine what shall be done with his own body."[7] The law of informed consent may vary to some degree from state to state, but regardless of the law of the state, each patient should be allowed an exchange of information with the physician before a procedure is done. Informed consent is not satisfied by merely having the patient sign a form. It is satisfied when consent was obtained after full disclosure of the risks, benefits, and alternatives of the procedure.

Many states use the "reasonable practitioner standard" to judge whether informed consent was obtained. This standard focuses on what a reasonable physician would disclose. The physician's duty is not to disclose all risks but primarily those that are significant or material. A risk is material depending on its likelihood of occurrence or the degree of harm it presents. The focus is on whether a reasonable person in the patient's position probably would attach significance to the specific risk. This is the "reasonable patient standard" that some state courts apply.

Moreover, to prevail on a claim for lack of informed consent, in most states the patient must still prove causation (i.e., that he or she would not have consented to the procedure if informed of the risk. As a practical matter, it is difficult for a patient to persuade a judge or jury that even though the surgery was needed to relieve pain or disease, he or she would not have consented if told of the risk of, for example, perforation of the colon. This is particularly true when a patient is told of much more severe risks such as death or paraplegia and agrees to the surgery. In that regard, the question to be answered by the judge or jury on an issue of informed consent is whether a reasonable patient in the plaintiff's position would have consented to the treatment or procedure even if the material information and risks were disclosed.

The following points should always be discussed with the patient:

- The nature of the ailment, condition, or diagnosis being treated
- The general nature of the proposed treatment or procedure
- The likely prospects for success of the treatment (but no guarantee)
- The risks of failing to undergo the treatment
- The alternative methods of treatment, if any, and their inherent risks

Suffice it to say that good rapport with the patient coupled with accurate and complete charting are the best tools to deter suits based on informed consent and to provide a heavy shield in defending them.

DOCUMENTATION

The importance of good communication and rapport with patients (i.e., treating patients as you would like to be treated) cannot be overemphasized in deterring lawsuits; however, complete and accurate documentation of patient care is invaluable to a defense of claims. In addition, good documentation may well nip in the bud a potential claim when the plaintiff attorney considering filing suit reviews the record and care is fully documented. Plaintiff attorneys are more likely to bring suit when the case is poorly documented, because they can more easily argue that what happened in the care of the patient was sinister and improper. Where documentation is clear and accurate, the plaintiff attorney may be deterred from filing suit because what happened is easily proved from the record. Thus judgment becomes the issue when documentation is accurate, and judgment used by physicians in most cases is easier to successfully defend than a vague, evasive, and poorly documented chart.

The following are some time-honored rules for charting that help defend against malpractice claims.

Charting

A. Thorough and accurate charting is your primary shield to liability.

B. If an event in which you are involved gives rise to litigation, chances are your testimony will not be taken for 1 or 2 years after the event. Accordingly, your chart will provide the content and guidelines for your testimony.

C. *Most important:* If it is not charted, it was not done, nor was it observed, administered, or reported. In *Smith v. State through Dept. of HHR,*[8] the court stated:

> The experts concluded that decedent's condition required continued monitoring and that charting should have been done on a regular basis. The experts also agreed that the lack of documentation indicated that no one was properly observing the decedent, based on the standard maxim *"not charted, not done."*
>
> . . . The evidence indicates that the decedent was not adequately monitored in this case. The nurses did not specifically recall the patient, and thus the *best evidence of their actions would have been the documentation of the chart* (emphasis added).

D. General guidelines
   1. If you are the treating or primary physician, make a daily entry on the chart.
   2. Chart at the earliest possible time.
   3. If the situation prevents you from charting until later, state why and that the recorded times are best estimates and not fully accurate.
   4. Always record the time (designate AM or PM) and the date of every entry.
   5. Chart all consultations.
   6. *Never* black out or white out any entry on a chart. Should you make a mistake in charting, place a single line through the erroneous entry and label the entry "error in charting." However, if a hospital policy exists that governs errors in charting, follow it. An addendum is acceptable if placed properly in sequence with the date and time it is made. An addendum squeezed between progress notes is inappropriate.
   7. Write legibly.
   8. Spell correctly.
   9. Chart professionally; do not impugn or insult the patient.
   10. *Never* alter the medical records.
   11. Do not insult, impugn, or criticize colleagues, co-workers, or support staff.
   12. *Always* designate the dose, site, route, and time of medication administration.

13. Sign your entries on the chart.
14. Do not chart an incident report in your notes.
15. Chart objectively, not subjectively; do not use ambiguous terms (examples below).

Subjective	Objective
Patient doing well.	Patient denies any complaints. Awake, alert, and oriented. Vital signs stable: BP, 100/70; P, 72; R, 18.
Breath sounds within normal limits (WNL).	Respirations regular and unlabored. Breath sounds clear and equal bilaterally on auscultation. No rales or rhonchi noted.
Circulation check WNL.	Pedal pulses noted bilaterally. Nail beds blanch quickly and toes warm to touch. Patient denies any pain or tingling.

16. Document use of all restraints and safeguards, and patient positioning (extremely important in surgery).
17. Document all patient noncompliance.
18. Document all patient education and discharge instructions, and patient responses.
19. Always document patient status on transfer or discharge.
20. Record the patient's name on each page of the medical chart.
21. Use accepted medical abbreviations.
22. Do not chart in advance.

E. Guidelines for charting in the ambulatory setting
   1. Always chart the return visit date and that the date was provided to the patient.
   2. Always chart all cancelled and missed appointments.
   3. Document all telephone conversations and their content.
   4. Chart all prescriptions and refills, as well as patient teaching regarding prescriptions.
   5. Chart all follow-up and discharge instructions. If possible, have the patient or his or her representative cosign these instructions.

ANATOMY OF A MALPRACTICE SUIT

Initial Phase

Once a patient initiates a claim for medical malpractice, the physician should immediately place a call to the risk manager or to the malpractice insurance carrier. An attorney will usually be selected, and the physician should insist that the appointed counsel be experienced and have a well-established reputation in the handling of malpractice cases.

Physicians should work closely with the defense attorney to review and analyze the allegations of the suit, with particular focus on the strengths and weaknesses of the case. This team effort can often substantially enhance the strength of the defense by educating the attorney on the medical aspects of the case.

Pretrial Discovery

During this stage, each side will discover the facts and opinions in the case. Written questions, or interrogatories, can usually be propounded to obtain written responses. Depositions usually follow the written discovery and are important to the overall outcome of the case. Before testifying by deposition or otherwise, it is advisable that the physician be thoroughly familiar with the facts, including previous and subsequent medical care of the patient and the allegations against the physician. This requires careful review of medical records, other depositions, and all medical data related to the case. A conference should be held with the attorney before the physician's deposition. The physician should allow ample time to confer with the defense attorney before testifying. Remember that the judicial system is adversarial, and the purpose of the deposition is not to convince the plaintiff attorney to understand the case is frivolous. The physician is there to answer the questions and defend the care administered, not to educate the plaintiff attorney.

The deposition is simply the physician's testimony, given under oath, before a court reporter, in an informal setting. Attorneys for both defendant and plaintiff are present. Any party to the lawsuit may be present, but often the physician is the only party present. The testimony is taken down in question-and-answer form. Under the laws of discovery, the plaintiff attorney has the right to ask the defendant physician proper questions. The physician is present simply to discharge a legal obligation to answer proper questions.

The physician's deposition is most important. A good effort is essential for an effective presentation. Close cooperation with the defense attorney in preparation is fundamental. Above all, a physician must be his or her own person.

Thorough preparation will assist physicians in giving a deposition with which they will be perfectly comfortable when they see the printed transcript, that is, one that will be easily defended, should any part of it later be challenged.

The following suggestions for giving testimony in depositions can be helpful to the physician:

1. Tell the truth; you must testify accurately.
2. Do not guess or speculate. If you do not know the answer to a question, say so.
3. If you are not certain of what the attorney is asking, ask that the question be clarified or repeated. Do not attempt to rephrase the question for the interrogator (e.g., "If you mean such and such,").
4. Keep your answers short and concise. Do not volunteer information. Answer only the question posed.

5. Be courteous. Avoid jokes and sarcasm.
6. Think about each question that is posed. Listen to each word. Formulate an answer, then give the answer. Do not permit yourself to become hurried.
7. Do not argue with opposing counsel. If an argument is necessary, your attorney will do it for you.
8. If you realize that you have given an incorrect answer to a previous question, stop at that moment and say so; then correct your answer.
9. Be aware of questions that involve distances and time. If you make an estimate, make sure everyone knows it is an estimate.
10. Do not lose your temper, no matter how hard pressed. This may be a deliberate ploy; do not fall for it.
11. Do not anticipate questions. Be sure to let the attorney completely finish the question before you begin to respond.
12. Do not exaggerate or brag.

Testing Your Memory of the Case

You have the right to refer to the chart or hospital records whenever you wish. Your memory is usually a composite of events you recall as jogged by your records. Watch for generalities, ploys, and tricky questions by the plaintiff attorney during the deposition.

Generalities. Often the plaintiff's attorney will begin with general questions, such as, "Doctor, how do you treat a patient when you suspect he has *X* disease?" In all likelihood, the lawsuit to which you are a party involves *X* disease or involves the plaintiff's attorney trying to make it *X* disease. You really cannot answer this question, and you should say just that. *X* disease probably occurs in various forms, and you have been given no particular information—no patient complaints, no patient history, no findings on physical examination, no results of laboratory studies, no clinical impression—all factors you must know to diagnose and treat intelligently. The question is simply too general.

A similar question might be "Doctor, what are the standards for making a diagnosis of *X* disease?" Again, you should advise that this question is too broad and defies rational response because no details have been given. You, as a physician, do not immediately diagnose *X* disease or any other disease. You evaluate all the data in light of your formal training and clinical experience in considering or making a diagnosis. Patient signs and symptoms are innumerable. You must have specifics. For example, in one doubtful clinical presentation, you may have to order a particular set of laboratory studies; in another, the evidence of a certain disease process may be more definitive and clear-cut from the history and clinical examination.

A proper question is, "Doctor, what are the characteristics of *X* disease?"

Particularly if your case involves *X* disease, you should know its characteristics, but you should also point out that they are general characteristics and most certainly will vary in specific instances.

The point is, you must avoid generalities. You must demand specifics. Try to make the questioner stick to the specific case.

Ploys

Question: "Doctor, you have no memory of events independent of your records, do you?"

Appropriate response: "I have an excellent recall of the events when I refer to the records."

Ploy: "Doctor, if an event is not noted in your records or in the hospital records, is it fair to say that event did not occur?"

Appropriate response: "That is incorrect. It is impossible for a physician to note everything that occurs. My records are for my own use, to jog my memory. Thus I note pertinent highlights, which when later reviewed give me the complete picture at the time in question."

Remember that physicians treat patients, not charts. You may properly testify to the following:

1. What you actually recall
2. What you recall with the assistance of your records
3. What is recorded
4. What your routine or standard procedure is, even when such is not recalled and not recorded

Tricky questions. Many plaintiff attorneys will use questions cleverly phrased to evoke a response that can later be used against the physician.

Possibilities. Questions phrased in terms of possibility invite speculation and are improper. The criterion is reasonable medical probability.

Question: "Doctor, isn't such and such possible?" or "Couldn't such and such have happened?"

Appropriate response: "Most improbable."

Doing things differently. Almost all malpractice cases involve the "retrospectroscope" or Monday morning quarterbacking to suggest the physician knew things beforehand that were only learned later or that the physician has 100% control over the healing process.

Question: "Doctor, is there anything you would do differently now if you had Mrs. White's case to treat again?"

Appropriate response: "My recommendations to Mrs. White were based on her complaints, her history, and findings at the time and on my clinical impression at that time. The course I recommended was appropriate on the basis of those factors."

Question: "Doctor, you did not intend for Mrs. White to have this complication, did you?"

Appropriate response: "Of course, no harm to Mrs. White was intended. At the time of my recommendations, there were good prospects for a good result. The procedure (or regimen) does have known complications, and that is why the risks were explained to her beforehand."

Many other factors are involved in preparing for and successfully testifying by deposition or at trial.[9] Suffice it to say that effective and sincere testimony is critical to a successful defense in malpractice cases. Ineffective testimony can render a defensible case indefensible. Many tricks and ploys may be used by the plaintiff attorney, and the physician who is prepared with a basic understanding of how to answer such questions can substantially enhance the defense.

Trial

After pretrial discovery, the physician should have a clear understanding of the evidence and witnesses, the experts in particular, to be used against him or her at trial. Working with the defense attorney to rebut this evidence and to assist with selection of expert witnesses to testify for the defense is strongly advised and helps the physician to prepare the defense.

At the trial, the physician is carefully observed at all times by the judge and jury, and the physician's trial testimony, mannerisms, and behavior are critical to a favorable verdict. A well-trained and educated physician who portrays a sincere, conscientious, and caring attitude about the patient's well-being greatly increases the chances of a favorable jury verdict, even where severe complications have occurred and there may be questions of the appropriateness of the course of treatment chosen.

CONCLUSION

The defense of medical malpractice claims is similar to the defense of criminal cases. The physician stands accused and reputation is usually an issue of great importance. The emotional costs to the physician are sometimes staggering. The physician should recognize that until some meaningful tort reform is enacted, these cases will likely continue to increase and should be dealt with as a regrettable aspect of the practice.[10] Under these circumstances, it is best to accept the reality of the medicolegal arena and use the best means available to aggressively defend and win the malpractice case.

REFERENCES

1. Entman SS, Glass CA, Hickson GB, Githens PB, Whetten-Goldstein K, Sloan FA. The relationship between malpractice claims history and subsequent obstetric care. JAMA 272: 1588-1591, 1994.

2. Hickson GB, Clayton EW, Githens PB, Sloan FA. Factors that prompted families to file medical malpractice claims following perinatal injuries. JAMA 267:1359-1363, 1992.
3. Carnegie D. How to Win Friends and Influence People. New York: Simon & Schuster, 1936.
4. Orlikoff J, Vanagunas A. Malpractice Prevention and Liability Control for Hospitals. Chicago: American Hospital Association, 1988.
5. Danzon PM. The frequency and severity of medical malpractice claims: New evidence. Law Contemp Probl 49:57-84, 1986.
6. Kern K. Medical malpractice involving colon and rectal disease: A 20-year review of United States civil court litigation. Dis Colon Rectum 36:531-539, 1993.
7. Schloendorff v. Society of New York Hospital, 2112 NY125, 105 NE 92,93 (1914).
8. Smith v. State, through Dept of HHR, 517 So2d 1072 (La App 3d Cir 1987).
9. Taraska JM. The physician as witness. In Legal Guide for Physicians. New York: Matthew Bender, 1994, pp 1-56.
10. Taraska JM. Tort reform. In Legal Guide for Physicians. New York: Matthew Bender, 1994, pp 1-64.

CHAPTER 30

Miscellaneous Conditions

FERAN AGACHAN
STEVEN D. WEXNER

In addition to the complications already discussed, pruritus ani, condyloma acuminatum, sexually transmitted diseases, and AIDS merit discussion.

PRURITUS ANI

Although there are many causes of pruritus ani, in the majority of patients there is no identifiable cause.[1] Despite the availability of a variety of alternative medical treatments, keeping the skin of the anal area clean, dry, and slightly acidic remains the most effective means of achieving a permanent cure for pruritus ani.[2] Dietary control, management of infections, dermatoses, systemic disorders, and avoidance of irritating oral and topical medications are also beneficial measures. Pruritus ani may occasionally be associated with fissures, fistulas, prolapsing hemorrhoids, anal mucosal prolapse, and a variety of isolated skin lesions. If a definable anatomic abnormality can be determined to be the sole cause of the pruritus, surgery may be appropriate. However, the vast majority of cases are idiopathic. Optimal management in these patients generally consists of instruction in diet and perianal hygiene. Acute exacerbation of pruritus ani can be treated with a short course of topical hydrocortisone; however, long-term use of topical fluorinated steroids may cause comedone formation and attenuation of skin, with exacerbation of symptoms. Other, more aggressive treatments have been suggested, many of which can produce significant complications.

Injection of alcohol, oil-soluble anesthetics, or methylene blue into the perianal skin or tattooing of the perianal skin with mercuric sulfide provide only temporary relief of intractable pruritus ani.[3,4] These procedures are associated with abscess formation in the subcutaneous tissue, necrosis of the skin, and sloughing of the perianal skin as a result of the extreme irritability of the solutions. These complications can be treated with local drainage, debridement of necrotic tissue, and broad-spectrum antibiotics. Because of the prohibitive morbidity and negligible success rates, injection therapy is not widely practiced.

Another treatment option for severe pruritis is surgical undercutting.[5] Although complete denervation of the skin may be accomplished, relief is usually short-lived. Moreover, sepsis and separation of the wounds may occur. Control of these complications is managed with the use of antibiotics and local drainage. Again, because morbidity outweighs the success, undercutting is not generally recommended.

Radiation therapy to the perianal region may provide complete and permanent relief. However, in most cases it is ineffective, and radiation burns of the perianal skin may be worse than the pruritis itself. In addition, when healing is achieved, radiation therapy may result in a narrowed, shortened, stenotic orifice. If a healed, fixed stricture develops, anoplasty may be possible if the radiation injury is not severe; alternatively, a stoma may be necessary. Therefore, radiation therapy is not advised for treatment of pruritus ani.

CONDYLOMA ACUMINATUM

Despite the availability of a huge variety of alternative procedures for the treatment of condyloma acuminatum, recurrence after treatment remains the most common complication. For this reason, in addition to treatment of the possible sources of autoinfections, patients should be advised as to how to avoid reinfection. Before complete eradication, genital or oropharyngeal autoinnoculation sources should be carefully excluded. All sexual partners should be treated at the same time. Common treatment options for condyloma acuminatum include excision, destruction, and immunotherapy.

Excision

Excision of condylomata allows for histopathologic evaluation and human papillomavirus (HPV) typing.[6] Early postoperative bleeding occurs in approximately 2% to 3% of patients after excision. When excising warts, the surgeon must take care to limit the damage to the surrounding normal skin. If adequate skin bridges are not preserved, the risk of reducing the circumference of the anal canal is increased and complications such as chronic fibrosis, chronic fissure formation, and fixed stricture may develop. Sitz baths are a routine part of postoperative care to reduce the risk of skin problems such as cellulitis and abscess.

Destruction

The risk of malignant transformation of condylomata (particularly in HPV types 16 or 18) requires complete histopathologic microscopic examination. Use of destruction for cure makes this evaluation impossible. Methods of destruction include use of podophyllin or bichloracetic acid–trichloracetic acid, electrocautery, cryotherapy, and laser. Each of these methods has associated complications.

Complications of podophyllin therapy range from severe local irritation to systemic toxicity. Local complications include skin necrosis, fistula in ano, dermatitis, anal stenosis, and histologic changes around this area that can mimic carcinoma in situ. Nausea, altered mental status, and bone marrow depression are possible systemic side effects.[7] Hepatic, renal, GI, respiratory, hematologic, and neurologic problems occur when large doses are used. Podophyllin is contraindicated in pregnancy.

Because of its caustic effects, inappropriate use of bichloracetic acid–trichloroacetic acid may lead to skin necrosis, fistula in ano, or anal stenosis. Inaccurate cauterization or fulgeration of the condyloma with electrocautery results in injury to the surrounding normal epithelium, with severe deep burns or fibrous scarring. The resultant scars may cause anal stenosis.

A limitation of cryotherapy is the difficulty in controlling the depth of tissue destruction. Its use may lead to injury to the surrounding normal tissue that can produce wide, deep wounds associated with delayed, painful tissue sloughing. Moreover, a foul-smelling discharge accompanies the sloughing ulcer.

The laser may cause circumferential burns and tissue loss that may then result in anal stenosis.[8] Abscesses from deep destruction, prolonged perianal drainage, and stricture formation can also lead to anal stenosis. As a result of the aerosolized viral particles, respiratory papillomas may develop in medical providers who apply laser treatment.[9]

Immunotherapy

Abcarian and Sharon[10] have studied the use of autologous vaccine taken from wart tissue. In this study, the mechanism of regression was undetermined, although humoral immunity was thought to play a role. Complications of this method are as yet unclear. Injection of interferon-2b, either intralesionally or intramuscularly, may cause complications such as fever, chills, myalgia, headache, fatigue, or leukopenia.[7]

SEXUALLY TRANSMITTED DISEASES

Sexually transmitted diseases are caused by bacteria, viruses, and parasites.[11,12] The treatment and potential complications are summarized in Table 30-1.

ACQUIRED IMMUNODEFICIENCY SYNDROME

HIV can be isolated from blood, semen, and saliva of anti-HIV–positive patients. A large percentage of patients have become infected by a sexual route, but increasing numbers of patients are becoming infected by other routes such as intravenous drug use. HIV infects the T helper-inducer lymphocytes, which lose their functional capacity and die prematurely. The defect of cellular immunity results in increased susceptibility to opportunistic infections and allows development of particular tumors such as Kaposi's sarcoma and non-Hodgkin's lymphoma. The

Table 30-1 Treatment and complications of sexually transmitted diseases

Disease	Treatment	Complications
Bacterial		
Gonorrhea	Ceftriaxone	Resistance
		Allergy (20% cross-reactivity with penicillin)
	Doxycycline	Fatty infiltration of liver, nephrotoxicity, nephrogenic diabetes insipidus
		GI reactions (e.g., diarrhea, pseudomembranous colitis)
		Resistance, cross reactivity with penicillin
		Photosensitivity and hypersensitivity reactions
		Pigmentation of teeth, bone growth retardation
		Vestibular disturbance
		Thrombophlebitis
Syphilis	Penicillin	Allergic reactions (immediate, accelerated, delayed)
		Resistance (high level)
		Neurologic toxicity
		Nerve and muscle injury, CNS procaine toxicity
		Interstitial nephritis
		Electrolyte disturbance
		Hematologic reactions
		Diarrhea; pseudomembranous colitis
		Jarisch-Herxheimer reaction
Chlamydia and lymphogranuloma venereum	Tetracycline	Resistance, cross-reactivity with penicillin
		Fatty infiltration of liver, nephrotoxicity, nephrogenic diabetes insipidus
		GI reactions
		Photosensitivity and hypersensitivity reactions
		Vestibular disturbance
		Pigmentation of teeth, bone growth retardation
Haemophilus ducreyi (chancroid)	Erythromycin	Resistance
		GI effects
		Hepatoxicity

Continued.

Table 30-1 Treatment and complications of sexually transmitted diseases–cont'd

Disease	Treatment	Complications
Bacterial–cont'd		
Granuloma inguinale	Tetracycline	Resistance, cross-reactivity with penicillin Fatty infiltration of liver, nephrotoxicity, nephrogenic diabetes insipidus GI reactions Photosensitivity and hypersensitivity reactions Vestibular disturbance Pigmentation of teeth, bone growth retardation
Hidradenitis suppurativa	Complete surgical excision	Recurrence Skin necrosis Fistula in ano Abscess Long perianal drainage
Viral		
Molluscum contagiosum	Excision	Bleeding Chronic fibrosis Chronic fissure
	Cryotherapy	Wide deep wounds from injury to the surrounding normal tissue
HPV	Destruction	See text
AIDS	AZT	Pancytopenia Neurotoxicity
	2',3' Dideoxycytidine or 2',3' Dideoxyadenosine	Painful peripheral neuropathy Rash symptom complex
Cytomegalovirus	Ganciclovir	Neutropenia CNS toxicity Catheter-related sepsis Skin necrosis Thrombosis
Herpes simplex virus	Acyclovir	Resistance CNS effects Catheter-related irritation Pruritis Edema Erythema

Table 30-1 Treatment and complications of sexually transmitted diseases—cont'd

Disease	Treatment	Complications
Parasitic		
Entamoeba histolytica	Metronidazole	Resistance GI effects CNS disorders Mutagenic and carcinogenic potential
Giardia lamblia	Metronidazole	Resistance GI effects CNS disorders Mutagenic and carcinogenic potential
Shigella	Trimethoprim-sulfamethoxazole	GI effects Skin rashes Vitamin B_{12} deficiency Reversible renal impairment
Campylobacter	Erythromycin	Resistance GI effects Hepatotoxicity
Cryptosporidia	Hydration	Electrolyte imbalance
Isospora	Trimethoprim-sulfamethoxazole	GI effects Skin rashes Vitamin B_{12} deficiency Reversible renal impairment
Mycobacterium avium-intracellulare	Antituberculosis agents	Recurrence Resistance Failure Drug-related complications

colorectal surgeon must be familiar with the anorectal and abdominal manifestations of AIDS and the complications related to medications used to manage the systemic effects of HIV infection. These are summarized in Table 30-2.

Anorectal Manifestations

HIV infection and its consequences on the immune defenses may affect every organ system. The GI tract is one of the most common sites of clinical expression, and all levels from the oral cavity to the anus are frequently involved. In approximately one third of patients, perirectal lesions may develop. A source of considerable concern is that many of these conditions are difficult to detect and refractory to therapy, although new diagnostic and therapeutic strategies are rapidly being developed.[10-16]

Table 30-2 Common colorectal manifestations of AIDS

Proctocolitides	Colorectal tumors	Anal and perianal disease
Viral	**Histoplasmoma**	**Malignant**
CMV	Lymphoma	Condyloma
Herpes simplex virus	Non-B-cell immunoblastic	Cloacogenic cancer
HIV	Burkitt's	Lymphoma
	Reticulosarcoma	Kaposi's sarcoma
Fungal and protozoan	Other	
Cryptosporidiosis	Kaposi's sarcoma	**Benign**
Isosporosis		Condyloma
Candidiasis		Histoplasmoma
Histoplasmosis		Lymphoma
		Tuberculoma
Bacterial		Ulcers and fissures
M. avium-intracellulare		Herpes simplex virus
HIV wasting syndrome		HIV
Amoebiasis		Other anorectal disease
Salmonellosis		Hemorrhoids
Shigellosis		Fistulas and abscesses
		Fissures

Most anorectal operations in patients with HIV infection are minor and elective. They are restricted to fistula in ano, fissure, hemorrhoids, transrectal biopsy, or drainage of small abscesses. Regardless of the type of operation, wounds in patients with symptomatic HIV infection often fail to heal. Patients with advanced disease (Walter Reed Classification System for HIV[17] [WR] stages 4 to 6; Centers for Disease Control Classification System[11] [CDC] groups 3 and 4) have significantly higher morbidity and mortality and less wound healing than do patients with early disease (WR stages 1 and 2, CDC groups 1 and 2). Thus, benign anorectal manifestations of AIDS must be treated cautiously. Evaluation must be thorough, including specific attention to HIV status, and treatment determined only after disease status has been established.[12] Benign anorectal conditions important in patients with AIDS include anal ulcers, abscesses, and fistulas; malignant conditions include Kaposi's sarcoma and anorectal lymphoma.

Anal ulcer. Misdiagnosis, recurrence, and failure to heal are the most common complications encountered with the treatment of anal ulcers. Treatment methods and their respective complications vary with the type of ulcer. Ulcers related to herpes simplex virus, cytomegalovirus (CMV), syphilis, and *Cryptococcus neoformans*[1] are usually treated medically.[18,19] Use of acyclovir can lead to resistance,

CNS effects, catheter-related irritation, pruritis, edema, or erythema. Gancyclovir therapy has been associated with neutropenia, CNS toxicity, and catheter-related sepsis. Penicillin-associated complications include resistance (high level), allergic reactions (immediate, accelerated, or delayed), neurologic toxicity, electrolyte imbalance, diarrhea, pseudomembranous colitis, hematologic reactions, interstitial nephritis, nerve and muscle injury, and CNS procaine toxicity. Chronic, symptomatic, nonhealing ulcers are best managed with surgery. Complications of surgical therapy include early postoperative bleeding, superinfections, prolonged drainage, delayed healing, and anal incontinence.

Perianal abscess and fistula in ano. In patients with CDC groups 3 and 4 disease, intersphincteric abscesses with or without fistulous connections, chronic abscesses, and complex fistulas seem to be more common. These conditions are managed with conventional surgery. Complications include nonhealing wounds, anal incontinence, progressive sepsis, and recurrence.

Kaposi's sarcoma. Recurrence and failure after treatment remain the most common problems in managing Kaposi's sarcoma. Each method of therapy has additional complications. Surgical excision can produce early postoperative bleeding, superinfections, long drainage time, delayed healing, and anal incontinence. Electrocautery can lead to severe burns, fibrous scarring, superinfection, or delayed healing. Radiation therapy can lead to severe burns, small bowel obstruction, or diarrhea. Immunotherapy with agents such as If-2a and 2b has been associated with fever, chills, myalgia, headache, fatigue, and leukopenia.

Several chemotherapeutic agents have been used to treat Kaposi's sarcoma. Complications of vincristine include hypersensitivity, paralytic ileus, intestinal necrosis or perforation, urinary retention, neuromuscular side effects, bronchospasm, skin irritation, and necrosis or cellulitis with extravasation of the intravenously administered drug. Death can occur if this drug is given intrathecally.

Perianal lymphoma. Misdiagnosis, recurrence, and failure after treatment remain the most common complications of lymphoma therapy. Treatment of perianal lymphoma includes irradiation and chemotherapy. Severe skin burns, small bowel obstruction, and diarrhea can be produced by radiation therapy. Complications associated with chemotherapy include a low complete response rate (33% to 50%), a high frequency of associated opportunistic infections, and high relapse and mortality rates.

Abdominal Manifestations of AIDS

The risk of complications in emergency colorectal operations in patients with AIDS is higher than for elective colorectal operations and includes sepsis, wound infection, wound dehiscence, anastomotic leakage, stoma necrosis, and postoperative small bowel obstruction. The use of diversion techniques decreases complication rates compared with use of primary anastomosis.[20-22]

CMV infection is found at autopsy in nearly 90% of patients with AIDS.[23,24] The sites of involvement are diverse and may include virtually any portion of the GI tract including the esophagus, stomach, small bowel, and colon. Colonic involvement is the most common. When complicated by ileocolitis or proctocolitis, CMV infection is the most frequent indication for colectomy. Bleeding and perforation of ulcers are the most common causes of surgical intervention. Other lesions such as lymphoma, Kaposi's sarcoma, and *M. avium-intracellulare* may occasionally lead to surgery. However, toxic megacolon, intussusception, obstruction, stricture, bleeding and perforation are emergent complications and require immediate surgery. Immunocompromised patients are not capable of withstanding additional complications, and the prognosis in these patients is generally dismal. These factors indicate cautious and conservative treatment.[18,22]

Complications With Systemic Treatment With AZT, ddC, or ddA

Although no series exists to document the efficacy of azidothymidine (AZT), dideoxycytidine (ddC), or dideoxyadenosine (ddA) in colorectal or anorectal surgery in patients with either AIDS or asymptomatic HIV-1 infection, their prophylactic use is recommended. Their application, however, may result in complications. AZT has been associated with pancytopenia, neurotoxicity, nausea, myalgia, insomnia, severe headaches, and seizures. Use of ddC and ddA can cause painful peripheral neuropathy and a rash symptom complex.

REFERENCES

1. Hicks TC, Opelka FG. Pruritus ani: Diagnosis and treatment. In Beck DE, Wexner SD, eds. Fundamentals of Anorectal Surgery. New York: McGraw-Hill, 1992, pp 157-169.
2. Wexner SD, Schottler JL. Pruritus ani: Differential diagnosis and management. Mod Med 96:102, 1989.
3. Stone HB. Pruritus ani. Treatment by alcohol injection. Surg Gynecol Obstet 42:565-566, 1926.
4. Turell R. Tattooing with mercury sulfide for intractable anal pruritis. Surgery 23:63, 1948.
5. Lockhart-Mummery JP. Diseases of the Rectum and Colon. London: Baillière, 1934.
6. Wexner SD. Sexually transmitted diseases of the colon, rectum and anus. Dis Colon Rectum 12:1048-1062, 1990.
7. Boot JM, Stolz E. Intralesional interferon-2b treatment of condylomata acuminata previously resistant to podophyllin resin application. Genitourin Med 65:50-53, 1983.
8. Krebs HB, Wheelock JB. The CO_2 laser for recurrent and therapy resistant condylomata acuminatum. J Reprod Med 30:489-492, 1985.
9. Volen D. Intact viruses in CO_2 laser plumes spur safety concern. Clin Laser Monthly 5:101-103, 1987.
10. Abcarian H, Sharon N. Long term effectiveness of immunotherapy of anal condyloma acuminatum. Dis Colon Rectum 10:648-651, 1982.

11. Centers for Disease Control. Classification system for human T-lymphotropic virus type III/lymphadenopathy associated virus infections. MMWR 35:334-339, 1986.
12. Wexner SD. AIDS: What the colorectal surgeon needs to know. Perspect Colon Rectal Surg 2:19-54, 1989.
13. Wexner SD, Smith WB, Wilson JW. The surgical management of anorectal disease in AIDS and pre-AIDS patients. Dis Colon Rectum 29:719-723, 1986.
14. Sim AJW. AIDS and the surgeon. Surgery 59:1396-1401, 1988.
15. Miles AJ, Mellor CH, Gazzard B, Allen-Mersh TG, Wastell G. Surgical management of anorectal disease in HIV-positive homosexuals. Br J Surg 77:869-871, 1990.
16. Beck DE, Jaso RG, Zajac RA. Proctologic management of the HIV positive patient. South Med J 81:511, 1988.
17. Redfield RR, Wright DC, Tramont EC. The Walter Reed Classification for HTLV-III/LAV infection. N Engl J Med 314:131-132, 1986.
18. Cohen SM, Schmitt SL, Lucas FV, Wexner SD. The diagnosis of anal ulcers in AIDS patients. Int J Colorect Dis 9:168-173, 1994.
19. Viamonte M, Dailey TH, Gottesman L. Ulcerative disease of the anorectum in the HIV positive patient. Dis Colon Rectum 36:801-805, 1993.
20. Burack JH, Mandel MS, Bizer LS. Emergency abdominal operations in the patient with AIDS. Arch Surg 124:285-286, 1989.
21. Zelnick R, Poulard JB, Auguste LJ, Vretakis G, Margolis IB. Surgery in the AIDS patient. AIDS Patients 1:10-14, 1991.
22. Macho JR. Gastrointestinal surgery in the AIDS patient. Gastroenterol Clin North Am 3: 563-571, 1988.
23. Welch K, Finkbeiner W, Alpers CE, Blumenfeld W, Davis RL, Smuckler EA, Beckstead JH. Autopsy findings in AIDS. JAMA 252:1152-1159, 1984.
24. Chachova A, Dietrich D, Krasinski K. 9(1,3-Dihydroxy-2-propoxymethyl) guanine (gancylovir) in the treatment of cytomegalovirus gastrointestinal disease in AIDS. Ann Intern Med •: 107-133, 1987.

Index

D

J

K

L

Q

R